ICSA Book Series in Statistics

Series Editors

Ding-Geng Chen, College of Health Solutions, Arizona State University, Phoenix, AZ, USA

Yichuan Zhao, Department of Mathematics & Statistics, Georgia State University, Atlanta, GA, USA

The ICSA Book Series in Statistics showcases research from the International Chinese Statistical Association that has an international reach. It publishes books in statistical theory, applications, and statistical education. All books are associated with the ICSA or are authored by invited contributors. Books may be monographs, edited volumes, textbooks and proceedings.

Yichuan Zhao • Ding-Geng Chen
Editors

Big Data Analytics in Biostatistics and Bioinformatics

Springer

Editors

Yichuan Zhao
Department of Mathematics & Statistics
Georgia State University
Atlanta, GA, USA

Ding-Geng Chen
College of Health Solutions
Arizona State University
Phoenix, AZ, USA

ISSN 2199-0980 ISSN 2199-0999 (electronic)
ICSA Book Series in Statistics
ISBN 978-3-032-06648-0 ISBN 978-3-032-06649-7 (eBook)
https://doi.org/10.1007/978-3-032-06649-7

Chen, C's work was supported by National Institutes of Health grants R01AG089377 and P30AG028747 and by the Johns Hopkins Institute for Clinical and Translational Research (ICTR) funded under grant 1UM1TR004926 from the National Center for Advancing Translational Sciences (NCATS) a component of the National Institutes of Health (NIH), and NIH Roadmap for Medical Research. The content of this paper is solely the responsibility of the authors and do not necessarily represent the official view of the Johns Hopkins ICTR, NCATS, or NIH.

This Springer imprint is published by the registered company Springer Nature Switzerland AG
The registered company address is: Gewerbestrasse 11, 6330 Cham, Switzerland

Preface

This book focuses on big data analytics in biostatistics and bioinformatics, providing a comprehensive overview of the theory, methods, and applications in this field. Its primary goal is to bring together leading experts to highlight the latest developments and challenges in this rapidly evolving area, while encouraging further exploration of related topics. The chapters feature contributions from outstanding researchers at outstanding universities, representing diverse backgrounds and expertise, reflecting the interdisciplinary nature of big data analytics research.

This book covers a wide range of topics in big data analytics for biostatistics and bioinformatics, including foundational concepts, statistical theory, deep learning and machine learning procedures, and their broad applications. It also explores areas such as transfer learning, neural networks, causal inference, ultrahigh-dimensional discriminant analysis, and sparse Bayesian clustering. Each chapter underwent a rigorous peer-review process, with multiple rounds of evaluation by two referees. The chapters present machine learning and statistical methods specifically tailored to biostatistics and bioinformatics. Timely and relevant in the AI era, this book has the potential to impact the fields of statistics, biostatistics, bioinformatics, neuroscience, public health, AI, and data science. Targeted at a broad audience including professionals, practitioners, researchers, and graduate students, this book provides valuable insights and guidance for AI-related research. Overall, this book serves as a comprehensive resource for anyone interested in data science.

The chapters of this book are organized into four parts: Part I serves as an introduction, providing an overview of big data analytics. Part II covers recent advancements in statistical and machine learning methods for gene expression data analysis, presented across five chapters. Part III focuses on integrating neural networks into machine learning and their applications to image data, also explored in five chapters. Part IV examines the use of joint modeling and survival analysis with clinical trial data across four chapters. Each chapter is self-contained, with references provided at the end for easy access. To support readers in applying the methods, this book includes computer programs and datasets, making implementation straightforward. Many of these codes are publicly available on the GitHub pages of the chapter authors, who are also open to requests for R scripts.

The timely publication of this book would not have been possible without the efforts and contributions of many individuals. We sincerely express our heartfelt gratitude to the chapter authors listed in the "List of Contributors" for their outstanding contributions. We also gratefully acknowledge the dedicated efforts of the reviewers listed in the "List of Chapter Reviewers," whose insightful comments greatly enhanced the clarity and quality of this book. We extend our sincere appreciation to Faith Su, Publishing Editor for the ICSA Book Series in Statistics at Springer, and Kesavy Sivasankaran, Production Editor at Springer Nature, for their guidance and unwavering support throughout the publication process. Their expertise was instrumental in the successful production of this book.

We welcome readers' feedback as part of our commitment to continuous improvement. If you notice any typos, errors, or have suggestions for enhancing this book, please do not hesitate to contact the editors, Drs. Yichuan Zhao and Ding-Geng Chen. Your insights are highly valued, and we look forward to hearing your comments/suggestions to help make this book even more useful.

Atlanta, GA, USA
Phoenix, AZ, USA
Pretoria, South Africa

Yichuan Zhao
Ding-Geng Chen

Contents

Editors and Contributors

About the Editors

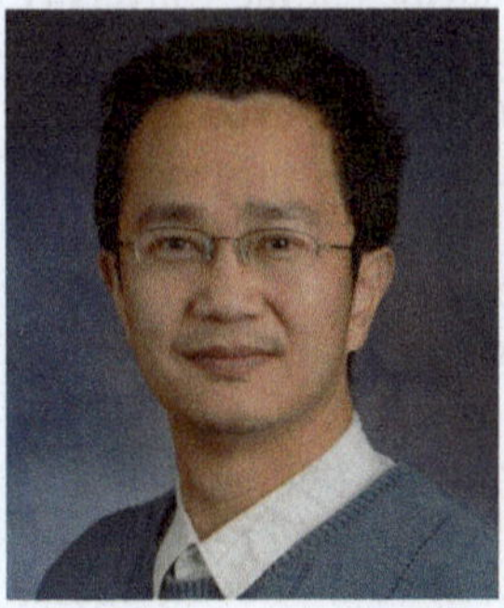

Yichuan Zhao is a Professor of Statistics at Georgia State University in Atlanta. He has a joint appointment as an associate member of the Neuroscience Institute and is also an affiliated faculty member of the School of Public Health at Georgia State University. His current research interest focuses on survival analysis, empirical likelihood methods, nonparametric statistics, analysis of ROC curves, bioinformatics, Monte Carlo methods, and statistical modeling of fuzzy systems. He has published more than 100 research articles in statistics and biostatistics, has co-edited seven books on statistics, biostatistics, and data science, and has been an invited speaker for more than 200 research talks nationally and internationally. Dr. Zhao has organized the Workshop Series on Biostatistics and Bioinformatics since its initiation in 2012. He also organized the 25th ICSA Applied Statistics Symposium in Atlanta as the chair of the organizing committee to great success. In addition, the 6th ICSA China Conference that he organized as the chair of both the organizing committee and program committee was a huge success. He currently serves as an associate editor or on the editorial board for several statistical journals, including the *Electronic Journal of Statistics* and the *Journal of Nonparametric Statistics*.

Dr. Zhao is a Fellow of the American Statistical Association and an elected member of the International Statistical Institute. He serves on the Board of Directors, ICSA, and is the Chair, Risk Analysis Section, the American Statistical Association.

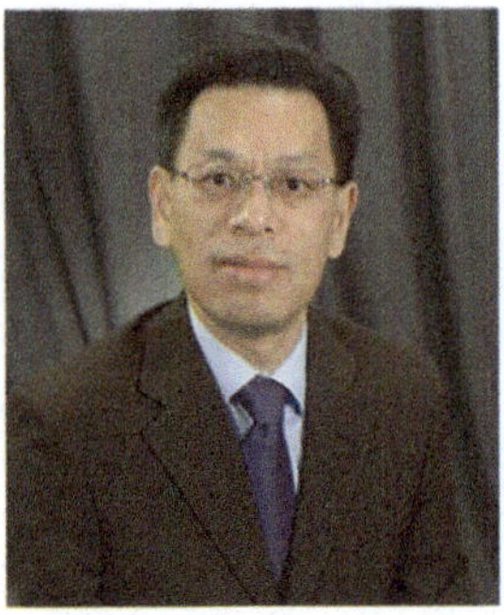

Ding-Geng Chen is an elected fellow of the American Statistical Association and currently serves as the Executive Director and Professor of biostatistics at the College of Health Solutions, Arizona State University. He is also an elected member of the Academy of Science of South Africa (MASSAf) (https://www.assaf.org.za/) and holds positions as an Extraordinary Professor and the SARChI Research Chair in Biostatistics at the University of Pretoria and an Honorary Professor at the University of KwaZulu-Natal, South Africa. Dr. Chen was a Professor of Biostatistics at the University of North Carolina at Chapel Hill, the University of Rochester Medical School, and held the Karl E. Peace Endowed Eminent Scholar Chair in Biostatistics at Georgia Southern University. He is a senior biostatistics consultant for biopharmaceuticals and government agencies, with extensive expertise in biostatistics, clinical trials, and public health statistics. Dr. Chen has more than 200 referred professional publications, co-authored 12 books, and co-edited 29 books on clinical trial methodology, meta-analysis, data science, causal inference, and public health research. This work is partially supported by the South African National Research Foundation (NRF) and South African Medical Research Council (SAMRC) (South African DST-NRF-SAMRC SARChI Research Chair in Biostatistics, Grant Number 114613).

Contributors

Karthik Bharath School of Mathematical Sciences, University of Nottingham, Nottingham, UK

Vladimir Bondarenko Department of Mathematics and Statistics, Georgia State University, Atlanta, GA, USA

Daniel Brumley Department of Mathematics & Statistics, University of Central Oklahoma, Edmond, OK, USA

Sounak Chakraborty Department of Statistics, University of Missouri, Columbia, MO, USA

Chixiang Chen Department of Epidemiology & Public Health, University of Maryland School of Medicine, Baltimore, MD, USA

Ding-Geng Chen College of Health Solutions, Arizona State University, Phoenix, AZ, USA
Department of Statistics, University of Pretoria, Pretoria, South Africa

Elynn Chen New York University, New York, NY, USA

Jianmin Chen University of Pennsylvania, Philadelphia, PA, USA

Li-Pang Chen Department of Statistics, National Chengchi University, Taipei City, Taiwan

Xiaohe Chen Department of Statistics, Florida State University, Tallahassee, FL, USA

Ye Jin Choi Department of Statistics, The Ohio State University, Columbus, OH, USA

Tyler Cook Department of Mathematics & Statistics, University of Central Oklahoma, Edmond, OK, USA

Halef Doğan Department of Biochemistry, Cumhuriyet University, Türkiye

Vahap Eldem Department of Biology, Faculty of Sciences, Istanbul University, Türkiye

Luella Fu Department of Mathematics, San Francisco State University, San Francisco, CA, USA

Bowen Gang Department of Statistics and Data Science, Fudan University, Shanghai, China

Yongli Han Biostatistics and Data Management, Daiichi Sankyo, Inc., NJ, USA

Gregory Hawk Dr. Bing Zhang Department of Statistics, University of Kentucky, Lexington, KY, USA

Jianliang He Department of Statistics and Data Science, Yale University, New Haven, CT, USA

Zhaowei Zoe Hua Servier Bio-Innovation, Boston, MA, USA

Chao Huang Department of Epidemiology and Biostatistics, University of Georgia, Athens, GA, USA

Funda İpekten Department of Biostatistics, Institute of Health Sciences, Erciyes University, Türkiye

Rishikesan Kamaleswaran Department of Surgery and Department of Anesthesiology, Duke University School of Medicine, Durham, NC, USA

Necla Koçhan Department of Mathematics, Izmir University of Economics, Türkiye

Sebastian Kurtek Department of Statistics, The Ohio State University, Columbus, OH, USA

Cai Li Department of Biostatistics, St. Jude Children's Research Hospital, Memphis, TN, USA

Jia Liang St. Jude Children's Research Hospital, Memphis, TN, USA

Menglu Liang Department of Epidemiology and Biostatistics, University of Maryland, MD, USA

Danping Liu Biostatistics Branch, Division of Cancer Epidemiology and Genetics, National Cancer Institute, Rockville, MA, USA

Rongjie Liu Department of Statistics, University of Georgia, Athens, GA, USA

Shuangge Ma Department of Biostatistics, Yale School of Public Health, New Haven, CT, USA

Qian Meng Servier Bio-Innovation, Boston, MA, USA

Ronald Moore Computer Science, Emory University, Atlanta, GA, USA

Chaan Ng Department of Abdominal Imaging, The University of Texas MD Anderson Cancer Center, Houston, TX, USA

Bimal Ray College of Veterinary Medicine, University of Missouri, Columbia, MO, USA

David Rice Department of Mathematics and Statistics, Washington State University, Pullman, WA, USA

Akshay Sharma Department of Bone Marrow Transplantation & Cellular Therapy, St. Jude Children's Research Hospital, Memphis, TN, USA

Weining Shen Department of Statistics, University of California, Irvine, CA, USA

Li Tang Department of Quantitative Health Sciences, Cleveland Clinic, Cleveland, OH, USA

Rui Sammi Tang Astellas Pharma, Cambridge, MA, USA

Zhaoyang Teng Astellas Pharma, Cambridge, MA, USA

Katherine Thompson Dr. Bing Zhang Department of Statistics, University of Kentucky, Lexington, KY, USA

Lucie Truffaut-Chalet Institut de Recherche International Servier, Gif-sur-Yvette, France

Hui-Shan Tsao Department of Statistics, National Chengchi University, Taipei City, Taiwan

Jiping Wang Department of Biostatistics, Yale School of Public Health, New Haven, CT, USA

Jiyu Wang National Renewable Energy Laboratory, Golden, CO, USA

Ming Wang School of Medicine, Case Western Reserve University, Cleveland, OH, USA

Rong Wang Department of Chronic Disease Epidemiology, Yale School of Public Health, Yale Cancer Outcomes, Public Policy and Effectiveness Research (COPPER) Center, New Haven, CT, USA

Tianying Wang Department of Statistics, Colorado State University, Fort Collins, CO, USA

Yuan Wang Department of Mathematics and Statistics, Washington State University, Pullman, WA, USA

Zhenyu Wang Pfizer Pharmaceuticals, Cambridge, MA, USA

Song Wei H. Milton Stewart School of Industrial and Systems Engineering, Georgia Institute of Technology, Atlanta, GA, USA

Jou-Chin Wu Department of Statistics, National Chengchi University, Taipei City, Taiwan

Yao Xie H. Milton Stewart School of Industrial and Systems Engineering, Georgia Institute of Technology, Atlanta, GA, USA

Yifan Yang Department of Population and Quantitative Health Sciences, School of Medicine, Case Western Reserve University, Cleveland, OH, USA

Gökmen Zararsız Department of Biostatistics, Faculty of Medicine, Erciyes University, Türkiye

Gözde Zararsız Department of Biostatistics, Faculty of Medicine, Erciyes University, Türkiye

Hanyu Zhang H. Milton Stewart School of Industrial and Systems Engineering, Georgia Institute of Technology, Atlanta, GA, USA

Zhiwei Zhang Biostatistics Branch, Biometric Research Group, Division of Cancer Treatment & Diagnosis, National Cancer Institute, Rockville, MD, USA

Yichuan Zhao Department of Mathematics and Statistics, Georgia State University, Atlanta, GA, USA

Yiwang Zhou Department of Biostatistics, St. Jude Children's Research Hospital, Memphis, TN, USA

Xiangqi Zhu College of Engineering, Oregon State University, Corvallis, OR, USA

List of Chapter Reviewers

Seungjun Ahn, Department of Population Health Science and Policy, Icahn School of Medicine at Mount Sinai, New York, NY, USA
Paul Bernhardt, Department of Mathematics and Statistics, Villanova University, Villanova, PA, USA
Guanqun Cao, Department of Statistics and Probability Michigan State University, East Lansing, MI, USA
Thierry Chekouo, Division of Biostatistics and Health Data Science, School of Public Health, The University of Minnesota Twin Cities, MN, USA
Ding-Geng Chen, College of Health Solutions, Arizona State University, Phoenix, USA, and Department of Statistics, University of Pretoria, South Africa
Yuehua Cui, Department of Statistics and Probability Michigan State University, East Lansing, MI, USA
Byron Gajewski, Department of Biostatistics and Data Science, University of Kansas Medical Center, Kansas City, KS, USA
Yuan Gao, Guanghua School of Management, Peking University, Beijing, China
Peisong Han, Department of Biostatistics, School of Public Health, University of Michigan, Ann Arbor, MI, USA
Guanyu Hu, Department of Biostatistics and Data Science, The University of Texas Health Science Center at Houston, Houston, TX, USA
Chiung-Yu Huang, Department of Epidemiology and Biostatistics, University of California, San Francisco, CA, USA
Yuan Ji, Department of Public Health Sciences, The University of Chicago, Chicago, IL USA
Joyce Jiang, Division of Epidemiology, Biostatistics, and Environmental Health School of Public Health, University of Memphis, Memphis, TN, USA
Anand Joshi, Electrical and Computer Engineering, University of California, Los Angeles, USA
Shantanu Joshi, Laboratory of Neuroimaging, University of California, Los Angeles, USA
Joshua Lambert, College of Nursing, University of Cincinnati, Cincinnati, OH, USA
Kyoungjae Lee, Department of Statistics, Sungkyunkwan University, Seoul, Korea

MinJae Lee, Division of Clinical & Translational Sciences, Department of Internal Medicine, McGovern Medical School, University of Texas Health Science Center at Houston: Houston, TX, USA
Liang Li, Department of Biostatistics, University of Texas MD Anderson Cancer Center, Houston, TX, USA
Sai Li, Institute of Statistics and Big Data, Renmin University of China, Beijing, China
Zhigang Li, Department of Biostatistics, University of Florida, Gainesville, FL, USA
Catherine Liu, Department of Data Science and Analytics, Hong Kong Polytechnic University, Hong Kong, China
Wodan Ling, Population Health Sciences, Weill Cornell Medical College, New York, NY, USA
Sheng Luo, Department of Biostatistics & Bioinformatics, Duke University, Durham, NC, USA
Chuoxin Ma, Department of Statistics and Data Science, Faculty of Science and Technology, Beijing Normal University-Hong Kong Baptist University United International College, Zhuhai, China
Suqi Ma, Department of Mathematics, China Agricultural University, Beijing, China
Matteo Pedone, Department of Statistics, Computer Science and Applications University of Florence, Florence, Italy
Zhimei Ren, Department of Statistics and Data Science, Wharton School, University of Pennsylvania, Philadelphia, PA, USA
Richard Riley, Department of Applied Health Sciences, University of Birmingham, Birmingham, UK
Fred Shi, Department of Biostatistics and Data Science, University of Kansas Medical Center, Kansas City, KS, USA
Shuoyang Wang, Department of Bioinformatics and Biostatistics, School of Public Health and Information Sciences, University of Louisville, Louisville, KY, USA
Lili Wu, Microsoft Research, New York, NY, USA
Xin Xing, Department of Statistics, Virginia Tech, Blacksburg, VA, USA
Yuehan Yang, School of Statistics and Mathematics, Central University of Finance and Economics, Beijing, China
Ying Yuan, Department of Biostatistics, University of Texas MD Anderson Cancer Center, Houston, TX, USA
Xian Zhang, School of Mathematical Science, Heilongjiang University, Harbin, China
Yichuan Zhao, Department of Mathematics and Statistics, Georgia State University, Atlanta, GA, USA
Jin Zhou, Department of Biostatistics, Fielding School of Public Health, University of California, Los Angeles, CA, USA

Part I
An Overview of Big Data Analytics in Biostatistics and Bioinformatics

Big Data Analytics in Biostatistics and Bioinformatics: The Past, the Current, and the Future

Yichuan Zhao and Ding-Geng Chen

Abstract This chapter provides a comprehensive roadmap of big data analytics in biostatistics and bioinformatics, from its historical development, current practices, and future directions. As a common goal for big data analytics, this chapter will focus on the introduction of the theory, methods, and applications covered in this book. It includes an overview of big data analytics in biostatistics and bioinformatics, statistical methods of Bayesian analysis and gene expression data, deep learning and neural network, clinical trials and survival analysis.

Keywords Artificial intelligence · Big data analytics · Transfer learning · Deep learning · Machine learning

1 The Roadmap from Big Data Analytics in Biostatistics and Bioinformatics

Big data in biostatistics and bioinformatics involves massive, heterogeneous datasets from sources such as genomics, clinical records, and medical imaging, often containing millions of variables. The primary objective is to develop robust analytical methods that can efficiently extract meaningful insights while addressing challenges such as noise, missing data, and biases inherent in these complex, high-dimensional datasets. This work is essential for advancing our understanding of intricate biological systems and disease mechanisms, ultimately contributing to improved public health outcomes.

Y. Zhao (✉)
Department of Mathematics and Statistics, Georgia State University, Atlanta, GA, USA
e-mail: yichuan@gsu.edu

D.-G. Chen
College of Health Solutions, Arizona State University, Phoenix, AZ, USA

Department of Statistics, University of Pretoria, Pretoria, South Africa

Y. Zhao, D.-G. Chen (eds.), *Big Data Analytics in Biostatistics and Bioinformatics*, ICSA Book Series in Statistics,
https://doi.org/10.1007/978-3-032-06649-7_1

Big data analytics in biostatistics and bioinformatics enables the identification of biomarkers by uncovering associations between genetic variations, molecular profiles, and disease phenotypes. Leveraging machine learning and statistical models on large-scale datasets allows researchers to predict disease progression, patient outcomes, and treatment effectiveness. These predictive capabilities are central to precision medicine, facilitating personalized interventions tailored to an individual's unique health profile, including specific disease risks and optimal treatment strategies, as detailed in our previous work [1]. Beyond individual care, insights from big data analysis inform population-level health strategies, supporting epidemiological research and guiding policy decisions for predicting disease outbreaks, and identifying high-risk groups.

Advancing precision medicine requires continued innovation in big data analytics within biostatistics and bioinformatics. Building on Zhao and Chen [1], this volume presents cutting-edge theories, methods, and applications for precision public health. It introduces new statistical and machine learning techniques, integrates survival analysis into clinical trials, and explores deep learning, neural networks, and transfer learning. These approaches support personalized medicine, enhance public health strategies, enable biomarker discovery, and strengthen predictive modeling.

This book is organized into four parts, each focusing on a core topic in big data analytics. The structure is designed to guide readers toward a comprehensive understanding of big data analysis, with particular emphasis on its applications in biostatistics and bioinformatics in the era of artificial intelligence.

2 Part I: An Overview of Big Data Analytics in Biostatistics and Bioinformatics (Chaps. 2, 3, 4 and 5)

Part I, comprising Chaps. 2, 3, 4 and 5, provides an in-depth exploration of new statistical and machine learning methods in the era of big data. This part offers a comprehensive overview of how complex, large-scale datasets are transforming the landscape of biostatistics and bioinformatics, enabling modern statistical and machine learning approaches to tackle real-world data analysis challenges.

In Chap. 2 of this book, titled "Navigating Sample Size Dilemmas in ML-based Predictive Analytics: A Comprehensive Review," Tang, Zhou, Li and Sharma deliver the comprehensive review of the advancements in machine learning (ML) methods due to their well-documented predictive performance in the modern era. There remains a noticeable dearth of literature addressing the formal planning of sample sizes by employing ML methods. This challenge becomes even more pronounced where limited resources can only support moderate sample sizes. This chapter studies existing methods for addressing this issue in the above scenarios. The authors explore the potential future direction for resolving the sample size dilemma in ML-based predictive analytics, making it a significant contribution to the book's content.

Chapter 3, titled "Moving Beyond Mean: Harnessing Big Data for Health Insights by Quantile Regression," authored by Wang, offers a comprehensive review of recent advances in quantile regression methods with a focus on biostatistical applications, highlighting the challenges for future research in this area. The era of big data has opened up new possibilities and these opportunities come with challenges due to data heterogeneity and the computational demands. Quantile regression in this chapter offers a powerful approach to these challenges, providing a flexible framework to handle the complexities of big data. This chapter can provide deeper insights into risk factors, and targeted interventions across different population groups when examining the full distribution of health outcomes in biostatistics.

Chapter 4, titled "Incorrect Model Selection Using R^2 and Akaike Information Criterion in Big Data Analyses," authored by Thompson and Hawk, explores the difficulty in choosing a scientifically correct model, and compares the performance of model selection with maximum R^2 or minimum Akaike Information Criterion (AIC) with that of more recent methods. The results in this chapter show that often the model with the largest R^2 or smallest AIC may not be the correct model. This chapter starts with the derivation of the probability of choosing the scientifically correct model in data sets as a function of regression model parameters when using R^2 or AIC. Then, a data analysis example in the chapter shows that these model selection criteria are outperformed by methods that produce multiple candidate models for researchers' consideration.

Chapter 5, titled "False Discovery Control in Multiple Testing: A Brief Overview of Theories and Methodologies," authored by He and Gang, delivers a comprehensive review of the latest developments in false discovery rate (FDR) control methodologies. In addition, this chapter develops a conceptual framework to better describe this vast literature; understands its intuition and key ideas; and provides guidance for the researcher interested in both the application and development of the methodology. As the volume and complexity of data continue to expand, the need for robust methods to account for the multiplicity of comparisons has grown widespread. A popular measure of type 1 error rate in multiple testing literatures is the FDR, which provides a powerful and practical approach to large-scale multiple testing. The various methods have been proposed to control the FDR.

3 Part II: Statistical Methods of Bayesian Analysis and Gene Expression Data (Chaps. 6, 7, 8, 9 and 10)

Part II, covering Chaps. 6, 7, 8, 9 and 10, focuses on the recent developments in statistical methods for gene expression data analysis. This part provides a rigorous overview of modern statistical and machine learning procedures, highlighting their relevance and application within Bayesian analysis. Below is a brief overview of the key topics addressed in this part.

Chapter 6, titled "Investigating and Assessing Diverse Strategies and Classification Techniques Applied in the Integration of Multi-Omics Data," authored by İpekten et al.., explores and employs various data integration methodologies and machine learning techniques on multi-omics data to predict disease classes. Integrating and analyzing various data sets will accurately diagnose the disease, and develop advanced treatment approaches. Many integration techniques have been developed, enabling researchers to reveal the complex patterns and underlying mechanisms behind biological occurrences.

Chapter 7, titled "Sparse Bayesian Clustering of Matrix Data," authored by Rice et al., introduces a novel Bayesian framework for probabilistic clustering of matrix valued data. The proposed approach models the number of clusters as a stochastic partition of the data and introduces a sparsity constraint on the covariance matrices using a beta shrinkage prior for the off-diagonal elements. In this chapter, the effectiveness and superiority of the proposed MCMC algorithm are demonstrated. The authors show the improved estimation of group structures compared to competing methods.

Chapter 8, titled "Bayesian Kernel Based Modeling and Selection of Genetic Pathways and Genes in Cancer Studies: A Step Toward Targeted Treatment Protocols," authored by Chakraborty, Wang, and Ray, presents a Bayesian kernel machine model which can incorporate existing information on genetic pathways and gene networks in the analysis of DNA microarray data. In this chapter, the overall effect of each pathway is modeled using a reproducing kernel Hilbert space. The pathway and the gene selection within a pathway are done with the help of mixture prior on the pathway indicator variables and the gene indicator variables. The proposed kernel-based method in this chapter provides a very flexible modeling framework to model both linear and nonlinear pathway effects. Within this chapter, the authors propose an efficient Markov Chain Monte Carlo algorithm to fit our proposed model.

Chapter 9, titled "Using Guided Regularized Random Forests to Identify Important Biological Pathways and Genes," authored by Cook, Brumley, and Chakraborty, proposes a novel method for identifying important biological pathways and genes for classification problems using guided regularized random forests (GRRF). This approach allows for ranking both pathways and genes, and the regularization of GRRF can help researchers select a compact set of features related to the biological outcome. The proposed methodology in the chapter can identify significant biological pathways and genes and achieve low misclassification rates.

Chapter 10, titled "Ultrahigh-Dimensional Discriminant Analysis and Its Application to Gene Expression Data," authored by Chen, Wu, and Tsao, extends the model free feature screening method to reduce the dimension of variables and detect possibly nonlinear pairwise dependence structure among variables to handle ultrahigh dimensionality in the sense that the dimension of variables is extremely larger than the sample size. This chapter adopts several graphical estimation methods to estimate the homogeneous or heterogeneous precision matrices and then implements the estimator to the discriminant function to improve classification. The authors conduct simulation studies to assess the performance of prediction for the proposed method.

4 Part III: Deep Learning and Neural Network (Chaps. 11, 12, 13, 14 and 15)

Part III, comprising Chaps. 11, 12, 13, 14 and 15, examines the integration of neural networks into machine learning and their applications to image data. This part explores the intersection of deep learning, transfer learning, causal inference, and classification for complex biological datasets. Below is a brief overview of the key topics addressed in this part.

Chapter 11, titled "Deep Image-on-scalar Regression Model with Hidden Confounders," authored by Chen, Liu, and Huang, proposes a novel model known as the deep image-on-scalar regression model with hidden confounders (DISRM-HC), which can simultaneously detect hidden confounders and learn primary effects from variables of interest by employing the functional surrogate variable analysis and deep neural networks. Compared to existing solutions, DISRM-HC can handle imaging heterogeneities and capture complex patterns of primary effects. This chapter established estimation procedures for both unknown varying coefficients and hidden confounders. The authors study asymptotic properties of the estimation procedures.

Chapter 12, titled "Transfer Learning for Causal Effect Estimation," authored by Wei et al., presents a transfer causal Learning (TCL) framework when target and source domains share the same covariate/feature spaces whereas the treatment assignment mechanisms might differ, aiming to improve causal/treatment effect estimation accuracy. The proposed method, named $\ell 1$-TCL, incorporates $\ell 1$ regularized transfer learning (TL) for nuisance models; the TL estimator of the nuisance parameters is plugged into downstream average treatment effect estimators. In this chapter, the authors establish non-asymptotic recovery guarantees for the $\ell 1$-TCL with generalized linear model (GLM) in the high-dimensional setting and demonstrate the empirical benefits of $\ell 1$-TCL for GLM and recent neural network nuisance models.

Chapter 13, titled "Hybrid Distance for Classification of Complex Biological Data Based on Elastic Shape Analysis of Curves and Topological Data Analysis of Point Clouds," authored by Choi, Bharath, and Kurtek, develops a hybrid distance for classification of complex biological data objects that can capture shape variation of disparate components. For the curve component, the authors leverage a shape distance originating from the elastic shape analysis framework. For the point cloud component, this chapter uses the bottleneck distance between persistence diagrams, which capture birth and death times of topological features, and this distance captures complementary shape features of the data objects. This chapter provides the utility of the proposed framework for classification using simulations and two real data scenarios.

Chapter 14, titled "Bifurcation Analysis of an Analog Hopfield Neural Network with Three Time Delays," authored by Bondarenko, studies an analog Hopfield neural network with excitatory and inhibitory connections and three-time delays. The neural networks show synchronous outputs shortly after the initial conditions. This chapter demonstrates that networks with inhibitory connections showed either decaying oscillations or growing oscillations until saturation of their amplitudes. Additionally, this chapter proves that an increase of time delay in one, two, or three inhibitory subnetworks leads to a variety of activities.

Chapter 15, titled "Advancing Information Integration through Empirical Likelihood: Selective Reviews and a New Idea," authored by Chen et al.., provides a comprehensive discussion of recent methodological developments in information integration via empirical likelihood, wherein only summary information is required. Moreover, the authors offer a new insight and a potentially promising framework that could broaden the application of information integration across a wider spectrum. Finally, this new framework proposed in this chapter offers computational convenience compared to classic empirical likelihood-based methods.

5 Part IV: Clinical Trials and Survival Analysis (Chaps. 16, 17, 18 and 19)

Part IV, comprising Chaps. 16, 17, 18, and 19, focuses on the integration of clinical trial data with joint modeling and survival analysis. This part examines the intersection of longitudinal data analysis, hierarchical modeling, recurrent event analysis, and survival data analysis. Below is a brief overview of the key topics covered in this part.

Chapter 16, titled "Hierarchical Semi-parametric Bayesian Modeling in Patient Screening and Enrollment Dynamic Prediction for Multicenter Clinical Trials," authored by Chen et al., offers the intricacies of screening and enrollment forecasting for trials involving various disease subtypes or biomarker-defined subgroups. In this chapter, the authors employ a hierarchical semi-parametric Bayesian approach to model recruitment dynamics, which allows for the accommodation of heterogeneity. In addition, the authors propose a dynamic prediction framework that offers continuous guidance for recruitment planning. This chapter provides an innovative tool, grounded in model-based and data-driven methodologies, which demonstrate notable flexibility and precision. Finally, this chapter efficiently identifies potential future risks.

Chapter 17, titled "Comparative Effectiveness Analysis of Lobectomy and Limited Resection for Elderly Non-Small Cell Lung Cancer Patients via Emulation," authored by Wang, Wang, and Ma, evaluates the relative effectiveness in terms of overall survival for elderly patients. This chapter conducts an emulation analysis of the Surveillance, Epidemiology, and End Results (SEER)-Medicare data, where the authors constructed an emulated "randomized clinical trial" with rigorously defined inclusion/exclusion criteria, treatment regimens. The authors found the lobectomy was to be superior in terms of overall survival for the elderly SEER-Medicare early-stage non-small cell lung cancer (NSCLC) patients. Therefore, this chapter provides new insight into surgical treatment of NSCLC.

Chapter 18, titled "Recent Developments in Joint Modeling for Recurrent Gap Times with a Terminal Event," authored by Wang et al., offers a comprehensive review of existing methods and discusses recently proposed ones for recurrent and terminal events with censoring to address these gaps, highlighting their advantages and disadvantages. Moreover, evaluating patient prognosis and dynamically predicting the risk of death are clinically significant, and utilizing developed models considering historical recurrent events is expected to enhance medical decisions and improve healthcare outcomes. In this chapter, these methods are illustrated using large-scale real datasets. Finally, the authors offer insight on current methodological gaps and propose directions for future research in clinical and observational studies.

Chapter 19, titled "A Conditional Modeling Approach for Dynamic Risk Prediction of a Survival Outcome Using Longitudinal Biomarkers with an Application to Ovarian Cancer," authored by Han et al., introduces an innovative conditional modeling approach for dynamic risk prediction of a survival outcome using longitudinal biomarkers. The new idea proposed in this chapter is to factor the joint density of the biomarkers and the survival time into the product of a conditional density of the biomarkers. Moreover, the authors develop a nonlinear mixed model that treats the survival time as an additional covariate via a smooth or latent change point kernel function. The proposed conditional modeling approach in this chapter makes less strict model assumptions and has more robust predictive performance.

6 Further Discussions

As the opening chapter of this book, our primary goal is to provide a comprehensive overview of the evolutionary journey from biostatistics to bioinformatics in the era of big data. We examine the historical roots, current developments, and future directions of these fields, highlighting emerging research opportunities. This chapter serves as an introduction, laying the groundwork for the theories, methodologies, and applications that will be explored in detail across the 18 contributed chapters.

Our focus encompasses several critical areas. First, in Chaps. 2, 3, 4 and 5 of Part I, we explore the landscape of big data analytics in biostatistics, highlighting how large-scale datasets have transformed modern data science. We discuss the pivotal roles of big data analytics, machine learning, and deep learning in shaping the future of both biostatistics and bioinformatics.

In Chaps. 6, 7, 8, 9 and 10 of Part II, we examine advances in Bayesian statistical methods applied to gene expression data, highlighting their importance in achieving accurate classification results. This discussion underscores the pivotal role of modern statistical approaches in advancing genetic pathway analysis and omics-based research, particularly in the context of cancer studies.

In Chaps. 11, 12, 13, 14 and 15 of Part III, we explore novel applications of machine learning in image analysis and causal inference. We demonstrate how deep learning and neural networks are poised to transform the classification of biological data and enhance the effectiveness of big data analytics.

Finally, in Chaps. 16, 17, 18 and 19 of Part IV, we examine the integration of data analysis with survival and longitudinal data, with a particular focus on risk prediction for cancer patients. By applying joint modeling in clinical trials, we provide readers with a deeper understanding of patient screening and dynamic prediction within clinical research.

In summary, this chapter serves as a key entry point into the fascinating world of big data analytics, tracing the path from biostatistics to bioinformatics. It sets the stage with a clear overview and fresh insights, providing a solid foundation for understanding the theories, concepts, methods, and applications that will be explored throughout the book.

Reference

1. Zhao, Y., Chen, D.G.: Statistics in Precision Health: Theory, Methods and Applications ICSA Book Series in Statistics. Springer (2024). https://doi.org/10.1007/978-3-031-50690-1

Navigating Sample Size Dilemmas in ML-Based Predictive Analytics: A Comprehensive Review

Li Tang, Yiwang Zhou, Cai Li, and Akshay Sharma

Abstract Machine learning (ML) methods have garnered increasing attention in the data science community due to their well-documented predictive performance and computational efficiency in the modern era. Many ML techniques also have robust statistical foundations and well-established operating characteristics. Despite their popularity, there remains a noticeable dearth of literature addressing the formal planning of sample sizes for predictive analytics studies employing ML methods, particularly in scenarios where access to extensive data sources is limited. This challenge becomes even more pronounced when designing prospective studies where limited resources can only support moderate sample sizes. In this comprehensive review article, we aim to examine existing methods for addressing this issue and explore potential future directions for resolving sample size dilemmas in ML-based predictive analytics.

Keywords Machine learning · Sample size · Study design · Predictive analytics · Data science

1 Introduction

The widespread agreement on the critical nature of sample size determination (SSD) spans various disciplines, significantly impacting the accuracy, credibility, and overall achievement of a study. SSD fundamentally tackles the question of the

L. Tang (✉)
Department of Quantitative Health Sciences, Cleveland Clinic Foundation, Cleveland, OH, USA
e-mail: TANGL4@ccf.org

Y. Zhou · C. Li
Department of Biostatistics, St. Jude Children's Research Hospital, Memphis, TN, USA

A. Sharma
Department of Bone Marrow Transplantation & Cellular Therapy, St. Jude Children's Research Hospital, Memphis, TN, USA

Y. Zhao, D.-G. Chen (eds.), *Big Data Analytics in Biostatistics and Bioinformatics*, ICSA Book Series in Statistics,
https://doi.org/10.1007/978-3-032-06649-7_2

necessary number of subjects to ensure results are both precise and replicable. Inaccuracies in SSD can either undermine research validity by impeding reproducibility or result in misallocation of resources and potential ethical concerns arising from overestimation [1].

The emergence of advanced machine learning (ML) techniques alongside the increase in data complexity has elevated the importance of ML-based studies, especially in the realm of predictive analytics [2–5]. Although informal empirical guidelines drawn from previous experiences are frequently utilized, formal research endeavors, particularly those seeking funding or addressing ethical concerns, necessitate a rigorously determined sample size. This is driven by the expectations of institutional scientific and ethics review boards and the escalating requirement from scholarly publications for comprehensive justifications of sample sizes within their method sections. The issue becomes more pronounced when designing prospective studies with limited access to extensive datasets, highlighting the deficiency in established protocols for ML-centric investigations.

This review seeks to underscore the critical role of SSD within the context of ML application studies, aligning with the emphasis seen in traditional studies. We aim to examine widely used approaches and criteria for choosing appropriate sample sizes, intentionally eschewing detailed computational techniques to prevent redundancy with existing information in the literature. By highlighting the unique challenges of SSD in ML projects, this review provides practical recommendations and suggests directions for future research. The discussion encompasses essential aspects of SSD, such as complexity of statistical models, prediction performance and accuracy, as well as tolerance of overfitting, fostering a detailed and pragmatic dialog among research teams. This conversation is vital for assessing the adequacy of sample size against research objectives, data availability, project timelines, and budget constraints. The goal is to improve the understanding and implementation of SSD in data science and ML research, focusing on methodological thoroughness and resource efficiency. The scope of this review is focused on model training and development rather than model validation. While validation is also critically important in practice, we believe that the essential components discussed here can offer insights relevant to sample size determination (SSD) for validation studies as well. Overview of Sample Size Determination (SSD).

1.1 Common Considerations in SSD

SSD hinges on the principle that a sample must accurately reflect the broader population it represents. This is particularly crucial in studies of rare diseases or situations where sampling is financially or operationally challenging, often leading to smaller sample sizes. Such small sample sizes may make findings hard to replicate and increase the risk of false negatives. Conversely, extensive samples may raise ethical concerns and overly elevate the likelihood of identifying statistically significant results for effects that are, in reality, trivial, thus potentially resulting in the misleading interpretation of findings. The ultimate goal of SSD is to ascertain a necessary sample size that strikes an optimal balance between ensuring sufficient statistical power to detect genuine effects and adhering to ethical standards [6].

The interplay between the selection of statistical analysis and the requisite sample size is pivotal [7] because the statistical analysis, inherently connected to the research design and objectives, determines the necessary sample size. Different analyses necessitate distinct sample sizes, meticulously customized to the study's requirements. The presence of diverse analytical methods requires a deep understanding of the underlying statistical principles pertinent to the research question to ensure a well-balanced sample size.

At the core of SSD, the concept of effect size [8] plays a crucial role, representing the anticipated impact of the intervention under investigation. Accurately determining the appropriate effect size is both complex and critical, as it enables the selection of a sample size capable of reliably identifying the true magnitude of the effect. As in traditional studies, estimations of effect size often rely on historical data, expert consensus, or early-phase studies, which collectively aid in making well-informed decisions.

In descriptive research focused on detailing variable distributions within a population without inferring causality, SSD hinges on achieving precise estimates of proportions or means. These sample size calculations depend on preset confidence intervals and specifications for the margin of error, often referencing existing studies for parameters such as standard deviations or anticipated proportions [9–11]. In the context of studies comparing variable distributions between groups, whether through observational or experimental designs, it is imperative to conduct thorough sample size calculations. This ensures sufficient power (i.e., 1-type II error) to uncover meaningful differences while controlling type I error (i.e., the rate of false positives). It is worth noting that contemporary methods are also shifting toward simulation-based sample size calculations, offering a more tailored solution for SSD. This approach underscores the importance of a strategic, well-informed process in determining the most effective sample size for a given study [12, 13], in addition to the aforementioned.

In summary, traditional SSD approaches hinge on several pre-determined factors: the nature of the study (descriptive or comparative), the chosen analytical technique, and the effect size, often presented as a standardized measure of a central tendency. Additionally, considerations of type I and type II errors are integral, particularly in comparative studies. It is essential to recognize that traditional studies typically specify either a hypothesis test or a margin of error to guide the SSD process. The specified hypothesis test may involve comparisons between different groups or against historical benchmarks. At the same time, the margin of error is instrumental in defining the precision of an estimate, which is particularly valuable in descriptive research.

1.2 Absence of Guidelines of SSD in ML-Centric Studies

Studies focused on ML algorithms, especially those aimed at developing predictive models, often confront unique challenges when applying traditional SSD methodologies. The inherent nature of ML research usually involves large datasets, which can diminish the perceived need for rigorous SSD due to the seemingly limitless availability of data. Nevertheless, as ML techniques are increasingly applied to studies with moderate or small sample sizes, the necessity for formal SSD becomes evident. For example, a recent review investigating the SSD methodologies for ML in medical imaging research revealed a notable lack of SSD discussion, with only 2.3% ($n = 4$) of 167 studies directly addressing it and an additional 10.8% ($n = 18$) of studies testing the impact of sample size on model performance as an exploratory aim [14]. It was noted that several identified studies operated with sample sizes in the hundreds [15–17], challenging the common perception that ML research invariably involves vast datasets. This discrepancy underscores a significant gap in the standardization of SSD practices and reporting, leading to considerable variability among studies.

Despite the absence of stringent SSD practices in ML studies, the influence of sample size on model accuracy remains paramount. Examination of this impact has been sporadic and varied across studies. Research conducted by Vabalas and colleagues demonstrated the varying effects of sample sizes, ranging from 20 to 1000, on the performance of algorithms like support vector machines (SVM) and logistic regression (LR). Their findings indicated that smaller datasets could achieve accuracy rates above 95%, whereas more extensive collections of 100 to 1000 samples tended to lower accuracy to between 60% and 70% [18]. In contrast, Cui and Gong's work showed that increasing the sample size from 20 to 700 improved predictive accuracy in MRI data analysis [19]. Moreover, Faber and Fonseca observed that beyond a certain point, enlarging the sample size does not markedly improve model performance [20]. These insights suggest that smaller sample sizes may inflate the accuracy of ML models, potentially due to overfitting or random variations. In contrast, studies on a larger scale definitely demand more resources and time. However, excessively large studies should not be mistaken as a straightforward solution or a substitute for substantive hypothesis testing [21]. Hence, identifying an appropriate sample size is vital for reliable and efficient ML research outcomes despite the notable absence of explicit guidelines for SSD.

1.3 Challenges in SSD for ML-Centric Studies

The complexities associated with SSD in ML-focused research can be attributed to several key factors:

1. *Exploratory Nature of Model Building*: The exploratory nature of constructing ML models complicates the initial definition of study objectives, which can be

either descriptive or comparative. Often, these models are employed to generate hypotheses rather than to test pre-specified ones [23]. This inherent ambiguity makes it challenging to determine whether the focus should be on estimating precision or comparing different models' performance.

2. *Diversity of ML Methods*: The diversity of ML methodologies poses a significant challenge, particularly when multiple methods are tested within a single project to identify the best performer. For instance, in studies aimed at binary classification, available options of ML algorithms include, but are not limited to, LR, k-nearest neighbors (KNN), Naïve Bayes (NB), SVM, random forests (RF), and neural networks (NN). Each method might necessitate a distinctly different sample size, yet there is a noticeable gap in solid theoretical guidance on how these choices affect SSD. Although there is empirical evidence indicating that different methods have varying data requirements [24], the absence of clear guidelines adds complexity to the SSD process in ML projects.
3. *Curse of Dimensionality*: The advancement of ML methods can largely be attributed to improved computational capabilities and the exponential growth in data dimensionality. In contrast to traditional studies, where the number of features is usually limited, ML techniques are frequently employed with dimensionality reduction and feature selection. Despite efforts to reduce dimensions, it is common to encounter scenarios where the number of features surpasses the sample size capacity from a traditional perspective. This has prompted discussions on identifying an optimal feature count within a given sample size constraint [25].
4. *Training, Tuning, and Validation Processes*: In ML research, the process typically involves separate stages for training, tuning, and validating models. This structured approach raises questions about the scope of SSD considerations, specifically whether they should apply to just the training set [26], the validation set [27], or both [28]. The complexity deepens with practices like cross-validation of trained models, leading to debates about the significance of SSD for internal versus external independent validation.

Navigating these challenges necessitates a sophisticated approach that acknowledges the distinct characteristics of ML research. A promising avenue involves the development of SSD frameworks that are more adaptable and flexible, capable of accommodating the inherently exploratory nature of ML projects, and the diverse range of ML techniques. Moreover, there is a pressing need for both empirical studies and theoretical advancements to enhance our understanding of how sample size influences model performance across various ML methodologies. Promoting transparency in how SSD decisions are made and reported in ML research will further improve the ability to compare and reproduce results, ultimately leading to more reliable and effective ML models for research purposes.

2 SSD in Modern Data Science: Focus on ML-Centric Studies

2.1 *Overview of Popular ML Models in Classification and Regressions*

ML algorithms have revolutionized data analysis by offering various methods suited for different types of outcomes, such as classification, regression, clustering, and dimensionality reduction (Fig. 1) [29]. This review primarily discusses classification algorithms widely used in predictive modeling, with a brief overview of regression methods. Although some classification methods can perform regression tasks, this distinction is not our primary concern. A typical machine learning predictive model undergoes at least two key phases: training on a dataset and validation on a separate set. Our emphasis is on simplifying the conversation around SSD, though it is crucial to recognize that similar SSD principles can be applied across all algorithm categories.

2.1.1 Classification Algorithms

Classification is a supervised ML technique to predict a class label for a given example. It involves creating a mapping function from input variables to discrete output categories. It can be further classified as binary or multi-class classification, with the former involving two possibilities in an outcome (e.g., "true/false") and the latter having an outcome with more than two categories [30].

Many ML algorithms are designed to address classification problems. LR is a probabilistic model used in machine learning for classification, employing a logistic function to predict probabilities. It excels with datasets that are linearly separable but may overfit when dealing with high-dimensional data [31], although regularization may help prevent overfitting [32]. However, its assumption of linearly separable variables is a drawback. NB utilizes Bayes' theorem, presuming feature

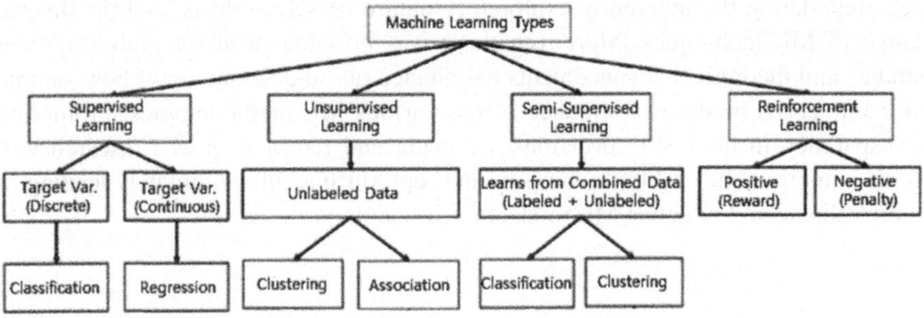

Fig. 1 An overall view of popular ML algorithm types. (Reprint from [29])

independence, to effectively classify data into binary or multi-class categories [33]. It performs well with minimal training data, offering a swift and robust model even in noisy conditions [32]. Despite its simplicity and speed, the assumption of independent features can restrict its performance. Linear Discriminant Analysis (LDA) operates as a linear classifier by fitting data to class-specific densities and employing Bayes' rule [33]. Evolving from Fisher's linear discriminant, LDA simplifies datasets to lower dimensions, thereby reducing model complexity and computational demands. It typically models classes with Gaussian distributions, assuming a shared covariance matrix among classes. The methodology of LDA aligns with principles of analysis of variance (ANOVA) and regression analysis, focusing on delineating a dependent variable through linear relationships with other variables. KNN is a type of nonparametric algorithm that avoids building a generalized model and instead retains all training instances in n-dimensional space [34]. It classifies new instances based on their proximity to the nearest neighbors, determined by similarity metrics like Euclidean distance. The classification outcome relies on the majority vote among their k closest neighbors. However, selecting the optimal number of neighbors (k) poses a significant challenge. SVM is another ML method effective for classification, regression, and other tasks, particularly in high-dimensional spaces [35]. It works by creating a hyperplane or multiple hyperplanes with the largest possible margin from the nearest data points across classes, thereby minimizing generalization error. Its performance and behavior can vary with different kernel functions, allowing it to adapt to various data structures. Decision Tree (DT) [36–38] operates by traversing from the root to leaf nodes, classifying instances based on attributes at each node. Splitting criteria commonly involve "gini" for Gini impurity and "entropy" for information gain, facilitating decision-making at each branch. Built upon DT, RF is a prominent ensemble technique, employing multiple decision trees on varied data subsets in parallel to improve accuracy and mitigate overfitting through majority voting or averaging [39]. By integrating boot-strap aggregation and random feature selection, RF enhances model reliability over single-tree models, effectively handling both classification and regression tasks for diverse data types [40] (Fig. 2 [29]). Adaptive Boosting (AdaBoost) is a meta-learning ensemble technique that iteratively corrects the mistakes of weak classifiers to form a robust predictive model. Introduced by Yoav Freund et al. [41], it sequentially combines weak learners, particularly decision trees, to enhance classification accuracy. Although highly effective, especially in binary classification, AdaBoost can be prone to overfitting and is sensitive to noise and outliers in the data. Extreme Gradient Boosting (XGBoost) is another ensemble method that refines models through gradient boosting, focusing on loss minimization with second-order gradient computations and regularization to curb overfitting. Notable for its efficiency and ability to manage large datasets, XGBoost improves generalization and performance by leveraging the principles of gradient descent and ensemble learning [32].

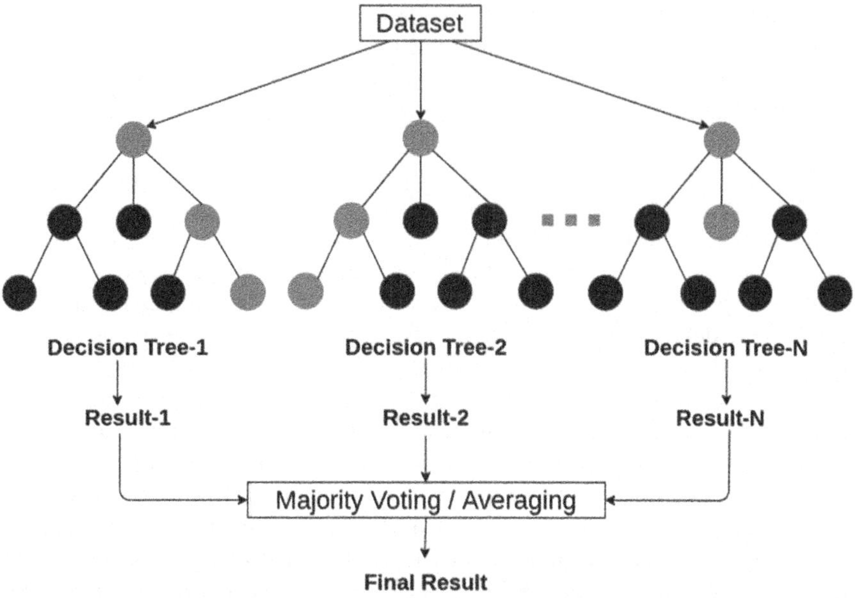

Fig. 2 An example of RF. (Reprint from [29])

2.1.2 Regression Algorithms

In ML, regression analysis typically encompasses methods that predict a continuous outcome variable based on one or more predictor variables, distinguishing itself from classification by forecasting continuous quantities rather than discrete class labels [30]. Key regression algorithms include linear regression, which establishes a linear relationship between dependent and independent variables through a best-fit line; polynomial regression, which models nonlinear relationships as polynomial degrees; and least absolute shrinkage and selection operator (LASSO) and ridge regression, which address the challenges of overfitting and feature selection in datasets with a high number of features. LASSO uses L1 regularization to potentially shrink some coefficients to zero, thus performing feature selection. In contrast, ridge regression applies L2 regularization to minimize coefficient sizes, effectively handling multicollinearity without eliminating variables. Collectively, these methodologies offer a robust framework for predictive modeling for continuous variables in various complex scenarios [42].

The summary provided in this review article is not exhaustive of all existing ML methods or does not mention deep learning (DL) methods but aims to give an overview of the diversity and scope of contemporary and widely used ML techniques. ML significantly boosts decision-making capabilities through predictive analytics, utilizing past data to predict future outcomes in numerous fields [29, 43]. For instance, in healthcare, these methods play a crucial role in diagnosis and outcome prediction, encompassing disease prediction, data analysis, and patient management [44].

2.2 Existing Methods of SSD in ML Applications and Limitations

While there have been extensive discussions on SSD for general study designs [45–47], this review emphasizes SSD within ML-based predictive modeling, noting the significant gap in standardized SSD guidelines despite their increasing application in predictive analysis [14]. A recent comparative analysis of traditional statistics and ML methods in breast cancer prognosis explicitly stated, "No standard method exists to estimate minimum sample size for our machine learning models of interest..." [48], highlighting the lack of robust SSD guidelines. The literature primarily discusses a limited range of SSD approaches, focusing mainly on LR, which is further detailed below.

2.2.1 "Rule-of-Thumb"

One commonly employed method is the "rule-of-thumb" approach, where a pre-determined number of events is specified for each candidate predictor to be included in the final model [49–55]. The final estimated sample size for patients with events is calculated by multiplying this pre-determined count with the total number of features incorporated in the final model. Subsequently, the sample size for individuals without events can also be calculated with the event rate. Despite its longstanding use, simplicity, and ease of implementation, there is no consensus on the appropriate number of events per variable (EPV) to be utilized [48].

Harrell et al. [50, 51] discuss the need for EPV in statistical models, suggesting a requirement of 10–20 EPV. In contrast, Peduzzi et al. [52] argue, based on simulation studies with real datasets, that an EPV range of 5–10 may be adequate. Through further simulation studies, Vittinghoff and McCulloch [53] concluded that a minimum of five EPV generally results in satisfactory confidence interval coverage and minimal relative bias. However, the effectiveness of adhering to 5, 10, or 20 EPV guidelines across various scenarios and data structures, evaluated against an extensive set of metrics, remains uncertain. Courvoisier et al. [55] pointed out the difficulties in LR with limited EPV, showing that achieving accurate parameter estimates is challenging even with an EPV above ten and that EPV alone does not guarantee model reliability [22]. also pointed out that EPV is not strongly related to predictive performance metrics and is therefore not an appropriate criterion for developing (binary) prediction models. Factors such as the number of predictors, the percentage of predictors that are highly correlated or non-null, the sizes of potential regression coefficients, and the sizes of predictor correlations play significant roles in the accuracy of estimates. Large regression coefficients and predictor correlations can hinder the estimation process, and a low EPV often leads to insufficient power, even with 20 EPV. Thus, it is critical to look beyond a single EPV threshold and consider these additional factors for determining the appropriate sample size for LR models. Austin and Steyer-berg [54] further investigated how EPV affects the accuracy of LR predictions using three validation methods: apparent performance, split-sample validation, and boot-strap optimism correction. They found that apparent performance overestimates accuracy, an issue that lessens with higher EPV. Boot-strap-corrected methods closely aligned with an independent validation sample when EPV reached at least 20, demonstrating its superior reliability. In contrast, split-sample validation was pessimistic and introduced significant uncertainty, effectively reducing the effective sample size.

This inconsistency in the applicability of EPV is not confined to LR but also affects other ML models, as examined in Fig. 3 [24]. This study compared the predictive accuracy of multiple modeling techniques in medical prediction tasks, investigating their dependence on sample size. Through simulations with clinical cohorts, this study assessed modern methods such as SVM, NN, and RF against LR. The study measured their performance via the area under the Receiver Operating

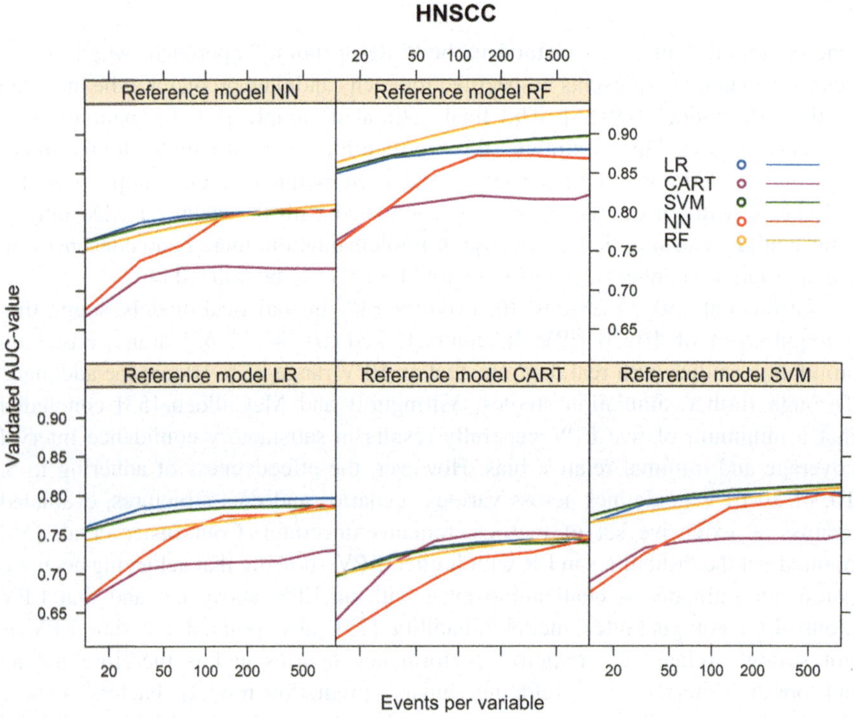

Fig. 3 Validated AUC-values vs. events per variable. (Reprint from [24])

Characteristic (ROC) curve (AUC). It found that while LR needed the fewest events per variable (20–50) for AUC stability, modern ML methods required more than ten times the number of events per variable. The findings suggest that modern ML techniques demand significantly larger datasets for reliable predictions than classical methods, recommending their use only in data-rich scenarios.

The primary concern with the "rule-of-thumb" or EPV approach stems from its lack of statistical precision and the absence of a universally agreed-upon minimum EPV. This number varies significantly based on the characteristics and goals of a study. As a result, relying on this method for SSD can be considered an oversimplification or a naïve strategy. It also seems inappropriate to apply a universal EPV requirement to all studies, as studies can vary across multiple factors that influence the appropriate sample size [67].

2.2.2 "Model-Based" SSD for Achieving Prediction Accuracy

In the realm of predictive modeling, striving for high accuracy is crucial, influencing the selection of sample size based on targeted accuracy levels. Among the various SSD strategies, "model-based" approaches are prevalent. An exemplary study [56] explored how to ascertain the ideal sample size for a training set intended for developing an efficient classifier, specifically within the context of microarray data, using a two-tiered model. The first tier involves pinpointing genes with differential expression (DE) between groups, focusing on those that offer valuable information while discarding the irrelevant ones. The next tier is dedicated to constructing the classifier from these identified genes with DE. This research proposes a model-based approach to SSD, which considers three pivotal factors: standardized fold change, class prevalence, and the number of genes or features. An example is given when having balanced numbers of patient samples across classes. By ensuring an equal selection from each class for the training set, the proposed sample size calculations proceed with an assumed prevalence of 50%. For instance, Fig. 4 [56] serves as a guide for planning classifier development projects, where the X-axis represents the standardized fold change, and the Y-axis indicates the tolerance level. The plotted lines correspond to various training set sizes, with half of the samples coming from each class. As depicted in Fig. 4, if the goal is to evenly select patients based on their recurrence status ± 2 years post-surgery for prognostic classification purposes, with an anticipated standardized fold change of 0.80 and a tolerance of 0.05, the requisite sample size is approximately 160 samples (80 per class). Although insightful, this SSD approach is mainly driven by simple models and is deemed too rudimentary for studies centered around ML techniques.

2.2.3 Learning Curve Fitting

A learning curve graphically represents the relationship between a classifier's performance and the sizes of training samples. Assuming the target performance

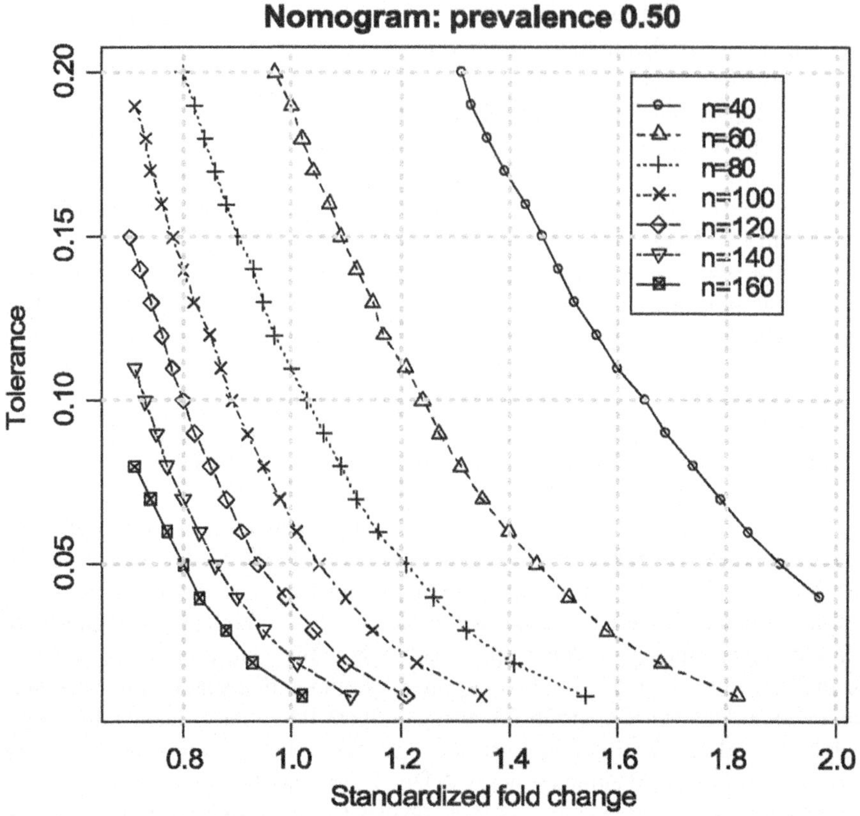

Fig. 4 How standardized fold change and tolerance levels impact sample size, assuming a 0.50 prevalence. The diagram features curved lines representing the total sample size n, with half of the samples allocated to each group, assuming the arrays contain 22,000 genes. (Reprint from [56])

measure is classification, a learning curve is typically generated by either describing the overall classification accuracy as a function of the training sample size using an inverse power law model or by learning the AUC value as a function of one over the training sample size through linear regression [14, 57]. Essentially, the process involves obtaining the data points (x_j, y_j) and creating and testing classifiers at increasing training set sizes n_j with a batch size k here $n_j = kj$, $j = 1, \ldots, m$ and m represents the number of batches. Learning curves are essential for gauging how classifier performance correlates with training data volume. Considering the curve of overall classification accuracy versus sample size as an example, a learning curve typically unfolds in three phases. The initial phase sees a marked improvement in performance as more data is added, highlighting the substantial effect of increased data on model accuracy. This early stage is critical, as even small additions of data can yield considerable performance boosts. As additional data is incorporated, the model enters a phase of diminishing returns, wherein each new

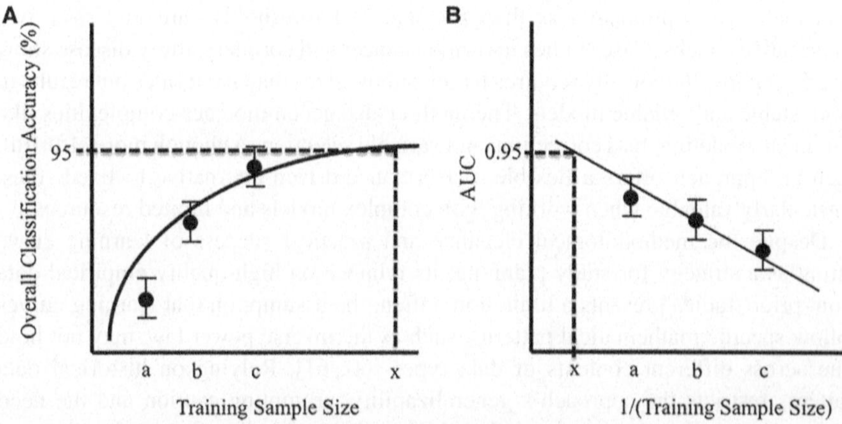

Fig. 5 Two general types of learning curve. (**a**) Overall classification accuracy versus training sample size; (**b**) AUC versus one over training sample size. (Reprint from [13])

data point contributes less to performance improvement, indicating that the model is approaching its performance ceiling. Eventually, the model reaches a plateau phase, where further additions of data cease to enhance performance significantly. This plateau suggests that the model has achieved optimal efficiency, and further improvements may require exploring alternative strategies like feature engineering or model architecture adjustments. Figure 5 [13] visually illustrates the two different types of learning curves and the learning curve stages for the first type, offering insights into the model development process.

Mukherjee et al. [58] delved into the potential of applying inverse power laws to empirical learning curves with the aim of predicting classifier performance for larger training sets. This approach sought to mathematically model how future additions to the training set might influence overall classifier accuracy. Additionally, they introduced a permutation test as a novel means to assess the statistical significance of classification performance concerning the dataset size. This methodological innovation opens new avenues for validating the robustness of classification performance improvements.

Expanding upon this concept, Boonyanunta et al. [59] applied curve fitting techniques to substantially larger datasets ($n = 1000$), adopting a nonlinear model that adheres to the inverse power law, and demonstrated the method's precision by reporting consistently low mean absolute errors. This advancement underscores the scalability of the approach and its applicability to datasets of varying sizes, enhancing its relevance for contemporary data-rich environments.

A recent case study [83] illustrates an adaptive sample size determination (SSD) approach for developing predictive logistic models. This adaptive method monitors model performance as data accumulate, adjusting the sample size to fit the modeling context. Starting with a small number of patients and adding a certain amount at a time, the model is updated until performance targets—calibration slope greater than and AUC optimism less than pre-specified thresholds—are met over two consecutive checks. Case studies in ovarian cancer and coronary artery disease show that this approach typically requires larger sample sizes than fixed rules but results in more stable and reliable models. The method also accommodates complexities like nonlinear modeling, bias correction, and variable selection. Although more effortful, such an approach offers a flexible, performance-driven alternative to fixed rules, particularly valuable when working with complex models and limited resources.

Despite the methodological elegance and practical success of learning curve fitting as a strategy for study planning, its reliance on high-quality empirical data from prior studies presents a limitation. Often, the assumption that learning curves follow specific mathematical patterns, such as the inverse power law, may not hold true across different contexts or data types [60, 61]. Relying on historical data patterns restricts the approach's generalizability, prompting caution and the need for broader empirical validation [15, 28]. Nonetheless, the ongoing exploration and refinement of learning curve methodologies continue to offer valuable insights into the nuanced relationship between data volume and model performance, guiding researchers in the efficient design and optimization of predictive models. It is also worth noting that the work in [83] does not provide a concrete tool for application, which may require additional effort from practitioners when implementing the method.

2.2.4 Simulation-Based Methods

Like traditional approaches in study design, simulation-based methods offer a sophisticated alternative for SSD, as evidenced in the literature [55, 62]. These methods have demonstrated the ability to provide more reliable outcomes than the conventional "rule-of-thumb" technique, especially when the simulation parameters closely resemble real-world scenarios. In such cases, their efficacy is anticipated to surpass other methodologies, including "learning curve fitting." Simulation-based SSD involves an in-depth process where researchers define a range of parameters—model specifications, correlations between predictors, effect sizes, and various other factors—to generate data that closely approximates actual data used in developing predictive models. This approach allows for a nuanced exploration of how different variables interact and affect the outcome, offering insights that better align with the complexities of real-world data.

The precision of these simulation-based methods is significantly influenced by the accuracy with which researchers can specify these parameters. The closer the simulation settings and parameters align with the actual data characteristics, the more likely the prediction model's performance is likely to be accurate. However, it's crucial to acknowledge that the success of these simulations is contingent upon the researcher's ability to accurately represent the real-world context within the simulation environment. This involves a thorough understanding of the underlying mechanisms of the study's subject matter, which may often require extensive preliminary research or access to detailed empirical data.

On the flip side, despite offering a range of benefits, simulation-based SSD methods come with their own sets of challenges. Depending on the complexity and the required depth of the simulation, this approach can be both time-consuming and computationally demanding. Researchers must balance the need for detailed, accurate simulations with the practical limitations of time and computational resources. This balancing act is crucial for ensuring that the simulation-based SSD method remains a viable and effective tool for study planning.

Hence, simulation-based methods for SSD represent a powerful and flexible tool in the researcher's toolkit, capable of providing detailed insights into the potential performance of prediction models. By facilitating the exploration of a wide range of scenarios and variables, these methods can significantly enhance the reliability and relevance of study designs. However, the effectiveness of simulation-based SSD relies heavily on the researcher's ability to accurately model the complexities of the real-world data, along with practical considerations of time and computational capacity. As such, while presenting a promising avenue for study design, simulation-based SSD requires careful planning and execution to harness its potential fully.

2.2.5 Riley's Framework

Riley et al. have recently developed a detailed parametric framework for SSD in predictive modeling, covering binary, continuous, and time-to-event outcomes, which has garnered significant interest [63–66]. This framework challenges the traditional "rule-of-thumb" method, which typically requires at least 10 EPV for predictive models, in line with findings from other studies [67], suggesting that such a rule may not always be applicable. According to their analysis, the adequacy of the EPV ratio can vary widely with context, influenced by several factors, including the total number of participants in the study, the incidence rate of the outcome in the population, and the expected predictive accuracy of the model [66]. Their approach emphasizes achieving a balance between obtaining precise estimates of model parameters and minimizing the risk of overfitting and optimism, proposing a more nuanced and tailored approach to SSD in various predictive modeling scenarios.

This method applies to various types of outcomes and unfolds in a four-step framework for any of the aforementioned outcomes.

Step 1: Determining the Sample Size for Precise Estimation of Overall Outcome Risk (binary or time-to-event outcome) or Mean Value (continuous outcome).

The first step focuses on determining the sample size required to accurately estimate the overall outcome risk for binary or time-to-event outcomes or the mean value for continuous outcomes. The aim is to achieve a sample size that allows for a small margin of error in estimating the intercept of a model with no predictors (the null model). For binary or time-to-event outcomes, this involves ensuring a margin of error within 0.05 for estimating any overall risk or proportion, with the necessity of specifying a key time point and event rate for time-to-event outcomes. In the case of continuous outcomes, the process is similar. Still, it requires providing the expected mean and variance of the outcome, along with the anticipated proportion of total variability explained by the model, known as R^2.

Step 2: Determining the Sample Size Needed for Predicted Values to Exhibit Minimal Mean Error Across All Individuals.

This step ensures minimal mean prediction error across the whole study. For binary outcomes, the calculation is designed to guarantee that newly developed prediction models will maintain a low prediction error in estimating outcome probabilities within the target population. This is quantified by the mean absolute prediction error (MAPE) within a pre-specified threshold, for example, 0.05. The formula necessitates predefining the number of potential predictor parameters and the expected outcome proportion in the target population. In the case of continuous outcomes, ensuring precise predictions across the range of predicted values entails accurately estimating the standard deviation of the residuals. Time-to-event outcomes proceed to step 3.

Step 3: Determining the Sample Size Needed to Achieve Minimal Required Shrinkage of Predictor Effects.

The third step involves identifying the sample size needed to minimize overfitting issues. It arises when a model's predictions for new data from the same target population are excessively extreme compared to what they should be [51]. The result is often an overly optimistic assessment of the model's predictive performance on the development dataset in the presence of overfitting, which doesn't hold when applied to new data. To combat overfitting, shrinkage (or penalization/regularization) methods [68–72] adjust the variability in the model's predictions, pulling extreme predictions toward the average. Riley et al. [63, 64] propose calculating the sample size and number of predictors to ensure a low desired shrinkage level ($\leq 10\%$) during model development. This involves pre-specifying the number of predictors and, for binary or time-to-event outcomes, the expected outcome proportion or rate in the target population. Additionally, an anticipated model performance measure, the Cox-Snell R^2 statistic [73], must be defined. In continuous outcomes, the Cox-Snell R^2 value represents the proportion of outcome variance the model explains, simply the coefficient of determination R^2.

Step 4: Ensuring Minimal Optimism in Model Fit Through Adequate Sample Size.

This step aims to select a sample size that guarantees minimal discrepancy between the model's apparent performance and its optimism-corrected fit, specifically regarding the Nagelkerke R^2, an indicator of overall model fit [74]. The apparent Nagelkerke R^2 reflects the model's performance based on the dataset used for its development. At the same time, the optimism-adjusted Nagelkerke R^2 offers a more accurate and nearly unbiased prediction of the model's fit within the target population. The calculations require an input of both the expected and the maximum Cox-Snell R^2.

Riley's approach has been garnering attention and finding broader applications. Because determining and setting prerequisites for different versions of the Cox-Snell R^2, based on prior studies or knowledge, is not always straightforward. Sometimes, these metrics may not be routinely reported or even computed. Alternatives include using the C-statistic [65] with details described below or assuming an R^2 Nagelkerke of 15%. Moreover, given that these metrics are specific to parametric models like LR, Riley's framework encounters limitations in its application to a wide range of nonparametric ML algorithms.

Building on their initial discussions of the framework, Riley et al. [66] recognize the challenge of specifying the Cox-Snell R^2. They suggest a method for approximating R^2 from the reported C-statistic (AUC) for existing models predicting binary outcomes through simulations. This method originates from the assumption that in an LR model, the linear combination of features is normally distributed, with a shared variance but distinct means for subjects with and without events. The difference in these means is related to the C-statistic [76, 77]. Drawing from this premise, a large, simulated dataset is generated, reflecting these two normal distributions for events and non-events while adjusting for the actual event prevalence in the target population. Subsequently, an LR model is applied to this dataset to obtain the Cox-Snell R^2 value.

While this SSD method covers a broad range of outcomes and can be conveniently applied through the "pmsampsize" R package, to the best of our understanding, there haven't been comprehensive simulation studies to validate the empirical effectiveness of this approach. Furthermore, it has not been formally compared with other methods, leaving its performance uncertain.

Nevertheless, we refer to the series of works by Riley et al. as the most relevant for clinical prediction model development in a broader sense, compared to other approaches. In particular, the "pmsampsize" R package provides practitioners with a convenient and reliable tool to plan SSD based on customized parameters.

In conclusion, although there has been progress in predictive analytics and associated SSD methodologies, a noticeable gap persists for those needing to plan sample sizes before deploying ML algorithms. Many existing methods originate from or mirror traditional statistical contexts, transitioning primarily to well-known parametric multivariate models. However, these approaches do not adequately cater to the diverse range of common ML techniques, which often diverge from traditional frameworks. For example, [24] suggests that the complexity of ML methods can lead to a larger minimally required sample size than estimates provided by the pmsampsize R package, highlighting the need for caution when applying existing approaches without accounting for the specific complexity of ML models. This study by Pate et al. [84] further investigates how sample size affects the stability of individual risk scores derived from cardiovascular disease (CVD) prediction models. Using data from a large primary care database, they developed models on varying sample sizes and examined how risk scores fluctuated across 1000 model replications. Their findings show that, even models meeting acceptable calibration and discrimination showed considerable variability when sample sizes were small. The authors conclude that larger sample sizes are essential to ensure stable and reliable individual risk predictions, especially when these models are used to guide clinical decisions, and they argue that sample size planning should explicitly consider risk score stability alongside traditional performance metrics. Taking all together, there remains a substantial need for further advancements in SSD strategies specifically designed for the vast array of popular ML methodologies, an area that is still seeking resolution.

3 Future Directions of SSD in ML Applications

3.1 The Role of SSD in ML-Focused Study Design

The assertion that ML-focused studies no longer adhere to traditional hypotheses, with many researchers favoring a "run first" approach, has sparked considerable controversy. This mindset appears to undermine the principles of SSD founded on classical experimental design and power analysis, generating widespread concern and debate within the academic community. Despite this shift, we maintain that SSD retains its importance in the realm of study design.

There is a prevalent belief that in studies involving vast datasets, SSD may seem to lose its relevance. Instead, the emphasis shifts toward extracting practically meaningful insights. While this perspective holds merit, we argue that issues like overfitting and the risk of false positives gain prominence in such scenarios. Thus, careful planning of study designs, ensuring appropriate size-to-feature ratios and signal-to-noise balances, becomes crucial, highlighting the continued relevance of SSD and design considerations.

The use of moderately sized or relatively small datasets for training ML models and making predictions or inferences is becoming increasingly common. For instance, studies on rare diseases might rely on single-center data comprising a few hundred events. The challenge then lies in ensuring that models trained on such datasets produce statistically sound and clinically meaningful results. Without a solid SSD rationale, the validity and reproducibility of these findings come into question. However, for studies of this scale, it is reasonable to adopt a design framework akin to traditional studies, albeit with ML models replacing conventional statistical models.

In conclusion, SSD remains a vital component in the era of "big data" and ML, underscoring the need for further research to uphold scientific integrity and robustness. As the landscape of data-driven research evolves, the integration of SSD into ML-based study designs will be crucial for ensuring the reliability and reproducibility of scientific discoveries.

3.2 Considerations of SSD Perspectives in ML Application Contexts

In this section, focusing on moderate or small scale studies and predictive modeling, we highlight crucial considerations for designing an ML-centric study.

3.2.1 Essentials s for SSD Calculations

Determining the appropriate metric for SSD, whether for precision or hypothesis testing, is vital. Despite various SSD methods, no consensus exists on the optimal measure. Riley et al.'s method [63–66], which focuses on various interpretations of Cox-Snell R^2 as a model fit and signal-to-noise ratio indicator, stands out. The diverse ML methods and performance metrics, however, may complicate this issue.

Riley et al. [66] highlight the AUC as a pivotal metric for evaluating classifier performance, which is widely acknowledged and thoroughly discussed in the scientific community for both parametric and nonparametric models [75–78].

Additionally, it is important to mention that several ML and DL methods not extensively covered in this article are nonparametric, making them particularly suited for high-dimensional data scenarios where the number of potential features significantly surpasses the number of subjects. For studies employing these methods in the primary analysis, there is a clear methodologic need to devise suitable predictive metrics that can support the SSD beyond just the AUC [79–82].

3.2.2 Training Vs. Validation

In ML studies, distinguishing between sample size considerations for training/model development and validation/testing is often blurred due to the iterative nature of ML model building. It is crucial to recognize the importance of both the training set size, which influences model quality and robustness and the validation set size, which determines test reliability. Insufficient training data undermines model credibility, while inadequate test data hampers model validation. In this review, we have focused on model development and SSD for the training set. We recommend involving cross-validation or resampling to facilitate internal validation first. External validation SSD requires additional and separate considerations. Riley et al. [84] focus on how to calculate appropriate sample sizes for external validation studies of clinical prediction models, emphasizing the limitations of traditional "rules of thumb". The authors argue that these general guidelines are often insufficient because they do not account for model-specific and population-specific factors that influence performance measures like calibration and discrimination. Instead, they propose tailored, performance-driven sample size calculations to achieve precise estimates of key metrics, including calibration-in-the-large, calibration slope, R^2, and net benefit. They present structured approaches for both continuous and binary outcomes, with worked examples demonstrating the impact of different assumptions on required sample sizes. The article highlights that many existing validation studies are underpowered, leading to imprecise estimates that can misguide clinical use. Tools like the "pmvalsampsize" package for Stata and R are introduced to implement these calculations. Ultimately, the authors stress the importance of careful sample size planning to ensure reliable and clinically useful external validation of prediction models..

4 Concluding Remarks

In conclusion, the evolving landscape of ML in research necessitates a reevaluation of traditional SSD methodologies. While ML offers unprecedented opportunities for predictive modeling, especially in datasets of moderate to small sizes, it also presents unique challenges that conventional SSD frameworks may not fully address. The shift toward ML-centric studies emphasizes the need for precision in model predictions. It underscores the importance of hypothesis testing, even in data-rich environments where the relevance of SSD could be questioned.

The complexities and nuances of SSD in ML-driven research point to the necessity for ongoing innovation and adaptation of SSD methodologies. As the field grows, so does the imperative for methods that can accommodate the diversity of ML algorithms and the specific demands of predictive modeling. The ongoing dialog among researchers, as evidenced by the work of Riley et al. [63–66], among others, is vital in paving the way for more nuanced, flexible, and effective SSD strategies that can support the integrity and robustness of ML applications in science.

Ultimately, while challenges persist in integrating traditional SSD concepts with the dynamic requirements of ML studies, the potential for advancing scientific knowledge through these methods is immense. Embracing complexity, fostering innovation, and maintaining a commitment to rigorous study design will be key to harnessing the full power of ML in research. As we move forward, it is evident that SSD will continue to play a critical role in the success of ML-centric studies, ensuring that they not only yield insightful predictions but also adhere to the highest standards of scientific validity and reproducibility.

Acknowledgments Y.Z., C.L., and A.S. are supported for their work at St Jude Children's Research Hospital by the American Lebanese Syrian Associated Charities and National Institutes of Health/National Cancer Institute grant (P30 CA021765). This work was partially supported by the American Society of Hematology (by a Scholar Award to A.S.) and a National Heart, Lung and Blood Institute/National Institutes of Health 1U01HL163983 award (to A.S.).

The content is solely the responsibility of the authors and does not necessarily represent the official views of the National Institutes of Health.

In the preparation of this manuscript, the authors utilized [OpenAI. (2024). *ChatGPT* (June 18 version) [Large language model]] for grammatical revisions. Following the use of this tool, the authors carefully reviewed and further refined the content where necessary, assuming full responsibility for the publication's final content.

Conflict of Interest A.S. has received consultant fees from Spotlight Therapeutics, Medexus Inc., Vertex Pharmaceuticals, Sangamo Therapeutics, and Editas Medicine. He is a medical monitor for an RCI BMT CSIDE clinical trial for which he receives financial compensation. He has also received research funding from CRISPR Therapeutics and honoraria from Vindico Medical Education. AS is the St. Jude Children's Research Hospital site principal investigator of clinical trials for genome editing of sickle cell disease sponsored by Vertex Pharmaceuticals/CRISPR Therapeutics (NCT03745287), Novartis Pharmaceuticals (NCT04443907), and Beam Therapeutics (NCT05456880). The industry sponsors provide funding for the clinical trial, which includes salary support paid to AS's institution. AS has no direct financial interest in these therapies.

References

1. Harrison, R.F., Kennedy, R.L.: Artificial neural network models for predicting acute coronary syndromes using clinical data from the time of presentation. Ann. Emerg. Med. **46**(5), 431–439 (2005). https://doi.org/10.1016/j.annemergmed.2004.09.012. PMID: 16271675
2. Ennis, M., Hinton, G., Naylor, D., Revow, M., Tibshirani, R.: A comparison of statistical learning methods on the gusto database. Stat. Med. **17**(21), 2501–2508 (1998)
3. Cutillo, C.M., Sharma, K.R., Foschini, L., Kundu, S., Mackintosh, M., Mandl, K.D., MI in Healthcare Workshop Working Group: Machine intelligence in healthcare-perspectives on trustworthiness, explainability, usability, and transparency. NPJ Digit Med. **3**, 47 (2020)
4. Obermeyer, Z., Emanuel, E.J.: Predicting the future—big data, machine learning, and clinical medicine. N. Engl. J. Med. **375**(13), 1216–1219 (2016)
5. Wilkinson, J., Arnold, K.F., Murray, E.J., van Smeden, M., Carr, K., Sippy, R., de Kamps, M., Beam, A., Konigorski, S., Lippert, C., Gilthorpe, M.S., Tennant, P.W.G.: Time to reality check the promises of machine learning-powered precision medicine. Lancet Digit. Health. **2**(12), e677–e680 (2020)
6. Chow, S.-C., Shao, J., Wang, H., Lokhnygina, Y.: Sample Size Calculations in Clinical Research. Chapman & Hall, CRC Press (2017)
7. Quinn, G.P., Keough, M.J.: Experimental Design and Data Analysis for Biologists. Cambridge University Press, Cambridge (2002)
8. Lenth, R.V.: Some practical guidelines for effective sample size determination. Am. Stat. **55**(3), 1–11 (2001)
9. Porta, M.: A Dictionary of Epidemiology, 6th edn. Oxford University Press, Oxford (2014)
10. Grimes, D.A., Schulz, K.F.: Descriptive studies: what they can and cannot do. Lancet. **359**, 145–149 (2002)
11. Mantel, N.: Rapid estimation of standard errors of means for small samples. Am. Stat. **5**(4), 26–27 (1951)
12. Schulz, K.F., Grimes, D.A.: Sample size calculations in randomised trials: mandatory and mystical. Lancet. **365**(9467), 1348–1353 (2005)
13. Wang, D., Bakhai, A.: Clinical Trials: a Practical Guide to Design, Analysis, and Reporting. Remedica, London (2006)
14. Balki, I., Amirabadi, A., Levman, J., Martel, A.L., Emersic, Z., Meden, B., Garcia-Pedrero, A., Ramirez, S.C., Kong, D., Moody, A.R., Tyrrell, P.N.: Sample-size determination methodologies for machine learning in medical imaging research: a systematic review. Can. Assoc. Radiol. J. **70**(4), 344–353 (2019)
15. Cho J, Lee K, Shin E, Choy G, Do S. How much data is needed to train a medical image deep learning system to achieve necessary high accuracy?. arXiv preprint arXiv:1511.06348. 2015
16. Sahiner, B., Chan, H.P., Petrick, N., Wagner, R.F., Hadjiiski, L.: Feature selection and classifier performance in computer-aided diagnosis: the effect of finite sample size. Med. Phys. **27**(7), 1509–1522 (2000 Jul)

17. Hitzl, W., Reitsamer, H.A., Hornykewycz, K., Mistlberger, A., Grabner, G.: Application of discriminant, classification tree, and neural network analysis to differentiate between potential glaucoma suspects with and without visual field defects. J. Theoret. Med. **5**(3–4), 161–170 (2003)
18. Vabalas, A., Gowen, E., Poliakoff, E., Casson, A.J.: Machine learning algorithm validation with a limited sample size. PLoS One. **14**(11), e0224365 (2019)
19. Cui, Z., Gong, G.: The effect of machine learning regression algorithms and sample size on individualized behavioral prediction with functional connectivity features. NeuroImage. **178**, 622–637 (2018)
20. Faber, J., Fonseca, L.M.: How sample size influences research outcomes. Dental Press J. Orthod. **19**(4), 27–29 (2014)
21. Ten, F.K.: Ironic rules for non-statistical reviewers. NeuroImage. **61**(4), 1300–1310 (2012)
22. van Smeden, M., Moons, K.G., de Groot, J.A., Collins, G.S., Altman, D.G., Eijkemans, M.J., Reitsma, J.B.: Sample size for binary logistic prediction models: beyond events per variable criteria. Stat. Methods Med. Res. **28**(8), 2455–2474 (2019 Aug)
23. Ludwig, J., Mullainathan, S.: Machine learning as a tool for hypothesis generation. Q. J. Econ., qjad055 (2024)
24. van der Ploeg, T., Austin, P.C., Steyerberg, E.W.: Modern modelling techniques are data hungry: a simulation study for predicting dichotomous endpoints. BMC Med. Res. Methodol. **22**(14), 137 (2014 Dec)
25. Hua, J., Xiong, Z., Lowey, J., Suh, E., Dougherty, E.R.: The optimal number of features as a function of sample size for various classification rules. Bioinformatics. **21**(8), 1509–1515 (2005)
26. Rajput, D., Wang, W.J., Chen, C.C.: Evaluation of a decided sample size in machine learning applications. BMC Bioinform. **24**(1), 48 (2023)
27. Goldenholz, D.M., Sun, H., Ganglberger, W., Westover, M.B.: Sample size analysis for machine learning clinical validation studies. Biomedicine. **11**(3), 685 (2023)
28. Rokem, A., Wu, Y., Lee, A.: Assessment of the need for separate test set and number of medical images necessary for deep learning: a sub-sampling study. BioRxiv, 196659 (2017)
29. Sarker, I.H.: Machine learning: algorithms, real-world applications and research directions. SN Comput Sci. **2**(3), 160 (2021)
30. Han, J., Pei, J., Kamber, M.: Data Mining: Concepts and Techniques. Elsevier, Amsterdam (2011)
31. LeCessie, S., Van Houwelingen, J.C.: Ridge estimators in logistic regression. J. R. Stat. Soc.: Ser. C: Appl. Stat. **41**(1), 191–201 (1992)
32. Pedregosa, F., Varoquaux, G., Gramfort, A., Michel, V., Thirion, B., Grisel, O., Blondel, M., Prettenhofer, P., Weiss, R., Dubourg, V., et al.: Scikit-learn: machine learning in python. J. Mach. Learn. Res. **12**, 2825–2830 (2011)
33. John, G.H., Langley, P.: Estimating continuous distributions in Bayesian classifiers. In: Proceedings of the Eleventh Conference on Uncertainty in Artificial Intelligence, pp. 338–345. Morgan Kaufmann Publishers Inc. (1995)
34. Aha, D.W., Kibler, D., Albert, M.: Instance-based learning algorithms. Mach. Learn. **6**(1), 37–66 (1991)
35. Keerthi, S.S., Shevade, S.K., Bhattacharyya, C., Radha Krishna, M.K.: Improvements to Platt's SMO algorithm for SVM classifier design. Neural Comput. **13**(3), 637–649 (2001)
36. Quinlan, J.R.: C4.5: Programs for Machine Learning. Morgan Kaufmann Publishers (1993)
37. Quinlan, J.R.: Induction of decision trees. Mach. Learn. **1**, 81–106 (1986)
38. Breiman, L., Friedman, J., Stone, C.J., Olshen, R.A.: Classification and Regression Trees. CRC Press (1984)
39. Breiman, L.: Random forests. Mach. Learn. **45**(1), 5–32 (2001)
40. Sarker, I.H., Watters, P., Kayes, A.S.M.: Effectiveness analysis of machine learning classification models for predicting personalized context-aware smartphone usage. J. Big Data. **6**(1), 1–28 (2019)
41. Freund, Y., Schapire, R.E., et al.: Experiments with a new boosting algorithm. ICML, Citeseer. **96**, 148–156 (1996)

42. James, G., Witten, D., Hastie, T., Tibshirani, R.: An Introduction to Statistical Learning: with Applications in R. Springer, New York (2013)
43. Cao, L.: Data science: a comprehensive overview. ACM Comput Surv (CSUR). **50**(3), 43 (2017)
44. Zhou, Y., Smith, J., Keerthi, D., Li, C., Sun, Y., Mothi, S.S., Shyr, D.C., Spitzer, B., Harris, A., Chatterjee, A., Chatterjee, S., Shouval, R., Naik, S., Bertaina, A., Boelens, J.J., Triplett, B.M., Tang, L., Sharma, A.: Longitudinal clinical data improve survival prediction after hematopoietic cell transplantation using machine learning. Blood Adv. **8**(3), 686–698 (2024)
45. Maxwell, S.E., Kelley, K., Rausch, J.R.: Sample size planning for statistical power and accuracy in parameter estimation. Annu. Rev. Psychol. **59**, 537–563 (2008)
46. Adcock, C.J.: Sample size determination: a review. J. R Stat. Soc.: Series D (The Statistician). **46**(2), 261–283 (1997)
47. Lenth, R.V.: Some practical guidelines for effective sample size determination. Am. Stat. **55**(3), 187–193 (2001)
48. Clift, A.K., Dodwell, D., Lord, S., Petrou, S., Brady, M., Collins, G.S., Hippisley-Cox, J.: Development and internal-external validation of statistical and machine learning models for breast cancer prognostication: cohort study. BMJ. **381**, e073800 (2023)
49. Moons, K.G., Royston, P., Vergouwe, Y., Grobbee, D.E., Altman, D.G.: Prognosis and prognostic research: what, why, and how? BMJ. **338**, 338 (2009)
50. Harrell Jr., F.E., Lee, K.L., Matchar, D.B., Reichert, T.A.: Regression models for prognostic prediction: advantages, problems, and suggested solutions. Cancer Treat. Rep. **69**(10), 1071–1077 (1985)
51. Harrell Jr., F.E., Lee, K.L., Mark, D.B.: Multivariable prognostic models: issues in developing models, evaluating assumptions and adequacy, and measuring and reducing errors. Stat. Med. **15**(4), 361–387 (1996)
52. Peduzzi, P., Concato, J., Kemper, E., Holford, T.R., Feinstein, A.R.: A simulation study of the number of events per variable in logistic regression analysis. J. Clin. Epidemiol. **49**(12), 1373–1379 (1996)
53. Vittinghoff, E., McCulloch, C.E.: Relaxing the rule of ten events per variable in logistic and Cox regression. Am. J. Epidemiol. **165**(6), 710–718 (2007)
54. Austin, P.C., Steyerberg, E.W.: Events per variable (EPV) and the relative performance of different strategies for estimating the out-of-sample validity of logistic regression models. Stat. Methods Med. Res. **26**(2), 796–808 (2017)
55. Courvoisier, D.S., Combescure, C., Agoritsas, T., Gayet-Ageron, A., Perneger, T.V.: Performance of logistic regression modeling: beyond the number of events per variable, the role of data structure. J. Clin. Epidemiol. **64**(9), 993–1000 (2011 Sep)
56. Dobbin, K., Zhao, Y., Simon, R.: How large a training set is needed to develop a classifier for microarray data? Clin. Cancer Res. **14**(1), 108–114 (2008)
57. Figueroa, R.L., Zeng-Treitler, Q., Kandula, S., Ngo, L.H.: Predicting sample size required for classification performance. BMC Med. Inform. Decis. Mak. **15**(12), 8 (2012 Feb)
58. Mukherjee, S., Tamayo, P., Rogers, S., Rifkin, R., Engle, A., Campbell, C., Golub, T.R., Mesirov, J.P.: Estimating dataset size requirements for classifying DNA microarray data. J. Comput. Biol. **10**(2), 119–142 (2003)
59. Boonyanunta, N., Zeephongsekul, P.: Predicting the Relationship Between the Size of Training Sample and the Predictive Power of Classifiers. Knowledge-Based Intelligent Information and Engineering Systems, vol. 3215, pp. 529–535. Springer, Berlin/Heidelberg (2004)
60. Fukunaga, K., Hayes, R.R.: Effects of sample size in classifier design. IEEE Trans. Pattern Anal. Mach. Intell. **11**(8), 873–885 (1989)
61. Cortes, C., Jackel, L.D., Solla, S.A., Vapnik, V., Denker, J.S.: Learning Curves: Asymptotic Values and Rate of Convergence. Morgan Kaufmann Publishers, VI, San Francisco (1994)
62. Snell, K.I., Archer, L., Ensor, J., et al.: External validation of clinical prediction models: simulation-based sample size calculations were more reliable than rules-of-thumb. J. Clin. Epidemiol. **135**, 79–89 (2021)

63. Riley, R.D., Snell, K.I.E., Ensor, J., Burke, D.L., Harrell Jr., F.E., Moons, K.G.M., Collins, G.S.: Minimum sample size for developing a multivariable prediction model: part I—continuous outcomes. Stat. Med. **38**(7), 1262–1275 (2019). https://doi.org/10.1002/sim.7993. Epub 2018 Oct 22. PMID: 30347470
64. Riley, R.D., Snell, K.I., Ensor, J., et al.: Minimum sample size for developing a multivariable prediction model: PART II-binary and time-to-event outcomes. Stat. Med. **38**(7), 1276–1296 (2019)
65. Riley, R.D., Van Calster, B., Collins, G.S.: A note on estimating the Cox-Snell R2 from a reported C statistic (AUROC) to inform sample size calculations for developing a prediction model with a binary outcome. Stat. Med. **40**(4), 859–864 (2021)
66. Riley, R.D., Ensor, J., Snell, K.I.E., Harrell Jr., F.E., Martin, G.P., Reitsma, J.B., Moons, K.G.M., Collins, G., van Smeden, M.: Calculating the sample size required for developing a clinical prediction model. BMJ. **18**(368), m441 (2020 Mar)
67. van Smeden, M., de Groot, J.A., Moons, K.G., et al.: No rationale for 1 variable per 10 events criterion for binary logistic regression analysis. BMC Med. Res. Methodol. **16**, 163 (2016)
68. Pavlou, M., Ambler, G., Seaman, S.R., et al.: How to develop a more accurate risk prediction model when there are few events. BMJ. **351**, h3868 (2015)
69. Van Houwelingen, J.C., Le Cessie, S.: Predictive value of statistical models. Stat. Med. **9**, 1303–1325 (1990)
70. Copas, J.B.: Regression, prediction and shrinkage. J R Stat Soc B. **45**, 311–5410 (1983)
71. Tibshirani, R.: Regression shrinkage and selection via the lasso. J R Stat Soc B. **58**, 267–8810 (1996)
72. Copas, J.B.: Using regression models for prediction: shrinkage and regression to the mean. Stat. Methods Med. Res. **6**, 167–183 (1997)
73. Cox, D.R., Snell, E.J.: The Analysis of Binary Data, vol. 46, 2nd edn. Chapman and Hall (1989)
74. Nagelkerke, N.: A note on a general definition of the coefficient of determination. Biometrika. **78**, 691–692 (1991)
75. Pencina, M.J., D'Agostino, R.B., Massaro, J.M.: Understanding increments in model performance metrics. Lifetime Data Anal. **19**(2), 202–218 (2013)
76. Su, J.Q., Liu, J.S.: Linear combinations of multiple diagnostic markers. J. Am. Stat. Assoc. **88**(424), 1350–1355 (1993)
77. Hanley, J.A., McNeil, B.J.: The meaning and use of the area under a receiver operating characteristic (ROC) curve. Radiology. **143**(1), 29–36 (1982)
78. Lee, C.Y.: Nested logistic regression models and ΔAUC applications: change-point analysis. Stat. Methods Med. Res. **30**(7), 1654–1666 (2021 Jul)
79. McNeil, B.J., Hanley, J.A.: Statistical approaches to the analysis of receiver operating characteristic (ROC) curves. Med. Decis. Mak. **4**(2), 137–150 (1984)
80. Lehmann, E.L.: Nonparametrics: Statistical Methods Based on Ranks. Prentice-Hall, Englkewood Cliffs, NJ (1998)
81. Mee, R. W. Confidence intervals for probabilities and tolerance regions based on a generalization of the Mann–Whitney statistic. J. Am. Stat. Assoc. 1990; 85: 793–800
82. Blume, J.D.: Bounding sample size projections for the area under a ROC curve. J Stat Plan Inference. **139**(1), 711–721 (2009)
83. Christodoulou, E., van Smeden, M., Edlinger, M., Timmerman, D., Wanitschek, M., Steyerberg, E.W., Van Calster, B.: Adaptive sample size determination for the development of clinical prediction models. Diagn. Progn. Res. **5**(1), 6 (2021)
84. Riley, R.D., Snell, K.I.E., Archer, L., Ensor, J., Debray, T.P.A., van Calster, B., van Smeden, M., Collins, G.S.: Evaluation of clinical prediction models (part 3): calculating the sample size required for an external validation study. BMJ. **22**(384), e074821 (2024 Jan)

Moving Beyond Mean: Harnessing Big Data for Health Insights by Quantile Regression

Tianying Wang

Abstract The era of big data has opened up new possibilities in predictive, preventive, and personalized medicine, especially in understanding complex genetic traits and disease mechanisms. However, these opportunities come with significant challenges, particularly due to data heterogeneity and the computational demands of analyzing such vast datasets. Traditional statistical methods often struggle with the diverse nature of big data, which can vary across population subgroups, measurement techniques, and study designs. This variability can make it difficult to uncover consistent patterns and draw reliable conclusions. Quantile regression offers a powerful approach to these challenges, providing a flexible and robust framework that can handle the complexities of big data. It is especially useful in biostatistics, where examining the full distribution of health outcomes can provide deeper insights into risk factors, treatment effects, and targeted interventions across different population groups. This chapter reviews recent advances in quantile regression methods with a focus on biostatistical applications, highlighting both the opportunities and challenges for future research in this area.

Keywords Quantile regression · Big data · Biostatistics · Heterogeneity · Distributional effects

1 Introduction

As an important component of public health, biostatistics includes methodological, collaborative, and translational research across multiple disciplines. It connects advanced theory and methods from statistics, machine learning, and data science with cutting-edge scientific applications in epidemiology, genetics, and genomics. Noteworthy examples include case-control designs [10, 83], cancer risk prediction

T. Wang (✉)
Department of Statistics, Colorado State University, Fort Collins, CO, USA
e-mail: Tianying.Wang@colostate.edu

Y. Zhao, D.-G. Chen (eds.), *Big Data Analytics in Biostatistics and Bioinformatics*, ICSA Book Series in Statistics,
https://doi.org/10.1007/978-3-032-06649-7_3

[38, 98], genome-wide association studies [91, 99], and studies on microbiome, metabolomic, and genetic markers [71, 81]. New technologies and the growing availability of large datasets, such as the UK Biobank[1] and All of Us,[2] provide invaluable resources for researching the causes of complex diseases [16, 88]. With data from over 500,000 participants, the UK Biobank offers extensive phenotypic and genotypic information, helping researchers understand complex conditions by integrating lifestyle, environmental, and genetic factors. Research utilizing the UK Biobank has provided insights into conditions like cardiovascular diseases and obesity [60, 124]. Another significant resource, the All of Us Research Program by the National Institutes of Health,[3] includes data from one million participants across the United States, covering aspects like environment, lifestyle, and biology. It is a giant database derived from multiple data sources and reflects the rich diversity of the United States. At the end of 2022, data involving electronic health records, surveys, physical measurements, genomics, and digital health data from Fitbit were released to researchers. More intensive data were released in 2023, including 245K+ whole genome sequencing data, 312K+ genotyping arrays, and Fitbit sleep data. Although there are currently fewer studies based on All of Us data compared to the UK Biobank, the gradual release of data suggests that research using All of Us will soon grow significantly [53]. Other large population-based studies with genetic and phenotype data available include BioBank Japan [39], TOPMed [90], H3Africa [97], Million Veteran Program [26], etc. In this chapter, we will focus on the advances, challenges, and opportunities in analyzing "big data," characterized by its large volume and diverse nature.

Big data, combined with emerging technologies and methods, is paving the way for new strategies in predictive, preventive, and personalized medicine. The vast amount of data in fields like epidemiology, genetics, and genomics has driven significant scientific advancements, leading to the development of innovative methods that reveal new discoveries. More than 5,700 genome-wide association studies (GWAS) have been conducted, shedding light on the genetic basis of complex traits and deepening our understanding of genotype-phenotype relationships [99, 113]. The growth of biobanks and large-scale population datasets has greatly facilitated GWAS analyses, leading to the development of numerous databases that compile GWAS summary statistics, including the GWAS Catalog [7], Pan UKBB,[4] and dbGaP.[5] Moreover, integrative approaches that combine diverse datasets, such as multi-omics analyses in cancer research, are evolving rapidly, providing deeper insights into disease mechanisms [11, 89]. The increasing availability of data from

---

[1] https://www.ukbiobank.ac.uk/

[2] https://www.researchallofus.org/

[3] https://allofus.nih.gov/

[4] https://pan.ukbb.broadinstitute.org/

[5] https://www.ncbi.nlm.nih.gov/gap/

resources like The Cancer Genome Atlas[6] and the Cancer Cell Line Encyclopedia[7] raises a key question: how can we leverage big data in biostatistics more efficiently and effectively to drive meaningful discoveries [41]? There are several well-known challenges for analyzing biobanks and large population-based data, including computational demands (e.g., storage, speed, data privacy), integrating multi-view data, and dealing with data heterogeneity that can undermine traditional statistical methods. Specifically, data heterogeneity can stem from a variety of factors, including unobserved variables, gene-environment interactions, model misspecification, or measurement errors, all of which complicate data analysis and interpretation [59, 62, 106, 107].

Numerous innovative approaches leveraging linear and generalized linear regression models have been extensively developed for a wide range of applications in public health, including association analysis, enrichment analysis, risk prediction analysis, and causal mediation analysis. See examples in genetics, such as GWAS and gene-set-based association tests for sequencing studies [5, 55, 121], transcriptome-wide association studies (TWAS) [28, 101], and Mendelian randomization [8, 20]. However, the rise of big data has shown that mean-based models often fall short of capturing the full spectrum of biological variability, proving inadequate in many cases. For instance, studies have shown that the FTO gene influences both the average and the variability of body mass index (BMI) [122]; variance quantitative trait loci (vQTLs) have been identified and related to unmodeled gene-environment interactions [68]. This highlights the need for more sophisticated models that go beyond simple linear frameworks to a more flexible approach to understanding complex diseases.

Quantile regression, initially introduced in economics by Koenker and Bassett Jr. [48], has gained widespread recognition across various fields. In the past decade, it has received growing attention in various disciplines, especially many research areas in public health [3]. Its strength comes from not relying on strict parametric assumptions, which makes it more robust and adaptable in real-world applications [106, 108]. Despite its proven effectiveness, quantile regression remains underexploited in biostatistics. In epidemiology, quantile regression has shown great promise for modeling complex health outcomes such as childhood BMI and maternal weight changes [96] and is instrumental in creating reference charts for monitoring child growth [116]. In genetics, quantile regression shows its invaluable ability to handle data heterogeneity and identify distribution-wise effects other than mean-based effects [68, 87, 106–108]. Furthermore, in genomics and bioinformatics, quantile regression has been used to analyze zero-inflated data and remove batch effects [57, 59]. The recognition of data heterogeneity due to unmeasured confounders or model misspecification, especially in genetics and genomics, highlights the need for more quantile regression-based methods, driving forward novel scientific discoveries.

[6] https://www.cancer.gov/ccg/research/genome-sequencing/tcga

[7] https://sites.broadinstitute.org/ccle/

In the era of big data, quantile regression stands out for its ability to handle diverse error distributions and data heterogeneity. This approach offers fresh perspectives on numerous topics, extending beyond traditional mean-based analyses. It is particularly adept at assessing effects at the distribution tails, vital for exploring rare diseases and related treatments [46]. In recent genetic studies, it has been reported that quantile regression can reveal expression quantitative trait loci (eQTL) with heterogeneous quantile effects that are closely related to strong GWAS enrichment [87], spurring a surge in biostatistics methodologies based on quantile regression. One of the key challenges of quantile regression lies in its non-differentiable loss function, which can make computation more difficult. Recent breakthroughs in computational methods have greatly enhanced the capabilities of quantile regression, offering efficient algorithms for estimation and variable selection in high-dimensional datasets [2, 78, 105, 120]. These advancements, along with new methods for handling missing data and measurement errors, have greatly expanded the scope and potential of quantile regression [115, 117]. The development of computational tools has propelled quantile regression into the forefront of statistical analysis, making it more accessible and applicable to large datasets. This progress allows for its application in sophisticated models across various domains, including genetics and epidemiology, where it is instrumental in analyzing the distributional effects of genetic variants and environmental factors on health outcomes [68, 106]. Innovations continue to evolve, addressing challenges such as censored and zero-inflated data [57, 58]. New statistical tests and inference techniques are making quantile regression even more reliable and robust in practice. Moreover, combining quantile regression with machine learning techniques is leading to the development of more refined and personalized predictive models, reaffirming its integral role in contemporary data analysis [35].

With the advent of larger datasets and diverse data sources, the field of biostatistics stands on the cusp of fully harnessing the capabilities of quantile regression. In the subsequent sections of this chapter, we will introduce the foundational aspects of quantile regression, covering model formulation, estimation techniques, and inferential methods. We will also explore its recent forays into epidemiology, genetics, and genomics, highlighting its practical applications and contributions to these fields. Concluding the chapter, we will examine the prospects and obstacles presented by the big data landscape, setting the stage for its broader adoption and innovation in biostatistics.

2 Core Concepts and Methods in Quantile Regression

In this section, we introduce the fundamental notations and concepts that form the basis of quantile regression. We start with the basic quantile linear regression model, which focuses on a fixed quantile level $\tau \in (0, 1)$. This model describes the τth quantile of the response variable as a linear combination of covariates. We will gradually expand this framework, adapting it to address various applied problems.

2.1 Basic Principles and Modeling

Let Y be a real-valued random variable with distribution function F. For a quantile level $\tau \in (0, 1)$, the τth quantile of Y can be written as

$$Q_\tau(Y) := F^{-1}(\tau) = \inf\{y : F(y) \geq \tau\}.$$

This quantile function encapsulates Y's distribution, allowing the τth sample quantile to be estimated via the empirical distribution of a sample. Introduced by Koenker and Bassett Jr. [48], quantile regression models the τth quantile of Y as a function of covariates $X \in \mathbb{R}^p$, which can be either continuous or discrete, where typically $p \ll n$. Assuming we have data for n subjects $\{Y_i, X_i\}_{i=1}^n$, we begin with the linear model:

$$Y_i = \beta_0 + X_i^\top \beta_1 + \epsilon_i, \tag{1}$$

where the errors ϵ_i are independent and identically distributed (iid). The conditional quantile of Y given X is

$$Q_{Y_i}(\tau \mid X_i) = \beta_0 + X_i^\top \beta_1 + F_\epsilon^{-1}(\tau), \tag{2}$$

with $F_\epsilon^{-1}(\tau)$ representing the τth percentile of ϵ. We consider a more general form of quantile regression as below

$$Q_{Y_i}(\tau \mid X_i) = \beta_0(\tau) + X_i^\top \beta_1(\tau), \tag{3}$$

where $\beta_0(\tau)$ and $\beta_1(\tau)$ are the unknown intercept and coefficients. Under the specific linear model in Eq. (2), we know that $\beta_0(\tau) = \beta_0 + F_\epsilon^{-1}(\tau)$ and $\beta_1(\tau) = \beta_1$. Though both Models (1) and (3) admit linear form, Model (3) is more general and encompasses a wider array of possible relationships between Y and X. For example, in a heteroscedastic model where the error term varies with X:

$$Y_i = \beta_0 + X_i^\top \beta_1 + \sigma(X_i)\epsilon_i, \tag{4}$$

where $\sigma(x) = x^\top \gamma$ and ϵ_i's are iid. Then, the conditional quantile function of Y can be written as

$$Q_{Y_i}(\tau \mid X_i) = \beta_0 + X_i^\top \beta_1 + \sigma(X_i) F_\epsilon^{-1}(\tau) = \beta_0(\tau) + X_i^\top \beta_1(\tau),$$

where $\beta_0(\tau) = \beta_0$ and $\beta_1(\tau) = \beta_1 + \gamma F_\epsilon^{-1}(\tau)$. In general, the explicit form of $\beta_0(\tau)$ and $\beta_1(\tau)$ is not assumed. Unlike traditional regression, quantile regression does not assume a particular distribution for the errors, which confers advantages such as robustness to outliers and non-Gaussian error terms.

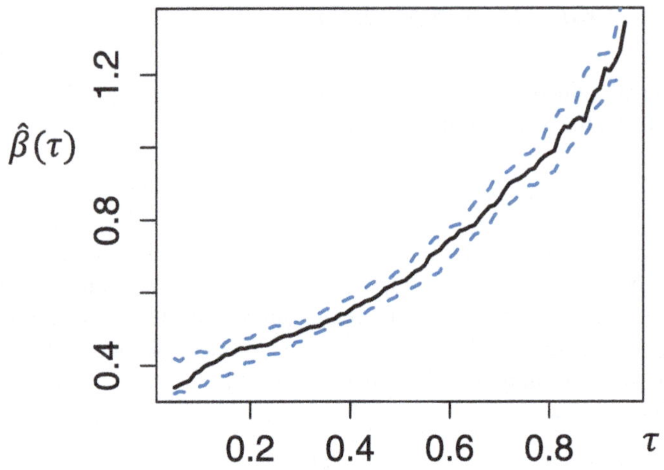

Fig. 1 Estimated $\beta(\tau)$ at different quantile levels. Blue dashed lines indicate 95% confidence intervals

The conditional distribution of Y can be estimated by fitting quantile regression for $\tau \in (0, 1)$. The model presented in Eq. (3) can be interpreted from a random coefficient viewpoint, as illustrated in Fig. 1. By assuming the model's validity across the entire range of $\tau \in (0, 1)$, we outline a stochastic process for the generation of the response variable Y. Specifically, given $X = x$, Y can be modeled by $Y = \beta_0(U) + x^\top \beta_1(U)$, where U is drawn from a Uniform[0, 1] distribution. This approach of employing estimated quantile regression coefficients to reconstruct Y's distribution is a well-established practice.

Focusing on Model (3), we estimate $\beta_0(\tau)$ and $\beta_1(\tau)$ by minimizing the quantile loss function $\rho_\tau(\cdot)$. The sample estimators are obtained as follows:

$$\hat{\beta}_0(\tau), \hat{\beta}(\tau) = \arg\min_{\beta_0, \beta} \sum_{i=1}^{n} \rho_\tau(y_i - \beta_0 - X_i^\top \beta), \quad \text{for} \quad \tau \in (0, 1), \tag{5}$$

where $\rho_\tau(u) = u(\tau - I(u < 0))$, illustrated in Fig. 2. Unlike the least squares method used in linear regression, the quantile regression loss function uses absolute deviations instead of squared errors, making it less sensitive to outliers and influential data points. Linear programming algorithms are employed to solve this loss function, yielding consistent estimators for β [43, 49]. The R package `quantreg` [47] provides various algorithms for quantile regression under different situations.

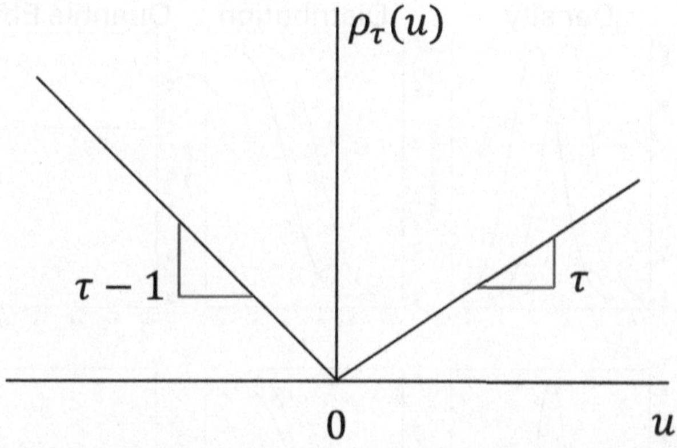

Fig. 2 Quantile regression loss function $\rho_\tau(u) = u(\tau - I(u < 0))$ for $\tau \in (0, 1)$

2.2 *Quantile Treatment Effects*

The quantile treatment effect (QTE) is defined by the relative displacement between two distribution functions, as characterized by Doksum [21], Koenker [46]. Consider two distributions F and G; the QTE is then expressed as the "horizontal distance" at each quantile level:

$$\Delta(\tau) = G^{-1}(\tau) - F^{-1}(\tau), \tag{6}$$

representing the discrepancy at the τth quantile between the distributions. The empirical counterpart of the QTE is given by

$$\hat{\Delta}(\tau) = \hat{G}_n^{-1}(\tau) - \hat{F}_n^{-1}(\tau),$$

where $\hat{G}_n$ and $\hat{F}_n$ are the empirical distribution functions from the treatment and control samples, respectively.

Moreover, the mean treatment effect (MTE) is the integral of the QTE over all quantiles $\tau \in (0, 1)$:

$$\bar{\Delta} = \int_0^1 \Delta(\tau)d\tau = \int G^{-1}(\tau)d\tau - \int F^{-1}(\tau)d\tau = \mu(G) - \mu(F),$$

with $\mu(G)$ and $\mu(F)$ denoting the means of the distributions G and F. This integral effectively summarizes the average effect across all quantiles.

Considering a dataset with n independent observations, let X_i denote a binary treatment indicator where $X_i = 1$ represents a treated subject and $X_i = 0$ indicates a control. With the assumption of random assignment and balance between the groups, the quantile effect model mirrors Eq. 3. This model acknowledges potential variations in the response variable Y's distribution across treatment and control

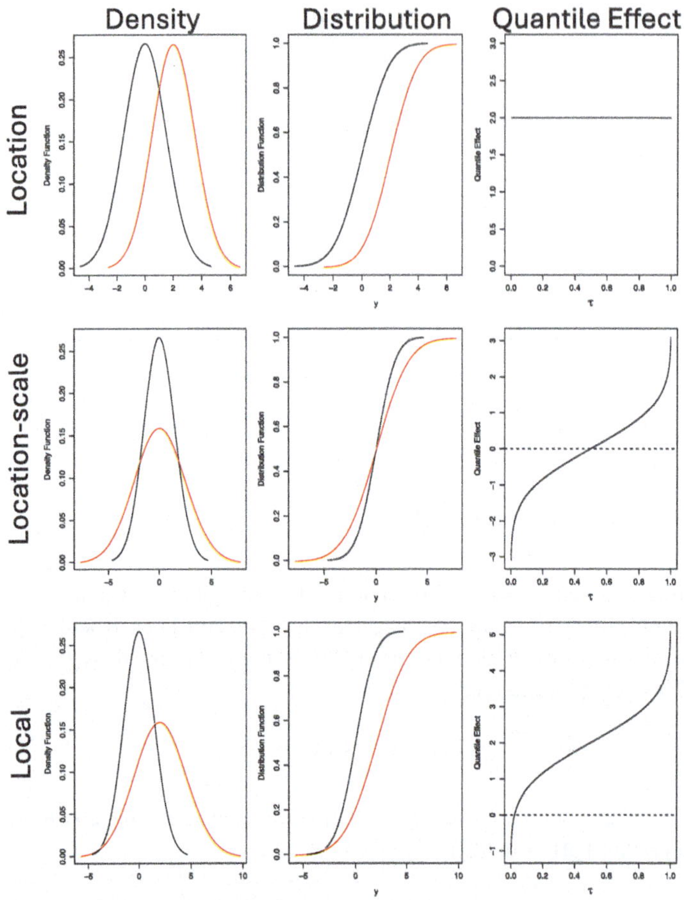

Fig. 3 Quantile effects in different models: location shift (**top** panel), location-scale (**middle** panel), and local (**bottom** panel) models. The three columns, from left to right, are the density function, distribution function, and quantile effect of two distributions under different models

groups through the parameters $\beta_0(\tau)$ and $\beta_1(\tau)$. Here, $\beta_0(\tau)$ characterizes the quantile function for the control group, while $\beta_1(\tau)$ quantifies the discrepancy in quantiles between treated and control subjects, defining the quantile treatment effect. This effect is analogous to the generalized mean treatment effect viewed from a distributional stance, as shown in Eq. (6).

For illustrative purposes, Fig. 3 depicts the quantile effects under various models: location shift, location-scale, and local. Notably, $\beta_1(\tau)$ varies with the quantile level τ in the location-scale and local models, suggesting that quantile regression captures a nuanced comparison between distributions. This aspect highlights its potential as a robust tool for assessing distributional similarities, such as comparing treatment versus control group outcomes.

Statistical inference for $\hat{\beta} = (\hat{\beta}_0, \hat{\beta}_1)$ is grounded in classical large-sample theory. Suppose that ϵ_i's are iid with a distribution function F_ϵ and a density function f_ϵ. Assume that $f_\epsilon(F_\epsilon^{-1}(\tau)) > 0$. Denote $Q_n = n^{-1}\sum_{i=1}^n \tilde{X}_i\tilde{X}_i^\top$ with $\tilde{X}_i = [1\ X_i]$. We assume that Q_n converges to a positive definite matrix Q_0. Under these conditions, the asymptotic behavior of $\hat{\beta}$ is characterized by

$$\sqrt{n}[\hat{\beta}(\tau) - \beta(\tau)] \rightsquigarrow N\left(0, \frac{\tau(1-\tau)}{f_\epsilon^2(F_\epsilon^{-1}(\tau))} Q_0^{-1}\right).$$

The density f_ϵ can be estimated using kernel methods, as suggested by Koenker [45]. From this foundation, a Wald-type test statistic is derived to facilitate hypothesis testing.

For quantile regression models applied across multiple levels $\{\tau_1, \cdots, \tau_K\}$, the joint asymptotic distribution of the estimators $\hat{\beta}^*_{Kp\times 1} = (\hat{\beta}^\top(\tau_1), \cdots, \hat{\beta}^\top(\tau_K))^\top$ is given by

$$\sqrt{n}[\hat{\beta}(\tau) - \beta(\tau)] \rightsquigarrow N\left(0, \Omega \bigotimes Q_0^{-1}\right),$$

where Ω is a $K \times K$ matrix with its (j, j') elements being

$$\Omega_{j,j'} = (\tau_j \wedge \tau_{j'} - \tau_j\tau_{j'})/\{f_\epsilon[F_\epsilon^{-1}(\tau_j)]f_\epsilon[F_\epsilon^{-1}(\tau_{j'})]\}.$$

This framework also extends to cover non-iid settings in the asymptotic distribution of $\hat{\beta}(\tau)$. As the error density is no longer identical for all observations, the asymptotic theory of $\hat{\beta}(\tau)$ is more complicated:

$$\sqrt{n}(\hat{\beta}(\tau) - \beta(\tau)) \rightsquigarrow N(0, \tau(1-\tau)H_n^{-1}Q_nH_n^{-1}),$$

where $H_n = \lim_{n\to\infty} n^{-1}\sum_{i=1}^n \tilde{X}_i\tilde{X}_i^\top f_{\epsilon,i}(F_{\epsilon,i}^{-1}(\tau))$. Note that $f_{\epsilon,i}(F_{\epsilon,i}^{-1}(\tau)$ denotes the conditional density of the response Y_i at the τth conditional quantile. In this case, the error density estimation is a more challenging task. More details can be found in [45, Section 3.2.3, 4.3].

2.3 *Rank-Based Inference Approaches*

While constructing Wald-type test statistics directly from the asymptotic distributions is straightforward, the rank score test is favored for its simplicity, as it bypasses the need to estimate the error density, requiring only the null model to be fitted. We will briefly introduce the regression rank scores and associated tests.

The essence of the quantile regression rank score lies in the linear programming approach to solving the quantile loss function $\rho_\tau(\cdot)$. For the quantile regression model in Eq. (3), an equivalent linear programming formulation is

$$
\begin{aligned}
&\tau \mathbf{1}_n^\top u^+ + (1-\tau)\mathbf{1}_n^\top u^- := \min \\
&\text{s.t.} \quad \tilde{X}\hat{\beta} + u^+ - u^- = Y \\
&\beta \in \mathbb{R}^{p+1}, \quad u^+, u^- \in \mathbb{R}_+^n, \quad \tau \in (0,1)
\end{aligned}
\tag{7}
$$

where $\tilde{X} = [1\ X]$, $\beta_{(p+1)\times 1} = (\beta_0, \beta_1^\top)^\top$, and $\mathbf{1}_n = (1, \cdots, 1)^\top \in \mathbb{R}^n$. This problem can be efficiently solved for all $\tau \in (0, 1)$ using parametric linear programming, offering $O_p(n \log n)$ distinct solutions [76]. The regression rank score is introduced by Gutenbrunner and Jurecková [29] through a dual program of Eq. (7)

$$
\begin{aligned}
&Y^\top \hat{a}(\tau) := \max \\
&\tilde{X}^\top \hat{a}(\tau) = (1-\tau)\tilde{X}^\top \mathbf{1}_n \\
&\hat{a}(\tau) \in [0,1]^n, \quad \tau \in (0,1),
\end{aligned}
\tag{8}
$$

where $\hat{a}(\tau)$ is the solution of this dual form of the linear program, namely, regression rank score. The regression rank score $\hat{a}_i$ for $i = 1, \cdots, n$ implies that

$$
\hat{a}_i(\tau) = \begin{cases} 1 & \text{if } Y_i > \tilde{X}_i^\top \hat{\beta}(\tau) \\ 0 & \text{if } Y_i < \tilde{X}_i^\top \hat{\beta}(\tau), \end{cases} \tag{9}
$$

and $\hat{a}_i(\tau)$ for $\{i \mid Y_i = \tilde{X}_i^\top \hat{\beta}(\tau)\}$ is determined by the equality constraints in Eq. (8). In short, in a location model, the regression rank score for the ith observation is one only when Y_i is above the τth quantile regression plane. Integrating $\hat{a}_i(\tau)$ over τ provides a rank vector for the sample, linking quantile regression rank scores with nonparametric tests like the Wilcoxon-Mann-Whitney test. Further details can be found in [86] and [29].

The related statistical inference can be built either on the rank score at a fixed τ (i.e., Eq. (9)) or an integrated rank score, which integrates $\hat{a}_i(\tau)$ over [0, 1]. Novel methods have been proposed based on a single τ rank score [87] and an integrated τ rank score [106]. We will review the details in the context in Sect. 4.

2.4 *Model Selection and Evaluation*

In addition to the Wald test and rank score test, quantile regression also has likelihood ratio tests, which are commonly used as a criterion for model fitting [51]. Consider the asymmetric Laplace density $f(u) = \tau(1-\tau)\exp\{-\rho_\tau(u)\}$, and assuming ϵ_i's follow this distribution, the log-likelihood becomes

$$l(\beta) = n \log(\tau(1-\tau)) - \sum_i \rho_\tau(Y_i - \tilde{X}_i^\top \beta).$$

The likelihood ratio statistic for comparing nested quantile regression models is given by

$$-2 \log \lambda(\tau) = 2\{l(\hat{\beta}(\tau)) - l(\tilde{\beta}(\tau))\} = 2(\tilde{V}(\tau) - \hat{V}(\tau)),$$

where $\hat{\beta}(\tau)$ and $\tilde{\beta}(\tau)$ are estimates from the full and nested models, respectively, with $\hat{V}(\tau)$ and $\tilde{V}(\tau)$ representing the corresponding minimized quantile loss values.

Expanding these hypothesis tests to encompass all quantile levels from 0 to 1 leads to the introduction of the Wald, rank score, and likelihood ratio processes. For a comprehensive discussion, [45] provides further insights.

2.5 Computational Techniques in Quantile Regression

Computational efficiency plays a crucial role in quantile regression. Estimating coefficients in quantile regression (Eq. (3)) is often solved by algorithms from three main categories: simplex, interior point, and smoothing [13]. The simplex algorithm solves the primary linear programming problem (i.e., estimating coefficients β) [1], but it can be computationally intensive for large datasets. In contrast, interior point algorithms, designed for extensive linear programming challenges, offer a more scalable solution [40]. Notably, an accelerated interior point method tailored for quantile regression at specific τ levels in large datasets was introduced by [78]. It is based on solving the equations to satisfy the Karush-Kuhn-Tucker conditions for optimality and is appealing for fitting the quantile regression model at a specific τ in large data. We refer to [119] for more details. The smoothing algorithm offers an alternative by approximating the non-differentiable quantile loss function $\rho_\tau(u)$ with a generalized Huber function $H_{\gamma,\tau}(u)$, defined piecewise as:

$$H_{\gamma,\tau}(u) = \begin{cases} u(\tau-1) - \frac{1}{2}(\tau-1)^2\gamma & \text{if } u \leq (\tau-1)\gamma \\ \frac{u^2}{2\gamma} & \text{if } (\tau-1)\gamma \leq u \leq \tau\gamma \\ u\tau - \frac{1}{2}\tau^2\gamma & \text{if } u \geq \tau\gamma \end{cases}. \qquad (10)$$

See Fig. 4 for a visualization. These computational strategies, particularly those encapsulated within the R package `quantreg`, are crucial for applying quantile regression across various scientific domains.

In a nutshell, while linear regression describes the conditional expectation $E(Y \mid X)$, quantile regression provides a unique perspective and describes the conditional quantile of $Y \mid X$. By modeling through all $\tau \in (0, 1)$, one models

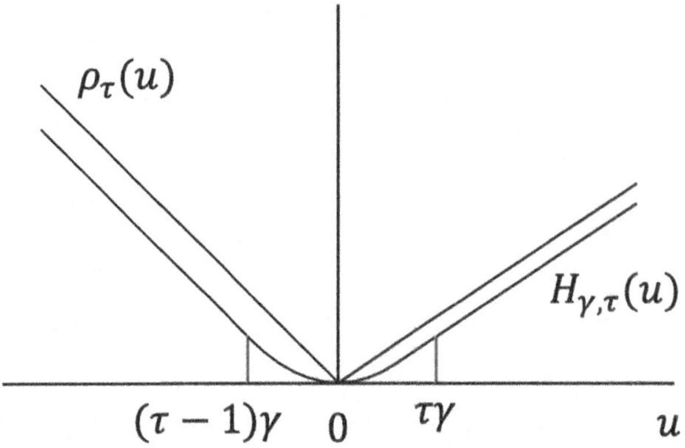

Fig. 4 Quantile loss function ρ_τ and the approximation function $H_{\gamma,\tau}$

the entire conditional distribution of Y. The basic features and characteristics we reviewed in this section have been exploited in many scientifically important applications [59, 87, 95]. The subsequent sections will review recent quantile regression advancements in fields like epidemiology, genetics, and genomics, highlighting their potential and challenges in the context of big data.

3 Empowering Epidemiological Insights: Quantile Regression in Time-Dependent Data

Quantile regression is gaining recognition in epidemiology for its capacity to model outcomes beyond the limitations of traditional linear regression. This approach reveals how exposures or treatments impact different parts of the outcome distribution, rather than focusing only on the mean. This is particularly important in epidemiology, where health outcomes often have skewed distributions or are shaped by extreme values, and where the effect of exposure can vary across different population groups. In environmental health studies, for instance, the impact of air pollution on lung function can vary widely among different segments of the population. Quantile regression can help identify how specific subgroups, such as children or the elderly, are affected differently at various levels of lung function. In nutritional epidemiology, the link between dietary factors and body mass index (BMI) may vary along the BMI scale, indicating that dietary interventions might be tailored to specific population groups [95]. In this section, we will explore the use of quantile regression in epidemiology, focusing on its applications in growth charts, longitudinal data analysis, and survival analysis.

3.1 *Quantile Regression in Growth Chart Development*

Reference centile charts serve as crucial epidemiological instruments for disease screening and evaluating health status. A well-known application is the use of growth charts to compare a child's growth with that of peers, a practice highlighted by Wei et al. [116] and recently expanded to include reference construction for rare diseases through natural history data [111]. In this subsection, we focus on a continuous variable of interest, denoted as Y, alongside time or age, represented by t. Typically, the analysis involves n independent subjects, each with observations Y_i, t_i, where i ranges from 1 to n. We will clarify whether the data comprises repeated or longitudinal measurements within the given context.

3.1.1 Development and Application of Growth Charts

The growth chart is a specific type of reference centile chart that is utilized by pediatricians to compare an individual's measurements against population norms. Since 1977, the National Center for Health Statistics (NCHS) in the United States developed the first version of pediatric growth chart[8] as a clinical tool for determining if the growth of a child is adequate. A growth chart consists of a set of curves describing how the response variable (e.g., weight or height) changes with covariates (e.g., age) at different population quantiles. Each curve on the chart illustrates how the response variable changes at a particular quantile τ. Common approaches for constructing reference centile charts include the LMS method [15] and various quantile regression methods. The LMS method, grounded in the Box-Cox power transformation [6], presupposes that the Box-Cox-transformed measurements of Y adhere to a normal distribution. It models the quantiles of Y as

$$Q(\tau \mid t) = \mu(t)(1 + \lambda(t)\sigma(t)\Phi^{-1}(\tau))^{1/\lambda(t)},$$

where the functions $\{\lambda(t), \mu(t), \sigma(t)\}$ evolve with age t. These functions are estimated by maximizing a penalized log-likelihood that incorporates the Box-Cox log-likelihood. Carey et al. [9] provides an extensive discussion of the estimation process. However, the assumption of normality post-Box-Cox transformation remains a point of contention.

Estimating a family of conditional quantile functions by solving a nonparametric quantile regression problem is a natural solution:

$$\min_{g \in \mathcal{G}} \sum_{i=1}^{n} \rho_\tau(Y_i - g(t_i)), \tag{11}$$

[8] https://www.cdc.gov/growthcharts/background.htm

where g is an unknown function within a set of candidate functions $\mathscr{G}$. The function $g(\cdot)$ can be approximated using B-spline bases. Model (11) describes *unconditional growth curves*, capturing the quantile of Y (such as height or BMI) based solely on age t. In contrast, *conditional growth curves* leverage longitudinal data to consider growth history and additional covariates. A detailed evaluation of quantile regression methods for both unconditional and conditional growth curve construction is discussed in [116]. When longitudinal data is collected, the conditional growth models can be formulated through a first-order autoregression model for quantile regression [116]:

$$Q_{Y_i(t_{i,j})}(\tau \mid t_{i,j}, Y_i(t_{i,j-1}), x_i) = g_\tau(t_{i,j}) + (\alpha(\tau) + \beta(t_{i,j} - t_{i,j-1}))Y_i(t_{i,j-1}) + x_i^\top \gamma(\tau),$$

where the measurements are $\{Y_i(t_{i,j}) : j = 1, \cdots, T_i, i = 1, \cdots, n\}$ on n individuals. The g_τ is nonparametric and can be expressed as a linear expansion of B-splines. Additional covariates can be incorporated into the model.

Growth charts map out population growth patterns over time and are pivotal for identifying atypical growth trajectories in individuals. For example, a shift from the 50th to the 30th percentile in a child's growth trajectory might signal the need for further medical investigation. Once established, these charts allow healthcare professionals to track a child's growth by overlaying their longitudinal measurements against the population benchmarks to detect any significant shifts in their growth percentile. Consider Fig. 5 as an illustration, where the curves delineate growth patterns for ages 6 to 10. Here, the growth paths of subjects 89 (circles)

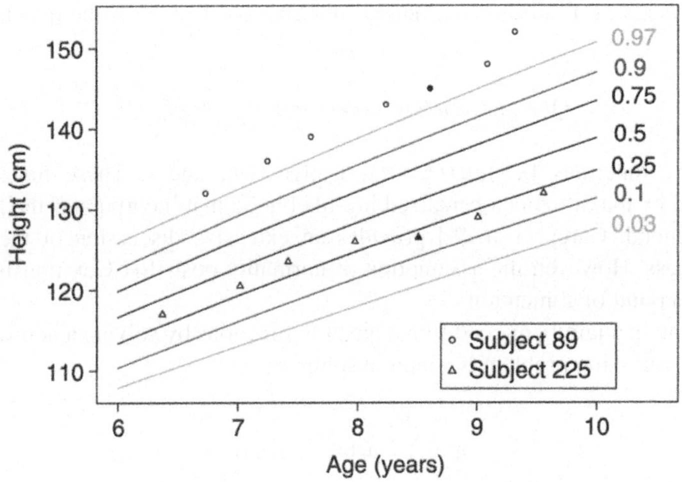

Fig. 5 An example of using a reference growth chart to screen individual growth paths (Figure 5 from [116])

and 225 (triangles) are juxtaposed with the reference curves. While both subjects have grown over time, their relative standings among peers have diverged: subject 89 remains consistently above the 97th percentile, while subject 225, initially at the median, descends to the 25th percentile post-age 8, indicating potential health concerns.

The advent of quantile regression has popularized and enhanced the development of growth charts in recent years, facilitating more nuanced and comprehensive growth assessments [70, 75]. Upcoming discussions will cover the adaptation of these methods to bivariate outcomes, such as height and weight.

3.1.2 Bivariate Models for Growth Assessment

Reference centile curves are traditionally univariate, but extending these to multivariate responses like height and weight simultaneously poses significant challenges due to the undefined rank of multivariate outcomes. Wei [114] introduces a two-stage method to estimate bivariate quantile functions, enhancing pediatric growth assessment by incorporating longitudinal data and multiple covariates. By leveraging quantile regression for longitudinal data, this new method expands the applicability of traditional growth charts to more application scenarios. The nonparametric estimation of the reference quantile contours, C_τ, involves a two-step procedure. Denote $\{\mathbf{y}_i = (y_{i1}, y_{i2})^\top, i = 1, \cdots, n\}$ as a random sample following the joint density of a random vector $\mathbf{Y}$. First, we standardize the data as

$$z_i = \hat{S}^{-1}(\mathbf{y}_i - \hat{\mu}),$$

where $\hat{\mu}$ is the vector of sample medians, and $\hat{S}$ is the diagonal matrix of sample median absolute deviations. Then, we estimate the τth reference quantile contour as a function of the polar angle, $g_\tau(\theta) : [0, 2\pi] \to \mathbb{R}$, subject to the constraint $g_\tau(0) = g_\tau(2\pi)$. This involves optimizing over a family of constrained smooth functions $G = \{g(\theta) : [0, 2\pi] \to \mathbb{R}\ s.t.\ g(0) = g(2\pi)\}$ to minimize the objective function:

$$\sum_{i=1}^{n}\sum_{k=1}^{2} \rho_{(\tau+1)/2}(r_{i,k} - g(\theta_{i,k})),$$

where $r_{i,k}$ and $\theta_{i,k}$ are the polar coordinates of the standardized data points z_i and ρ_τ is the quantile regression loss function. Then, the stratified quantile regression models are proposed for the marginal and conditional distributions. Consider a dataset $\{\mathbf{Y}_{ij}, t_{ij}, X_{ij}\}$ collected from $i = 1, \cdots, n$ subjects and $j = 1, \cdots, m_i$ longitudinal measurements for the ith subject. The distribution of $\mathbf{Y}$ is modeled given t and X through two stratified quantile models. For the marginal model for Y_{ij1}:

$$Q_\tau(Y_{ij1}) = g_1(\tau; t_{ij}, X_{ij}),$$

where g_1 represents the quantile function for the first outcome variable $\mathbf{Y}_{ij1}$ (e.g., height) given time t_{ij} and covariates X_{ij}. Then, we consider the conditional model for Y_{ij2} given Y_{ij1}:

$$Q_\tau(Y_{ij2}|Y_{ij1}) = g_2(\tau; t_{ij}, X_{ij}, Y_{ij1}),$$

where g_2 represents the quantile function for the second outcome variable $\mathbf{Y}_{ij2}$ (e.g., weight) given the first outcome variable, time, and covariates. The estimated quantile functions $\hat{g}_{n1}(\tau)$ and $\hat{g}_{n2}(\tau)$ are obtained by minimizing the quantile regression loss function:

$$\hat{g}_{n1}(\tau) = \arg \min_{g_1 \in G_1} \rho_\tau(Y_{ij1} - g_1(t_{ij}, X_{ij})),$$

$$\hat{g}_{n2}(\tau) = \arg \min_{g_2 \in G_2} \rho_\tau(Y_{ij2} - g_2(t_{ij}, X_{ij}, Y_{ij1})),$$

where ρ_τ is the check function for quantile τ, and G_1, G_2 are families of measurable functions for g_1 and g_2, respectively.

This innovative methodology is particularly applied to constructing bivariate age-dependent growth charts, providing a more comprehensive assessment of children's growth and health status than traditional univariate charts. The paper demonstrates the utility of this approach through a simulation study and an application to US children's growth data, highlighting its potential for more informative and adaptive bivariate growth charts and other multivariate applications.

Besides extending traditional growth chart into multivariate responses, a new method, motivated by modeling natural history data containing a significant portion of zeros, has been proposed as a two-part modeling approach that jointly models the zeros and positive responses [111]. Essentially, quantile regression (Eq. (3)) requires a continuous response. However, excessive zeros are widely observed in the research-interested responses in many applications. The authors show that the proportion of zeros in the response (e.g., a disease-related measurement), in rare diseases, is varying over time (age) and should not be ignored. This method addresses the challenge of directly using such data as external control due to age-dependent distributions and the possibility of an absorbing state of zero in disease progression. By applying zero-inflated kernel quantile (ZIKQ) estimation to Duchenne Muscular Dystrophy data, the paper demonstrates how these charts can enhance treatment efficacy evaluation and patient enrollment strategies in rare disease clinical development. We will skip the technical details here and introduce how to model zero-inflated responses in Sect. 5.

3.2 *Other Longitudinal Data Analysis with Quantile Regression*

Quantile regression techniques, like the empirical likelihood method, excel in analyzing longitudinal data by adeptly managing within-subject correlations and cases where participants drop out for reasons tied to the study [44, 103]. These methods shine in biostatistical analyses, where non-normal data distributions and dropout events are frequent in longitudinal medical studies. They provide a robust framework for efficient and accurate data analysis without requiring assumptions about the true correlation structure, making them suitable for a wide range of applications in medical research.

The work by Geraci and Bottai [24] introduces a novel approach using the asymmetric Laplace distribution for quantile regression in longitudinal studies. This method allows for a detailed examination of the conditional quantiles of a response variable, accommodating the complexities of repeated measurements over time, which is essential for understanding the dynamics of medical outcomes and treatment effects. He et al. [31] focus on median regression for longitudinal data, presenting a methodology that is particularly useful for skewed data distributions. This approach is robust to outliers in response measurements, providing a more reliable analysis of central tendencies in biomedical research. Similarly, [34] tackles the estimation of large covariance matrices in longitudinal data using basis function approximations, addressing the challenge of modeling the correlation structure in repeated measurements from the same subject. The work of [54] enhances the efficiency of quantile regression estimations for longitudinal data through smoothing combined estimating equations, offering a more accurate depiction of the conditional distribution of the response variable across different quantiles. Lu and Fan [63] further contribute to this field by introducing weighted quantile regression, which accounts for the varying reliability of observations within longitudinal datasets. This method allows for a nuanced analysis of the conditional distribution of the response variable, providing insights into the effects of treatments or exposures across the entire distribution of outcomes. Together, these papers represent significant progress in the application of quantile regression methods to longitudinal data, offering powerful statistical tools for the nuanced analysis required in biostatistics and epidemiological research.

For censored longitudinal data, [102] presents a novel approach to censored quantile regression for longitudinal data, addressing challenges in biomedical research with censored outcomes. It introduces a semi-parametric model, avoiding strict distributional assumptions, and proposes a rank score test for large-sample inference. This methodology is significant for its ability to analyze the impact of predictors across various points of a response variable's conditional distribution, which is particularly beneficial for skewed and censored data, offering a more comprehensive understanding of treatment effects and medical outcomes. In addition, [104] presents partially linear varying coefficient models in the context of quantile regression for longitudinal data. It presents a semi-parametric approach that enhances model flexibility without stringent assumptions on error distributions. By utilizing basis function approximations, the paper offers robust estimations of functional coefficients, which are crucial for understanding complex relationships in biomedical data. The work also provides comprehensive statistical tests for evaluating model hypotheses, significantly contributing to the field by allowing more nuanced analyses of conditional quantile curves, which are pivotal for discerning the effects of treatments or exposures across diverse population segments.

These contributions mark significant strides in applying quantile regression to longitudinal data, equipping researchers with sophisticated statistical instruments for the detailed analysis essential in biostatistics and epidemiology. The field has seen notable advancements in quantile regression for longitudinal data, enriching biostatistics with robust analytical tools for complex medical and health research datasets. For scenarios with missing data, an inverse probability weighting approach has been introduced to mitigate bias from nonrandom participant dropout.

3.3 *Survival Analysis with Quantile Regression*

Unlike longitudinal data, which tracks repeated measures over time, survival analysis specifically deals with time-to-event data, making it a fundamental tool in epidemiological research. Quantile regression in survival analysis provides a flexible approach for exploring how covariates affect survival outcomes at different points of the outcome distribution. By moving beyond the traditional focus on mean effects or proportional hazards models like the Cox model, quantile regression offers a richer view of the dynamics of survival data, supporting more informed policy decisions, better-targeted interventions, and personalized treatment strategies.

In survival analysis, a standard quantile regression model considers the conditional quantile of the transformed survival time $Y = \log(T)$ given covariates Z. This model is expressed as:

$$Q_Y(\tau \mid Z) = Z^\top \beta_0(\tau), \quad \tau \in [\tau_L, \tau_U],$$

where $\beta_0(\tau)$ represents regression coefficients that vary with the quantile level τ. By allowing $\beta_0(\tau)$ to change across quantiles, this model captures how covariate effects differ across the survival time distribution, revealing patterns that might be missed by models focused solely on mean outcomes. Thus, quantile regression is particularly useful for handling skewed or heavy-tailed distributions, which are often seen in survival data. For example, [50] used quantile regression to study the lifespan of Mediterranean fruit flies, showing how the effects of covariates differed across various survival percentiles—findings that would be overlooked by mean-based methods. This ability to detect different effects across subgroups makes quantile regression a powerful tool in guiding personalized treatment plans and targeted interventions.

One significant advantage of quantile regression over traditional survival models is its ability to relax assumptions like proportional hazards, which the Cox model relies on [73]. This flexibility is crucial in medical research or policy evaluations, where the impact of covariates may vary over time. Studies by Peng [73], Peng and Huang [74] and others have demonstrated how quantile regression can effectively handle right-censored data using techniques like Kaplan-Meier integrals and reweighting, making it a robust choice for analyzing survival outcomes in real-world settings.

In recent decades, developments in quantile regression for survival analysis have focused on overcoming the challenges of censored data. One key breakthrough came with the introduction of censored quantile regression (CQR), pioneered by authors like [77] and [79]. These methods incorporated specialized reweighting or imputation strategies to handle right-censoring, ensuring that estimation remained unbiased even when some events were only partially observed. Additionally, [74] developed a martingale-based method that directly targets survival quantiles without relying on proportional hazards assumptions, allowing for a more detailed analysis of heterogeneous effects across the survival distribution.

In addition to improving estimation methods, recent contributions have focused on expanding the utility and interpretability of quantile regression models for survival analysis in real-world applications. For instance, [50] demonstrated the effectiveness of quantile-based methods in biological settings by applying these techniques to analyze medfly longevity, showing how contrasting patterns of effects on different survival quantiles could uncover important biological insights missed by hazard-based methods. Similarly, in more recent works [73], the emphasis on nonproportional effects in survival analysis highlighted the limitations of conventional models and spurred innovation in inferential tools for survival quantile estimation. These developments significantly improve the flexibility and robustness of survival modeling, particularly in complex datasets where the assumption that covariates have uniform effects on survival times may not hold, pushing the boundaries beyond proportional hazards models and enabling more nuanced policy and clinical decision-making.

4 Deciphering Genetic Complexities: Quantile Regression in Genetic and Genomic Association Studies

Over the past decade, an explosive growth of genetics and genomics research, driven by advancements in sequencing technologies, has remarkably improved our understanding of genetic regulations and their roles in complex human diseases. Researchers developed numerous novel statistical and machine learning methods to decode the intricate genetic structures and their complex associations with diverse traits, from rare diseases to drug responses. Genotype data with larger sample sizes and more advanced sequencing technologies, such as the UK Biobank introduced before, have become easily accessible. Research on association studies, such as genome-wide association studies (GWAS) and transcriptome-wide association studies (TWAS), has played an important role in identifying genetic variants that influence different levels of expression. For instance, GWAS identified many significant pairs of SNP-phenotype associations and expression quantitative trait loci (eQTLs), which are genetic variants that influence the gene expression level. Most studies focus on identifying mean effects by examining the marginal linear association. However, the distribution of the trait can be regulated by genetic variants in a heterogeneous fashion. For example, [122] discovered that the gene FTO, which is well-known to be associated with fat mass and obesity, was associated with not only the mean of BMI but also the variance of BMI. More evidence of heterogeneous associations is reported in [68, 87, 107].

In this section, we review the recently developed methods in statistical genetics that are based on quantile regression, which investigates heterogeneous associations and reveals genetic effects at different quantiles of the response other than the mean. We interchangeably use the terms "SNP" and "genetic variant" and use the term "SNP-trait test" to refer to the marginal test in GWAS. The trait can be a phenotype (e.g., height, BMI) or a quantity measure during regulation (e.g., gene expression level). We group the methods based on the type of tests, namely, the SNP-trait association test, gene-trait association test, variance-based test, and two-sample test. Computational adaptation to large sample sizes and high-dimensional genotype matrix, when a gene is considered as a unit, will be discussed.

4.1 SNP-Trait Association Studies

As a counterpart to the classical linear regression model for the SNP-trait test, [87] proposed a rank test based on quantile regression to identify genetic variants that affect the expression level of a gene, i.e., expression quantitative trait loci (eQTLs). By combining test results at multiple quantile levels, [87] identified unique eQTLs that are associated with the conditional quantile functions of gene expression. Figure 6 describes the example of heterogeneous genetic associations reported in [87]: (a) is an insignificant SNP, (b) is a significant SNP identified by both the linear model ("LR") and quantile model ("QRank"), (c) is an SNP that is only identified by Qrank, and (d) shows an SNP that has been identified by both LR and QRank. The SNPs presented in Fig. 6 suggest different heterogeneous association patterns. In Fig. 6c, the associations for the three groups (SNP $= 0/1/2$) are crossing, indicating that a higher mutation burden increases the lower quantile of that gene expression level and decreases the upper quantile. In Fig. 6d, the genetic effect is heterogeneous across different quantiles but unidirectional, in the sense that the group with a higher mutation burden will consistently have a higher gene expression level across all quantiles. Compared to the homogeneous genetic effect that similarly impacts all quantiles (Fig. 6b), heterogeneous effects are better captured by the quantile rank score test.

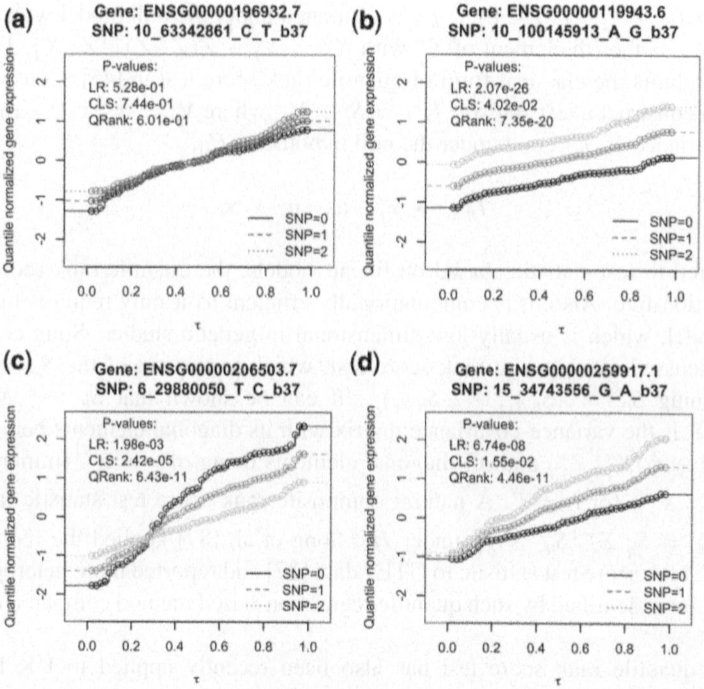

Fig. 6 An example of estimated conditional distribution functions of gene expression for SNP-gene pairs in thyroid tissue (Figure 3 from [87])

To briefly introduce the quantile rank score test, we assume that the dataset consists of n subjects, with their gene expressions measured on K genes for M SNPs in total. Denote $Y_{n\times K}$ as the gene expression matrix and $X_{n\times M}$ as the genotype matrix. For the ith subject, denote $Y_{i,k}$ as his/her kth gene expression level, $x_{i,j}$ as the jth genotype, and z_i as the corresponding covariates to be adjusted (e.g., age, gender, genetic principal components). For a specific gene, SNPs within ±1 Mb of the pre-defined transcriptional start site of that gene are considered as a candidate set for further examination. For each SNP-gene pair (j, k) within the candidate set, [87] employed the following model:

$$Y_{i,k} = z_i^\top \alpha_{jk,\tau} + x_{i,j}\beta_{jk,\tau} + \epsilon_{i,k}, \quad \tau \in (0, 1)$$

where $\epsilon_{i,k}$ is the random error term with the assumption of its τth quantile $Q_{\epsilon_i,k}(\tau \mid z_i, x_{i,j}) = 0$.

The primary interest of analysis is $H_0 : \beta_{jk,\tau} = 0$. For a specific quantile level $\tau \in (0, 1)$, the rank score function in quantile regression is formulated as

$$S_{n,\tau} = n^{-1/2} \sum_{i=1}^{n} \phi_\tau\{y_{i,k} - z_i^\top \hat{\alpha}_{jk,\tau}\} x^*_{i,j},$$

where $\phi_\tau(u) = \tau - I(u < 0)$, $\hat{\alpha}_{jk,\tau}$ is estimated under the null model with $\beta_{jk,\tau} = 0$, and $x^*_{i,j}$ is the ith element of X^*_j with $X^*_j = X_j - Z(Z^\top Z)^{-1}Z^\top X_j$. The form of $S_{n,\tau}$ admits the classical form of quantile rank score test in [45]. Consequently, one can construct a test statistic $T_{n,\tau} = S^2_{n,\tau}/V_n$, where $V_n = n^{-1}\tau(1-\tau)X^{*\top}_j X^*_j$ is the variance of $S_{n,\tau}$, and under the null hypothesis H_0,

$$T_{n,\tau} \to \chi^2_1 \quad \text{as} \quad n \to \infty.$$

Compared to test statistics based on linear models, the quantile rank score test is distribution-free. Also, it is computationally efficient as it only requires fitting the null model, which is usually low-dimensional in genetic studies. Song et al. [87] also discussed a composite rank score test, which tests a set of the $S_{n,\tau}$ together by defining $S_n = (S_{n,\tau_1}, \cdots, S_{n,\tau_\ell})^\top$. It can be shown that $S_n \to N(0, \Sigma)$, where Σ is the variance-covariance matrix with its diagonal elements being $\sigma_{l,l} = n^{-1}\tau_l(1-\tau_l)X^{*\top}_{j,l} Z^*_{j,l}$ and off-diagonal elements being $\sigma_{l,l'} = n^{-1}(\min(\tau_l, \tau_{l'}) - \tau_l\tau_{l'})X^{*\top}_{j,l} X^{*\top}_{j,l'}$ for $l \neq l'$. A natural composite rank score test statistic takes the form $T_\ell = S_n^\top \Sigma^{-1} S_n \sim \chi^2_\ell$ under H_0. Song et al. [87] applied the (composite) quantile rank score test statistic to GTEx data [27] and reported more heterogeneous associations identified by such quantile regression-based method compared to linear models.

The quantile rank score test has also been recently applied to UK Biobank data [107]. Though nonlinear regression techniques have been rarely explored in the context of GWAS, their work suggests that quantile regression helps uncover unmodeled gene-environment interactions and provides insightful discoveries to understand genotype-phenotype correlations.

4.2 *Gene-Trait Association Studies*

Gene-based testing is a prevalent strategy in genetic association studies, yet the complexity of gene-trait associations—due to factors like population heterogeneity and gene-environment interactions—often failed to be captured by existing mean-based tests [55, 66, 80, 121]. These traditional tests can miss or underestimate higher-order associations, which might hold significant scientific interest. To more effectively accommodate the nuanced nature of complex associations, [106] introduce a new family of gene-level association tests that leverage the quantile rank score process for identifying rare variants associated with complex diseases by constructing integrated quantile rank scores over the entire quantile process. Suppose a dataset contains n independent individuals with (Y_i, z_i, x_i) for $i = 1, \cdots, n$, where z_i is a set of covariates, x_i is a p-dimensional genotype vector in a region (e.g., a gene), and Y_i is a continuous response variable, such as BMI and cholesterol. For $\forall\tau \in (0, 1)$, the following model is considered:

$$Q_{Y_i}(\tau \mid z_i, x_i) = \alpha_0(\tau) + z_i^\top \alpha(\tau) + x_i^\top \beta(\tau).$$

The model is similar to the model considered in [87] except that x_i is a vector instead of a univariate variant here. More important, the null hypothesis is $H_0 : \beta(\tau) = 0$ for all $\tau \in (0, 1)$ instead of a fixed τ being tested in [87]. The integrated test statistic is built on integrating the classical rank score test statistic over the entire quantile process:

$$S^{\varphi} = n^{-1/2} \sum_{i=1}^{n} x_i^{*\top} \int_0^1 (1\{Y_i \le z_i \hat{\alpha} + \hat{\alpha}_0\} - \tau) d\varphi(\tau),$$

where $\hat{\alpha}$ and $\hat{\alpha}_0$ are estimated under the null model, and $\varphi(\cdot)$ is a prespecified square-integrable weighting function. In their study, Wang et al. [106] explored the adaptation of the weighting function φ to meet the unique scientific goals of different research projects. For instance, they recommend the Lehmann weighting function $\phi(\tau) = -\log(1 - \tau) - 1$ for the phenotype BMI, highlighting its focus on the upper quantiles of BMI to enhance test power. The introduced integrated quantile rank test statistics are expressed in the quadratic form of S^{φ}, with a predetermined weight matrix W applied to genetic variants. [106] have shown that the proposed test statistics follow a mixture of independent chi-square variables with a degree of freedom of one. The proposed method iQRAT offers several advantages: efficiency in detecting both homogeneous and heterogeneous associations, utility in risk stratification, distribution-free statistics accommodating various underlying distributions, and computational efficiency. The method's effectiveness is demonstrated through simulations and applications to the Metabochip data on lipid traits and GTEx data for identifying eGenes, showcasing its potential in enhancing the analysis of gene-trait associations. Figure 7 demonstrates how varying mutation burdens affect different parts of the triglyceride distribution: variants in the gene LPL predominantly influence the upper quantiles, whereas variants in ZPR1 affect the distribution more uniformly. This analysis, highlighted by the clinical threshold for high triglycerides, offers insights into the potential clinical relevance of these

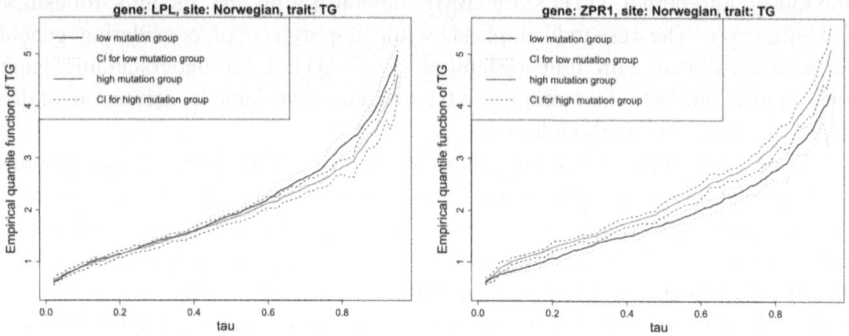

Fig. 7 An example of genes with tail effect (**left**) and homogeneous effect (**right**) associated with triglycerides in the Metabochip data (Figure 1 from [106])

associations, suggesting how genetic mutations might impact the risk of high cholesterol.

4.3 Extensions

In addition to examining the distribution-wise heterogeneous genetic effect, quantile regression has been extended to estimate genetic effects on trait variability. A quantile integral linear model (QUAIL) to detect genetic variants associated with the variance of complex traits (i.e., variance quantitative trait loci, vQTLs) [68]. The QUAIL method is structured around the concept of vQTL mapping, aiming to identify single-nucleotide polymorphisms (SNPs) that exhibit differential variability of a quantitative trait across genotype groups. This variability is quantified without conditioning on the environment, leveraging the conditional quantile function of a response variable given its predictors. QUAIL assumes a linear quantile regression model between the trait Y and the SNP G: $Q_Y(\tau \mid G = g) = g\beta_\tau$. For an SNP considered a vQTL for a trait, the slope, β_τ, changes at different quantile levels τ. Thus, the authors introduced a quantile-integrated effect:

$$\beta_{QI} = \int_0^{0.5} (\beta_{1-\tau} - \beta_\tau) d\tau,$$

and the hypothesis test of interest is $H_0 : \beta_{QI} = 0 \quad versus \quad H_a : \beta_{QI} \neq 0$. For practical implementation, especially in genome-wide analyses, QUAIL simplifies the computational process by transforming the phenotype into an integrated quantile rank score using only trait values and covariates. Then, it regresses this transformed phenotype on covariate-adjusted SNP residuals, avoiding the need to fit regressions for multiple quantile levels. This approach requires only two linear regressions per SNP, significantly enhancing computational efficiency.

By applying the proposed method to UK Biobank data, the study identifies previously unreported vQTLs for BMI, demonstrating the model's robustness and efficiency. The research emphasizes the importance of considering genetic variants associated with trait variability (i.e., vQTLs) for understanding gene-environment interactions, aiming to advance gene-environment interaction studies with its findings and methodologies.

As the availability of GWAS summary statistics online grows, transcriptome-wide association studies (TWAS) have emerged as a significant method for unraveling the genetic underpinnings of various traits and diseases. By leveraging gene expression data, TWAS provides insights that enhance and complement GWAS findings, thereby offering a more detailed understanding of disease mechanisms. To address the limitations of traditional TWAS approaches, which primarily focus on linear associations and might miss complex biological interactions, a novel quantile transcriptome-wide association study framework has been proposed [109]. This framework uses quantile regression to investigate the nonlinear and diverse nature of gene-trait relationships, thereby enriching our comprehension of how variations in gene expression affect phenotypes. This approach is demonstrated to be effective through simulations and applications to real-world data, providing insights into the genetic basis of various traits and diseases.

5 Decoding Microbial Complexities: Zero-Inflated Quantile Regression

Metagenomics involves analyzing genetic material directly from environmental samples, which includes studying the diverse communities of microorganisms present in different habitats, such as the human gut, soil, or oceans. As an important component, microbiome studies focus on understanding the composition and function of these microbial communities, their interactions with their environment, and their impact on health and disease. The importance of microbiome studies is highlighted by their ability to identify bacterial taxa associated with diseases, exposures, and other variables, thereby offering a deeper understanding of microbes' roles in various conditions.

Traditional statistical methods for association testing with microbiome data often fail to accommodate the unique characteristics of these data, such as differential read depth and distributional peculiarities, leading to a loss of power or inflated false positives. Further, excessive zeros, or so-called zero inflation, in microbiome data also cause many challenges. The zero-inflated feature of microbiome data refers to the characteristic where a significant portion of the data consists of zeros, alongside nonzero values that follow a positive distribution (e.g., negative binomial, log-normal, beta, and gamma distributions). This feature arises due to the sparsity of microbiome datasets, where many microbial taxa are not detected in a given sample, resulting in zero counts. Zero-inflated models are proposed to account for this sparsity by modeling the data as a mixture of zeros and a positive continuous or discrete distribution. The zero-inflated negative binomial (ZINB) model is commonly used in microbiome studies to account for excess zeros and overdispersion in count data. The ZINB model combines a negative binomial distribution for count data with a point mass at zero to model the excess zeros, which is suitable for overdispersed data [64]. Other distribution-based methods are zero-inflated beta model [32], zero-inflated generalized Dirichlet-multinomial model [94], and beta-binomial framework [67].

Quantile regression-based methods emerge in genomic studies, from hypothesis testing to batch effect removal. Though not as popular as linear regression models, it has been discovered recently that quantile regression has unique advantages in hypothesis testing and model fitting of genomic data due to its free-of-distribution characteristic.

5.1 Association Tests

A series of works has been developed for estimation and inference on zero-inflated data with quantile regression [56–59]. We first introduce the common two-part modeling technique for zero-inflated data. Suppose the data collected in microbiome studies can be described as $\{Y_i, X_i, Z_i\}$ for n samples. Suppose Y_i represents a taxon of interest, X_i is the clinical variable under investigation, and Z_i denotes a set of other covariates, including the intercept. The proposed two-part quantile regression model considers the probability of observing nonzero and zero outcomes separately, also called the two-part modeling strategy. First, the probability of observing a nonzero is modeled by a logistic regression

$$\text{logit}\{P(Y_i > 0 \mid Z_i, X_i)\} = \gamma X_i + Z_i^{\top}\zeta,$$

where ζ and γ are the true unknown logistic coefficients and can be estimated by classical logistic regression. Then, conditioning on the positive outcomes $Y_i > 0$, a quantile regression is constructed

$$Q_{Y_i}(\tau \mid Z_i, X_i, Y_i > 0) = Z_i^{\top}\alpha(\tau) + \beta(\tau)X_i,$$

where $\alpha(\tau)$ and $\beta(\tau)$ are the true unknown quantile-specific coefficients and can be estimated from solving quantile regression loss function in the positive outcomes only:

$$(\hat{\alpha}(\tau), \hat{\beta}(\tau)) = \arg\min_{\alpha,\beta} \sum_{i=1}^{n} \rho_\tau\{Y_i - Z_i^{\top}\alpha + \beta X_i\} I(Y_i > 0).$$

Zero-inflated quantile regression has also been extended to semiparametric models. For example, [112] introduced a zero-inflated quantile single-index model, which employs a more flexible single-index approach for modeling positive outcomes $(Y_i > 0)$ in overdispersed data.

For hypothesis testing, a testing procedure based on the two-part zero-inflated quantile regression (ZINQ) modeling is proposed in [57]. The main goal is to detect whether there is an association between the clinical variable of interest X and the taxon Y. Thus, the global null hypothesis is

$$H_0 : \gamma = 0 \quad \& \quad \beta(\tau) = 0, \quad \forall \tau \in (0, 1).$$

The alternative hypothesis is $H_a : \gamma \neq 0$ or $\beta(\tau) \neq 0$ for a $\tau \in (0, 1)$. The test combines the p values from the logistic regression and the quantile regression on a sequence of τ via the Cauchy combination method [61]. The method allows for covariate adjustment and does not rely on distributional assumptions, making it robust and broadly applicable to various types of normalized data. Compared to existing methods based on parametric distributions such as ZINB and zero-inflated poisson, the zero-inflated quantile approach enjoys several merits. First, it can accurately account for the large proportion of zeros through the utilization of logistic regression and quantile regression. Also, ZINQ does not rely on specific distributional assumptions about the data, making it broadly applicable to various types of microbiome data, regardless of their underlying distribution. Most importantly, it has shown improved type I error control and enhanced power for detecting complex associations beyond mean differences by examining multiple quantiles of nonzero abundance.

5.2 *Batch Effect Removal*

Incorporating a two-part modeling strategy similar to the one discussed earlier, [59] developed a method, referred to as ConQuR. It utilizes the aforementioned two-part zero-inflated quantile regression model to address the batch effect issue that arises from the differential processing of specimens, which can lead to false-positive discoveries and obscure true signals. We consider the two-part modeling described in Sect. 5.1. Denote the variable of interest X as an indicator of the batch. After estimating the coefficients from the logistic regression and quantile regression, a quantile curve that combines the two-part models is constructed (denoted as $\hat{Q}^0$). Then, another quantile curve that removes the batch effects (e.g., removing the term of $X^\top \beta(\tau)$) is constructed, denoted as $\hat{Q}^c$. A matching step between $\hat{Q}^0$ and $\hat{Q}^c$ is then proceeded. Assume one can find a unique quantile level in $\hat{Q}^0$ such that $Y_i = \hat{Q}^0(\hat{\tau})$. Then the corrected value is $Y_i^c (Y_i^c = \hat{Q}^c(\hat{\tau}))$. As Y_i is read counts, an adjustment is described in [59] when multiple quantiles in $\hat{Q}^0$ are equal to the observed Y_i. Figure 8 presents the principal coordinate analysis (PCoA) plots that are clustered by batch ID, with each color representing a different batch. These

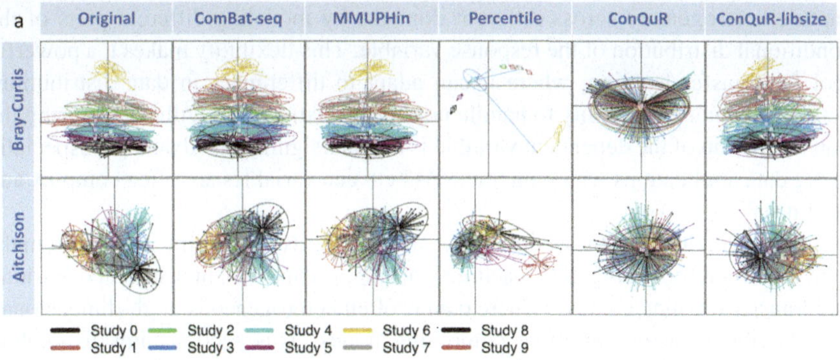

Fig. 8 Comparing the batch effect removal results from different methods. "ConQuR" is the method from [59] (Figure 3(a) from [59])

plots are based on the Bray-Curtis and Aitchison dissimilarities, respectively. The better alignment of the ellipses across batches by ConQuR suggests a successful minimization of batch effects and a more accurate depiction of the inherent sample similarities and differences, unconfounded by batch variations.

The two-part zero-inflated quantile model has been extended to other omics data, including differential analysis in single-cell RNA-seq data, as demonstrated by Zhang et al. [126]. By accounting for the unique distributional patterns in omics data, quantile regression-based approaches are opening up new possibilities for understanding the complex omics factors underlying various traits and diseases.

6 Advancements in Quantile Regression for Modern Statistical Challenges

In modern big data applications, machine learning approaches, including distributed learning and transfer learning, have gained increasing attention. A key challenge in these massive datasets is data heterogeneity, which often arises from variations in sampling and data collection processes. This inherent diversity complicates data analysis and statistical inference. Quantile regression is increasingly gaining popularity due to its robustness and less restriction to parametric assumptions.

Quantile regression plays a vital role in big data machine learning, including distributed learning and transfer learning, due to several key advantages. First, quantile regression is less sensitive to outliers in the response measurements than traditional mean regression. This robustness is particularly beneficial in big data settings where outliers and extreme values are more common due to the vast amount of data. In addition, it provides a more comprehensive analysis by estimating the conditional median and other quantiles of the response variable, providing a more complete view of the relationship between variables. This is especially useful in distributed learning, where the data might be coming from diverse sources with different distributions. Another appealing feature is that quantile regression can capture heterogeneity across different domains by modeling different parts of the conditional distribution of the response variable. This flexibility makes it a powerful tool for transfer learning, where it can adapt to differences in data distributions between domains. Its ability to handle nonlinear relationships without requiring the transformation of the dependent variable is another significant advantage, especially in big data applications where interactions between variables are often complex and nonlinear.

In essence, the robustness, flexibility, and scalability of quantile regression make it an important tool in big data machine learning, particularly in distributed learning and transfer learning contexts where data is often heterogeneous, high-dimensional, and distributed across multiple computing nodes. This section aims to explore quantile regression-based methodologies designed for large-scale data analysis and highlights the future opportunities and challenges in this evolving field.

6.1 Addressing Data Storage and Privacy: Distributed Quantile Regression

Distributed learning is a common strategy when the dataset is separately stored on multiple machines, due to storage or privacy concerns when sending raw data. As the communication in the network can be slower than local communications, fast and communication-efficient algorithms are desired. Methods for high-dimensional linear regression are developed based on subsampling [42, 65], divide-and-conquer, or the one-shot methods [14, 36, 37, 52]. Among them, divide-and-conquer methods are popular as they are computationally fast and easily implemented. Yet, their direct application to quantile regression remains challenging due to the non-smooth nature of its loss function, raising questions about their theoretical validity.

To tackle the challenges posed by massive heterogeneous datasets in the statistical analysis due to their complex structure and computer memory limitations, [33] extended the communication-efficient surrogate likelihood [37] to quantile regression by transferring the subgradients of quantile loss functions between local machines and the master machine and estimating parameters by solving the surrogate loss function on the master machine. Specifically, [33] consider the simple linear quantile regression model (Eq. (3)) and define the surrogate loss function by replacing the gradient in [37] by a subgradient from quantile regression loss function. They employed an alternating direction method of multipliers (ADMM) algorithm to navigate the computational intricacies introduced by the non-smooth loss function.

The communication-constrained distributed quantile regression has also been studied by Tan et al. [92]. The authors developed a double-smoothing approach applied to both local and global objective functions in distributed settings, which facilitates interpretation while maintaining parametric characteristics. They established a finite-sample theoretical framework for distributed quantile regression estimators and proposed confidence set constructions based on Wald and score-type tests, resampling techniques, and detailing improvements for extreme quantile coefficients. The non-smooth nature of the quantile regression loss function, which invalidates existing methods for linear models, is resolved through a double-smoothing technique. The paper demonstrates that the distributed penalized quantile regression estimator achieves the global convergence rate after a minimal number of communication rounds, backed by extensive simulation studies.

The distributed inference of the quantile regression process has been studied in [100]. The authors proposed a comprehensive approach that considers not just a single quantile level but multiple quantile levels to obtain a fuller picture of the conditional distribution of the response variable given the predictors. This is significant because analyzing a single quantile might provide limited insights, whereas considering multiple quantiles can offer a more detailed understanding of the underlying distribution, capturing various aspects like the center, spread, and tail behaviors. The method described involves estimating the conditional quantile function at several quantile levels, which is computationally demanding because each new quantile estimation necessitates running the algorithm from the start. To manage this computational load, the paper introduces a two-step quantile projection algorithm. In the first step, the divide-and-conquer algorithm computes $\beta(\tau_1), \cdots, \beta(\tau_K)$ for a grid of quantile values $\tau_1, \cdots, \tau_K$. Then, in the second step, a matrix derived from these β values is used to estimate the quantile projection estimator $\beta(\tau)$ for any τ, enabling the estimation of the conditional distribution function without needing to access the original dataset again. This approach significantly reduces the computational burden while providing a method to analyze the conditional distribution across a range of quantiles.

6.2 Revealing Rewards and Penalties: Quantile Reinforcement Learning

Quantile regression is increasingly used in reinforcement learning (RL), particularly within the domain of distributional reinforcement learning. This approach addresses the variability in long-term returns stemming from sampled state transitions, rewards, and actions, offering robustness against outliers and avoiding strict parametric assumptions. It enables a more thorough analysis by estimating various quantiles of the response variable, thus providing a more comprehensive understanding of the relationship between variables.

A notable advancement in this field is the introduction of the Quantile Regression Deep Q-Network (QR-DQN), which incorporates quantile regression to model the quantile function of the return distribution rather than its probability mass function [18]. This shift allows for a more accurate prediction of returns that can vary significantly across different states. Then, the implicit quantile networks (IQN) are proposed as an advancement in distributional reinforcement learning [17], extending previous methods like QR-DQN by learning the full quantile function for state-action return distributions. This approach allows for a continuous mapping from probabilities to returns, forming an implicit distribution that can approximate any return distribution given sufficient network capacity. IQN was developed to overcome the limitations of earlier algorithms that assigned probabilities to a fixed set of possible returns, offering a more flexible way to understand return distributions. By learning the full quantile function, IQN offers a more flexible and comprehensive approach that can adapt to various quantile levels, enhancing the understanding and utilization of the return distribution. This flexibility allows for developing risk-sensitive policies and a better analysis of their impact on reinforcement learning. The introduction of IQN represents a significant step forward in distributional reinforcement learning, offering a more flexible, efficient, and comprehensive approach to understanding and leveraging the return distribution in reinforcement learning tasks.

To improve the approximation of the true distribution of returns, [123] proposed a fully parameterized quantile function that estimates both the quantile fractions and quantile values, which allows for a better representation of the randomness inherent in RL environments. This dual parameterization allows for a more accurate approximation of the true return distribution, which is crucial for effective decision-making in RL. The authors propose a fraction proposal network to generate quantile fractions and a quantile value network to yield corresponding values, with both networks being jointly trained. This results in a more flexible and precise model that can better adapt to the randomness inherent in RL environments. This comprehensive approach to distributional reinforcement learning, with its focus on quantile regression, marks a significant advancement in the field, enabling the development of risk-sensitive policies and a deeper exploration of policy effects in reinforcement learning tasks. Moreover, the non-crossing constraints in quantile regression have also been studied in the context of RL [125].

6.3 *Robust Transferring of Knowledge: Quantile Transfer Learning*

Quantile regression in transfer learning is an approach that leverages the robustness and flexibility of quantile regression models to enhance performance in target tasks by utilizing information from source domains. This method is particularly effective in handling high-dimensional data characterized by heterogeneity and heavy tails, which are common challenges in modern big data applications. Transfer learning with quantile regression aims to learn the conditional quantiles of a target population by incorporating data from related source populations, which share the same set of features and responses. This process involves identifying source models that are sufficiently similar to the target model, which can then provide valuable supplementary information for the target task. The approach includes developing estimation procedures that incorporate both target and source data, potentially leading to improved estimators by considering transferable source domains. This method also addresses the creation of valid confidence intervals and hypothesis testing for quantile regression coefficients, further enhancing its applicability and effectiveness in transfer learning scenarios.

A transfer learning framework specifically tailored for high-dimensional quantile regression is proposed in [35]. The core idea is to enhance the estimation of quantile regression at the target domain by using auxiliary data from related source domains. This approach is particularly innovative because it addresses three types of heterogeneity often encountered in transfer learning scenarios: feature distributions, model coefficients, and error distributions. The proposed method has four key steps. Assuming the informative sources are known, transfer learning is executed through a four-step process: single-source modeling, response surrogation, fusion learning, and debiasing. This structured approach allows for the incorporation of valuable information from sources similar to the target, thereby improving the estimator's accuracy for the target model. For single-source modeling, each source, including the target, is modeled individually using L_1 penalized quantile regression. This step ensures that the unique characteristics of each source are captured, which is crucial for the subsequent fusion of information. Then, to simplify the quantile regression problem, surrogate responses are constructed. This step transforms the quantile regression into a more manageable linear regression problem, facilitating the integration of information from various sources. At the fusion learning stage, the information from all sources, including the target, is combined through L_1 penalized regression with the surrogate responses. This step is pivotal in synthesizing the diverse insights gleaned from individual sources to enhance the target model. Finally, debiasing is performed using only the target data to refine the estimator further, ensuring that the final model is as accurate and unbiased as possible. This method stands out for its ability to effectively handle the complexities associated with high-dimensional data and quantile regression. By acknowledging and addressing the heterogeneities in the data, the method provides a robust framework for improving quantile estimation in the target domain, thereby offering significant advantages over traditional models that rely solely on target data or naively combine all available information.

Another noteworthy contribution is the paper on transfer learning for high-dimensional quantile regression via convolution smoothing [127]. This study addresses the challenges of high-dimensional data and multiple source integration in quantile regression by proposing a smoothed two-step estimator. The methodology is grounded in the principles of transfer learning, aiming to leverage related source datasets to improve prediction accuracy for a target dataset. The paper establishes theoretical foundations for this approach, including estimation error bounds and the consistency of detecting transferable sets, demonstrating its potential through simulated data and empirical analysis of Genotype-Tissue Expression (GTEx) data.

6.4 Tackling High-Dimensional Challenges: Sparse Quantile Regression

High-dimensional data has become increasingly common in biostatistics, especially with the rise of omics technologies like genomics, transcriptomics, proteomics, and metabolomics. Recent advancements in quantile regression for high-dimensional data have seen a variety of innovative approaches aimed at improving estimation accuracy, computational efficiency, and robustness to data heterogeneity and sparsity. For example, [85] introduced an additive nonlinear quantile regression method that employs B-splines to better model complex relationships within high-dimensional datasets, incorporating a nonconvex group penalty for simultaneous estimation and variable selection, which is particularly effective in handling heteroscedasticity and outliers. In another development, [19] proposed a high-dimensional variable selection method using a spike-and-slab lasso penalty within a variational Bayesian framework, enhancing computational efficiency while allowing for the quantification of randomness. The "conquer" estimator, proposed by He et al. [31], offers a solution for large-scale data inference by smoothing the quantile loss function, facilitating faster optimization and statistical inference with less stringent requirements on predictor dimensions. Fei et al. [23] tackled the challenge of censored quantile regression in high-dimensional settings, proposing a novel procedure for inference on high-dimensional predictors, which is particularly useful in survival analysis and the study of heterogeneous effects of genetic biomarkers. Also focused on censored quantile regression, [30] introduces a smoothed martingale-based sequential estimating equation approach, addressing challenges in computation and statistical inference for large-scale, high-dimensional data, and improving the uniform convergence rate while providing a valid multiplier bootstrap method for inference in sparse settings. Lastly, [110] explored the incorporation of graphical structures among predictors in sparse quantile regression, which significantly improves parameter estimation, model selection, and prediction accuracy by leveraging the inherent relationships among variables. These methods make important progress in tackling the challenges of quantile regression in high-dimensional data by offering more nuanced and computationally feasible approaches.

7 Summary of Advancements and Challenges of Quantile Regression for Big Data

Beyond topics covered so far in previous chapters, quantile regression has been fruitfully applied across various domains, including secondary analysis with case-control data [118], imputation on missing data [117], high-dimensional statistical inference [93, 105], treatment effects [25, 72], mediation analysis [4], etc. Recent research has made great progress in combining quantile regression with machine learning. One such development is the exploration of flexible model aggregation for quantile regression [22], which focuses on combining different quantile regression models to improve prediction accuracy and model robustness. This approach is particularly relevant in fields requiring precise uncertainty quantification, such as epidemiological prediction and cost estimation. This progress highlights the development and growth of quantile regression over time, from its early statistical roots to its modern application in machine learning, including developments in kernel machines, additive models, and high-dimensional regression. The rise of artificial intelligence has further propelled progress in quantile regression, allowing for more advanced modeling of conditional quantile functions, such as conformal quantile regression [82, 84]. These studies exemplify the ongoing efforts to enhance quantile regression techniques through machine learning, offering new tools and methodologies for more nuanced and robust statistical analyses across various domains.

Despite significant advances in statistical methodology, coefficient estimation for quantile regression remains computationally challenging due to the absence of a closed-form solution [12, 13]. Even quantile rank score tests, which only require fitting under the null model, face difficulties when applied to large-scale biomedical data, where weak signal-to-noise ratios and high computational demands pose additional challenges. As reported in [107], quantile regression is computationally more expensive than linear regression. They demonstrated that for the trait BMI in UK Biobank with 324,306 individuals and 8,572,925 variants, GWAS based on linear models took 92 hours of CPU time using `PLINK`, while quantile regression with the `QRank` package in `R` took 9,534 hours of CPU time. Besides quantile regression inference at a single quantile level, novel statistical methods based on integrating multiple quantile levels or the quantile process are suggested to have substantial power gain [87, 106, 109]. Specifically, calculating the quantile process is computationally much more expensive with a large number of sample size, as the number of distinct solutions to Eq. (3) is $O_p(n \log(n))$ [76]. There are many researchers devoted to addressing computational challenges and enhancing the precision of quantile regression analysis in big data contexts; for example, the work of [69] provides robust statistical guarantees and introduces efficient algorithms suited for high-dimensional composite quantile regression in large datasets. However, there is still an urgent need to develop a fast algorithm to serve the genome-wide association tests based on quantile regression.

Selecting an appropriate quantile level for analysis poses another question, especially in genetic and genomic association studies where the target quantile is less clear compared to fields like economics, where quantile levels often align with specific research goals. For example, to analyze the relationship between annual income and a set of demographic variables, one would consider the "rich group" as the 80th or 90th quantile of annual income and the "poor group" as the 10th or 20th quantile of annual income. However, in the context of genetic and genomic association studies, how to define a target quantile is an open question owing to our limited knowledge. In epidemiological studies, upper quantiles (e.g., 80th or 90th percentiles) are considered for BMI when the research interest is obesity [3, 96]. But in genetics and genomics, the choice of quantile level is less straightforward, making the use of integrated quantile levels an attractive option [68, 106]. Future research should aim to perform unified tests while effectively selecting quantile levels.

Model interpretation of quantile regression in biostatistical studies presents unique challenges, as health sciences often require results that are more confirmative, easily interpretable, and unidirectional. On the one hand, quantile regression offers a powerful framework for uncovering gene-trait associations by addressing data heterogeneity and revealing associations across different quantiles. For instance, [107] demonstrated that quantile regression can detect genotype-phenotype associations that might result from unmodeled gene-environment interactions, while [109] identified novel gene-trait associations in TWAS using quantile regression. On the other hand, the complexity of varying directions and magnitudes of effects across quantiles can make it difficult for clinicians and biologists to design experiments based on quantile regression results, whereas linear models often yield clear hypotheses with specific magnitudes and directions through interpreting estimated linear regression coefficients. To address these challenges, tools such as decision trees or machine learning-based quantile forests could enhance model interpretability, helping to distill quantile regression results into actionable conclusions. Additionally, direct experimental validation and standardized pipelines for model validation are essential to increase confidence in quantile regression findings and facilitate broader adoption within the genomic research community. For example, experimental validation might involve testing gene-trait associations detected by quantile regression through functional genomic assays or CRISPR-based experiments.

In summary, quantile regression has emerged as a versatile and powerful tool, extending its utility beyond traditional applications to embrace the complexities of high-dimensional data, particularly within genetic and genomic studies. The innovative methodologies highlight the adaptability and potential of quantile regression to unravel intricate relationships in data characterized by heterogeneity and sparsity. Despite the methodological leaps, the computational intensity and the challenges in model interpretation and validation in large-scale applications highlight areas ripe for further innovation. The ongoing efforts to refine computational algorithms and enhance interpretability promise to broaden the applicability of quantile regression, potentially unlocking new insights into the genetic underpinnings of traits and diseases.

Acknowledgments The author is grateful to the editors and referees for their insightful and constructive comments, which have improved the clarity of this chapter.

References

1. Barrodale, I., Roberts, F.D.: An improved algorithm for discrete l_1 linear approximation. SIAM J. Numer. Anal. **10**(5), 839–848 (1973)
2. Belloni, A., Chernozhukov, V.: ℓ1-penalized quantile regression in high-dimensional sparse models. Ann. Stat. **39**(1), 81–130 (2011)
3. Beyerlein, A., von Kries, R., Ness, A.R., Ong, K.K.: Genetic markers of obesity risk: stronger associations with body composition in overweight compared to normal-weight children. Plos One **6**(4), e19057 (2011)
4. Bind, M.-A., VanderWeele, T., Schwartz, J., Coull, B.: Quantile causal mediation analysis allowing longitudinal data. Stat. Med. **36**(26), 4182–4195 (2017)
5. Bomba, L., Walter, K., Soranzo, N.: The impact of rare and low-frequency genetic variants in common disease. Gen. Biol. **18**(1), 1–17 (2017)
6. Box, G.E., Cox, D.R.: An analysis of transformations. J. R. Stat. Soc. Ser. B: Stat. Methodol. **26**(2), 211–243 (1964)
7. Buniello, A., MacArthur, J.A.L., M. Cerezo, Harris, L.W., J. Hayhurst, C. Malangone, A. McMahon, J. Morales, E. Mountjoy, E. Sollis, et al.: The NHGRI-EBI GWAS catalog of published genome-wide association studies, targeted arrays and summary statistics 2019. Nucleic Acids Res. **47**(D1), D1005–D1012 (2019)
8. Burgess, S., Small, D.S., Thompson, S.G.: A review of instrumental variable estimators for mendelian randomization. Stat. Methods Med. Res. **26**(5), 2333–2355 (2017)

9. Carey, V., Yong, F., Frenkel, L., McKinney, R.: Growth velocity assessment in paediatric aids: smoothing, penalized quantile regression and the definition of growth failure. Stat. Med. **23**(3), 509–526 (2004)
10. Carroll, R.J., Gail, M.H., Lubin, J.H.: Case-control studies with errors in covariates. J. Am. Stat. Assoc. **88**(421), 185–199 (1993)
11. Chakraborty, S., Hosen, M.I., Ahmed, M., Shekhar, H.U.: Onco-multi-omics approach: a new frontier in cancer research. BioMed Res. Int. **2018:9836256** (2018)
12. Chen, C.: A finite smoothing algorithm for quantile regression. J. Comput. Graph. Stat. **16**(1), 136–164 (2007)
13. Chen, C., Wei, Y.: Computational issues for quantile regression. Sankhyā: Indian J. Stat. **67**(2), 399–417 (2005)
14. Chen, X., Xie, M.-g.: A split-and-conquer approach for analysis of extraordinarily large data. Stat. Sin. **24**(4), 1655–1684 (2014)
15. Cole, T.J.: Fitting smoothed centile curves to reference data. J. R. Stat. Soc. Ser. A: Stat. Soci. **151**(3), 385–406 (1988)
16. Collins, R.: What makes UK biobank special? Lancet **379**(9822), 1173–1174 (2012)
17. Dabney, W., Ostrovski, G., Silver, D., Munos, R.: Implicit quantile networks for distributional reinforcement learning. In: International Conference on Machine Learning, pp. 1096–1105. PMLR (2018)
18. Dabney, W., Rowland, M., Bellemare, M., Munos, R.: Distributional reinforcement learning with quantile regression. In: Proceedings of the AAAI Conference on Artificial Intelligence, vol. 32 (2018)
19. Dai, D., Tang, A., Ye, J.: High-dimensional variable selection for quantile regression based on variational bayesian method. Mathematics **11**(10), 2232 (2023)
20. Davey Smith, G., Hemani, G.: Mendelian randomization: genetic anchors for causal inference in epidemiological studies. Hum. Mol. Genet. **23**(R1), R89–R98 (2014)
21. Doksum, K.: Empirical probability plots and statistical inference for nonlinear models in the two-sample case. Ann. Stat., **2**(2), 267–277 (1974)
22. Fakoor, R., Kim, T., Mueller, J., Smola, A., Tibshirani, R.J.: Flexible model aggregation for quantile regression. J. Mach. Learn. Res. **24**, 1–45 (2023)
23. Fei, Z., Zheng, Q., Hong, H., Li, Y.: Inference for high-dimensional censored quantile regression. J. Am. Stat. Assoc. **118**, 898–912 (2021)
24. Geraci, M., Bottai, M.: Quantile regression for longitudinal data using the asymmetric laplace distribution. Biostatistics **8**, 140–154 (2007)
25. Giessing, A., Wang, J.: Debiased inference on heterogeneous quantile treatment effects with regression rank scores. J. R. Stat. Soc. Ser. B: Stat. Methodol. **85**(5), 1561–1588 (2023)
26. Giri, A., Hellwege, J.N.., Keaton, J.M., Park, J., Qiu, C., Warren, H.R., Torstenson, E.S., Kovesdy, C.P., Sun, Y.V., Wilson, O.D., et al.: Trans-ethnic association study of blood pressure determinants in over 750,000 individuals. Nat. Genet. **51**(1), 51–62 (2019)
27. GTEx Consortium: The GTEx consortium atlas of genetic regulatory effects across human tissues. Science **369**(6509), 1318–1330 (2020)
28. Gusev, A., Ko, A., Shi, H., Bhatia, G., Chung, W., Penninx, B.W., et al.: Integrative approaches for large-scale transcriptome-wide association studies. Nat. Genet. **48**(3), 245–252 (2016)
29. Gutenbrunner, C., Jurecková, J.: Regression rank scores and regression quantiles. Ann. Stat. **20**(1), 305–330 (1992)
30. He, X., Pan, X., Tan, K.M., Zhou, W.-X.: Scalable estimation and inference for censored quantile regression process. Ann. Stat. **50**(5), 2899–2924 (2022)
31. He, X., Pan, X., Tan, K.M., Zhou, W.-X.: Smoothed quantile regression with large-scale inference. J. Econ. **232**(2), 367–388 (2023)
32. Hu, T., Gallins, P., Zhou, Y.-H.: A zero-inflated beta-binomial model for microbiome data analysis. Stat. **7**(1), e185 (2018)
33. Hu, A., Jiao, Y., Liu, Y., Shi, Y., Wu, Y.: Distributed quantile regression for massive heterogeneous data. Neurocomputing **448**, 249–262 (2021)

34. Huang, J., Liu, L., Liu, N.: Estimation of large covariance matrices of longitudinal data with basis function approximations. J. Comput. Graph. Stat. **16**, 189–209 (2007)
35. Jin, J., Yan, J., Aseltine, R.H., Chen, K.: Transfer learning with large-scale quantile regression. Technometrics 1–30 (2024). Just-accepted
36. Jordan, M.I.: On statistics, computation and scalability. Bernoulli **19**(4), 1378–1390 (2013)
37. Jordan, M.I., Lee, J.D., Yang, Y.: Communication-efficient distributed statistical inference. J. Am. Stat. Assoc. **114**, 668–681 (2018)
38. Kachuri, L., Graff, R.E., Smith-Byrne, K., Meyers, T.J., Rashkin, S.R., Ziv, E., Witte, J.S.., Johansson, M.: Pan-cancer analysis demonstrates that integrating polygenic risk scores with modifiable risk factors improves risk prediction. Nat. Commun. **11**(1), 6084 (2020)
39. Kanai, M., Akiyama, M., Takahashi, A., Matoba, N., Momozawa, Y., Ikeda, M., Iwata, N., Ikegawa, S., Hirata, M., Matsuda, K., et al.: Genetic analysis of quantitative traits in the Japanese population links cell types to complex human diseases. Nat. Genet. **50**(3), 390–400 (2018)
40. Karmarkar, N.: A new polynomial-time algorithm for linear programming. In: Proceedings of the Sixteenth Annual ACM Symposium on Theory of Computing, pp. 302–311 (1984)
41. Kinkorová, J., Topolčan, O.: Biobanks in the era of big data: objectives, challenges, perspectives, and innovations for predictive, preventive, and personalised medicine. EPMA J. **11**(3), 333–341 (2020)
42. Kleiner, A., Talwalkar, A., Sarkar, P., Jordan, M.I.: A scalable bootstrap for massive data. J. R. Stat. Soc. Ser. B Stat Methodol. **76**(4), 795–816 (2014)
43. Koenker, R.: Confidence intervals for regression quantiles. In: Asymptotic Statistics: Proceedings of the Fifth Prague Symposium, Held from September 4–9, 1993, pp. 349–359. Springer, Berlin (1994)
44. Koenker, R.: Quantile regression for longitudinal data. J. Multivar. Anal. **91**(1), 74–89 (2004)
45. Koenker, R.: Quantile Regression, vol. 38. Cambridge University Press, Cambridge (2005)
46. Koenker, R.: Rank tests for heterogeneous treatment effects with covariates. In: Nonparametrics and Robustness in Modern Statistical Inference and Time Series Analysis: A Festschrift in honor of Professor Jana Jurečková, vol. 7, pp. 134–143. Institute of Mathematical Statistics, Beachwood (2010)
47. Koenker, R.: quantreg: Quantile Regression. R package version 5.97 (2023)
48. Koenker, R., Bassett, Jr. G.: Regression quantiles. Econ. J. Econ. Soc. **46**(1), 33–50 (1978)
49. Koenker, R.W., d'Orey, V.: Computing regression quantiles. Appl. Stat. **36**(3), 383–393 (1987)
50. Koenker, R., Geling, O.: Reappraising medfly longevity: a quantile regression survival analysis. J. Am. Stat. Assoc. **96**(454), 458–468 (2001)
51. Koenker, R., Machado, J.A.: Goodness of fit and related inference processes for quantile regression. J. Am. Stat. Assoc. **94**(448), 1296–1310 (1999)
52. Lee, J.D., Liu, Q., Sun, Y., Taylor, J.E.: Communication-efficient sparse regression. J. Mach. Learn. Res. **18**(1), 115–144 (2017)
53. Lee, T.C., Radha-Saseendrakumar, B., Delavar, A., Gordon, Y.Y., Ting, M.A., Topilow, N.J., Bass, J., Korn, B.S., Kikkawa, D.O., Baxter, S.L., et al.: Evaluation of depression and anxiety in a diverse population with thyroid eye disease using the nationwide NIH all of us database. Ophthalmic Plast. Reconstr. Surg. **39**(3), 281–287 (2023)
54. Leng, C., Zhang, W.: Smoothing combined estimating equations in quantile regression for longitudinal data. Stat. Comput. **1**, 123–136 (2014)
55. Li, B., Leal, S.M.: Methods for detecting associations with rare variants for common diseases: application to analysis of sequence data. Am. J. Hum. Genet. **83**(3), 311–321 (2008)
56. Ling, W., Zhang, W., Cheng, B., Wei, Y.: Zero-inflated quantile rank-score based test (ZIQRank) with application to scRNA-seq differential gene expression analysis. Ann. Appl. Stat. **15**(4), 1673 (2021)
57. Ling, W., Zhao, N., Plantinga, A.M., Launer, L.J., Fodor, A.A., Meyer, K.A., Wu, M.C.: Powerful and robust non-parametric association testing for microbiome data via a zero-inflated quantile approach (ZINQ). Microbiome **9**(1), 1–19 (2021)

58. Ling, W., Cheng, B., Wei, Y., Willey, J.Z., Cheung, Y.K.: Statistical inference in quantile regression for zero-inflated outcomes. Stat. Sin. **32**(3), 1411 (2022)
59. Ling, W., Lu, J., Zhao, N., Lulla, A., Plantinga, A.M., Fu, W., Zhang, A., Liu, H., Song, H., Li, Z., et al.: Batch effects removal for microbiome data via conditional quantile regression. Nat. Commun. **13**(1), 5418 (2022)
60. Littlejohns, T.J., Sudlow, C., Allen, N.E., Collins, R.: UK biobank: opportunities for cardiovascular research. Euro. Heart J. **40**(14), 1158–1166 (2019)
61. Liu, Y., Xie, J.: Cauchy combination test: a powerful test with analytic p-value calculation under arbitrary dependency structures. J. Am. Stat. Assoc. **115**, 393–402 (2019)
62. Liu, Z., Ye, T., Sun, B., Schooling, M., Tchetgen Tchetgen, E.: Mendelian randomization mixed-scale treatment effect robust identification and estimation for causal inference. Biometrics **79**(3), 2208–2219 (2023)
63. Lu, X., Fan, Z.: Weighted quantile regression for longitudinal data. Comput. Stat. **30**, 569–592 (2015)
64. Lutz, K.C., Jiang, S., Neugent, M.L., De Nisco, N.J., Zhan, X., Li, Q.: A survey of statistical methods for microbiome data analysis. Front. Appl. Math. Stat. **8**, 884810 (2022)
65. Ma, P., Mahoney, M., Yu, B.: A statistical perspective on algorithmic leveraging. In: International Conference on Machine Learning, pp. 91–99. PMLR (2014)
66. Madsen, B.E., Browning, S.R.: A groupwise association test for rare mutations using a weighted sum statistic. PLoS Genet. **5**(2), e1000384 (2009)
67. Martin, B.D., Witten, D., Willis, A.D.: Modeling microbial abundances and dysbiosis with beta-binomial regression. Ann. Appl. Stat. **14**(1), 94 (2020)
68. Miao, J., Lin, Y., Wu, Y., Zheng, B., Schmitz, L.L., Fletcher, J.M., Lu, Q.: A quantile integral linear model to quantify genetic effects on phenotypic variability. Proc. Natl. Acad. Sci. **119**(39), e2212959119 (2022)
69. Moon, H., Zhou, W.-X.: High-dimensional composite quantile regression: optimal statistical guarantees and fast algorithms. Electron. J. Stat. **17**(2), 2067–2119 (2023)
70. Muggeo, V.M., Sciandra, M., Tomasello, A., Calvo, S.: Estimating growth charts via nonparametric quantile regression: a practical framework with application in ecology. Environ. Ecol. Stat. **20**, 519–531 (2013)
71. Namkung, J.: Machine learning methods for microbiome studies. J. Microbiol. **58**, 206–216 (2020)
72. Panigrahi, S., Wang, J., He, X.: Treatment effect estimation with efficient data aggregation. Preprint. arXiv:2203.12726 (2022)
73. Peng, L.: Quantile regression for survival data. Ann. Rev. Stat. Its Appl. **8**(1), 413–437 (2021)
74. Peng, L., Huang, Y.: Survival analysis with quantile regression models. J. Am. Stat. Assoc. **103**(482), 637–649 (2008)
75. Peterson, M.D., Krishnan, C.: Growth charts for muscular strength capacity with quantile regression. Am. J. Prevent. Med. **49**(6), 935–938 (2015)
76. Portnoy, S.: Asymptotic behavior of the number of regression quantile breakpoints. SIAM J. Scient. Stat. Comput. **12**(4), 867–883 (1991)
77. Portnoy, S.: Censored quantile regression. J. Am. Stat. Assoc. **98**(464), 1001–1012 (2003)
78. Portnoy, S., Koenker, R.: The Gaussian hare and the laplacian tortoise: computability of squared-error versus absolute-error estimators. Stat. Sci. **12**(4), 279–300 (1997)
79. Powell, J.L.: Censored regression quantiles. J. Econ. **32**(1), 143–155 (1986)
80. Price, A.L., Kryukov, G.V., de Bakker, P.I., Purcell, S.M., Staples, J., Wei, L.-J., Sunyaev, S.R.: Pooled association tests for rare variants in exon-resequencing studies. Am. J. Hum. Genet. **86**(6), 832–838 (2010)
81. Ritz, B.R., Chatterjee, N., Garcia-Closas, M., Gauderman, W.J., Pierce, B.L., Kraft, P., Tanner, C.M., Mechanic, L.E., McAllister, K.: Lessons learned from past gene-environment interaction successes. Am. J. Epidemiol. **186**(7), 778–786 (2017)
82. Romano, Y., Patterson, E., Candes, E.: Conformalized quantile regression. Adv. Neural Inf. Proces. Syst. **32** (2019)

83. Schulz, K.F., Grimes, D.A.: Case-control studies: research in reverse. Lancet **359**(9304), 431–434 (2002)
84. Sesia, M., Candès, E.J.: A comparison of some conformal quantile regression methods. Stat. **9**(1), e261 (2020)
85. Sherwood, B., Maidman, A.: Additive nonlinear quantile regression in ultra-high dimension. J. Mach. Learn. Res. **23**, 63:1–63:47 (2022)
86. Sidak, Z., Sen, P.K., Hajek, J.: Theory of Rank Tests. Elsevier, Amsterdam (1999)
87. Song, X., Li, G., Zhou, Z., Wang, X., Ionita-Laza, I., Wei, Y.: Qrank: a novel quantile regression tool for eQTL discovery. Bioinformatics **33**(14), 2123–2130 (2017)
88. Sudlow, C., Gallacher, J., Allen, N., Beral, V., Burton, P., Danesh, J., Downey, P., Elliott, P., Green, J., Landray, M., et al.: UK biobank: an open access resource for identifying the causes of a wide range of complex diseases of middle and old age. PLoS Med. **12**(3), e1001779 (2015)
89. Sun, Y.V., Hu, Y.-J.: Integrative analysis of multi-omics data for discovery and functional studies of complex human diseases. Adv. Genet. **93**, 147–190 (2016)
90. Taliun, D., Harris, D.N., Kessler, M.D., Carlson, J., Szpiech, Z.A., Torres, R., Taliun, S.A.G., Corvelo, A., Gogarten, S.M., Kang, H.M., et al.: Sequencing of 53,831 diverse genomes from the nhlbi topmed program. Nature **590**(7845), 290–299 (2021)
91. Tam, V., Patel, N., Turcotte, M., Bossé, Y., Paré, G., Meyre, D.: Benefits and limitations of genome-wide association studies. Nat. Rev. Genet. **20**(8), 467–484 (2019)
92. Tan, K.M., Battey, H., Zhou, W.-X.: Communication-constrained distributed quantile regression with optimal statistical guarantees. J. Mach. Learn. Res. **23**(1), 12456–12516 (2022)
93. Tan, K.M., Wang, L., Zhou, W.-X.: High-dimensional quantile regression: convolution smoothing and concave regularization. J. R. Stat. Soc. Ser. B: Stat. Methodol. **84**(1), 205–233 (2022)
94. Tang, Z.-Z., Chen, G.: Zero-inflated generalized dirichlet multinomial regression model for microbiome compositional data analysis. Biostatistics **20**(4), 698–713 (2019)
95. Terry, M.B., Wei, Y., Esserman, D.: Maternal, birth, and early-life influences on adult body size in women. Am. J. Epidemiol. **166**(1), 5–13 (2007)
96. Terry, M., Wei, Y., Esserman, D., McKeague, I., Susser, E.: Pre-and postnatal determinants of childhood body size: cohort and sibling analyses. J. Dev. Orig. Health Dis. **2**(2), 99–111 (2011)
97. The H3Africa Consortium: Enabling the genomic revolution in africa: H3africa is developing capacity for health-related genomics research in Africa. Science **344**, 1346 (2014)
98. Tyrer, J., Duffy, S.W., Cuzick, J.: A breast cancer prediction model incorporating familial and personal risk factors. Stat. Med. **23**(7), 1111–1130 (2004)
99. Uffelmann, E., Huang, Q.Q., Munung, N.S., De Vries, J., Okada, Y., Martin, A.R., Martin, H.C., Lappalainen, T., Posthuma, D.: Genome-wide association studies. Nat. Rev. Methods Primers **1**(1), 59 (2021)
100. Volgushev, S., Chao, S.-K., Cheng, G.: Distributed inference for quantile regression processes. Ann. Stat. **47**(3), 1634–1662 (2019)
101. Wainberg, M., Sinnott-Armstrong, N., Mancuso, N., Barbeira, A.N., Knowles, D.A., Golan, D., et al.: Opportunities and challenges for transcriptome-wide association studies. Nat. Genet. **51**(4), 592–599 (2019)
102. Wang, H.J., Fygenson, M.: Inference for censored quantile regression models in longitudinal studies. Ann. Stat. **37**(2), 756–781 (2009)
103. Wang, H.J., Zhu, Z.: Empirical likelihood for quantile regression models with longitudinal data. J. Stat. Plan. Infer. **141**(4), 1603–1615 (2011)
104. Wang, H.J., Zhu, Z., Zhou, J.: Quantile regression in partially linear varying coefficient models. Ann. Stat. **37**(68), 3841–3866 (2009)
105. Wang, L., Wu, Y., Li, R.: Quantile regression for analyzing heterogeneity in ultra-high dimension. J. Am. Stat. Assoc. **107**(497), 214–222 (2012)
106. Wang, T., Ionita-Laza, I., Wei, Y.: Integrated quantile rank test (iQRAT) for gene-level associations. Ann. Appl. Stat. **16**(3), 1423–1444 (2022)

107. Wang, C., Wang, T., Kiryluk, K., Wei, Y., Aschard, H., Ionita-Laza, I.: Genome-wide discovery for biomarkers using quantile regression at biobank scale. Nat. Commun. **15**(1), 6460 (2024)
108. Wang, T., Ling, W., Plantinga, A.M., Wu, M.C., Zhan, X.: Testing microbiome association using integrated quantile regression models. Bioinformatics **38**(2), 419–425 (2022)
109. Wang, T., Ionita-Laza, I., Wei, Y.: A unified quantile framework for nonlinear heterogeneous transcriptome-wide associations. Ann. Appl. Stat. **19**(2), 967–985 (2025)
110. Wang, Z., Liu, X., Tang, W., Lin, Y.: Incorporating graphical structure of predictors in sparse quantile regression. J. Bus. Econ. Stat. **39**, 783–792 (2020)
111. Wang, T., Zhang, W., Wei, Y.: ZIKQ: an innovative centile chart method for utilizing natural history data in rare disease clinical development **35**, 2451–2468 (2025)
112. Wang, Z., Wang, T.: A semiparametric quantile single-index model for zero-inflated outcomes. Stat. Sin. (2024). https://doi.org/10.5705/ss.202024.0104
113. Watanabe, K., Stringer, S., Frei, O., Umićević Mirkov, M., de Leeuw, C., Polderman, T.J., van der Sluis, S., Andreassen, O.A., Neale, B.M., Posthuma, D.: A global overview of pleiotropy and genetic architecture in complex traits. Nat. Genet. **51**(9), 1339–1348 (2019)
114. Wei, Y.: An approach to multivariate covariate-dependent quantile contours with application to bivariate conditional growth charts. J. Am. Stat. Assoc. **103**(481), 397–409 (2008)
115. Wei, Y., Carroll, R.J.: Quantile regression with measurement error. J. Am. Stat. Assoc. **104**(487), 1129–1143 (2009)
116. Wei, Y., Pere, A., Koenker, R., He, X.: Quantile regression methods for reference growth charts. Stat. Med. **25**(8), 1369–1382 (2006)
117. Wei, Y., Ma, Y., Carroll, R.J.: Multiple imputation in quantile regression. Biometrika **99**(2), 423–438 (2012)
118. Wei, Y., Song, X., Liu, M., Ionita-Laza, I., Reibman, J.: Quantile regression in the secondary analysis of case–control data. J. Am. Stat. Assoc. **111**(513), 344–354 (2016)
119. Wright, S.J.: Primal-Dual Interior-Point Methods. SIAM, Philadelphia (1997)
120. Wu, Y., Liu, Y.: Variable selection in quantile regression. Stat. Sin. **19**(2), 801–817 (2009)
121. Wu, M.C., Lee, S., Cai, T., Li, Y., Boehnke, M., Lin, X.: Rare-variant association testing for sequencing data with the sequence kernel association test. Am. J. Hum. Genet. **89**(1), 82–93 (2011)
122. Yang, J., Loos, R.J., Powell, J.E., Medland, S.E., Speliotes, E.K., Chasman, D.I., Rose, L.M., Thorleifsson, G., Steinthorsdottir, V., Mägi, R., et al.: FTO genotype is associated with phenotypic variability of body mass index. Nature **490**(7419), 267–272 (2012)
123. Yang, D., Zhao, L., Lin, Z., Qin, T., Bian, J., Liu, T.-Y.: Fully parameterized quantile function for distributional reinforcement learning. Adv. Neural Inf. Proces. Syst. **32** (2019)
124. Yates, T., Razieh, C., Zaccardi, F., Davies, M.J., Khunti, K.: Obesity and risk of covid-19: analysis of uk biobank. Prim. Care Diabetes **14**(5), 566–567 (2020)
125. Zhou, F., Wang, J., Feng, X.: Non-crossing quantile regression for distributional reinforcement learning. Adv. Neural Inf. Proces. Syst. **33**, 15909–15919 (2020)
126. Zhang, W., Wei, Y., Zhang, D., Xu, E.Y.: ZIAQ: a quantile regression method for differential expression analysis of single-cell RNA-seq data. Bioinformatics **36**(10), 3124–3130 (2020)
127. Zhang, Y., Zhu, Z.: Transfer learning for high-dimensional quantile regression via convolution smoothing. Preprint. arXiv:2212.00428 (2022)

Incorrect Model Selection Using R^2 and Akaike Information Criterion in Big Data Analyses

Katherine L. Thompson and Gregory S. Hawk

Abstract Although recent attention has focused on improving predictive models, less consideration has been given to variability introduced into models through incorrect variable selection. Here, the difficulty in choosing a scientifically correct model is explored theoretically, computationally, and practically, and the performance of model selection with maximum R^2 or minimum Akaike information criterion (AIC) is compared with that of more recent methods. The results in this paper show that often the model with the largest R^2 (or adjusted R^2) or smallest AIC may not be the scientifically correct model, suggesting that these model selection techniques may not be appropriate when data sets contain a large number of explanatory variables. This work starts with the derivation of the probability of choosing the scientifically correct model in data sets as a function of regression model parameters when using R^2 or AIC. Next, a data analysis example shows that these model selection criteria are outperformed by methods that produce multiple candidate models for researchers' consideration. These results are demonstrated in simulation studies and through the analysis of a National Health and Nutrition Examination Survey data set.

Keywords Linear regression · Logistic regression · Model selection · Subset selection · Variable selection

1 Introduction

One of the crucial aspects of building a regression model is the identification of scientifically correct variables impacting a response variable. Addressing this question becomes increasingly challenging as data set sizes increase. First, checking relationships among combinations of variables becomes impractical as the number

K. L. Thompson (✉) · G. S. Hawk
Dr. Bing Zhang Department of Statistics, University of Kentucky, Lexington, KY, USA
e-mail: katherine.thompson@uky.edu; greg.hawk@uky.edu

Y. Zhao, D.-G. Chen (eds.), *Big Data Analytics in Biostatistics and Bioinformatics*, ICSA Book Series in Statistics,
https://doi.org/10.1007/978-3-032-06649-7_4

of variables grows. For instance, in a data set containing 20,000 variables, an exhaustive search of pairwise combinations of variables in the data set to identify the statistically optimal model (e.g., the model with the greatest R^2 or smallest Akaike information criterion, or AIC) requires fitting almost 200 million models. In fact, in one genetics example, even using a supercomputer with 4,096 nodes, checking all combinations of three genetic factors is estimated to take more than 5.8 years [12]. Based on a 2022 review of a variety of methods, computational times for some genetic analyses have lasted more than 10 days or were infeasible (see Table 2 in [21]), particularly when interactions of more than two single nucleotide polymorphisms are considered. Second, the statistically optimal combination may or may not be the scientifically correct relationship. According to comments on work by Efron [5], errors in variable selection for a model are highly underrepresented in the literature. The work in this manuscript is motivated by the latter of these two challenges.

In fact, the probability of identifying the correct relationship in a given data set can be calculated as a function of the regression coefficients, the design matrix, and the variance of the error terms of the model. Although the distribution of R^2 for a single model was derived more than four decades ago [16] and the mean and variance of R^2 have been derived for three decades [4], properties of R^2 when comparing multiple models have been more limited. Interestingly, the distribution of maximal R^2 across all models with a fixed number of predictors was derived in the case that no linear relationship exists in the data, but the distribution of R^2 in the case that a relationship is present in a data set was not considered [8]. This limitation of the existing literature motivates the methods developed in this manuscript.

In this work, for each of two model selection criteria, the probability of selecting the correct predictor variable set for a linear or logistic regression model is derived as a function of the design matrices of the prospective models, the true vector of regression coefficients, and the variance of the error terms (for linear regression). Note that the results in this manuscript focus on choosing models with a fixed number of explanatory variables, so that all results from R^2 extend directly to metrics such as adjusted R^2 as well. However, some work comparing models of different orders is presented here. Not only does this work show that the chance of an error in model selection is high under very reasonable parameter settings, but it also illustrates the need for researchers to consider multiple models to reduce the probability of selecting an incorrect variable set for a model (when correct predictors are contained in the data set).

Next, Sect. 2 outlines some of the existing methods for model selection. Sections 3 and 4.1 demonstrate through theoretical work and simulation studies that the chance of a researcher selecting the correct set of variables to predict a response, by choosing the model with the greatest R^2 (linear regression) or lowest AIC value (logistic regression), is very low (less than 35% with R^2 and less than 5% with AIC) for medium effect sizes. Moreover, the chance of selecting the correct model can be improved by using algorithms that produce more than one possible set of predictors for consideration, thereby increasing the probability of a researcher selecting the correct model during data analysis (e.g., see those in [14, 20]). These results are supported by the data analysis example in Sect. 4.2.

2 Background

One of the central goals of model selection is to identify explanatory variables that truly relate to a response variable. Although recent literature has focused carefully on predictive modeling (see, e.g., [17]), others have pointed out that although the practice of ignoring variability due to variable selection is common, this practice also could result in incorrect inferences [5]. Often ignored in model selection, but crucial for accurate results [3], this challenge stymies methodology developers. Moreover, a discussion by Tibshirani [23] references the need for statisticians to focus on developing methods that help collaborators in other fields, rather than creating methods for the sole purpose of their creation. Developing methods with a focus on usefulness is even more present in the growing predictive modeling landscape, as impactful methods are developed with an understanding of how or why they are well-suited for particular data types or subject areas. Understanding the underpinnings of new methods is essential for appropriate application of predictive models in broader contexts. To address these limitations in variable selection methodology, the probability of obtaining the correct variables using subset selection is both derived theoretically and explored in practice.

Current methods for identification of relationships within model building include model selection or subset selection using maximum R^2 or minimum AIC, penalized regression methods, and regression tree techniques. In these model selection methods, a researcher fits all possible models with p explanatory variables and chooses the "best" model by optimizing some specified criterion. Examples of these criteria include R^2, adjusted R^2, prediction sum of squares (PRESS) statistic [1], AIC, or Bayesian information criterion (BIC), among others (see, e.g., those in [18]). For example, one early approach takes a Bayesian perspective to improving prediction using model selection [9]. In another example with financial applications, [7] found improved model selection performance over standard stepwise selection methods by considering interaction effects and modifying other aspects of stepwise selection. However, subset selection methods have been criticized due to their sensitivity to small changes in the data [10]. Here, this sensitivity is explored by simulating multiple data sets and calculating the probability that subset selection will produce the correct model.

In penalized regression methods, such as ridge regression or least absolute shrinkage and selection operator (LASSO) [22], the residual sum of squares is subject to some penalty during minimization [6, 13]. Lastly, in regression tree methods, explanatory variables are used to partition subjects into groups that have less variability in the response variable [17]. These methods produce results in which effects of individual predictors are unable to be parsed and interpreted in a scientific context.

Thus, the former model selection techniques are widely used and easily interpreted. Penalized regression methods may leave researchers with a large quantity of explanatory variables, often complicating interpretations through the consideration of large numbers of effects, when compared to traditional models with fewer explanatory variables identified by subset selection. While tree-based methods are built from simple decision rules, understanding the contributions of the underlying variables selected may not be straightforward when (1) many variables are selected or (2) multiple trees are built. Variable importance measures do provide an overall contribution of each variable to the prediction but may not yield one or two actionable risk factors in the form of explanatory variables. In the case of even simple tree-based methods, cutoff values are created for quantitative explanatory variables. These cutoffs ease interpretability but rely on the cutoff value rather than the observed quantitative value. Regression-based methods address this limitation by providing both a list of actionable risk factor(s) and the magnitude of the relationship of said risk factor(s) with an outcome in the presence of other covariate(s). One more recently developed method, the Feasible Solution Algorithm (FSA) [14, 19, 20], provides a direct comparison with model selection using maximum R^2 or minimum AIC to identify the "best" predictor set and is tested alongside model selection in the data analysis example in Sect. 4.2.

In the following section, the probability that a researcher identifies the scientifically correct model in a data set is derived in the context of linear regression (using R^2) or logistic regression (using AIC). Next, both simulation and data analyses are used to compare the performance of model selection techniques using maximum R^2 or minimum AIC in obtaining true models. In particular, simulation studies demonstrate changes in the probability of identification of the scientifically correct model as the regression parameters change, while the data set analysis example tests method performance in the presence of real-world variability.

3 Methods

In this section, some notation is introduced for both linear and logistic regression models. Next, the probability a researcher obtains the correct linear regression model using R^2 as a criterion is derived. Lastly, the probability a researcher identifies the correct logistic regression model using AIC as a criterion is derived.

3.1 Notation

Suppose one's interest in a particular data set lies in identifying relationships between explanatory variables and either a quantitative or binary response variable using n independent observations. Then potential data sets will have the following form:

$$\boldsymbol{Y} = \begin{bmatrix} Y_1 \\ Y_2 \\ \vdots \\ Y_n \end{bmatrix} \text{ and } \boldsymbol{X} = \begin{bmatrix} X_{11} & X_{12} & \dots & X_{1p} \\ X_{21} & X_{22} & \dots & X_{2p} \\ \vdots & \vdots & \ddots & \vdots \\ X_{n1} & X_{n2} & \dots & X_{np} \end{bmatrix} \tag{1}$$

Note that X_{i1} may be equal to 1 for $i \in \{1, 2, \dots, n\}$ if the model of interest contains an intercept. As a convention, let $\boldsymbol{X_j} \equiv [X_{1j}\ X_{2j}\ \dots\ X_{nj}]^T$ throughout this manuscript. Suppose the true linear relationship underlying the quantitative response variable, $\boldsymbol{Y}$, is

$$\boldsymbol{Y} = \boldsymbol{X_0\beta} + \boldsymbol{\epsilon}, \text{ where } \boldsymbol{\epsilon} \sim N_n(\boldsymbol{0}, \sigma^2\boldsymbol{I}) \tag{2}$$

Here, $\boldsymbol{X_0}$ contains p_0 columns from $\boldsymbol{X}$, meaning $\boldsymbol{X_0}$ has dimension $n \times p_0$, where $p_0 < p$. In the case that Y is a binary response variable, a logistic regression model is

$$logit(\pi_i) = \log\left(\frac{\pi_i}{1 - \pi_i}\right) = \boldsymbol{x_{i0}^T\beta}, \text{ for } i \in \{1, 2, \dots, n\} \tag{3}$$

where $\pi_i = P(Y_i = 1)$ and $\boldsymbol{x_{i0}^T}$ is the ith row of $\boldsymbol{X_0}$, which contains p_0 columns from $\boldsymbol{X}$. This means that $\boldsymbol{X_0}$ has dimension $n \times p_0$, where $p_0 < p$.

If the specified model is that with statistically optimal criterion value (e.g., largest R^2 or smallest AIC), there are exactly $\binom{p}{p_0} - 1$ combinations of explanatory variables that will yield incorrectly specified models. The overarching goal of this manuscript is to find the probability that all of these $\binom{p}{p_0} - 1$ combinations of explanatory variables will produce a model with a lower R^2 (linear regression) or higher AIC (logistic regression) than the correct design matrix, $\boldsymbol{X_0}$. However, in order to calculate the probability of interest, this work begins by comparing a single correctly specified model with a single one of the $\binom{p}{p_0} - 1$ incorrectly specified models. These probabilities are derived in Sects. 3.2.1 and 3.3.1 and then are extended to the cases of interest with comparison of many incorrectly specified models in Sects. 3.2.2 and 3.3.2.

For example, Table 1 contains a data set with n observations, a quantitative response variable (y), and $p = 4$ possible explanatory variables (X_1, X_2, X_3, X_4) to describe Y. Here, $\boldsymbol{X} = [\boldsymbol{X_1}\ \boldsymbol{X_2}\ \boldsymbol{X_3}\ \boldsymbol{X_4}]$. If we are interested in models with $p_0 = 2$ predictors without an intercept, a true linear regression model may be:

$$Y = \beta_1\boldsymbol{X_1} + \beta_2\boldsymbol{X_2} + \boldsymbol{\epsilon},\ \boldsymbol{\epsilon} \sim N(\boldsymbol{0}, \sigma^2\boldsymbol{I}) \tag{4}$$

Table 1 Example data set with n observations and $p = 4$ possible explanatory variables. This table shows an example data set with n observations (column 1), observed values of the response variable (column 2), $\boldsymbol{y}$, and four explanatory variables: $\boldsymbol{X_1}$, $\boldsymbol{X_2}$, $\boldsymbol{X_3}$, and $\boldsymbol{X_4}$ (columns 3–6), respectively

Observation	y	X_1	X_2	X_3	X_4
1	4.2	5.3	1.2	5.6	4.3
2	3.8	4.4	0.8	3.5	4.0
$\vdots$	$\vdots$	$\vdots$	$\vdots$	$\vdots$	$\vdots$
n	1.7	1.2	1.1	2.6	3.9

In this case, $\boldsymbol{X_0} = [\boldsymbol{X_1}\ \boldsymbol{X_2}]$. However, it may be that X_3 and X_4 (or $\boldsymbol{U} = [\boldsymbol{X_3}\ \boldsymbol{X_4}]$) produce a model with a higher R^2 than the model containing X_1 and X_2. In other words, it may be that $R^2_{X_0} < R^2_U$, even though $\boldsymbol{X_0}$ is the correct design matrix in the model to describe $\boldsymbol{Y}$. The probability that the correct model is obtained, or that $R^2_{X_0} > R^2_U$, is derived in Sect. 3.2.1. Moreover, we are interested in the probability that *any* combination of columns of $\boldsymbol{X}$ produce a model with a higher R^2 value than the model with $\boldsymbol{X_0}$. By defining the following: $\boldsymbol{U_1} = [\boldsymbol{X_1}\ \boldsymbol{X_3}]$, $\boldsymbol{U_2} = [\boldsymbol{X_1}\ \boldsymbol{X_4}]$, $\boldsymbol{U_3} = [\boldsymbol{X_2}\ \boldsymbol{X_3}]$, $\boldsymbol{U_4} = [\boldsymbol{X_2}\ \boldsymbol{X_4}]$, and $\boldsymbol{U_5} = [\boldsymbol{X_3}\ \boldsymbol{X_4}]$, the probability that $R^2_{X_0} > R^2_{U_j}\ \forall j \in \{1, 2, 3, 4, 5\}$ can be derived (see Sect. 3.2.2).

In these cases, since inequalities with R^2 can be written as a ratio of quadratic forms, the following theorem from [2] will be helpful. This theorem expresses the cumulative distribution function (cdf) of a ratio of quadratic forms as the cdf of a sum of independent weighted noncentral χ^2 random variables.

Theorem 1 *Let, for* $\boldsymbol{Z} \sim N(\boldsymbol{\mu}, \boldsymbol{\Sigma})$, $\boldsymbol{\Sigma} > 0$. *For symmetric matrices* $\boldsymbol{A^*}$ *and* $\boldsymbol{B^*}$, *where* $\boldsymbol{B^*}$ *is positive semidefinite with at least one eigenvalue strictly greater than zero, then*

$$P\left(\frac{\boldsymbol{Z^T A^* Z}}{\boldsymbol{Z^T B^* Z}} \leq r\right) = P\left(\boldsymbol{W^T \Lambda W} \leq 0\right) \tag{5}$$

where $\boldsymbol{W} \equiv \boldsymbol{P^T \Sigma^{-1/2} Z} \sim N(\boldsymbol{P^T \Sigma^{-1/2} \mu}, \boldsymbol{I_n})$. *Also,* $\boldsymbol{P \Lambda P^T}$ *denotes the spectral decomposition of* $(\boldsymbol{A} - r\boldsymbol{B})$, *where* $\boldsymbol{A} = \boldsymbol{\Sigma}^{1/2}\boldsymbol{A^*}\boldsymbol{\Sigma}^{1/2}$ *and* $\boldsymbol{B} = \boldsymbol{\Sigma}^{1/2}\boldsymbol{B^*}\boldsymbol{\Sigma}^{1/2}$. *Note that* $\boldsymbol{W^T \Lambda W}$ *can be written as the weighted sum of n independent noncentral* χ^2 *random variables,* $\sum_{i=1}^n \lambda_i W_i^2$, *where* $W_i^2 \overset{ind}{\sim} \chi_1^2(\nu_i^2)$ *for* $i = 1, \ldots, n$. *Here,* $\boldsymbol{\nu} = \boldsymbol{\Sigma^{-1/2} P^T \mu}$ *and* $\lambda_1, \lambda_2, \ldots, \lambda_n$ *are the diagonal elements of* $\boldsymbol{\Lambda}$.

This theorem will be used to derive the probability in Theorem 2 as a function of random variables with known distributions.

3.2 Model Selection Using R^2 in Multiple Linear Regression

Consider a linear regression analysis in which a data set such as that in (1) is being analyzed. In this case, the columns of $\boldsymbol{X}$ that are truly in the regression model ($\boldsymbol{X_0}$ in (2)) would produce the scientifically correct regression model. In Sect. 3.2.1, the probability of choosing the correct model between two candidate models is derived. In Sect. 3.2.2, this result is extended to derive the probability a researcher chooses the correct subset of p_0 explanatory variables from a data set containing p explanatory variables, thereby identifying the scientifically correct regression model. Note that these results also apply to adjusted R^2, assuming models contain a fixed number of predictors. Otherwise, these results can be extended to adjusted R^2 by deriving the analogous probability, shown in Corollary 1.

3.2.1 Comparing True Model to One Proposed Model

Suppose that two candidate models exist: the scientifically correct model and a scientifically incorrect model. The following theorem states that the probability that a researcher chooses the correct linear regression model, when selecting one of two potential models using R^2, can be expressed as a weighted sum of independent noncentral χ^2 random variables with noncentrality parameters that depend on the design matrices of the two candidate models, the vector of regression coefficients, and the variance of the error terms in the model.

Theorem 2 *Suppose that the scientifically correct model is given by (2). Let $\boldsymbol{H_U}$ and $\boldsymbol{H_{X_0}}$ be the projection matrices for two design matrices of candidate models, $\boldsymbol{U}$ and $\boldsymbol{X_0}$, respectively, where $\boldsymbol{H_U}$ follows the conditions given of $\boldsymbol{B}^*$ in Theorem 1. Let R^2_U and $R^2_{X_0}$ be the values of R^2 from fitting these two linear regression models with $\boldsymbol{Y}$ as the response variable. Then,*

$$P\left(R^2_{X_0} > R^2_U\right) = P\left(\sum_{i=1}^{n} \lambda_i W_i^2 < 0\right), \tag{6}$$

where $W_i^2 \overset{ind}{\sim} \chi_1^2(\nu_i^2)$ and $\boldsymbol{\nu} = \boldsymbol{P}^T \boldsymbol{X_0}\boldsymbol{\beta}/\sigma$. Further, $\boldsymbol{P}$ is the matrix of eigenvectors and $\lambda_1, \lambda_2, \ldots, \lambda_n$ are the eigenvalues of $\sigma^2(\boldsymbol{H_U} - \boldsymbol{H_{X_0}})$.

Proof See Appendix section "Proof of Theorem 2".

The probability in (22) is not analytically tractable, but can be estimated using computation *via* Monte Carlo integration [11]. In this case, sampling from the distributions of $W_1^2, W_2^2, \ldots, W_n^2$ is straightforward.

This theorem provides a way for analysts to explore the properties of using R^2 as a model selection criterion, even in the conservative case that there are only two models being considered. Deriving this probability yields the setup for use in

Sect. 3.2.2 in order to better understand how often scientists correctly identify a model using a subset of variables from a data set.

Note that if the models fit using $\boldsymbol{X_0}$ and $\boldsymbol{U}$ contain the same number of parameters, finding the optimal model using R^2 and using adjusted R^2 are equivalent. However, in the case that the numbers of regression parameters in the two models are different, the following corollary gives the probability of choosing the scientifically correct model using adjusted R^2.

Corollary 1 *Suppose that the scientifically correct model is given by (2). Let* $\boldsymbol{H_U}$ *and* $\boldsymbol{H_{X_0}}$ *be the projection matrices for two design matrices of candidate models,* $\boldsymbol{U}$ *and* $\boldsymbol{X_0}$*, respectively, where* $(\boldsymbol{I} - \boldsymbol{H_U})$ *follows the conditions given of* $\boldsymbol{B^*}$ *in Theorem 1. Let* R^2_{aU} *and* $R^2_{aX_0}$ *be the values of adjusted* R^2 *from fitting these two linear regression models with* $\boldsymbol{Y}$ *as the response variable, respectively. Then:*

$$P\left(R^2_{aX_0} > R^2_{aU}\right) = P\left(\sum_{i=1}^{n} \lambda_i W_i^2 \leq 0\right), \tag{7}$$

where $W_i^2 \overset{ind}{\sim} \chi_1^2(\nu_i^2)$ *and* $\boldsymbol{\nu} = \boldsymbol{P^T X_0 \beta}/\sigma$*. Further,* $\boldsymbol{P}$ *is the matrix of eigenvectors and* $\lambda_1, \lambda_2, \ldots, \lambda_n$ *are the eigenvalues of* $\sigma^2(r\boldsymbol{H_U} - \boldsymbol{H_{X_0}} + (1-r)\boldsymbol{I})$*, where* $r = (n - p_{X_0})/(n - p_U)$*. Let* p_{X_0} *and* p_U *denote the numbers of regression coefficients in the models from* $\boldsymbol{X_0}$ *and* $\boldsymbol{U}$*, respectively.*

The proof of Corollary 1 is analogous to the proof of Theorem 2. Thus, if a researcher is interested in using adjusted R^2 as a criterion for model fit, the probability of choosing the correct model given a set of potential explanatory variables can be calculated using methods analogous to those in Sect. 3.2.2.

3.2.2 Comparing True Model to Many Proposed Models

Although Theorem 2 shows the probability that a researcher chooses the correct linear regression model when presented with two candidate models, a realistic data analysis involves choosing among any $\binom{p}{p_0}$ models in the data set. In addition to the correct model, $k \equiv \binom{p}{p_0} - 1$ incorrect design matrices (called $\boldsymbol{U_1}, \boldsymbol{U_2}, \ldots, \boldsymbol{U_k}$) are considered, each containing p_0 columns from $\boldsymbol{X}$.

The following theorem gives the probability that the explanatory variables contained in *all* of these $\boldsymbol{U_i}$'s will produce models with smaller R^2 values than the true (correct) model. Further, this probability is expressed as the probability that the maximum of k weighted sums of independent noncentral χ^2 random variables is at most zero. The noncentrality parameters of the noncentral χ^2 random variables, along with the weights, depend on the design matrices of the two candidate models, the vector of regression coefficients, and the variance of the error terms in the model.

Theorem 3 *Let* $R^2_{U_1}, R^2_{U_2}, \ldots, R^2_{U_k}$*, and* $R^2_{X_0}$ *be the values of* R^2 *from fitting the linear regression models with* $\boldsymbol{Y}$ *as the response variable and* $\boldsymbol{U_1}, \boldsymbol{U_2}, \ldots, \boldsymbol{U_k}$*,* *and* $\boldsymbol{X_0}$*, respectively, as the design matrices for the k incorrect and single correct models, respectively. Then,*

$$P\left(R^2_{X_0} > R^2_{U_j}\ \forall j \in \{1, 2, \ldots, k\}\right) =$$

$$= P\left(\max_{j=1,2,\ldots,k}\left[\boldsymbol{W}_j^T \boldsymbol{\Lambda}_j \boldsymbol{W}_j\right] \le 0\right) \qquad (8)$$

where $\boldsymbol{P}_j \boldsymbol{\Lambda}_j \boldsymbol{P}_j^T$ *is the spectral decomposition of* $\sigma^2(\boldsymbol{H}_{U_j} - \boldsymbol{H}_{X_0})$ *and* $\boldsymbol{W}_j^T \boldsymbol{\Lambda}_j \boldsymbol{W}_j = \sum_{i=1}^n \lambda_{ij} W_{ij}^2$*. Note that* W_{ij}^2 *are independent random variables that follow* $\chi_1^2(\nu_{ij}^2)$ *distributions with* $\boldsymbol{\nu}_j = \boldsymbol{P}_j^T \boldsymbol{X}_0 \boldsymbol{\beta}$*.*

Proof See Appendix section "Proof of Theorem 3".

Once again, this quantity, although analytically intractable, can be estimated using Monte Carlo techniques by sampling noncentral χ_1^2 random variables with the noncentrality parameter as stated. This probability provides an analytical method for researchers to study the behavior of model selection with maximum R^2 in a variety of parameter settings, in order to better understand how often the scientifically correct model is also the statistically optimal model as a function of effect sizes. The behavior of this probability under different parameter settings is further explored in Sect. 4.1.

3.3 Model Selection Using *AIC* in Multiple Logistic Regression

Consider a logistic regression analysis in which a data set such as that in (1) is being analyzed. In this case, the columns of $\boldsymbol{X}$ that are truly in the regression model ($\boldsymbol{X}_0$ in (3)) would produce the scientifically correct regression model. In Sect. 3.3.1, the probability of choosing the correct model between two candidate models is derived. In Sect. 3.3.2, this result is extended to derive the probability a researcher chooses the correct subset of p_0 explanatory variables from a data set containing p explanatory variables, thereby identifying the scientifically correct regression model. Note that the results of these theorems also apply to BIC if n and p_0 are the same across models being compared. Otherwise, extensions of Theorems 4 and 5 will produce analogous probabilities for the cases in which n or p_0 varies across candidate models.

3.3.1 Comparing True Model to One Proposed Model

The following theorem states that, when presented with two candidate logistic regression models for a data set, the probability that a researcher chooses the correct model from two candidate models using AIC as a criterion can be expressed as a function of the response variable and the design matrices of the two candidate models (along with the maximum likelihood estimators, or MLEs, of their parameters).

Theorem 4 *Suppose a scientifically correct model is given by (3). Let AIC_U and AIC_{X_0} be the values of AIC from fitting the logistic regression models with $\mathbf{Y}$ as the response variable and $\mathbf{U}$ and $\mathbf{X_0}$, respectively, as two design matrices. Let $\mathbf{u}_i^T$ and $\mathbf{x}_{i0}^T$ be the ith rows of $\mathbf{U}$ and $\mathbf{X_0}$, respectively. Then the probability the correct model has a lower AIC than the incorrect model is:*

$$P\left(AIC_{X_0} < AIC_U\right) =$$

$$= P\left(\sum_i Y_i(\mathbf{x}_{0i}^T\hat{\boldsymbol{\beta}} - \mathbf{u}_i^T\hat{\boldsymbol{\beta}}_U) > \sum_i \log\left[\frac{1+\exp\left(\mathbf{x}_{0i}^T\hat{\boldsymbol{\beta}}\right)}{1+\exp\left(\mathbf{u}_i^T\hat{\boldsymbol{\beta}}_U\right)}\right]\right), \tag{9}$$

where $\hat{\boldsymbol{\beta}}_U$ and $\hat{\boldsymbol{\beta}}$ are MLEs of the parameter vector, $\boldsymbol{\beta}$, from the fitted models including $\mathbf{U}$ and $\mathbf{X_0}$, respectively.

Proof See Appendix section "Proof of Theorem 4".

Although this probability is not analytically tractable, Monte Carlo integration can be used to estimate it for different design matrices and parameter settings. Thus, in Sect. 4.1.4, data are simulated under the true model in (3) and the probability in (32) is calculated.

This probability is the foundation of the work in Sect. 3.3.2, in which a probability of choosing the correct model using minimum AIC as criterion is derived, given any potential set of explanatory variables is being considered in a model.

3.3.2 Comparing True Model to Many Proposed Models

The following theorem extends the result of Theorem 4 and gives the probability that all the $k \equiv \binom{p}{p_0} - 1$ incorrect candidate models produce higher values of AIC than that from the correct candidate model.

Theorem 5 *Let $AIC_{U_1}, AIC_{U_2}, \ldots, AIC_{U_k}$, and AIC_{X_0} be the values of AIC from fitting the logistic regression models with $\mathbf{Y}$ as the response variable and $\mathbf{U_1}, \mathbf{U_2}, \ldots, \mathbf{U_k}$ and $\mathbf{X_0}$ as the design matrices for the k incorrect and single correct models, respectively. Let $\mathbf{u}_{ij}^T$ and $\mathbf{x}_{i0}^T$ be the ith rows of $\mathbf{U}_j$ and $\mathbf{X_0}$, respectively. Then,*

$$P\left(\bigcap_{j=1}^{k}\{AIC_{X_0} < AIC_{U_j}\}\right) =$$

$$= P\left(\bigcap_{j=1}^{k}\left\{\sum_i Y_i(\boldsymbol{x}_{0i}^T\hat{\boldsymbol{\beta}} - \boldsymbol{u}_{ij}^T\hat{\boldsymbol{\beta}}_j) > \sum_i \log\left[\frac{1+\exp\left(\boldsymbol{x}_{0i}^T\hat{\boldsymbol{\beta}}\right)}{1+\exp\left(\boldsymbol{u}_{ij}^T\hat{\boldsymbol{\beta}}_j\right)}\right]\right\}\right) \tag{10}$$

where $\hat{\boldsymbol{\beta}}_j$ and $\hat{\boldsymbol{\beta}}$ are the MLEs of $\boldsymbol{\beta}$ from the logistic regression models with design matrices $\boldsymbol{U}_j$ and $\boldsymbol{X}_0$, respectively.

Proof See Appendix section "Proof of Theorem 5".

This resulting probability is not analytically tractable, but Monte Carlo integration can be used to estimate this probability for different design matrices. Thus, this theorem can be used to understand the behavior of model selection using minimum AIC in the presence of varied effect sizes. In Sects. 4.1.5–4.1.7, data are simulated under the true model in (3) and the probability in (34) is studied for varied parameter settings.

4 Results

In this section, we will explore the probabilities described above as functions of the design matrices, true model parameters, and variability in the model errors. This exploration will be performed through simulation studies and followed by a data analysis example.

4.1 *Simulation Study*

Simulation results are shown below to illustrate the the probability of choosing the correct model. These analyses include model selection with R^2 and AIC as criteria in linear and logistic regression frameworks, respectively.

4.1.1 Comparing X_0 and U Using R^2 as a Model Selection Criterion

In the first simulation study, the probability of choosing the scientifically correct model from two possible design matrices is estimated using Monte Carlo integration. Specifically, the design matrix takes the following form:

$$\boldsymbol{X} = \begin{bmatrix} 1 & X_{11} & X_{12} \\ 1 & X_{21} & X_{22} \\ \vdots & \vdots & \vdots \\ 1 & X_{n1} & X_{n2} \end{bmatrix} \tag{11}$$

where $X_{ij} \overset{iid}{\sim} Unif(-1, 1)$ for $i = 1, 2, \ldots, n$ and $j = 1, 2$. Here, $\boldsymbol{X_1}$ represents the correct explanatory variable for a regression model, and $\boldsymbol{X_2}$ represents an irrelevant variable in the data set. Thus, the following linear regression model is assumed:

$$Y_i = \beta_0 + \beta_1 X_{i1} + \epsilon_i \tag{12}$$

where $\epsilon_i \overset{ind}{\sim} N(0, \sigma^2)$ for $i = 1, 2, \ldots, n$. Here, $n = 100$ observations are under study, β_0 is set to 10, and values of β_1 between 0.25 and 1 are considered for $\sigma^2 = 1$. In order to calculate the probability of selecting the correct simple linear regression model, 1 million simulations were performed using Theorem 2 with each simulated design matrix.

This process is repeated using a model with two explanatory variables both without and with an interaction effect as follows:

$$Y_i = \beta_0 + \beta_1 X_{i1} + \beta_2 X_{i2} + \epsilon_i \tag{13}$$

$$Y_i = \beta_0 + \beta_1 X_{i1} + \beta_2 X_{i2} + \beta_{12} X_{i1} X_{i2} + \epsilon_i \tag{14}$$

All distribution and parameter settings are the same as in the simple linear regression case above. Note that β_1 is set equal to β_2 and β_{12} is varied in this simulation.

4.1.2 Comparing Theoretical and Simulated Probabilities of Correct Model Identification

In addition to the probabilities calculated theoretically described in the previous section, probabilities were simulated using 1 million response variable vectors simulated under the model given above for the matrix, $\boldsymbol{X}$, containing the two potential models for the analyst to choose. Then, the proportion of replications that the correct model used to generate the data had a higher value of R^2 than the incorrect model was recorded for each parameter setting.

These results are presented alongside the theoretical probabilities in Fig. 1. In each plot, the regression coefficients are 0.25 (black circles), 0.50 (red triangles), 0.75 (green plus signs), and 1.00 (blue $\times$'s). In each case, the large symbols show the means of the probabilities from the corresponding parameter settings, and the gray line shows the case in which the simulated and theoretical probabilities are the same. In (a)–(c), we see that the theoretical probability derived in Theorem 2 agrees with simulation results in simple linear regression, multiple linear regression (two variables), and multiple linear regression (two variables with an interaction). As expected, for large effects, the simulated and theoretical probabilities are close to one. Since these simulations confirm the accuracy of the probability from Theorem 2, we next explore the theoretical probability under several parameter settings.

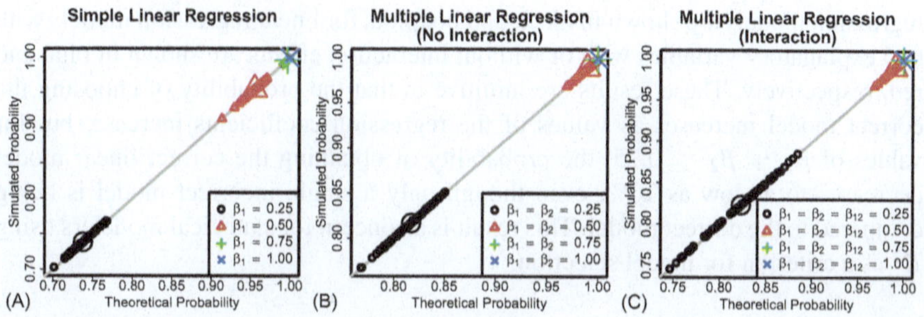

Fig. 1 Plot comparing theoretical and simulated probabilities. (**a**)–(**c**) show the estimated probability from simulated data sets plotted against the theoretical probability calculated using Theorem 2 for simple linear regression, multiple linear regression with two main effects, and multiple linear regression with two main effects and their interaction, respectively. Within each plot, values of the regression coefficients equal to 0.25, 0.50, 0.75, and 1.00 are shown in black circles, red triangles, green plus signs, and blue ×'s, respectively. The larger symbols show the mean probabilities for each regression coefficient. These plots show that the simulated and theoretical probabilities are accurate under all tested parameter settings, as shown by the gray line

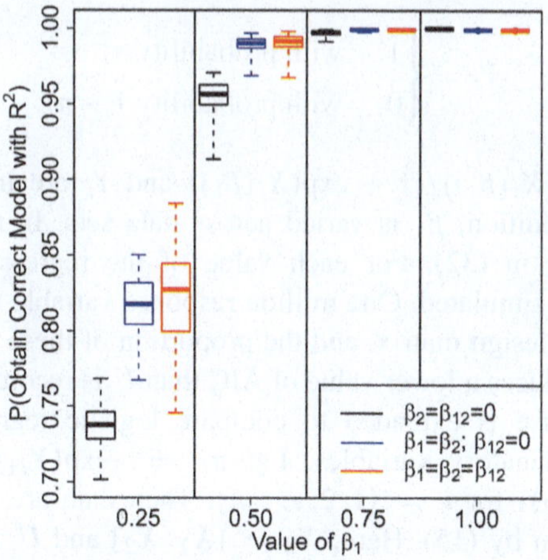

Fig. 2 Plot of probability that the correct model is identified using R^2 as the model selection criterion between two potential variable sets. In this figure, the probabilities calculated using Theorem 2 are shown in boxplots for 100 data sets at each value of β_1. In addition, boxplots for simple linear regression models are shown in black, boxplots for linear models with two explanatory variable models are shown in blue, and boxplots for linear models with two explanatory variables and their interaction are shown in red

4.1.3 Considering Theoretical Probability of Correct Model Identification

Figure 2 depicts the theoretical probabilities calculated using Theorem 2 in boxplots for 100 design matrices at varied values of the regression parameters, with design matrices simulated as described in Sect. 4.1.1. In addition, boxplots for simple linear regression models are shown in black and boxplots for linear regression models with two explanatory variables with or without interaction effects are shown in blue and red, respectively. These results are intuitive in that the probability of choosing the correct model increases as values of the regression coefficients increase, but for values of $\beta_1 = \beta_2 \leq 0.25$, the probability of obtaining the correct linear model decreases to as low as 70%, even though only a single incorrect model is being compared to the correct model. This result is a concern for statistical modelers using R^2 as a criterion for model selection.

4.1.4 Comparing X_0 and U Using AIC as a Model Selection Criterion

Next, data sets are simulated with a binary response variable in order to calculate the probability in Theorem 4 under multiple parameter settings. Covariate data were simulated as in the previous simulation study in Sect. 4.1.1. Response variable data are simulated under a logistic regression model with $\beta_0 = 0$ and the design matrix is defined as in (11). The true model for this simulation is, for $i = \{1, 2, \ldots, n\}$,

$$Y_i = \begin{cases} 1, & \text{with probability } \pi_i \\ 0, & \text{with probability } 1 - \pi_i \end{cases} \tag{15}$$

where $\pi_i = (\exp(X_{i1}\beta_1))/(1 + \exp(X_{i1}\beta_1))$ and Y_i are independent for $i = \{1, 2, \ldots, n\}$. In addition, β_1 is varied across data sets. In this scenario, $\boldsymbol{X_0} = \boldsymbol{X_1}$ and $\boldsymbol{U} = \boldsymbol{X_2}$ in (32). For each value of the regression coefficient, 100 design matrices are simulated. One million response variable data vectors are then simulated for each design matrix, and the proportion of these vectors in which the model with $\boldsymbol{X_0}$ produces a lower value of AIC than $\boldsymbol{U}$ is recorded.

Next, this premise is extended to compare logistic regression models each including two explanatory variables. Let $\pi_i = (\exp(X_{i1}\beta_1 + X_{i2}\beta_2))/(1 + \exp(X_{i1}\beta_1 + X_{i2}\beta_2))$ for $i = \{1, 2, \ldots, n\}$. Then data are simulated under the correct model, given by (15). Here, $\boldsymbol{X_0} = [\boldsymbol{X_1}\ \boldsymbol{X_2}]$ and $\boldsymbol{U} = [\boldsymbol{X_3}\ \boldsymbol{X_4}]$ in (34). Parameter settings and simulation setup are the same as in the previous single variable case, with $\beta_1 = \beta_2$.

In the analogous logistic regression model, now including an interaction effect, data are simulated under the correct model given by (15) with $\pi_i = \exp(X_{i1}\beta_1 + X_{i2}\beta_2 + X_{i1}X_{i2}\beta_{12})/(1 + \exp(X_{i1}\beta_1 + X_{i2}\beta_2 + X_{i1}X_{i2}\beta_{12}))$. Here, $\boldsymbol{X_0} = [\boldsymbol{X_1}\ \boldsymbol{X_2}\ \boldsymbol{X_1}\boldsymbol{X_2}]$ and $\boldsymbol{U} = [\boldsymbol{X_3}\ \boldsymbol{X_4}\ \boldsymbol{X_3}\boldsymbol{X_4}]$ in (34), where the ith element of $\boldsymbol{X_j}\boldsymbol{X_m}$ is $X_{ij}X_{im}$. Parameter settings and simulation setup are the same as in the previous two-variable case, where $\beta_1 = \beta_2$ and β_{12} is varied.

Figure 3 includes boxplots of these probabilities for each of the design matrices for varied values of the true regression coefficients. For small effects, the probability of obtaining the scientifically correct model using AIC is as low as 60% for a simple logistic regression model. As expected, the probability increases with the value of the regression parameters. However, even for medium or large effects ($\beta_1 \leq 0.75$

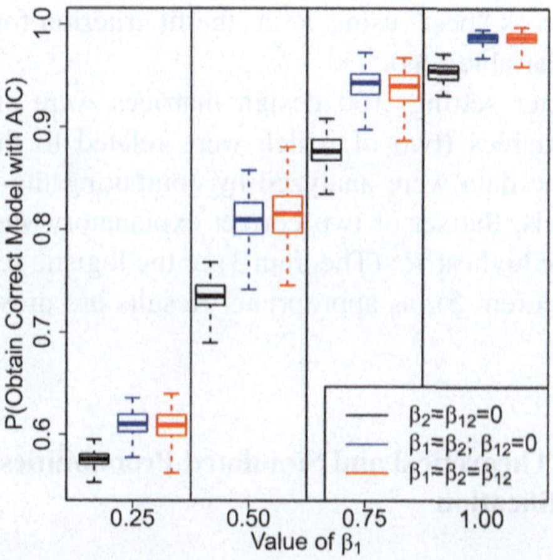

Fig. 3 Plot of probability that the correct model is identified using *AIC* as the model selection criterion between two potential variable sets. In this figure, the probabilities calculated using Theorem 4 are shown in boxplots for 100 data sets at each value of β_1. In addition, boxplots for simple logistic regression models are shown in black, boxplots for logistic regression models with two explanatory variable models are shown in blue, and boxplots for logistic regression models with two explanatory variables and their interaction are shown in red

for models with two explanatory variables and even $\beta_1 = 1$ for the simple logistic regression model), the probability is lower than 0.95, implying that even in the case of comparing one correct simple logistic regression model and one incorrect simple logistic regression model, researchers are likely to misidentify a relationship in a data set. In the presence of an interaction effect, the probability of a researcher selecting the correct logistic regression model is similar to the case without this added model complexity.

Together, these findings show that in the simplified case of choosing between two possible models, one correct and one incorrect, subset selection techniques with R^2 and AIC have difficulty in selecting the correct models. Next, the realistic case of analyzing a data set with more than two potential models is considered.

4.1.5 Testing Performance of R^2 and AIC in Model Selection

Here, we test the performance of model selection using R^2 or AIC in the more realistic framework in which a researcher fits all possible models to his/her data set and chooses the best model in terms of R^2 or AIC. In particular, rather than comparing two mutually exclusive sets of variables as in Sects. 4.1.1–4.1.4, comparisons are made between methods when considering all possible models containing two explanatory variables from a data set. Monte Carlo integration with 1,000 replications is used to estimate the probability that the scientifically correct model will be chosen as "best" using R^2 as the fit criterion for each of 100 design matrices (predictor variable sets).

For each parameter setting, 100 design matrices were simulated, each with 100 explanatory variables (two of which were related to the response variable of interest). Next, the data were analyzed by computing the probability that, out of all possible models, the set of two correct explanatory variables produced the linear model with the highest R^2 (Theorem 3) or the logistic regression model with the lowest AIC (Theorem 5), as appropriate. Results are presented in Sects. 4.1.6 and 4.1.7.

4.1.6 Comparing Theoretical and Simulated Probabilities of Correct Model Identification

In addition to the probabilities calculated theoretically as described above, probabilities were estimated using 1,000 response variable vectors simulated under the linear regression model given above for the matrix, $\boldsymbol{X}_1$. Then, all possible models were fit (to all combinations of two variables or two variables and an interaction) to the data sets. In each replication, the proportion of times the model used to generate the data had a higher value of R^2 than all other potential variable sets was recorded for each parameter setting. These results are presented alongside the theoretical probabilities in Fig. 4. In Fig. 4a–b, the regression coefficients are 0.25 (black ×'s), 0.50 (red circles), 0.75 (green triangles), and 1.00 (blue plus signs). Again, the large symbols show the means of the probabilities from the corresponding parameter settings, and the gray line shows the case in which the simulated and theoretical probabilities are the same. In all cases, the theoretical probability derived in Theorem 3 agrees with simulation results in multiple linear regression (two variables and two variables with an interaction), even in the case of small effect sizes. This provides evidence that the probability derived holds in a variety of parameter settings.

4.1.7 Considering Theoretical Probability of Correct Model Identification

Next, the theoretical probabilities calculated are more fully explored. First, Fig. 5 shows boxplots of the probability of obtaining the correct linear regression model using maximum R^2 in model selection. In the case without an interaction effect, model selection performance improves as the effect sizes of the regression parameters increase (Fig. 5a). For moderate to large regression coefficients and any interaction effect, choosing the model with the largest R^2 tends to perform reasonably well in terms of identifying the correct model. For a variety of interaction effect sizes in Fig. 5b–d, and small regression coefficients ($\beta_1 \leq 0.5$), model selection methods are limited by a low probability of detecting the scientifically correct linear regression model in a data set. This result is startling given the prevalent use of these techniques in practice.

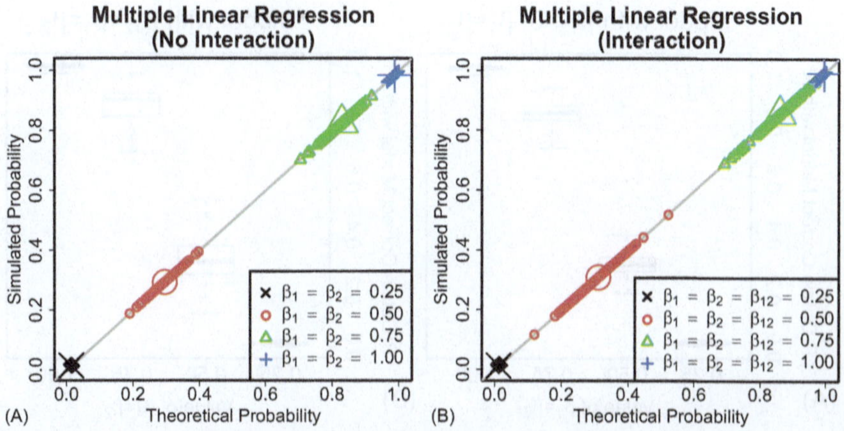

Fig. 4 Plot comparing theoretical and simulated probabilities in model selection with maximum R^2. (**a**) and (**b**) show the estimated probability from simulated data sets plotted against the theoretical probability calculated using Theorem 3 for multiple linear regression with two main effects and multiple linear regression with two main effects and their interaction, respectively. Within each plot, values of the regression coefficients equal to 0.25, 0.50, 0.75, and 1.00 are shown in black ×'s, red circles, green plus signs, and blue plus signs, respectively. The larger symbols show the mean probabilities for each regression coefficient. These figures show that the simulated and theoretical probabilities are accurate under all tested parameter settings, as shown by the gray line

Second, Fig. 6 shows boxplots of the probability of obtaining the correct logistic regression model with AIC using traditional model selection. For small to moderate regression coefficients and no interaction effect in Fig. 6a, AIC is limited by a small probability of detection of the underlying correct model (less than 40% in all cases). For increased interaction effect sizes (see Fig. 6b–d for values of $\beta_1 \geq 0.5$), model selection with AIC shows an improved probability of detecting the scientifically correct logistic regression model in some data sets, but only in the case of large effect sizes.

4.2 *Data Analysis Example*

The data set used in this work was from the National Health and Nutrition Examination Survey (NHANES) and has been previously analyzed in [15]. Data included 5038 observations from 174 potential predictors, of which 4473 observations are nonmissing in the response variable, high-density lipoprotein (HDL) cholesterol level. Other variables that measured cholesterol levels, categorical variables, variables lacking variation, or variables with more than 50% missing data in this data set were excluded from analysis, leaving 109 potential explanatory variables for inclusion in a linear model describing HDL level. Here, the analysis

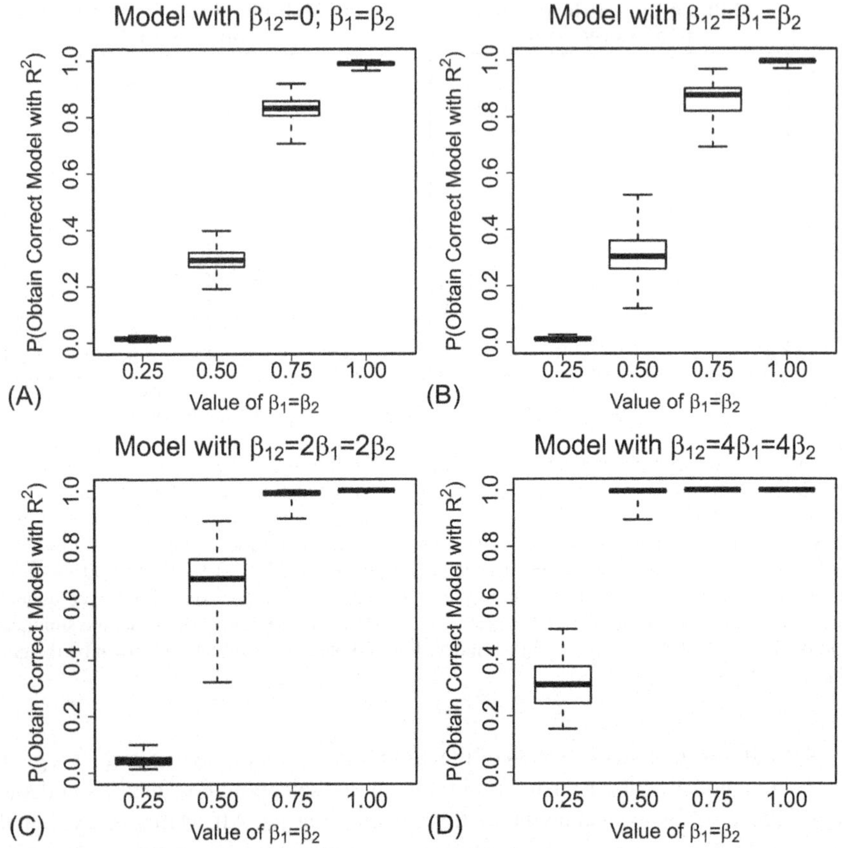

Fig. 5 Plot of probability that the correct model is identified using R^2 as the model selection criterion when considering all possible models. For each of 100 design matrices (each containing $p = 100$ explanatory variables), the probability that model selection with maximum R^2 identifies the correct model is shown when considering all $\binom{p}{p_0}$ models in analysis. (**a**)–(**d**) show the results when $\beta_{12} = 0$, $\beta_{12} = \beta_1$, $\beta_{12} = 2\beta_1$, and $\beta_{12} = 4\beta_1$, respectively

considered combinations of two predictors and, in some cases, their interaction effect.

In this work, the NHANES data set was modified to remove all pairwise variable effects, and a known relationship was placed in the data set (more detail is given in Sect. 4.2.2). The performance of model selection with maximum R^2 was then compared to the performance of the Feasible Solution Algorithm (FSA) in the case of the known, but hidden, relationships in the NHANES data. A brief description of FSA is provided next, followed by a description of the NHANES data analysis results.

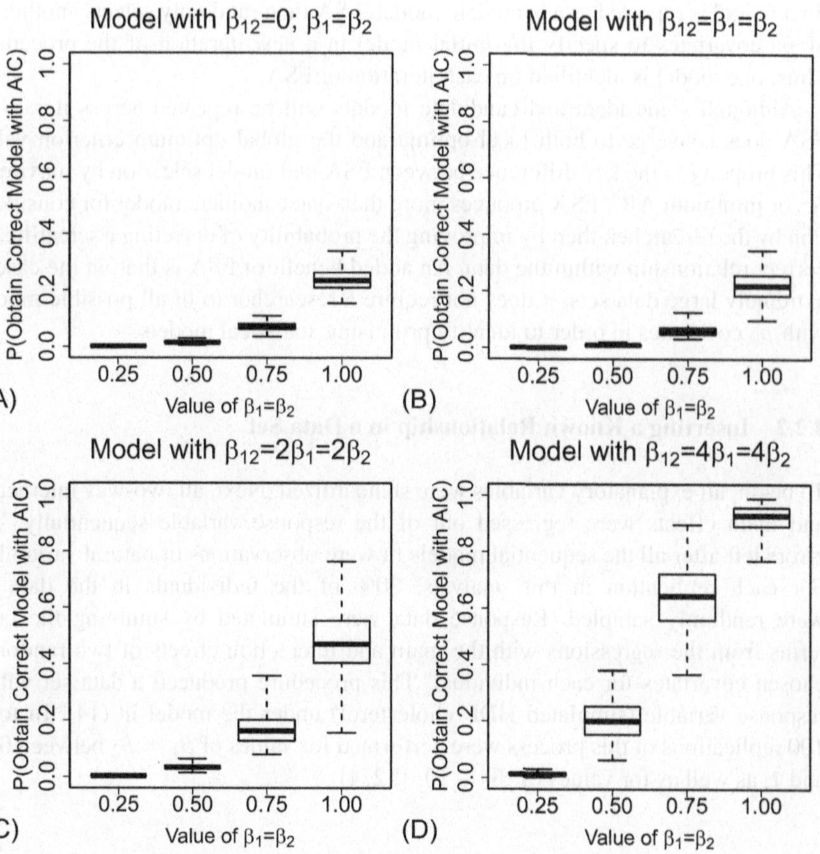

Fig. 6 Plot of probability that the correct model is identified using minimum AIC as the model selection criterion when considering all possible models. For each of 100 design matrices (each containing $p = 100$ explanatory variables), the probability that model selection with minimum AIC identifies the correct model is shown when considering all $\binom{p}{p_0}$ models in analysis. **(a)–(d)** show the results when $\beta_{12} = 0$, $\beta_{12} = \beta_1$, $\beta_{12} = 2\beta_1$, and $\beta_{12} = 4\beta_1$, respectively

4.2.1 Feasible Solutions Algorithm

The Feasible Solution Algorithm (FSA) is a fast, flexible method that aims to search a data set for potential relationships and produce multiple candidate models for further consideration by the analyst [14, 20]. To implement FSA, users specify an appropriate type of model for their data (along with a model fit criterion), a number of covariates desired in the model (p_0), and whether or not interactions among terms should be included in the model [19]. The algorithm randomly selects a set of p_0 covariates from the data set and fits the first model. Next, the algorithm makes particular exchanges of the explanatory variables in the model for the other covariates in the data set until no better model is identified with a new exchange. The final model is reported as a candidate model. FSA then randomly selects another set of p_0 covariates to specify the initial model in a new iteration of the procedure. Thus, one model is identified on each iteration of FSA.

Although some identified candidate models will be repeated across iterations, FSA does converge to both local optima and the global optimum criterion value. This property is the key difference between FSA and model selection by maximum R^2 or minimum AIC. FSA produces more than one candidate model for consideration by the researcher, thereby improving the probability of detecting a scientifically correct relationship within the data. An added benefit of FSA is that, in the case of extremely large data sets, it does not require a researcher to fit all possible models with p_0 covariates in order to identify promising statistical models.

4.2.2 Inserting a Known Relationship in a Data Set

To begin, all explanatory variables were standardized. Next, all two-way interaction and main effects were regressed out of the response variable sequentially. The errors left after all the sequential models fit were observations of natural variability. For each replication in this analysis, 80% of the individuals in the data set were randomly sampled. Response data were simulated by summing the error terms from the regressions with the main and interaction effects of two randomly chosen covariates for each individual. This procedure produced a data set with a response variable (simulated HDL cholesterol) under the model in (14). In total, 100 replications of this process were performed for values of $\beta_1 = \beta_2$ between 0.25 and 1, as well as for values of $\beta_{12} \in \{0, 1, 2, 4\}$.

4.2.3 Analyzing a Known Relationship in a Data Set

In this analysis, linear regression was performed with R^2 as the criterion function. Both model selection with maximum R^2 and FSA (with $m = 200$ random starts) were used to search for combinations of two explanatory variables (along with their interaction effect) to model the simulated HDL cholesterol data. In particular, FSA (implemented in the R package, `rFSA` Version 0.9.1 [19]) was run (with 200 random starts) for each data set replication, and the percentage of replications that FSA successfully identified both explanatory variables used to simulate HDL cholesterol level, meaning that it identified the scientifically correct model as one of its (possibly multiple) candidate models, was recorded. Similarly, the percentage of replications that model selection with maximum R^2 correctly identified both explanatory variables used to simulate HDL cholesterol level was recorded. We note that the model selected by maximum R^2 is a single model, while FSA can produce a set of candidate models that can include the correct explanatory variable set. This core feature of FSA allows subject area experts to consider multiple candidate models and select a final predictive model based on their expertise, when appropriate.

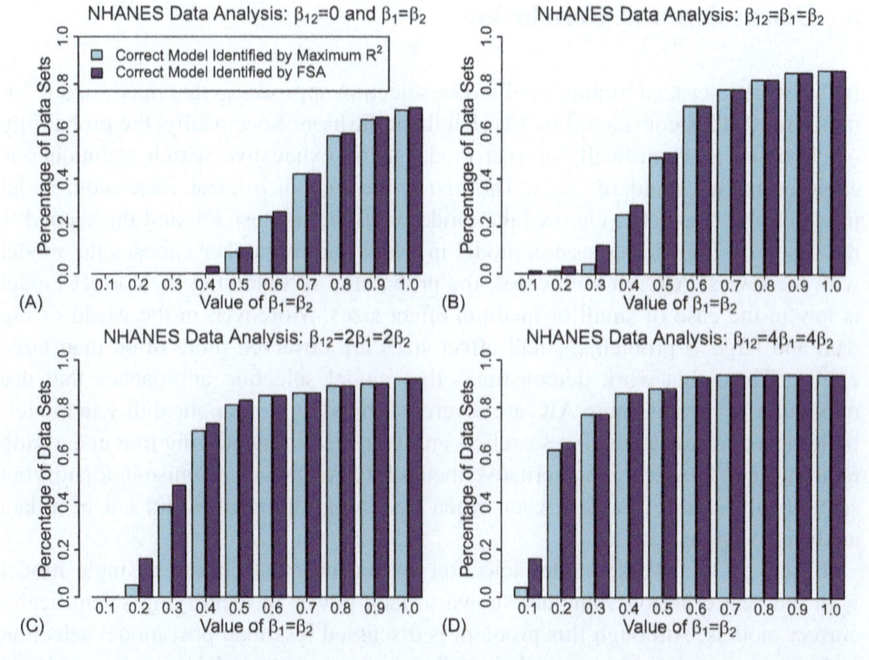

Fig. 7 Bar chart of percentages of data sets in which the correct model is identified using R^2 as the model selection criterion when considering all possible models or FSA. The percentages of 100 randomly sampled data sets that each of model selection with maximum R^2 (light blue bars) and FSA (purple bars) identified the correct two variables related to HDL cholesterol when considering all $\binom{109}{2}$ models in analysis are shown as a function of the regression coefficents, $\beta_1 = \beta_2$. (**a**)–(**d**) show the results when $\beta_{12} = 0$, $\beta_{12} = \beta_1$, $\beta_{12} = 2\beta_1$, and $\beta_{12} = 4\beta_1$, respectively

Figure 7 shows these results for all parameter settings. For small effects (see, for instance, when $\beta_1 = \beta_2 < 0.4$ and $\beta_{12} = 0$ in Fig. 7a), neither model selection with maximum R^2 nor FSA were able to identify the correct model. For moderate effects (when $\beta_{12} > 0$ and $\beta_1 = \beta_2$ are between 0.1 and 0.5), FSA outperforms model selection using R^2 in the identification of the correct model. For large effects (for all values of β_{12} and large $\beta_1 = \beta_2$), both FSA and model selection with maximum R^2 were able to identify the correct model in a large percentage of simulated data sets. Thus, in the presence of natural variation and small and large effect sizes, model selection using maximum R^2 and FSA perform similarly. However, for data with small to medium regression coefficient magnitudes, FSA outperformed model selection by identifying the correct model more often, suggesting that users of model selection with maximum R^2 fail to identify the correct model in practice when alternative approaches may show better performance.

5 Discussion and Conclusion

In this work, a crucial limitation of model selection approaches that maximize R^2 or minimize AIC is considered in a probabilistic fashion. Specifically, the probability of obtaining a scientifically correct model using exhaustive search techniques is explored in two standard cases. The first is the case of a linear regression model in which the researcher chooses the model with the highest R^2, and the second is the case of a logistic regression model in which the researcher chooses the model with the lowest AIC. In both cases, the probability of obtaining the correct model is low in the case of small or medium effect sizes. Moreover, in the world of big data and large p problems, small effect sizes are observed more often than large effects. Thus, this work demonstrates that model selection approaches that use maximum R^2 or minimum AIC are severely limited in their applicability in model-building exercises in which researchers are interested in identifying true underlying relationships. However, an alternative method, FSA, showed promise in identifying scientifically correct models, even when traditional approaches did not in a data analysis example.

Based on this work, model selection approaches that choose a single model with the best criterion value are shown to lack power in identifying scientifically correct models. Although this problem is discussed less than post model selection techniques, its importance is only growing in the presence of larger data sets and increased interest in analytics, and this work provides a theoretical foundation to continue addressing these practical questions. This theoretical work addresses the severe limitations of model selection with maximum R^2 or minimum AIC and shows that alternatives that produce multiple candidate models may improve the probability of a researcher obtaining a scientifically correct model during analysis.

Supplemental Materials
Supplemental materials, including code and figures, are available here: https://github.com/katherinelthompson/BBDABB-Thompson-Hawk-2025.

Acknowledgments The authors gratefully acknowledge both the University of Kentucky College of Arts and Sciences and the University of Kentucky High Performance Computing Center for the use of their computing resources for simulation data analysis. The authors thank Dr. Joshua Lambert for the use of the R package as well as Corrine Elliot for her manuscript comments. Lastly, the authors would like to thank Dr. Arnold Stromberg and Dr. Constance Wood for their insightful comments during this work.

Appendix

Proof of Theorem 2

Proof Let R_U^2 and $R_{X_0}^2$ be the values of R^2 from fitting the linear regression models with $\boldsymbol{Y}$ as the response variable and $\boldsymbol{U}$ and $\boldsymbol{X_0}$, respectively, as the design matrices. Note that $\boldsymbol{H_U}$ follows the conditions given of $\boldsymbol{B^*}$ in Theorem 1. Then,

$$P\left(R_{X_0}^2 > R_U^2\right) = P\left(1 - \frac{SSE_{X_0}}{SSTO} > 1 - \frac{SSE_U}{SSTO}\right) \tag{16}$$

where SSE_{X_0} and SSE_U are the sums of squared errors from the linear regressions of $\boldsymbol{Y}$ on $\boldsymbol{X_0}$ and $\boldsymbol{U}$, respectively. Note that $SSTO$ is the total sum of squares and does not change based on the terms in the linear model fit. Then:

$$P\left(R_{X_0}^2 > R_U^2\right) = P\left(SSE_{X_0} < SSE_U\right) \tag{17}$$

$$= P\left(\boldsymbol{Y^T}(\boldsymbol{I} - \boldsymbol{H_{X_0}})\boldsymbol{Y} < \boldsymbol{Y^T}(\boldsymbol{I} - \boldsymbol{H_U})\boldsymbol{Y}\right) \tag{18}$$

where $\boldsymbol{H_{X_0}} = \boldsymbol{X_0}(\boldsymbol{X_0^T X_0})^{-1}\boldsymbol{X_0^T}$ and $\boldsymbol{H_U} = \boldsymbol{U}(\boldsymbol{U^T U})^{-1}\boldsymbol{U^T}$. Then,

$$P\left(R_{X_0}^2 > R_U^2\right) = P\left(\frac{\boldsymbol{Y^T H_U Y}}{\boldsymbol{Y^T H_{X_0} Y}} < 1\right) \tag{19}$$

However, since the quantity in the probability statement in (19) is a ratio of quadratic forms, Theorem 1 from [2] applies.

Using Theorem 1 [2] with $\boldsymbol{A} = \sigma^2\boldsymbol{H_U}$, $\boldsymbol{B} = \sigma^2\boldsymbol{H_{X_0}}$, $\boldsymbol{\mu} = \boldsymbol{X_0\beta}$, $\boldsymbol{\Sigma} = \sigma^2\boldsymbol{I}$, $\boldsymbol{Z} = \boldsymbol{Y} \sim N_n(\boldsymbol{X_0\beta}, \sigma^2\boldsymbol{I})$, and $r = 1$, the spectral decomposition of $(\boldsymbol{A} - r\boldsymbol{B})$ is required:

$$(\boldsymbol{A} - r\boldsymbol{B}) = \sigma^2(\boldsymbol{H_U} - \boldsymbol{H_{X_0}}) \equiv \boldsymbol{P\Lambda P^T}, \tag{20}$$

where $\boldsymbol{\Lambda} = diag(\lambda_1, \lambda_2, \ldots, \lambda_n)$ is a diagonal $n \times n$ matrix containing the eigenvalues of $(\boldsymbol{A} - r\boldsymbol{B})$, denoted $(\lambda_1, \lambda_2, \ldots, \lambda_n)$, and $\boldsymbol{P}$ is an $n \times n$ matrix with columns given by the eigenvectors of $(\boldsymbol{A} - r\boldsymbol{B})$. Define $\boldsymbol{W} = \boldsymbol{P^T Y}/\sigma \sim N_n(\boldsymbol{\nu}, \boldsymbol{I})$ where

$$\boldsymbol{\nu} = \boldsymbol{P^T X_0 \beta}/\sigma \tag{21}$$

Then it follows that:

$$P\left(\frac{\boldsymbol{Y^T H_U Y}}{\boldsymbol{Y^T H_{X_0} Y}} < 1\right) = P\left(\boldsymbol{W^T \Lambda W} \leq 0\right) \tag{22}$$

where $\boldsymbol{W}^T \boldsymbol{\Lambda} \boldsymbol{W} = \sum_{i=1}^n \lambda_i W_i^2$, and $P(\sum_{i=1}^n \lambda_i W_i^2 = 0) = 0$, since $W_i^2 \overset{ind}{\sim} \chi_1^2(\nu_i^2)$ with $\boldsymbol{\nu}$ as defined in (21). □

Proof of Theorem 3

Proof Note that

$$P\left(R^2_{X_0} > R^2_{U_j}\ \forall j \in \{1, 2, \ldots, k\}\right) = P\left(\bigcap_{j=1}^{k}\left[R^2_{X_0} > R^2_{U_j}\right]\right) \tag{23}$$

$$= P\left(\bigcap_{j=1}^{k}\left[\frac{\boldsymbol{Y}^T \boldsymbol{H}_{\boldsymbol{U}_j} \boldsymbol{Y}}{\boldsymbol{Y}^T \boldsymbol{H}_{\boldsymbol{X}_0} \boldsymbol{Y}} < 1\right]\right) \tag{24}$$

Each of these ratios of quadratic forms takes the same form as in Sect. 3.2.1 with $\boldsymbol{U}_j$ in place of $\boldsymbol{U}$. Using the same procedure as above, this probability statement can be simulated using the following:

$$P\left(\bigcap_{j=1}^{k}\left[R^2_{X_0} > R^2_{U_j}\right]\right) = P\left(\bigcap_{j=1}^{k}\left[\frac{\boldsymbol{Y}^T \boldsymbol{H}_{\boldsymbol{U}_j} \boldsymbol{Y}}{\boldsymbol{Y}^T \boldsymbol{H}_{\boldsymbol{X}_0} \boldsymbol{Y}} < 1\right]\right) \tag{25}$$

$$= P\left(\bigcap_{j=1}^{k}\left[\boldsymbol{W}_j^T \boldsymbol{\Lambda}_j \boldsymbol{W}_j < 0\right]\right) \tag{26}$$

where $\boldsymbol{W}_j^T = \boldsymbol{P}_j^T \boldsymbol{Y}/\sigma \sim N_n(\boldsymbol{\nu}_j, \boldsymbol{I})$, and $\boldsymbol{\nu}_j = \boldsymbol{P}_j^T \boldsymbol{X}_0 \boldsymbol{\beta}/\sigma$. Thus,

$$P\left(\bigcap_{j=1}^{k}\left[R^2_{X_0} > R^2_{U_j}\right]\right) = P\left(\max_{j=1,2,\ldots,k}\left[\boldsymbol{W}_j^T \boldsymbol{\Lambda}_j \boldsymbol{W}_j\right] \leq 0\right) \tag{27}$$

Here, note that $\boldsymbol{P}_j \boldsymbol{\Lambda}_j \boldsymbol{P}_j^T$ is the spectral decomposition of $\sigma^2(\boldsymbol{H}_{\boldsymbol{U}_j} - \boldsymbol{H}_{\boldsymbol{X}_0})$. As in Sect. 3.2.1, $\boldsymbol{W}_j^T \boldsymbol{\Lambda}_j \boldsymbol{W}_j = \sum_{i=1}^n \lambda_{ij} W_{ij}^2$, where W_{ij}^2 are independent random variables following $\chi_1^2(\nu_{ij}^2)$ distributions. Thus,

$$P\left(\max_{j=1,2,\ldots,k}\left[\boldsymbol{W}_j^T \boldsymbol{\Lambda}_j \boldsymbol{W}_j\right] = 0\right) = 0$$

in (27). □

Proof of Theorem 4

Proof Let AIC_U and AIC_{X_0} be the values of AIC from fitting the logistic regression models with $\boldsymbol{Y}$ as the response variable and $\boldsymbol{U}$ and $\boldsymbol{X_0}$, respectively, as the design matrices. Then we know that:

$$P\left(AIC_{X_0} < AIC_U\right) = P\left(-2\hat{l}_{X_0} + 2p_0 < -2\hat{l}_U + 2p_0\right), \tag{28}$$

where l_U and l_{X_0} are log-likelihoods of the parameter vector, $\boldsymbol{\beta}$, and response variable, $\boldsymbol{Y}$, when the fitted model includes $\boldsymbol{U}$ and $\boldsymbol{X_0}$, respectively. Note that, according to notation used in [18]:

$$l_{X_0}(\hat{\boldsymbol{\beta}}) = \sum_i Y_i \boldsymbol{x}_{0i}^T \hat{\boldsymbol{\beta}} - \sum_i \log\left(1 + \exp\left[\boldsymbol{x}_{0i}^T \hat{\boldsymbol{\beta}}\right]\right), \tag{29}$$

where $\boldsymbol{x}_{0i}^T$ is the ith row of $\boldsymbol{X}_{i0}$. In the analogous case,

$$l_U(\hat{\boldsymbol{\beta}}_U) = \sum_i Y_i \boldsymbol{u}_i^T \hat{\boldsymbol{\beta}}_U - \sum_i \log\left(1 + \exp\left[\boldsymbol{u}_i^T \hat{\boldsymbol{\beta}}_u\right]\right), \tag{30}$$

where $\boldsymbol{u}_i^T$ is the ith row of $\boldsymbol{U}$. When comparing two models with the same number of parameters,using (29) and (30), the following holds:

$$P\left(AIC_{X_0} < AIC_U\right) = P\left(l_U(\hat{\boldsymbol{\beta}}_U) < l_{X_0}(\hat{\boldsymbol{\beta}})\right) \tag{31}$$

$$= P\left(\sum_i Y_i(\boldsymbol{x}_{0i}^T\hat{\boldsymbol{\beta}} - \boldsymbol{u}_i^T\hat{\boldsymbol{\beta}}_U) > \sum_i \log\left[\frac{1 + \exp\left(\boldsymbol{x}_{0i}^T\hat{\boldsymbol{\beta}}\right)}{1 + \exp\left(\boldsymbol{u}_i^T\hat{\boldsymbol{\beta}}_U\right)}\right]\right) \tag{32}$$

Proof of Theorem 5

Proof Consider $\boldsymbol{U}_1, \boldsymbol{U}_2, \ldots, \boldsymbol{U}_k$, where each matrix contains p_0 columns from $\boldsymbol{X}$. Let AIC_{U_j} (for $j \in \{1, 2, \ldots, k\}$) and AIC_{X_0} be the values of AIC from fitting the logistic regression models with $\boldsymbol{Y}$ as the response variable and $\boldsymbol{U}_j$ and $\boldsymbol{X_0}$, respectively, as the design matrices. Then, from (29) and (30), we have that:

$$P\left(\bigcap_{j=1}^{k}\{AIC_{X_0} < AIC_{U_j}\}\right) = P\left(\bigcap_{j=1}^{k}\left\{l_{X_0}(\hat{\boldsymbol{\beta}}) > l_{U_j}(\hat{\boldsymbol{\beta}}_j)\right\}\right) \tag{33}$$

$$= P\left(\bigcap_{j=1}^{k}\left\{\sum_i Y_i(\boldsymbol{x}_{0i}^T\hat{\boldsymbol{\beta}} - \boldsymbol{u}_{ij}^T\hat{\boldsymbol{\beta}}_j) > \sum_i \log\left[\frac{1+\exp\left(\boldsymbol{x}_{0i}^T\hat{\boldsymbol{\beta}}\right)}{1+\exp\left(\boldsymbol{u}_{ij}^T\hat{\boldsymbol{\beta}}_j\right)}\right]\right\}\right) \tag{34}$$

where $\hat{\boldsymbol{\beta}}_j$ and $\hat{\boldsymbol{\beta}}$ are the MLEs of the parameter vector, $\boldsymbol{\beta}$, from the fitted models including $\boldsymbol{U}_j$ and $\boldsymbol{X}_0$, respectively, and $\boldsymbol{u}_{ij}^T$ is the ith row of $\boldsymbol{U}_j$ for $i \in \{1, 2, \ldots, n\}$. □

References

1. Allen, D.M.: The relationship between variable selection and data agumentation and a method for prediction. Technometrics **16**(1), 125–127 (1974)
2. Broda, S., Paolella, M.S.: Evaluating the density of ratios of noncentral quadratic forms in normal variables. Comput. Stat. Data Analy. **53**(4), 1264–1270 (2009)
3. Buckland, S.T., Burnham, K.P., Augustin, N.H.: Model selection: an integral part of inference. Biometrics **53**(2), 603–618 (1997)
4. Cramer, J.S.: Mean and variance of R^2 in small and moderate samples. J. Econ. **35**(2–3), 253–266 (1987)
5. Efron, B.: Estimation and accuracy after model selection. J. Am. Stat. Assoc. **109**(507), 991–1007 (2014)
6. Fan, J., Li, R.: Variable selection via nonconcave penalized likelihood and its oracle properties. J. Am. Stat. Assoc. **96**(456), 1348–1360 (2001)
7. Foster, D.P., Stine, R.A.: Variable selection in data mining: Building a predictive model for bankruptcy. J. Am. Stat. Assoc. **99**(466), 303–313 (2004)
8. Foster, F.D., Smith, T., Whaley, R.E.: Assessing goodness-of-fit of asset pricing models: The distribution of the maximal r2. J. Finance **52**(2), 591–607 (1997)
9. Geisser, S., Eddy, W.F.: A predictive approach to model selection. J. Am. Stat. Assoc. **74**(365), 153–160 (1979)
10. George, E.I.: The variable selection problem. J. Am. Stat. Assoc. **95**(452), 1304–1308 (2000)
11. Givens, G.H., Hoeting, J.A.: Computational Statistics. Wiley, Hoboken (2005)
12. Goudey, B., Abedini, M., Hopper, J.L., Inouye, M., Makalic, E., Schmidt, D.F., Wagner, J., Zhou, Z., Zobel, J., Reumann, M.: High performance computing enabling exhaustive analysis of higher order single nucleotide polymorphism interaction in genome wide association studies. Health Inf. Sci. Syst. **3**(S1), S3 (2015)
13. Hastie, T., Tibshirani, R., Friedman, J.: The Elements of Statistical Learning: Data Mining, Inference, and Prediction. Springer, Berlin (2009)
14. Hawkins, D.M.: The feasible solution algorithm for least trimmed squares regression. Comput. Stat. Data Analy. **17**(2), 185–196 (1994)
15. Hofe, C.R., Feng, L., Zephyr, D., Stromberg, A.J., Hennig, B., Gaetke, L.M.: Fruit and vegetable intake, as reflected by serum carotenoid concentrations, predicts reduced probability of polychlorinated biphenyl–associated risk for type 2 diabetes: national health and nutrition examination survey 2003-2004. Nutrit. Res. **34**(4), 285–293 (2014)
16. Koerts, J., Abrahamse, A.: The correlation coefficient in the general linear model. Eur. Econ. Rev. **1**(3), 401–427 (1970)
17. Kuhn, M., Johnson, K.: Applied Predictive Modeling. Springer, Berlin (2013)
18. Kutner, M.H., Nachtsheim, C.J., Neter, J., Li, W.: Applied Linear Statistical Models. McGraw-Hill/Irwin, Columbus (2004)
19. Lambert, J., Gong, L., Elliott, C.: rFSA: Feasible Solution Algorithm for Finding Best Subsets and Interactions. R package version 0.9.1 (2018)

20. Miller, A.J.: Selection of subsets of regression variables. J. R. Stat. Soc. Ser. A (General) **147**(3), 389–425 (1984)
21. Pudjihartono, N., Fadason, T., Kempa-Liehr, A.W., O'Sullivan, J.M.: A review of feature selection methods for machine learning-based disease risk prediction. Front. Bioinf. **2**, 927312 (2022)
22. Tibshirani, R.: Regression shrinkage and selection via the lasso. J. R. Stat. Soc. Ser. B (Methodological) **58**(1), 267–288 (1996)
23. Tibshirani, R.: Regression shrinkage and selection via the lasso: a retrospective. J. R. Stat. Soci. Ser. B (Stat. Methodol.) **73**(3), 273–282 (2011)

False Discovery Control in Multiple Testing: A Brief Overview of Theories and Methodologies

Jianliang He, Bowen Gang, and Luella Fu

Abstract As the volume and complexity of data continue to expand across various scientific disciplines, the need for robust methods to account for the multiplicity of comparisons has grown widespread. A popular measure of type 1 error rate in multiple testing literature is the false discovery rate (FDR). The FDR provides a powerful and practical approach to large-scale multiple testing and has been successfully used in a wide range of applications. The concept of FDR has gained wide acceptance in the statistical community and various methods have been proposed to control the FDR. In this work, we review the latest developments in FDR control methodologies. We also develop a conceptual framework to better describe this vast literature, understand its intuition and key ideas, and provide guidance for the researcher interested in both the application and development of the methodology.

Keywords Multiple testing · False discovery rate · Type 1 error rate · Multiple comparisons · E-value

1 Introduction

In modern scientific research, massive and complex datasets with thousands or even millions of variables are collected routinely by governments, researchers, organizations, small businesses, and large enterprises. If not adequately addressed,

---

J. He
Department of Statistics and Data Science, Yale University, New Haven, CT, USA
e-mail: jianliang.he@yale.edu

B. Gang (✉)
Department of Statistics and Data Science, Fudan University, Shanghai, China
e-mail: bgang@fudan.edu.cn

L. Fu
Department of Mathematics, San Francisco State University, San Francisco, CA, USA
e-mail: luella@sfsu.edu

Y. Zhao, D.-G. Chen (eds.), *Big Data Analytics in Biostatistics and Bioinformatics*, ICSA Book Series in Statistics,
https://doi.org/10.1007/978-3-032-06649-7_5

multiplicity in large-scale studies may precipitate substantial issues in the reproducibility of findings, the emergence of publication bias, and the susceptibility to p-hacking within the scientific research community [34, 37]. Goodman et al. [33] claimed that multiplicity, combined with incomplete reporting, might be the largest contributor to the non-reproducibility or falsity of published claims.

Potential issues in error rate control arising from multiplicity have long been acknowledged. In 1953, to address the problem of multiplicity, John Tukey introduced the notion of family-wise error rate (FWER) which is the probability of making one or more false discoveries. When the number of hypotheses under consideration is large, FWER is usually too restrictive. To increase testing power, it is more reasonable to control the false discovery rate (FDR) [11], which is defined as the expected proportion of false discoveries among all discoveries. Since its introduction in 1995, FDR has become a central concept in modern statistics, and the literature has grown beyond what can reasonably be synthesized in this review. The choice of topics and cited references in our work is not intended to serve as an appraisal of their respective importance or contributions. Instead of striving for an exhaustive survey, which is an impractical endeavor, we have deliberately focused on a selection of subjects that we believe can be articulated with clarity and are likely to be highly relevant to those in the field of practice.

In this review, we give a generic framework for FDR control and show how some of the most popular FDR methods conform to this framework. We also consider methods that incorporate auxiliary information and methods that are valid under dependence. Both frequentist and Bayesian perspectives are considered.

In Sect. 2, we formally present the FDR control problem for multiple testing. In Sect. 3, we discuss the celebrated Benjamini-Hochberg (BH) procedure [11] and its variations. In Sect. 4, we review the Sun-Cai (SC) procedure [68] and its variations. In Sect. 5, the discussion is centered on the control of the FDR in the context of dependent data. Concluding the review in Sect. 6, we identify and highlight further topics pertinent to FDR control that may be of interest to the reader.

Notation Throughout the paper, we denote $\mathcal{M}$ or $[m] = \{1, \ldots, m\}$ as the index set of all hypotheses being simultaneously tested. Let $\mathbb{1}(\cdot)$ denote the indicator function that returns 1 if the condition in $(\cdot)$ is satisfied and 0 otherwise, and $|\mathcal{A}|$ denotes the cardinality of set $\mathcal{A}$. We use $a \vee b$ to denote $= \max\{a, b\}$.

2 Problem Formulation

Suppose we want to test m null hypotheses $H_{0,1}, \ldots, H_{0,m}$ simultaneously and are given corresponding summary statistics $X_1, \ldots, X_m$. Further assume the null distributions of the summary statistics are known. For example, if $X_1, \ldots, X_m$ are p-values we assume they follow Unif[0, 1] under the null. A multiple testing procedure examines these summary statistics and decides which null hypotheses to reject. Let $\mathcal{H}_0 = \{i : H_{0,i} \text{ is true}\}$ be the index set of true null hypotheses and $\mathcal{H}_1 = \mathcal{M}/\mathcal{H}_0$ as the index set of non-null hypotheses. Denote δ_i as the decision for $H_{0,i}$ with $\delta_i = 0$ indicating non-rejection of $H_{0,i}$ and 1 indicating rejection. Denote $\mathcal{R} = \{i : H_{0,i} \text{ is rejected}\}$ as the rejection set. Denote $\theta_i = \mathbb{1}(i \in \mathcal{H}_0)$ as the true state of the i-th hypotheses. A selection error, or false positive, occurs if the practitioner asserts that $H_{0,i}$ is false when it is not. In multiple testing problems, such false-positive decisions are inevitable if we wish to discover interesting effects with reasonable power. Instead of aiming to avoid any false positives, a practical goal is to keep the false discovery rate (FDR) small. The FDR is the expectation of the false discovery proportion (FDP) among all rejections:

$$\text{FDR}(\mathcal{R}) = \mathbb{E}\left[\text{FDP}(\mathcal{R})\right] \text{ where } \text{FDP}(\mathcal{R}) = \frac{|\mathcal{R} \cap \mathcal{H}_0|}{|\mathcal{R}| \vee 1}. \tag{1}$$

We use the true discovery rate (TDR) to measure the power of a testing procedure. It is defined as the expectation of true discovery proportion.

$$\text{TDR}(\mathcal{R}) = \mathbb{E}\left[\text{TDP}(\mathcal{R})\right] \text{ where } \text{TDP}(\mathcal{R}) = \frac{|\mathcal{R} \cap \mathcal{H}_1|}{|\mathcal{H}_1| \vee 1}. \tag{2}$$

The goal is to devise a testing procedure that has high TDR while ensuring that FDR is below a predetermined level α.

We mention two popular variants of FDR. One is the marginal FDR (mFDR) [65] defined as

$$\text{mFDR}(\mathcal{R}) = \frac{\mathbb{E}\left[|\mathcal{R} \cap \mathcal{H}_0|\right]}{\mathbb{E}\left[|\mathcal{R}|\right]}. \tag{3}$$

It was shown in [31] that under weak conditions mFDR and FDR are asymptotically equivalent. We provide the precise statement in the next proposition.

Proposition 1 *Let $\mathcal{R}$ be the rejection set concerning m null hypotheses following a specific decision rule, then* $\text{FDR}(\mathcal{R}) = \text{mFDR}(\mathcal{R}) + o(1)$ *as $m \to \infty$ if the following two conditions hold: 1) there exists an absolute constant $\eta > 0$ such that $m^{-1}\mathbb{E}[|\mathcal{R}|] \geq \eta$; 2)* $\text{Var}(|\mathcal{R}|) = o(m^2)$.

One attractive feature of mFDR is its ability to be "combined." Specifically, if we apply two testing rules that control mFDR at level α on two separate sets of null hypotheses, then the overall mFDR on the union of the two sets of null hypotheses is still controlled at level α. However, [11] point out that it is sometimes impossible to control mFDR. One such setting is where all null hypotheses are true, in which case the mFDR will either be undefined or equal to 1.

Another popular variant of FDR is the positive false discovery rate (pFDR), defined as:

$$\text{pFDR}(\mathcal{R}) = \mathbb{E}\left[\text{FDP}(\mathcal{R}) | \mathcal{R} > 0\right] = \text{FDR}(\mathcal{R}) / \mathbb{P}(\mathcal{R} > 0).$$

pFDR has a natural Bayesian interpretation, as illustrated in [66]. It is also shown in [66] that under some weak assumptions, pFDR is equivalent to mFDR.

2.1 A Generic Framework for FDR Control

We first outline a generic framework for FDR control. The vast majority of methodologies developed to control FDR in offline analyses adhere to the three-step framework outlined below:

Step 1 **(Ranking)** Construct a suitable summary statistics T_i for each $H_{0,i}$ and rank the null hypotheses according to T_i.

Step 2 **(FDP Estimation)** For any given t estimate, the FDP of the decision rule $\delta(t) = \{\delta_1(t), \ldots, \delta_m(t)\}$, where $\delta_i(t) = \mathbb{1}(T_i \leq t)$. Denote the estimate as $\widehat{\text{FDP}}(t)$.

Step 3 **(Thresholding)** For a given target FDR level α, define $t_\alpha = \sup\{t \in \mathcal{T} : \widehat{\text{FDP}}(t) \leq \alpha\}$. Reject $H_{0,i}$ if and only if $T_i \leq t_\alpha$.

Innovation within the FDR literature predominantly resides in the formulation of more informative summary statistics (Step 1) and the design of sharper estimators for the FDP (Step 2). In the next two sections, we examine several prominent methodologies for FDR control, elucidating their alignment with the three-step framework delineated above.

3 The BH Procedure and Its Variations

Introduced by Benjamini and Hochberg [11], the BH procedure inaugurated the control of the false discovery rate (FDR) and continues to be one of the most seminal and prevalently applied methodologies in multiple hypothesis testing. In this section we provide an overview of the BH procedure and its variations.

3.1 The BH Procedure

The BH procedure takes p-values $P_1, \ldots, P_m$ and target FDR level α as inputs. It computes threshold $P_{(k)}$ where

$$k = \max\left\{j : P_{(j)} \leq \frac{\alpha j}{m}\right\}, \quad P_{(1)} \leq \ldots \leq P_{(m)}.$$

Then it rejects $H_{0,i}$ if and only if $P_i \leq P_{(k)}$. In the framework of Sect. 2.1, the BH procedure uses the p-value as the ranking statistic and estimates the FDP at threshold t by

$$\widehat{\text{FDP}}(t) = \frac{mt}{\sum_{i=1}^{m} \mathbb{1}(P_i \leq t)}. \tag{4}$$

The denominator in (4) is the number of hypotheses rejected at threshold t. Note that if $P_{(j)}$ is the threshold then $\sum_{i=1}^m \mathbb{1}(P_i \leq P_{(j)}) = j$. The numerator is the estimated number of false rejections in the worst case where all the null hypotheses are true. The theoretical guarantee of the BH procedure is given in the next theorem.

Theorem 1 *Assume the p-values are independent under the null. Then, the BH procedure controls FDR at level* $\alpha|\mathcal{H}_0|/m$.

There are two elementary proofs for Theorem 1 (details are in [74]): one proof employs the concept of martingales, while the other utilizes a technique known as "leave-one-out." Both proofs are fundamental, serving as pivotal inspirations for the development of numerous sophisticated testing procedures.

3.2 π_0-Adaptive BH Procedure

From Theorem 1 we see that the BH procedure tends to be conservative as it controls FDR at level $(|\mathcal{H}_0|/m) \cdot \alpha$ instead of α. One remedy for this conservativeness is to estimate the null proportion $\pi_0 := |\mathcal{H}_0|/m$ and replace the target FDR level in the input of BH procedure by $\alpha/\hat{\pi}_0$. The problem of estimating π_0 has been discussed extensively in the literature [e.g., 15, 38, 52, 65]. The most popular estimator of π is the one proposed in [67], which is computed as

$$\hat{\pi}_0(\lambda) = \frac{1 + \sum_{i=1}^m \mathbb{1}(P_i \geq \lambda)}{m(1-\lambda)}. \tag{5}$$

The intuition behind Storey's null proportion estimator $\hat{\pi}_0(\lambda)$ in (5) is that

$$\begin{aligned} \hat{\pi}_0(\lambda) = \frac{1 + \sum_{i=1}^m \mathbb{1}(P_i \geq \lambda)}{m(1-\lambda)} &\geq \frac{\sum_{i\in\mathcal{H}_0} \mathbb{1}(P_i \geq \lambda)}{|\mathcal{H}_0| \cdot (1-\lambda)} \cdot \frac{|\mathcal{H}_0|}{m} \\ &\approx \pi_0 \cdot \frac{\mathbb{P}(P_i \geq \lambda \mid i \in \mathcal{H}_0)}{1-\lambda} = \pi_0, \end{aligned} \tag{6}$$

where "≈" comes from the law of large numbers. We can see from the above calculation that $\hat{\pi}_0(\lambda)$ tends to overestimate π_0 for any choice of λ. This is desirable as it makes the testing procedure conservative. There is an inherent bias-variance trade-off in the choice of λ. The "≥" in (6) is sharper when λ is bigger. However, a bigger λ also results in larger variance for $\hat{\pi}_0(\lambda)$. As λ shrinks, the bias of $\hat{\pi}_0(\lambda)$ grows larger, but the variance becomes smaller. The choice of proper λ has been studied in the literature. For example, [65, 66] proposed a bootstrapping and a spline-smoothing method, respectively. Langaas et al. [39] developed a class of estimators based on nonparametric maximum likelihood estimates (MLEs).

For any given λ, we can estimate the FDP by

$$\widehat{\mathrm{FDP}}_\lambda(t) = \frac{\hat{\pi}_0(\lambda) \cdot mt}{\sum_{i=1}^m \mathbb{1}(P_i \le t)}. \tag{7}$$

Define $t_\alpha^\lambda = \sup\{t \in (0, 1-\lambda] : \widehat{\mathrm{FDP}}_\lambda(t) \le \alpha\}$. It was shown in [67] that the procedure which rejects $H_{0,i}$ if and only if $p_i \le t_\alpha^\lambda$ asymptotically controls FDR at the target level. Recently, [30] proposed a new framework for choosing λ in a data-dependent fashion and demonstrated that the associated BH procedure controls the FDR in finite samples.

3.3 Mirror Sequence and Statistic

The problem of determining λ can be avoided entirely if we allow λ to vary. To see this recall that

$$\widehat{\mathrm{FDP}}_\lambda(t) = \frac{\hat{\pi}_0(\lambda) \cdot mt}{\sum_{i=1}^m \mathbb{1}(P_i \le t)} = \frac{1 + \sum_{i=1}^m \mathbb{1}(P_i \ge \lambda)}{m(1-\lambda)} \frac{mt}{\sum_{i=1}^m \mathbb{1}(P_i \le t)}.$$

Suppose we take $\lambda = 1 - t$ then the above reduces to

$$\widehat{\mathrm{FDP}}_{1-t}(t) = \frac{1 + \sum_{i=1}^m \mathbb{1}(1 - P_i \le t)}{\sum_{i=1}^m \mathbb{1}(P_i \le t)}. \tag{8}$$

In essence, (8) is exploiting the symmetry of $1 - P_i$ and P_i as both are Unif[0, 1] under the null. For this reason $1 - P_i$ is sometimes called the *mirror sequence* [43]. The methods developed in [42, 43] and [79] all rely on this crucial idea. If (8) is used to estimate the FDP, the threshold should be modified as

$$t_\alpha = \sup\{t \in (0, 0.5] : \widehat{\mathrm{FDP}}_{1-t}(t) \le \alpha\}. \tag{9}$$

We have the following theoretical guarantee, the proof of which uses martingale theory. Details can be found in [43].

Theorem 2 *The procedure that rejects $H_{0,i}$ if and only if $P_i \le t_\alpha$ where t_α is as defined in* (9) *controls FDR at level α.*

The technique of using symmetry to estimate FDP is not restricted to mirror sequence. Another approach is to utilize mirror statistic. While mirror sequences rely on the pairing symmetry of existing test statistics such as P_i and $1 - P_i$, mirror statistics involve the transformation or creation of test statistics to exhibit mirror-like properties. Barber and Candès [6, 7] introduced the "knockoff" technique for FDP estimation within the framework of variable selection in regression analysis. The key idea is to construct "knockoff" variants of the initial variables that maintain the intrinsic correlation structure of the original dataset while ensuring the knockoffs have no association with the response variable. Consequently, the distribution of the coefficients corresponding to these knockoff variables is symmetric about zero. Employing this symmetry, the knockoff filter is able to control the FDR. The idea of constructing mirror statistics and using that symmetry to control FDR was also explored in [17] and [18].

3.4 Weighted BH Procedure

In many applications relevant domain knowledge, such as carefully constructed auxiliary sequences from the same dataset [13, 50] and external covariates or prior data from secondary data sources [24, 35, 61, 79], are often available alongside the primary dataset. These elements of prior knowledge can be exploited to improve the performance of testing procedures. A pragmatic approach to integrating such prior knowledge is p-value weighting. This technique adjusts the significance of each test based on a priori information, thereby enhancing the sensitivity and interpretability of the overall testing procedure. P-value weighting was studied by Genovese et al. [32], Cai et al. [14], Durand [19] and many others.

The generic framework for p-value weighting is as follows: given positive weights $w_1, \ldots, w_m$ that are independent of $P_1, \ldots, P_n$ conditional on $\theta_1, \ldots, \theta_m$, compute the weighted p-values $Q_1, \ldots, Q_m$ where $Q_i = P_i/w_i$. We consider procedures that reject $H_{0,i}$ if and only if $Q_i \leq t$ for some t. For such procedures, the FDP can be estimated by

$$\widehat{\mathrm{FDP}}^{\mathrm{wBH}}(t) = \frac{\sum_{i=1}^{m} w_i t}{\sum_{i=1}^{m} \mathbb{1}(Q_i \leq t)}. \tag{10}$$

$H_{0,i}$ is rejected if and only if $Q_i \leq t_\alpha$ where $t_\alpha = \max\{t : \widehat{\mathrm{FDP}}^{\mathrm{wBH}}(t) \leq \alpha\}$. When the weighted BH procedure was first studied in [32] the authors set $\sum_{i=1}^{m} w_i \leq m$. Under this condition, the aforementioned procedure is equivalent to applying the BH procedure to the weighted p-values $Q_1, \ldots, Q_m$, hence the name. It was shown in [32] that the weighed BH procedure controls the FDR at level α.

In numerous instances, the weights are not provided explicitly; instead, side information denoted as s_i accompanies each p-value P_i. This auxiliary data can include various types of domain-specific knowledge, such as gene expression levels in genomic studies, demographic information in clinical trials, or historical performance metrics in economic forecasting. The motivation for using this side information to define weights lies in its potential to improve the power and accuracy of the BH procedure by incorporating relevant contextual information. For example, in genomic studies, genes known to be involved in certain biological pathways might be assigned higher weights, reflecting their higher prior probability of being significant.

To integrate this side information into the testing procedure, [14, 44] suggested constructing weights that reflect the prior probabilities $\pi_0(s_i) := \mathbb{P}(\theta_i = 0|s_i)$. One way of estimating $\pi_0(s_i)$ is to use a generalization of (5)

$$\hat{\pi}_0(s) = \frac{\sum_{i=1}^{m} K_h(s_i - s)\mathbb{1}(P_i > \lambda)}{(1-\lambda)\sum_{i=1}^{m} K_h(s_i - s)}, \tag{11}$$

where $K_h(t) = h^{-1}K(t/h)$ and K, a kernel function, satisfies $\int K(t)dt = 1$, $\int tK(t)dt = 0$ and $\int t^2K(t)dt < \infty$. Li and Barber [44] proposed using $1/(1 - \hat{\pi}_0(s_i))$ as weights, whereas [14] recommended using $\hat{\pi}_0(s_i)/(1 - \hat{\pi}_0(s_i))$ instead to mimic the optimal ranking. Ignatiadis et al. [36] proposed using e-values (see Definition 3) as weights. It is shown in [36] that if the w_i's are e-values, then the condition $\sum_{i=1}^{m} w_i \leq m$ is no longer necessary for the validity of the weighted BH procedure.

4 The SC Procedure and Its Variations

The BH procedure and its variations take a frequentist view of FDR where θ_i are regarded as fixed and the expectation is taken with respect to the randomness induced by $(P_i)_{i\in\mathcal{H}_0}$. In this section we re-examine the multiple testing problem from a Bayesian perspective and review the SC procedure [68] and its variations.

4.1 The SC Procedure

Suppose the underlying truths θ_i are random and the summary statistics X_i are modeled using the following hierarchical model:

$$\theta_i \overset{\text{iid}}{\sim} \text{Bernoulli}(\pi), \quad X_i \overset{\text{ind}}{\sim} (1-\theta_i)f_0 + \theta_i f_1, \quad \forall i \in \mathcal{M}, \tag{12}$$

where the null distribution f_0 is assumed to be known. In the Bayesian framework, the expectation in the definition of FDR and mFDR is taken with respect to both X_i and θ_i. Sun and Cai [68] showed that the optimal testing procedure for controlling mFDR at level α is a thresholding procedure on the local false discovery rate (Lfdr), defined as

$$\text{Lfdr}(X_i) := \mathbb{P}(\theta_i = 0|X_i) = \frac{(1-\pi)f_0(X_i)}{(1-\pi)f_0(X_i) + \pi f_1(X_i)}. \tag{13}$$

For procedures that reject $H_{0,i}$ if and only if $\mathrm{Lfdr}_i \leq t$, the SC procedure proposed by Sun and Cai [68] uses the following to estimate the FDP:

$$\widehat{\mathrm{FDP}}^{\mathrm{SC}}(t) = \frac{\sum_{i=1}^{m} \mathrm{Lfdr}(X_i)\mathbb{1}(\mathrm{Lfdr}(X_i) \leq t)}{\sum_{i=1}^{m} \mathbb{1}(\mathrm{Lfdr}(X_i) \leq t)}.$$

In practice, parameters that comprise the Lfdr values must be estimated from the data. The non-null proportion π can be estimated using the methods mentioned in Sect. 3.2. The marginal distribution $(1-\pi)f_0(X_i)+\pi f_1(X_i)$ can be estimated using standard density estimation techniques [47, 48, 64]. It can be shown that as long as the estimator $\widehat{\mathrm{Lfdr}} \xrightarrow{p} \mathrm{Lfdr}$ the SC procedure with $\mathrm{Lfdr}(X_i)$ replaced by its estimator $\widehat{\mathrm{Lfdr}}(X_i)$ in the definition of $\widehat{\mathrm{FDP}}^{\mathrm{SC}}(t)$ controls both FDR and mFDR and is optimal asymptotically. A key innovation of the SC procedure lies in its reliance on the Bayesian Lfdr rather than the frequentist p-value. This enables the development of an optimal multiple testing procedure that outperforms the optimal p-value-based procedure, because it captures more information about the alternative distribution.

4.2 *SC Procedure with Side Information*

If, in addition to the primary statistics X_i, a covariate s_i that encodes side information is also available, then the knowledge from s_i can be easily incorporated into the Lfdr statistic. Consider the following model for X_i:

$$\theta_i | s_i \overset{\text{iid}}{\sim} \mathrm{Bernoulli}(\pi(s_i)), \quad X_i | s_i \overset{\text{ind}}{\sim} (1-\theta_i) f_{0,s_i} + \theta_i f_{1,s_i}, \quad \forall i \in \mathcal{M}.$$

Define the conditional Lfdr as

$$\mathrm{Clfdr}_i = \mathbb{P}(\theta_i = 0 | X_i, s_i) = \frac{(1-\pi(s_i)) f_{0,s_i}(X_i)}{(1-\pi(s_i)) f_{0,s_i}(X_i) + \pi(s_i) f_{1,s_i}(X_i)}. \tag{14}$$

It was shown in [27] and [13] that the optimal testing procedure for controlling the mFDR is a thresholding rule based on the Clfdr. If Clfdr_i can be estimated consistently, then the SC procedure applied on $\widehat{\mathrm{Clfdr}}_i$ can control both FDR and mFDR and is optimal asymptotically. This is indeed the approach taken in [27] and [13]. However, the Clfdr_i is extremely difficult to estimate when the dimension of s_i exceeds two. To address this problem [43] proposed to use a formula similar to (8) to estimate the FDP. More specifically, [43] used a beta-mixture model to construct an assessor function $a(\cdot, \cdot)$ to approximate the Clfdr. However, the FDR guarantee of the ZAP method proposed in [43] needs no assumption on the accuracy of the approximation. Define $c_i(t) = \mathbb{P}(a(X_i, s_i) \le t|\theta_i = 0)$, then the FDP of tests that reject $H_{0,i}$ when $a(X_i, s_i) \le t$ can be estimated by

$$\widehat{\text{FDP}}^{\text{zap}}(t) = \frac{1 + \sum_{i=1}^{m} \mathbb{1}(c_i(a(X_i, s_i)) \ge 1 - c_i(t))}{\sum_{i=1}^{m} \mathbb{1}(a(X_i, s_i) \le t)}.$$

The key idea is to use $a(X_i, s_i)$ for ranking and the mirror sequence $c_i(a(X_i, s_i))$ for estimating the number of false rejections. In practice, the beta-mixture model's parameters are derived from the data, leading to a dependency among the test statistics $a(X_i, s_i)$. Nonetheless, [43] showed that the beta-mixture model parameters converge towards certain fixed values. Consequently, the $a(X_i, s_i)$ values can be regarded as asymptotically independent. A different tactic for confronting the challenges related to the accuracy of $\widehat{\text{Clfdr}}$ was investigated in [28], where a formula similar to (10) is used to estimate the FDP.

5 FDR Control Under Dependence

Up to this point, our discussion has proceeded under the implicit assumption that the summary statistics X_i are independent given the true state of affairs encapsulated by θ_i. Nonetheless, real-world observations frequently deviate from such an assumption of conditional independence. While the BH procedure retains its capacity to control the false discovery rate (FDR) at the predetermined level under specific forms of dependence [12, 22, 56], detailed below, confronting general dependence requires innovative approaches to ensure the FDR is maintained. This section aims to present an overview of some of the latest advances related to dependence in the context of FDR control.

5.1 Positive Regression Dependence Set (PRDS)

In this subsection, we focus on a specific type of dependence structure called a positive regression dependence set (PRDS), defined below.

Definition 1 A set $A \subseteq \mathbb{R}^m$ is said to be increasing if $\mathbf{x} \in A$ implies $\mathbf{y} \in A$ for all $\mathbf{y} \ge \mathbf{x}$. We say $\mathbf{X} = (X_1, \ldots, X_m)$ has a positive regression dependence on the subset $\mathcal{I}_0 \subseteq \mathcal{M}$ (PRDS) if for any $i \in \mathcal{I}_0$ and increasing set $A \subseteq \mathbb{R}^m$, the function $x \mapsto \mathbb{P}(\mathbf{X} \in A \mid X_i \le x)$ is increasing.

The PRDS property is a demanding form of positive dependence which can be interpreted, loosely speaking, as saying all pairwise correlations are positive. We remark that the original definition proposed in [12] requires that the function $\mathbb{P}(\mathbf{X} \in A \mid X_i = x)$ be increasing, which is stronger than the condition in

Definition 1. This version of PRDS was first used by Finner et al. [22]. The BH procedure controls FDR under PRDS dependence as the next theorem illustrates.

Theorem 3 *If p-values* $(P_i)_{i\in\mathcal{M}:\theta_i=0}$ *are PRDS, the BH procedure controls FDR at* $\alpha|\mathcal{H}_0|/m$.

Below we give two examples of PRDS dependence.

Example 1 Let $\mathbf{X} = (X_1, \ldots, X_m)$ be a random vector from multivariate normal distribution $\mathcal{N}(\mu, \Sigma)$. $\mathbf{X}$ is PRDS on $\mathcal{I}_0 \subseteq \mathcal{M}$ if and only if $\Sigma_{ij} > 0$ for all $i \in \mathcal{H}_0$ or $j \in \mathcal{H}_0$.

Consider testing $H_{0,i} : \mu_i = 0$ versus $H_{1,i} : \mu_i > 0$ for $\mathbf{X} \sim \mathcal{N}(\mu, \Sigma)$ with $\Sigma_{i,j} \geq 0$ for all $i, j \in \mathcal{M}$. Following Example 1, one-sided p-values $P_i = \Phi(X_i)$ are PRDS on $\mathcal{H}_0$ as $\Phi(x)$ is monotone increasing, thus allowing for valid application of the BH procedure.

The next example is related to conformal inference [9, 46, 51, 63]. A key concept in the conformal inference literature is the exchangeable distribution, which we define below.

Definition 2 Consider random variables $Z_1, \ldots, Z_N$. Suppose that for any collection of N values, the $N!$ different orderings are equally likely. Then we say that $Z_1, \ldots, Z_N$ are exchangeable.

Example 2 Let $X_1, \ldots, X_n$ be samples from a null distribution f_0. Call these the training data. Further assume we have testing data $X_{n+1}, \ldots, X_{n+m}$ such that $\{X_i : i = 1, \ldots, n+m, X_i \sim f_0\}$ are exchangeable. Then it was shown in [9] that the conformal p-values $\{P_i\}_{i=1,\ldots,m,X_i\sim f_0}$ are PRDS, where

$$P_i = \frac{1 + |\{j = 1, \ldots, n : X_j \leq X_i\}|}{n+1}.$$

Example 2 carries considerable importance because it facilitates the control of the FDR within the scope of novelty detection problems (a summary of research can be found in [54]), particularly in instances where the null distribution is not clearly defined or remains undetermined.

5.2 *Other Dependence Structures*

The PRDS condition is quite strong and often difficult to verify in practice. Nevertheless, FDR control under other forms of dependence has been widely studied in the literature. For instance, [67, 76], and [16] have shown that, in the asymptotic sense, the BH procedure remains valid under weak dependence, Markovian dependence, and linear process models, respectively. Furthermore, [14] demonstrated that their weighted p-value procedure can control FDR asymptotically under certain forms of weak dependence.

Intuitively, if the dependence structure among tests is known, it can be exploited to aggregate weak signals from individual tests, thereby increasing the signal-to-noise ratio. This concept is explored in works such as [10, 69], and [70], where the incorporation of functional, spatial, and temporal correlations into inference methods has been shown to improve both the power and interpretability of existing techniques.

However, the studies by Owen [53] and Finner et al. [22] revealed that high correlation can lead to increased variability in testing outcomes. To mitigate this issue, [41] and [26] investigated multiple testing under factor models and demonstrated that subtracting common factors can substantially weaken the dependence structure. Additionally, [20] and [21] discussed methodologies for incorporating the dependence structure to obtain more accurate FDR estimates for a given p-value threshold. Lastly, [18] introduced an innovative approach that bypasses the p-value calculation step entirely, using mirror statistics for FDR control.

5.3 General Dependence

The pioneering method for controlling the FDR under general dependence was introduced by Benjamini and Yekutieli [12]. The authors demonstrated that the BH procedure can maintain FDR control at level αS_m where $S_m = \sum_{i=1}^{m} \frac{1}{i} \approx \log m$. Based on these findings, a logical step is to recalibrate the initial BH target FDR level to α / S_m. The factor S_m is known as the BY correction in the literature.

Another methodological innovation, termed the dependence-adjusted BH procedure (dBH), was put forward by Fithian and Lei [23] to control the FDR under general dependence. The key technical idea is to decompose the FDR according to the additive contribution of each hypothesis and use conditional inference to adaptively calibrate a separate rejection rule for each hypothesis to directly control its FDR contribution. More precisely, we can write the FDR as

$$\mathrm{FDR} = \mathbb{E}\left(\frac{|\mathcal{R} \cap \mathcal{H}_0|}{|\mathcal{R}| \vee 1}\right) = \sum_{i \in \mathcal{H}_0} \mathbb{E}\left(\frac{\mathbb{1}(p_i \leq \tau_i)}{|\mathcal{R}| \vee 1}\right).$$

The FDR can be controlled if we can ensure each individual summand in the above equation is bounded by α / m. This is usually achieved by conditioning each term on a set of suitable statistics to block the influence of most or all of the nuisance parameters on the conditional analysis. This conditional FDR calibration can be much more powerful than the BY correction, but this advantage comes at a practical cost. In general, conditional FDR calibration is more of a versatile theoretical blueprint than a practical algorithm. However, conditional FDR calibration turns out to be practical and intuitive to implement in integrative conformal p-values [46].

The final approach in this review of FDR control under arbitrary dependence acts through a concept called the e-value.

Definition 3 An e-value is a nonnegative random variable satisfying $\mathbb{E}[E] \leq 1$ under the null hypothesis.

If E is an e-value, then, using the Markov inequality, it is straightforward to show that $1/E$ follows a super-uniform distribution, and hence is a special case of the p-value. Properties of the e-value and its relation to the p-value were studied extensively in [73]. Given e-values $E_1, \ldots, E_m$ we can simply apply the BH procedure on $1/E_1, \ldots, 1/E_m$. Such a procedure is called e-BH. A significant breakthrough associated with the e-BH procedure, shown in [75], is its capability to control the FDR under conditions of arbitrary dependence among the e-values.

A natural question is why one should care about e-values given the widespread use of p-values in the sciences. One important reason is that e-values can be constructed through martingales and betting scores, which arise naturally in sequential analysis [62, 75]. Moreover, e-values are more amenable to evidence aggregation [73]. For instance, when dealing with stages of data collection, if in the first stage we obtain an e-value E_1 and in the second stage another e-value E_2, the two e-values can be combined by simply taking their product, provided that $\mathbb{E}(E_2|E_1) \leq 1$, or their arithmetic mean, providing a straightforward method for cumulative evidence integration. This is particularly advantageous in adaptive designs and online learning scenarios, where data arrive in streams and decisions need to be updated continually.

Additionally, by Ville's inequality [72], e-values maintain their validity under optional stopping, a property that p-values do not generally possess. This means that researchers can conduct interim analyses and make decisions based on accumulating data without inflating the type I error rate, which is a significant benefit for real-time data monitoring and sequential testing frameworks. A more comprehensive discussion on the merits of e-values can be found in [75].

If we are only interested in the multiple testing problem, then $E_1, \ldots, E_m$ are only required to be generalized e-values for FDR control [59, 75],

Definition 4 We say $(E_i)_{i \in \mathcal{M}}$ is a set of generalized e-values if $\sum_{i \in \mathcal{H}_0} \mathbb{E}[E_i] \leq m$.

One interesting fact about generalized e-values is that the decision sequence of a FDR controlling method can be converted into generalized e-values, which was demonstrated in [5, 59] and [45]. More specifically, if a FDR controlling procedure is used to test $H_{0,1}, \ldots, H_{0,m}$ at target FDR level α and the decision sequence is $(\delta_1, \ldots, \delta_m)$, then it is straightforward to check that $\{e_i\}_{i=1}^m$ with $e_i = m\delta_i/(\alpha \sum_{i=1}^m \delta_i)$ is a generalized e-value. This fact can be leveraged for de-randomization [8, 59] and meta-analysis [5].

In terms of power, neither e-BH nor BY correction strictly dominates the other. Both methods are quite conservative in practice. It is essential to recognize that e-values typically utilize less information compared to p-values. While p-values necessitate a complete specification of the distributions of the test statistics, e-values only rely on the information about a known mean. A comparison between e-BH and BY correction can be found in [75]. Recently, [78] showed that the power of e-BH can be improved via randomization. Lee and Ren [40] pointed out that it is possible to improve the power of e-BH through conditioning. The field of e-values is quite new and rapidly evolving, and readers are encouraged to consult the latest literature for detailed discussions. The recent book [55] provides an excellent reference for e-values.

6 Discussions and Other Topics

This article offers a survey of certain recent developments in the realm of FDR control. Nevertheless, we would like to highlight that this overview is not exhaustive and does not represent the full breadth of the latest progress in this field. Due to space constraints, we must omit the influence of FDR on problems other than multiple testing. For example, FDR has proven to be a highly useful concept in sparse vector estimation [1], covariance matrix regularization [4], and graphical model estimation [49]. FDR has also found wide acceptance in variable selection problems [6, 7, 17, 71, 77]. Additionally, a series of recent papers pioneered the application of multiple testing schemes in machine learning problems such as multi-label classification [3, 51].

In this chapter we consider the problem of offline testing, where all summary observations are received at once, and all decisions must be made simultaneously. However, it is often at odds with modern data-driven decision-making processes requiring sequential decision-making. This has led to the development of online multiple testing procedures, which have been extensively studied in recent years [2, 25, 29, 57, 58]. Readers interested in online FDR control are encouraged to consult the review by Robertson et al. [60].

References

1. Abramovich, F., Benjamini, Y., Donoho, D.L., Johnstone, I.M.: Adapting to unknown sparsity by controlling the false discovery rate. Ann. Stat. **34**, 584–653 (2005)
2. Aharoni, E., Rosset, S.: Generalized α-investing: definitions, optimality results and application to public databases. J. R. Stat. Soc. Ser. B: Stat. Methodol. **76**(4), 771–794 (2014)
3. Angelopoulos, A.N., Bates, S., Candès, E.J., Jordan, M.I., Lei, L.: Learn then test: Calibrating predictive algorithms to achieve risk control. Ann. Appl. Stat. **19**(2), 1641–1662 (2025)
4. Bailey, N., Pesaran, M.H., Smith, L.V.: A multiple testing approach to the regularisation of large sample correlation matrices. J. Econ. **208**(2), 507–534 (2019)
5. Banerjee, T., Gang, B., He, J.: Harnessing the collective wisdom: fusion learning using decision sequences from diverse sources. Biometrika, asaf080 (2025)
6. Barber, R.F., Candès, E.J.: Controlling the false discovery rate via knockoffs. Ann. Stat. **5**, 2055–2085 (2015)
7. Barber, R.F., Candès, E.J.: A knockoff filter for high-dimensional selective inference. Ann. Stat. **47**(5), 2504–2537 (2019)
8. Bashari, M., Epstein, A., Romano, Y., Sesia, M.: Derandomized novelty detection with FDR control via conformal e-values. Adv. Neural Inf. Process. Syst. **36**, 65585–65596 (2023)
9. Bates, S., Candès, E., Lei, L., Romano, Y., Sesia, M.: Testing for outliers with conformal p-values. Ann. Stat. **51**(1), 149–178 (2023)

10. Benjamini, Y., Heller, R.: False discovery rates for spatial signals. J. Am. Stat. Assoc. **102**(480), 1272–1281 (2007)
11. Benjamini, Y., Hochberg, Y.: Controlling the false discovery rate: a practical and powerful approach to multiple testing. J. R. Stat. Soc.: Ser. B (Methodol.) **57**(1), 289–300 (1995)
12. Benjamini, Y., Yekutieli, D.: The control of the false discovery rate in multiple testing under dependency. Ann. Stat. **29**, 1165–1188 (2001)
13. Cai, T., Sun, W., Wang, W.: Covariate-assisted ranking and screening for large-scale two-sample inference. J. R. Stat. Soc. Ser. B: Stat. Methodol. **81**(2), 187–234 (2019)
14. Cai, T.T., Sun, W., Xia, Y.: Laws: a locally adaptive weighting and screening approach to spatial multiple testing. J. Am. Stat. Assoc. **117**(539), 1370–1383 (2022)
15. Chen, X.: Uniformly consistently estimating the proportion of false null hypotheses via lebesgue–stieltjes integral equations. J. Multivar. Anal. **173**, 724–744 (2019)
16. Clarke, S., Hall, P.: Robustness of multiple testing procedures against dependence. Ann. Stat. **37**, 332–358 (2009)
17. Dai, C., Lin, B., Xing, X., Liu, J.S.: False discovery rate control via data splitting. J. Am. Stat. Assoc. **118**(544), 2503–2520 (2023)
18. Du, L., Guo, X., Sun, W., Zou, C.: False discovery rate control under general dependence by symmetrized data aggregation. J. Am. Stat. Assoc. **118**(541), 607–621 (2023)
19. Durand, G.: Adaptive p-value weighting with power optimality. Electr. J. Stat. **13**, 3336–3385 (2019)
20. Efron, B.: Correlation and large-scale simultaneous significance testing. J. Am. Stat. Assoc. **102**, 93–103 (2007)
21. Fan, J., Han, X., Gu, W.: Estimating false discovery proportion under arbitrary covariance dependence. J. Am. Stat. Assoc. **107**(499), 1019–1035 (2012)
22. Finner, H., Dickhaus, T., Roters, M.: On the false discovery rate and an asymptotically optimal rejection curve. Ann. Stat. **37**, 596–618 (2009)
23. Fithian, W., Lei, L.: Conditional calibration for false discovery rate control under dependence. Ann. Stat. **50**(6), 3091–3118 (2022)
24. Fortney, K., Dobriban, E., Garagnani, P., Pirazzini, C., Monti, D., Mari, D., Atzmon, G., Barzilai, N., Franceschi, C., Owen, A.B., et al.: Genome-wide scan informed by age-related disease identifies loci for exceptional human longevity. PLoS Genet. **11**(12), e1005728 (2015)
25. Foster, D.P., Stine, R.A.: α-investing: a procedure for sequential control of expected false discoveries. J. R. Stat. Soc. Ser. B: Stat. Methodol. **70**(2), 429–444 (2008)
26. Friguet, C., Kloareg, M., Causeur, D.: A factor model approach to multiple testing under dependence. J. Am. Stat. Assoc. **104**(488), 1406–1415 (2009)
27. Fu, L., Gang, B., James, G.M., Sun, W.: Heteroscedasticity-adjusted ranking and thresholding for large-scale multiple testing. J. Am. Stat. Assoc. **117**(538), 1028–1040 (2022)
28. Gang, B., Qin, S., Xia, Y.: A unified and optimal multiple testing framework based on rho-values. Preprint. arXiv:2310.17845 (2023)
29. Gang, B., Sun, W., Wang, W.: Structure–adaptive sequential testing for online false discovery rate control. J. Am. Stat. Assoc. **118**(541), 732–745 (2023)
30. Gao, Z.: Adaptive storey's null proportion estimator. Preprint. arXiv:2310.06357 (2023)
31. Genovese, C., Wasserman, L.: Operating characteristics and extensions of the false discovery rate procedure. J. R. Stat. Soc. Ser. B: Stat. Methodol. **64**(3), 499–517 (2002)
32. Genovese, C.R., Roeder, K., Wasserman, L.: False discovery control with p-value weighting. Biometrika **93**(3), 509–524 (2006)
33. Goodman, S.N., Fanelli, D., Ioannidis, J.P.: What does research reproducibility mean? Sci. Transl. Med. **8**(341), 341ps12–341ps12 (2016)
34. Head, M.L., Holman, L., Lanfear, R., Kahn, A.T., Jennions, M.D.: The extent and consequences of p-hacking in science. PLoS Biol. **13**(3), e1002106 (2015)
35. Ignatiadis, N., Klaus, B., Zaugg, J.B., Huber, W.: Data-driven hypothesis weighting increases detection power in genome-scale multiple testing. Nat. Methods **13**(7), 577–580 (2016)
36. Ignatiadis, N., Wang, R., Ramdas, A.: E-values as unnormalized weights in multiple testing. Biometrika **111**(2), 417–439 (2024)

37. Ioannidis, J.P.: Why most published research findings are false. PLoS Med. **2**(8), e124 (2005)
38. Jin, J., Cai, T.T.: Estimating the null and the proportion of nonnull effects in large-scale multiple comparisons. J. Am. Stat. Assoc. **102**(478), 495–506 (2007)
39. Langaas, M., Lindqvist, B.H., Ferkingstad, E.: Estimating the proportion of true null hypotheses, with application to dna microarray data. J. R. Stat. Soc. Ser. B: Stat. Methodol. **67**(4), 555–572 (2005)
40. Lee, J., Ren, Z.: Boosting e-bh via conditional calibration. Preprint. arXiv:2404.17562 (2024)
41. Leek, J.T., Storey, J.D.: A general framework for multiple testing dependence. Proc. Natl. Acad. Sci. **105**(48), 18718–18723 (2008)
42. Lei, L., Fithian, W.: Adapt: an interactive procedure for multiple testing with side information. J. R. Stat. Soc.: Ser. B (Stat. Methodol.) **80**(4), 649–679 (2018)
43. Leung, D., Sun, W.: Zap: z-value adaptive procedures for false discovery rate control with side information. J. R. Stat. Soc. Ser. B: Stat. Methodol. **84**(5), 1886–1946 (2022)
44. Li, A., Barber, R.F.: Multiple testing with the structure-adaptive Benjamini–Hochberg algorithm. J. R. Stat. Soc. Ser. B: Stat. Methodol. **81**(1), 45–74 (2019)
45. Li, G., Zhang, X.: E-values, multiple testing and beyond. Preprint. arXiv:2312.02905 (2023)
46. Liang, Z., Sesia, M., Sun, W.: Integrative conformal p-values for out-of-distribution testing with labelled outliers. J. R. Stat. Soc. Ser. B: Stat. Methodol. **86**, qkad138 (2024)
47. Lindsey, J.K.: Comparison of probability distributions. J. R. Stat. Soc.: Ser. B (Methodol.) **36**(1), 38–47 (1974)
48. Lindsey, J.K.: Construction and comparison of statistical models. J. R. Stat. Soc.: Ser. B (Methodol.) **36**(3), 418–425 (1974)
49. Liu, W.: Gaussian graphical model estimation with false discovery rate control. Ann. Stat. **41**, 2948–2978 (2013)
50. Liu, W.: Incorporation of sparsity information in large-scale multiple two-sample t tests. Preprint. arXiv:1410.4282 (2014)
51. Marandon, A., Lei, L., Mary, D., Roquain, E.: Adaptive novelty detection with false discovery rate guarantee. Ann. Stat. **52**(1), 157–183 (2024).
52. Meinshausen, N., Rice, J.: Estimating the proportion of false null hypotheses among a large number of independently tested hypotheses. Ann. Stat. **34**(1), 373–393 (2006)
53. Owen, A.B.: Variance of the number of false discoveries. J. R. Stat. Soc. Ser. B: Stat. Methodol. **67**(3), 411–426 (2005)
54. Pimentel, M.A., Clifton, D.A., Clifton, L., Tarassenko, L.: A review of novelty detection. Sig. Proces. **99**, 215–249 (2014)
55. Ramdas, A., Wang, R.: Hypothesis testing with e-values. Preprint. arXiv:2410.23614 (2024)
56. Ramdas, A., Barber, R.F., Wainwright, M.J., Jordan, M.I.: A unified treatment of multiple testing with prior knowledge using the p-filter. Ann. Stat. **47**, 2790–2821 (2017)
57. Ramdas, A., Yang, F., Wainwright, M.J., Jordan, M.I.: Online control of the false discovery rate with decaying memory. Adv. Neural Inf. Proces. Syst. **30**, 5655–5664 (2017)
58. Ramdas, A., Zrnic, T., Wainwright, M., Jordan, M.: Saffron: an adaptive algorithm for online control of the false discovery rate. In: International Conference on Machine Learning, pp. 4286–4294. PMLR (2018)
59. Ren, Z., Barber, R.F.: Derandomised knockoffs: leveraging e-values for false discovery rate control. J. R. Stat. Soc. Ser. B Stat. Methodol. **86**(1), 122–154 (2024)
60. Robertson, D.S., Wason, J.M.S., Ramdas, A.: Online multiple hypothesis testing. Stat. Sci. **38**(4), 557–575 (2023)
61. Scott, J.G., Kelly, R.C., Smith, M.A., Zhou, P., Kass, R.E.: False discovery rate regression: an application to neural synchrony detection in primary visual cortex. J. Am. Stat. Assoc. **110**(510), 459–471 (2015)
62. Shafer, G.: Testing by betting: a strategy for statistical and scientific communication. J. R. Stat. Soc. Ser. A: Stat. Soc. **184**(2), 407–431 (2021)
63. Shafer, G., Vovk, V.: A tutorial on conformal prediction. J. Mach. Learn. Res. **9**(3), 371–421 (2008)

64. Silverman, B.W.: Density Estimation for Statistics and Data Analysis. Routledge, Oxfordshire (2018)
65. Storey, J.D.: A direct approach to false discovery rates. J. R. Stat. Soc.: Ser. B (Stat. Methodol.) **64**(3), 479–498 (2002)
66. Storey, J.D.: The positive false discovery rate: a bayesian interpretation and the q-value. Ann. Stat. **31**(6), 2013–2035 (2003)
67. Storey, J.D., Taylor, J.E., Siegmund, D.: Strong control, conservative point estimation and simultaneous conservative consistency of false discovery rates: a unified approach. J. R. Stat. Soc. Ser. B: Stat. Methodol. **66**(1), 187–205 (2004)
68. Sun, W., Cai, T.T.: Oracle and adaptive compound decision rules for false discovery rate control. J. Am. Stat. Assoc. **102**(479), 901–912 (2007)
69. Sun, W., Cai, T.: Large-scale multiple testing under dependence. J. R. Stat. Soc. Ser. B: Stat. Methodol. **71**(2), 393–424 (2009)
70. Sun, W., Wei, Z.: Multiple testing for pattern identification, with applications to microarray time-course experiments. J. Am. Stat. Assoc. **106**(493), 73–88 (2011)
71. van de Geer, S.A., Buhlmann, P., Ritov, Y., Dezeure, R.: On asymptotically optimal confidence regions and tests for high-dimensional models. Ann. Stat. **42**, 1166–1202 (2013)
72. Ville, J.: Etude critique de la notion de collectif. Gauthier-Villars, Paris (1939)
73. Vovk, V., Wang, R.: E-values: calibration, combination and applications. Ann. Stat. **49**(3), 1736–1754 (2021)
74. Wang, R.: Elementary proofs of several results on false discovery rate. Preprint. arXiv:2201.09350 (2022)
75. Wang, R., Ramdas, A.: False discovery rate control with e-values. J. R. Stat. Soc. Ser. B: Stat. Methodol. **84**(3), 822–852 (2022)
76. Wu, W.B.: On false discovery control under dependence. Ann. Stat. **36**, 364–380 (2008)
77. Xing, X., Zhao, Z., Liu, J.S.: Controlling false discovery rate using gaussian mirrors. J. Am. Stat. Assoc. **118**(541), 222–241 (2023)
78. Xu, Z., Ramdas, A.: More powerful multiple testing under dependence via randomization. Preprint. arXiv:2305.11126 (2023)
79. Zhang, X., Chen, J.: Covariate adaptive false discovery rate control with applications to omics-wide multiple testing. J. Am. Stat. Assoc. **117**(537), 411–427 (2022)

Part II
Statistical Methods of Bayesian Analysis and Gene Expression Data

Investigating and Assessing Diverse Strategies and Classification Techniques Applied in the Integration of Multi-Omics Data

Funda İpekten, Necla Koçhan, Gözde Ertürk Zararsiz, Halef Okan Doğan, Vahap Eldem, and Gökmen Zararsiz

Abstract High-throughput technologies have recently attracted much attention in academia. These technologies enable gathering information from various biological datasets, including genomics, transcriptomics, proteomics, and metabolomics data. Integrating and analyzing various datasets will allow us to accurately diagnose the disease, deepen our understanding of biological processes, and develop advanced treatment approaches. Numerous integration techniques have been developed for this aim, enabling researchers to unravel the complex patterns and underlying mechanisms behind biological occurrences, including those associated with illnesses. This study aims to explore and employ various data integration methodologies and machine-learning techniques on multi-omics data to predict disease classes using real datasets.

Supplementary Information The online version contains supplementary material available at https://doi.org/10.1007/978-3-032-06649-7_6.

F. İpekten
Department of Biostatistics, Institute of Health Sciences, Erciyes University, Kayseri, Türkiye

Department of Biostatistics, Faculty of Medicine, Adiyaman University, Adiyaman, Türkiye

N. Koçhan
Department of Mathematics, Izmir University of Economics, Izmir, Türkiye

G. E. Zararsiz · G. Zararsiz (✉)
Department of Biostatistics, Faculty of Medicine, Erciyes University, Kayseri, Türkiye
e-mail: gokmenzararsiz@erciyes.edu.tr

H. O. Doğan
Department of Biochemistry, Cumhuriyet University, Sivas, Türkiye

V. Eldem
Department of Biology, Faculty of Sciences, Istanbul University, Istanbul, Türkiye

Y. Zhao, D.-G. Chen (eds.), *Big Data Analytics in Biostatistics and Bioinformatics*, ICSA Book Series in Statistics,
https://doi.org/10.1007/978-3-032-06649-7_6

Keywords Multi-omics · Data integration · Machine learning · System biology · Precision medicine

1 Introduction

The emergence of advanced high-throughput technologies has enabled the acquisition of diverse omics data, including genomics, transcriptomics, proteomics, metabolomics, and epigenomics. Integrating these multiple layers of omics data has become a crucial focus in biomedical research, particularly in diagnostics, drug discovery, and precision medicine, because it plays a pivotal role in comprehending the underlying mechanisms of complex diseases.

Numerous studies highlight the significant impact of combining omics data in biomedical research [1–3]. Integrating these omics data is essential to improving the accuracy of predictions, diagnosis, and prognosis within medical and clinical settings. For instance, Tao et al. showed that a multi-omics approach rather than single omics data yields better results while classifying breast cancer patients [4]. The integration also facilitates the analysis of complex diseases, such as cancer [5, 6]. Furthermore, it can help identify disease-associated biomarkers, facilitating the development of more targeted and personalized diagnostic and therapeutic strategies that can be found across multiple layers of omics data. Many articles cover the importance of integrating different omics datasets from different perspectives [7–9].

Data integration aims to create a meaningful representation of the biological information contained in each omics data preserving the information content in each data. However, it is not easy to integrate these diverse omics datasets as their high dimensionality and complexity lead to significant computational and statistical difficulties for the downstream analysis. Numerous algorithms have been proposed and developed to integrate diverse omics datasets effectively to address these challenges. These algorithms can be categorized as unsupervised and supervised. In the unsupervised approach, there are no class labels in the data. In multi-omics data integration using the unsupervised approach, one tries to discover hidden structures in the observed data. However, in the supervised approach, the class labels are known. Here, the aim is to develop learning rules by integrating different omics data and thus predict the class labels of new observations. The algorithms discussed in this paper are limited to supervised approaches only.

"Model-based integration," one of the methods used in integrating multi-omics datasets, involves compiling a training set from various data types, including genomics, proteomics, transcriptomics, and more. This method generates multiple models during the training phase and subsequently combines these models into a unified model incorporating interactions between different omics structures [10]. One of the advantages of this method is that considerate considers the interaction between different omics structures associated with a specific disease or genotype. Additionally, it offers increased predictive power compared to the models built only on single omics data [8]. Also, it is reliable and effective in capturing the complexity of the underlying biological system. On the other hand, the "model-based integration" methods depend on the assumption about data distribution and violation of this assumption can lead to inaccurate results [11]. Additionally, one cannot observe the variables contributing to the final model. Therefore, it becomes challenging to identify the specific genes associated with the disease. The model-based integration strategy can amalgamate prediction models derived from various data kinds. This may facilitate the integration of data sets wherein each data type is sourced from distinct patient cohorts, although all patients share the same disease [10]. Therefore, the training phase is performed independently for each -omics data. In this process, cross-validation method can be used to reduce overfitting [12].

Another approach employed for integrating multi-omics datasets is "concatenate-based integration." This method combines measurements of individual omics structures into a multidimensional matrix before modeling, facilitating downstream analysis. An advantage of this approach is its simplicity once the determination of how variables will be combined in the matrix is made, allowing the use of various machine-learning methods for analyzing quantitative or categorical data. However, a challenge in data integration arises from variations in the number of biomarkers across omics datasets, given their diverse sizes. To address this issue, it is recommended that block scaling factors be applied to the omics datasets [11]. This helps eliminate problems arising due to differences in the number of biomarkers in the model, ensuring that each biomarker carries equal weight in the analysis. Moreover, omics datasets having varying dimensions and are obtained from different technologies, exhibiting diverse structures, unexpected values, distinct noise distributions, and disparate variances [13]. Managing these differences is crucial for successful concatenate-based integration and subsequent multi-omics data analysis.

The "transformation-based integration" method is introduced to transform individual omics data into a common shared format or representation such as a graph or kernel matrix [14]. Graph-based algorithms consider subjects as nodes and their relationships as edges, whereas kernel-based algorithms generate a classifier in feature space. Recently, Yang et al. [15] used kernel fusion, which leverages the similarities between subjects, to integrate multilevel heterogeneous omics datasets. While the transformation aids in integrating datasets with varying scales and measurement units, facilitating their utilization in machine-learning algorithms for subsequent analysis, this approach has several drawbacks. One limitation is the possibility of information loss from the original datasets due to the employed transformation technique. In this method, the original data is converted into a new data matrix format where the diagonal elements are zero, and the off-diagonal elements display the correlations between variables. However, issues such as singularity or a non-invertible variance-covariance matrix may lead to inaccuracies and/or challenges [16]. Therefore, selecting an appropriate transformation method becomes pivotal, as it can significantly influence the outcomes of integrated analysis.

While data integration methodology plays a pivotal role in integrating diverse datasets and creating common models for comprehensive analyses, it is essential to highlight that integration itself may not be sufficient for robust disease diagnosis and treatment strategies. Beyond integration, the analysis of integrated omics data using powerful machine-learning algorithms, such as Random Forest (RF), Nearest Shrunken Centroids (NSC), and Support Vector Machines (SVMs), is crucial for understanding the underlying mechanisms of diseases and for accurate disease classification and diagnosis. In 2015, Taskesen et al. showed that the results derived from integrated data surpass those obtained from single omics datasets [17]. Specifically, integrating gene expression and DNA methylation datasets significantly enhanced the prediction accuracy of the known molecular subtype of acute myeloid leukemia.

However, to the best of our knowledge, there has not been a comprehensive study that systematically compares the performance of classification algorithms along with data integration methods. This gap in the existing literature highlights the need for further research to thoroughly evaluate and compare the effectiveness of various classification algorithms along with different data integration strategies. Therefore, in this study, we aimed to investigate and implement the three data integration approaches described earlier, along with machine-learning algorithms, on multi-omics data to forecast disease subtypes using real datasets. We first integrated multi-omics data employing various strategies. We then applied diverse machine-learning algorithms for further analysis. Specifically, Multiple Kernel Learning (MKL), NSC, RF, and SVM algorithms were selected for application to the integrated data, obtained through concatenate-based and model-based integration techniques. Furthermore, we explored the performance of Composite Association Network (CANetwork), Relevance Vector Machine (RVM) and Ada-boost RVM algorithms for the data integrated using a transformation-based integration approach.

2 Materials and Methods

2.1 Datasets

This study used three different real cancer data sets were used: colon, kidney, and thyroid. Colon cancer datasets: The LinkedOmics platform provided the colon cancer miRNA, proteome, and RNA-Seq datasets. The dataset has two distinct classes including colon cancer and non-colon with 20 and 75 class sizes, respectively. From 95 samples, miRNA 989, the proteome 8.058, and RNA-Seq 13,482 have features.

Kidney cancer datasets The LinkedOmics platform provided the kidney cancer methylation, miRNA, and RNA-Seq datasets. The dataset has two distinct classes including kidney papillary renal cell carcinoma and kidney clear cell renal carcinoma with 73 and 16 class sizes, respectively. From 89 samples, methylation 13,744, the miRNA 799, and RNA-Seq 20,190 has features.

Thyroid cancer datasets The LinkedOmics platform provided the kidney cancer methylation, miRNA, and RNA-Seq datasets. The dataset has two distinct classes including thyroid papillary carcinoma and not thyroid papillary carcinoma with 142 and 354 class sizes, respectively. From 496 samples, methylation 20,118, the miRNA 808, and RNA-Seq 19,927 have features.

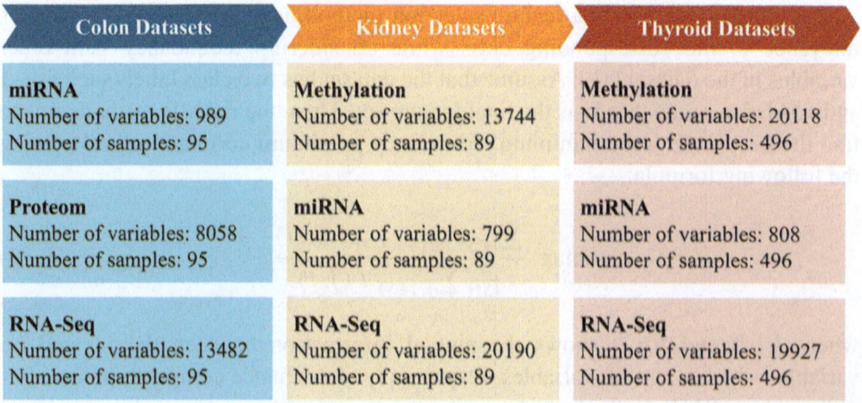

Fig. 1 Datasets used in this study

Information about these datasets is provided in Fig. 1. These datasets were downloaded from the web application resource "LinkedOmics," developed by Vasaikar et al. in 2018 [18]. LinkedOmics encompasses omics data and clinical information from 11,158 patients across 32 cancer types within the The Cancer Genome Atlas (TCGA) program/project. We used the "reduce()" and "lapply()" functions in the R programming language to organize data and extract matching samples for the same patient across individual omics datasets (e.g., transcriptomics, proteomics), ensuring consistency for further analysis. The data was split into 80% training set and 20% test set in order to be standard for the integration strategies and classification models to be described in the following subsections. All models were trained, and parameters were optimized on the training set and performance evaluation was performed on the test set. All datasets and software codes are available from https://github.com/gokmenzararsiz/Multi-Omics-Chapter-Files .

2.2 *Feature Selection*

In the classification problems, certain variables may significantly influence the outcome, while others may have negligible effects. Including variables without impact in the model can lead to unnecessary complexity and issues such as variable crowding. On the other hand, if feature selection is not done, processing such large data will require significant computational resources and time for accurate modeling and analysis.

Feature selection helps mitigate unnecessary complexity by identifying and including only the most relevant variables in the model. In our study, we employed the minimum Redundancy Maximum Relevance (mRMR) feature selection method [19]. This method was chosen based on a literature review, and it is widely recognized for its applicability in pooled data scenarios [20, 21].

The mRMR method is a feature selection method used to measure a variable's relevance to the corresponding class while considering redundancy with other variables in the dataset [19]. Assume that the dataset has two class labels such as -1 and 1. Also, assume that $S*$ is the final feature set. Then, the mRMR method aims to find the best $S*$ with the minimum redundancy maximum correlation level solving the following formula:

$$\max_{S^*} \frac{\sum_{i \in S^*, h \in \{+1,-1\}} I(h, i)}{\frac{1}{|S^*|} \sum_{i,j \in S^*} I(j, i)} \tag{1}$$

where $I(j, i)$ and $I(h, i)$ shows the mutual information between the jth and ith variables and hth and ith variables, respectively. To enhance computational performance, the mRMR method employs a recursive and additive approach to construct the final $S*$ by transforming Eq. [1] into the following equation:

$$\max_{i \in \Omega_{S^*}} \frac{I(+1, i) + I(-1, i)}{\frac{1}{|S^*|} \sum_{i,j \in S^*} I(i, j)} \tag{2}$$

where Ω is the whole variable set and $\Omega_S = \Omega - S$. See [16] for more information on the mRMR method.

2.3 *Dimension Reduction*

Despite the utilization of feature selection methods, there is still a possibility of having a high number of variables, potentially leading to increased complexity and challenges in interpretation. One approach to address these challenges is implementing principal component analysis (PCA) after performing feature selection. PCA reduces the number of variables in a dataset while retaining as much of the variability in the data as possible. The first principal component accounts for the maximum variance in the data. Subsequent components capture the remaining variance in decreasing order. PCA was performed using the "*prcomp()*" function in R.

2.4 *Integration Methods*

In this study, we focused on three distinct integration methods: (i) "model-based integration" methods, (ii) "concatenate-based integration" methods, and (iii) "transformation-based integration" methods. Each approach offers a unique way to combine and analyze multi-omics datasets.

The "model-based integration" method generated individual prediction models using each dataset. Subsequently, a final forecasting model was constructed by combining and utilizing the outcomes derived from these individual estimation models [8]. We employed the **caret** package in R for the "model-based integration" method.

The "concatenate-based" method involves merging three different datasets into a single matrix. However, using this combined matrix directly for classification could lead to inaccuracies. This is because the data, when directly merged into a single matrix, carries the risk of unequal weighting of variables due to varying variable sizes in each dataset. As Spicker et al. proposed, block scaling was implemented according to each dataset to address this issue [13]. The block scaling was performed using the "*blockscal()*" function in the **rnirs** package. In this process, the test matrix was derived by scaling the block scaling through the square root of the sum of variances for each column within the block of the reference matrix. This approach ensured that the variables used in the model carried equal weight, overcoming the challenge posed by different variable sizes in the original datasets. The subsequent classification analyses were conducted using this appropriately scaled test matrix.

The "transformation-based integration" is an approach that combines multiple datasets after transforming the dataset into a shared format, such as a graph or kernel matrix, before creating the model. This approach involves a mapping or data transformation tailored to the data type, aiming to retain the data type-specific features [10]. In the "transformation-based integration" process, the distance between datasets was calculated using the "*gausskernel()*" function in the **KRLS** package.

Various strategies were explored in the downstream analysis for the TCGA datasets obtained from "LinkedOmics." These strategies were investigated under two main categories: strategies tailored for single omics data and strategies falling under integration methods. Before applying the strategies mentioned in the next step, the data set should be pre-processed with methods specific to the relevant-omics data. These data preprocessing steps may include steps such as normalization, data transformation, etc. Therefore, before applying the following models, the data should be normalized and transformed into a data set which is ready for classification modeling. For instance, in RNA-sequencing data, systematic variations in the data can be removed with methods such as DESeq2, TMM (Trimmed Mean of M-values) normalization. In addition, data can be transformed by methods such as voom transformation, variance stabilizing transformation (VST) or rlog transformation. Details on preprocessing steps in omics data can be found in [22–25].

The strategies for single omics data (Fig. 2) can be further investigated in three scenarios:

(i) *Raw data:* This involves considering raw omics datasets separately. Subsequently, machine-learning algorithms were applied to these datasets. What is meant by raw data here is that no data integration has been made. We would like to state that this should be a data set that has passed preprocessing steps such as data normalization and data transformation and is ready for modeling.

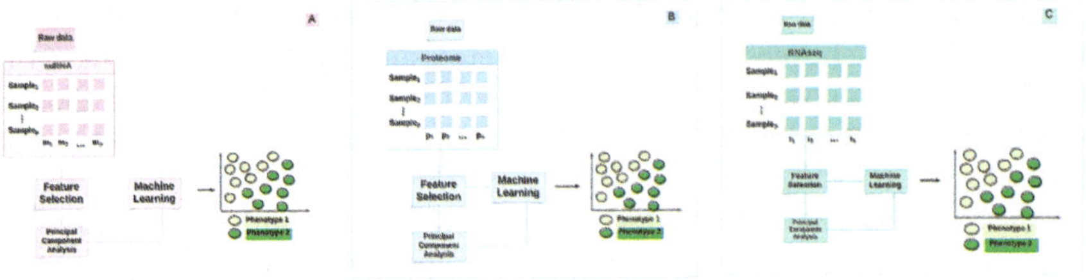

Fig. 2 The workflow of disease diagnosis using single omics data separately. We note here that the labels depicted with yellow and green may vary for each method

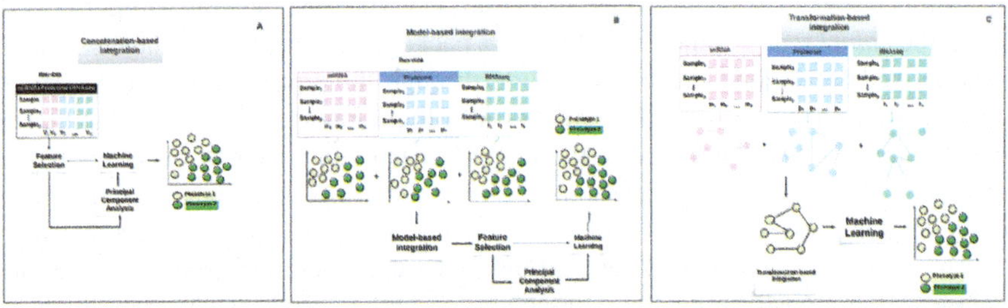

Fig. 3 The workflow of disease diagnosis with different data integration approaches. This figure outlines the main steps involved in disease diagnosis, highlighting the various approaches used for integrating different omics datasets

Raw data + feature selection: In this scenario, the mRMR approach, the feature selection method, was applied to raw omics data prior to implementing machine-learning algorithms.

(ii) *Raw data + feature selection + dimension reduction:* Here, dimension reduction is employed following mRMR feature selection. Machine-learning algorithms were then implemented to compare the classification performances.

The strategies falling under integration methods investigated in the following scenarios:

(i) *Integrated raw data:* This scenario entails integrating raw omics datasets and implementing machine-learning algorithms (Fig. 3).

(ii) *Integrated raw data + feature selection:* Raw omics datasets were initially integrated, followed by the application of the mRMR feature selection and machine-learning algorithms, respectively (Fig. 3).

(iii) *Integrated raw data + feature selection + dimension reduction:* In this scenario, dimension reduction is applied in addition to the mRMR feature selection method. Machine-learning algorithms are then applied (Fig. 3).

(iv) *Integrated data with applied feature selection method:* Here, feature selection, mRMR, is initially applied to raw single omics data separately. Then, these datasets are integrated and used in the classification process (Fig. 4). We note

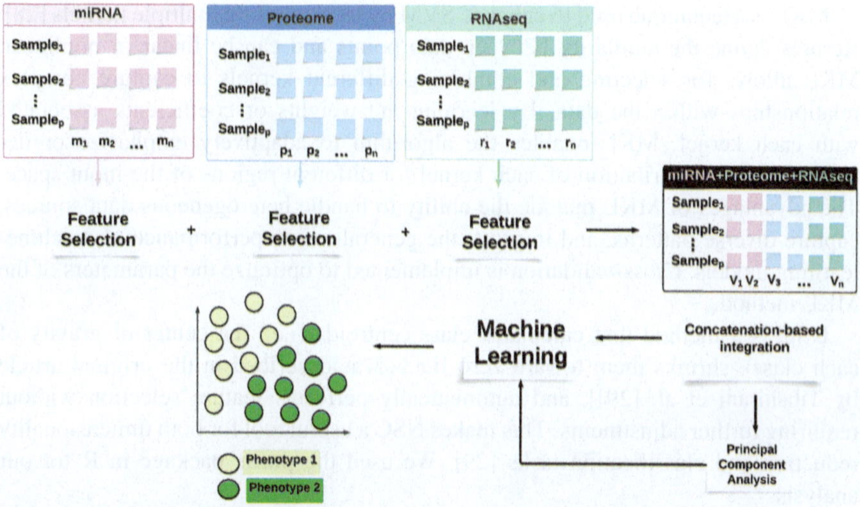

Fig. 4 The workflow of disease diagnosis with concatenate-based integration method. The workflow illustrates disease diagnosis, with concatenate-based integration employed after applying feature selection to each omics dataset

here that only the "concatenate-based integration" method is employed within this strategy.

(v) *Integrated data with applied feature selection method + dimension reduction:* In this scenario, after integrating the data that have undergone the feature selection method, precisely the mRMR method, PCA is performed. Machine learning is then implemented as the ultimatestep (Fig. 4). Similar to the fourth strategy, only the "concatenate-based integration" method is employed within this scenario.

2.5 *Classification Methods*

Following integrating multi-omics datasets, we proceeded the downstream analysis using machine-learning algorithms. Our approach involved implementing several machine-learning algorithms, including MKL, SVM, NSC, RF, CANetwork, RVM, and Ada-boost RVM. We note here that MKL, SVM, NSC, and RF algorithms were applied to model-based and concatenate-based integrated data, whereas CANetwork, RVM, and Ada-boost RVM algorithms were used for the data combined via transformation-based integration technique [14, 19, 26]. SVM is a supervised machine-learning algorithm widely used for classification and regression tasks [27]. Classification aims to find a hyperplane (a.k.a decision boundary) that best separates different classes (groups) of data points. We employed the "*gausskernel()*" function in our analyses.

MKL is a technique used to enhance SVM by incorporating multiple kernels [28]. Kernels define the similarity between data points and can be linear or nonlinear. MKL allows for selecting and combining different kernels to capture complex relationships within the data. By learning the weights or coefficients associated with each kernel, MKL enables the algorithm to adaptively emphasize or de-emphasize the contribution of each kernel for different regions of the input space. The advantages of MKL include the ability to handle heterogeneous data sources, capture diverse patterns, and improve the generalization performance of machine-learning models. Cross-validation is implemented to optimize the parameters of the MKL method.

NSC is a method that calculates class centroids (i.e., the center of gravity of each class), shrinks them toward zero [i.e., Δ as described in the original article by Tibshirani et al. [29]], and automatically performs feature selection without requiring further adjustments. This makes NSC a useful tool for both dimensionality reduction and classification tasks [29]. We used the **pamr** package in R for our analysis.

RF, known as ensemble learning, is one of the frequently used machine-learning algorithms as it is to implement. Moreover, it is a powerful and robust classification algorithm with two parameters to be optimized: the number of variables used in each node and the number of trees to be generated [30]. To implement RF, we used the **caret** package.

RVM and Ada-boost RVM are kernel-based machine-learning algorithms. These approaches use kernel functions to map input data into a higher-dimensional space, capturing complex relationships within the data [14]. The parameters, resampling size and the maximum number of iterations, were fine-tuned using cross-validation. The training of the models was executed using the *"ParaRVM()"* function, and the integration of omics datasets was achieved through the utilization of the *"RVMInt()"* function from the **MDIntegration** package.

The CANetwork graph-based method is another machine-learning approach used for high-dimensional data. This approach initially estimates the correlation matrices. Then, it uses the function *AFcorMI()* from the **WGCNA** package, which computes a predicted weighted mutual information adjacency matrix from a given correlation matrix [14]. Ultimately, the function *CANetwork()* from **MDIntegration** package integrates weighted mutual information adjacency correlation matrices obtained for each dataset. In the classification step, the classification models were constructed independently, employing various machine-learning algorithms on the training data. In the training step, specific parameters for each classification method were fine-tuned to optimize their performance. Furthermore, to ensure robustness and validity, the models underwent a resampling process five times, and the data were cross-validated five times within each of the ten resampled datasets. The performance of the models was ultimately assessed using the test data based on the metrics elaborated in Sect. 2.6.

All analyses were conducted using the R programming language (version 3.6.2) on the Centos Enterprise 7.3 Linux operating system. The computational resources utilized for these analyses were part of the TRUBA resources available at the TÜBİTAK ULAKBİM High Performance and Grid Computing Center.

2.6 Model Performance Evaluation

The Area Under Curve (AUC), accuracy, F1-score, and Matthew Correlation Coefficient (MCC) were used to evaluate the performance of classification methods. These metrics are calculated by comparing the predicted disease status with the actual disease status in the dataset (Table 1).

Area under the curve (AUC) is commonly used performance metric in classification problems to measure the performance of a classification model. It is the area under the receiver operating characteristic (ROC) curve illustrating the trade-off between sensitivity (true positive rate) and 1-specificity (false positive rate). Additionally, accuracy and F1-score offer quantitative measures that capture various aspects of model performance, ensuring a comprehensive evaluation. Also, Matthews Correlation Coefficient (MCC) is a powerful performance measure, especially for imbalanced data sets in binary classification problems. MCC is calculated by taking into account the true positive (TP), true negative (TN), false positive (FP), and false negative (FN) values. MCC takes a value between −1 and +1. +1 indicates perfect classification, −1 indicates completely incorrect classification, and 0 indicates random guess. The calculation for the MCC measure is as follows [31] (Table 2)

Table 1 Confusion matrix

		TRUE CLASS	
		Positive	**Negative**
PREDICTED CLASS	**Positive**	True positive (TP)	False positive (FP)
	Negative	False negative (FN)	True negative (TN)

Table 2 Model performance metrics

Metrics	Formula
Sensitivity	$\frac{TP}{TP+FN}$
Specificity	$\frac{TN}{TN+FP}$
Accuracy	$\frac{TP+TN}{TP+TN+FP+FN}$
F1-score	$2 * \left(\frac{TP}{2} * TP + FP + FN\right)$
MCC	$(TP * TN) - \frac{FP*FN}{TP+FP} * (TP + FN) * (FP + TN) * (FN + TN)$
AUC	$\int_{0}^{1} TPR(x)d\,(FPR(x))$

MCC Matthew correlation coefficients, *AUC* area under the curve, *TPR* true positive rate (sensitivity), *FPR* false positive rate (1-specificity)

3 Results for Real Datasets

The performance of the models under different scenarios is detailed separately, along with the corresponding processing times for each model. Comprehensive results for all real datasets are available in the **Supplementary File.**

3.1 Results for Kidney Cancer Dataset

The results for the kidney cancer dataset revealed that, when considering the raw data, the performance metrics of SVM methods applied to methylation and miRNA raw data were found to surpass those of NSC and RF methods (Table 3). However, in the RNA-Seq raw data, the RF method's performance was superior to that of the NSC and SVM methods. The SVM method exhibited a higher classification performance when examining concatenated-based integrated data than the NSC and RF methods. In model-based integrated data, the NSC method's classification performance was higher than that of the RF and SVM methods. Notably, the NSC method applied to model-based integrated data achieved the highest performance among the integration methods. When we use the "transformation-based integration" method, the highest performance was obtained with RVM (Table 4).

'Table 5 presents the results obtained from applying mRMR feature selection to the kidney cancer dataset. It can be seen from Table 5 that the best performance was obtained when MKL classification was applied to the concatenated-based integrated data, and mRMR feature selection was implemented after the integration. The performance of the SVM method was observed to be higher than the performance of MKL and RF methods when single miRNA and RNA-Seq data were utilized. On the other hand, the performance of the MKL method was observed to be higher than the performance of RF and SVM methods when methylation data was used. For concatenated-based integrated data, the classification performance of the MKL method was superior to the classification performance of RF and SVM methods. In the model-based integrated data, the SVM performed better than the RF. For the data where first mRMR and then the integration method is applied, the performance of the MKL was higher than that of RF and SVM methods.

Table 6 provides the results after applying mRMR and PCA to the kidney. The highest performance was achieved by applying SVM to the model-based integrated data with mRMR and PCA.

3.2 Results for Thyroid Cancer Dataset

According to the results of thyroid cancer dataset, the performance of NSC method used in miRNA and RNA-Seq raw data was higher than that of RF and SVM meth-

Table 3 The results of NSC, RF, and SVM methods on raw kidney cancer dataset

	Raw data			Concatenate-based integrated raw data	Model-based integrated raw data
Performance metrics	Methylation	miRNA	RNA-Seq	Methylation + miRNA+ RNA-Seq	Methylation + miRNA+ RNA-Seq
NSC					
AUC	0.919(0.007)	0.941(0.006)	0.910(0.007)	0.915(0.011)	**0.987(0.009)**
Accuracy	0.955(0.004)	0.969(0.003)	0.941(0.004)	0.951(0.006)	**0.995(0.003)**
F1-score	0.972(0.002)	0.981(0.002)	0.962(0.003)	0.969(0.004)	**0.997(0.002)**
MCC score	0.857(0.012)	0.903(0.010)	0.823(0.012)	0.845(0.019)	**0.983(0.012)**
RF					
AUC	0.883(0.008)	0.909(0.008)	**0.929(0.008)**	0.890(0.013)	0.947(0.016)
Accuracy	0.948(0.003)	0.958(0.004)	**0.972(0.003)**	0.958(0.005)	0.981(0.006)
F1-score	0.969(0.002)	0.974(0.002)	**0.983(0.002)**	0.974(0.003)	0.989(0.003)
MCC score	0.817(0.014)	0.863(0.012)	**0.906(0.010)**	0.857(0.017)	0.932(0.020)
SVM					
AUC	**0.922(0.003)**	**0.971(0.002)**	0.926(0.003)	**0.927(0.006)**	0.960(0.015)
Accuracy	**0.960(0.001)**	**0.988(0.001)**	0.967(0.001)	**0.969(0.003)**	0.986(0.005)
F1-score	**0.975(0.001)**	**0.993(0.001)**	0.980(0.001)	**0.981(0.002)**	0.992(0.003)
MCC score	**0.873(0.005)**	**0.962(0.003)**	0.888(0.005)	**0.900(0.009)**	0.949(0.018)

The number of features is given as mean (standard error)
Bold values indicate the best performances
AUC area under the curve, *MCC* Matthew correlation coefficient, *NSC* nearest Shrunken centroids, *RF* random forest, *SVM* support vector machine

Table 4 The results of RVM, Ada-boost, and CANetwork methods on transformation-based integrated kidney cancer dataset

Performance metrics	Kidney cancer dataset Methylation + miRNA+ RNA-Seq
RVM	
AUC	**0.927(0.022)**
Accuracy	**0.974(0.008)**
F1-score	**0.985(0.004)**
MCC score	**0.904(0.029)**
Ada-boost RVM	
AUC	0.885(0.023)
Accuracy	0.958(0.008)
F1-score	0.975(0.005)
MCC score	0.845(0.030)
CANetwork	
AUC	0.746(0.030)
Accuracy	0.875(0.015)
F1-score	0.926(0.009)
MCC score	0.537(0.060)

The number of features is given as mean (standard error)
Bold value indicates the best performance
AUC area under the curve, *MCC* Matthew correlation coefficient, *RVM* relevance vector machine, *Ada-boost RVM* adaptive-boosting relevance vector machine, *CANetwork* composite association network

ods. On the other hand, the performance of the SVM method was observed to be higher than that of NSC and RF methods in methylation raw data (**Supplementary File, Table S1**). For concatenated-based integrated data, the classification performance of the NSC method was higher than the classification performance of RF and SVM methods. Similarly, when the model-based integrated data was used in the classification, the performance of the NSC method was better than that of RF and SVM methods. If omics data were integrated using a 'transformation-based integration' method, CANetwork was identified as the most effective classification algorithm, demonstrating the highest classification performance (**Supplementary File, Table S2**). The results after applying mRMR feature selection for the thyroid cancer dataset are given in **Supplementary File, Table S3**. Like in the kidney cancer dataset, the best performance was obtained when MKL classification was applied to the concatenate-based integrated data where mRMR feature selection was implemented after the integration. The performance of the MKL method was observed to be higher than the performance of the RF and SVM methods when single miRNA and methylation data were utilized.

When concatenated-based integrated data was used, the classification performance of the SVM method was superior to the classification performance of MKL and RF methods. Similar results were obtained in the kidney cancer dataset when the data were integrated using "model-based integration," where SVM outperformed RF. Additionally, for the data where mRMR was applied first and then the

Table 5 The results of MKL, RF, and SVM methods on FS applied kidney cancer dataset across different integration methods

	FS applied single data			FS applied concatenate-based integrated data	FS applied model-based integrated data	Integrated data after applying FS to each single omics data
Performance metrics	Methylation	miRNA	RNA-Seq	Methylation + miRNA+ RNA-Seq	Methylation + miRNA+ RNA-Seq	Methylation + miRNA+ RNA-Seq
MKL						
AUC	**0.916(0.019)**	0.913(0.004)	0.802(0.006)	**1.000(0.000)**	–	**0.940(0.011)**
Accuracy	**0.965(0.007)**	0.965(0.002)	0.911(0.003)	**1.000(0.000)**	–	**0.974(0.005)**
F1-score	**0.978(0.004)**	0.978(0.001)	0.947(0.002)	**1.000(0.000)**	–	**0.984(0.026)**
MCC score	**0.884(0.024)**	0.885(0.005)	0.703(0.010)	**1.000(0.000)**	–	**0.921(0.012)**
RF						
AUC	0.853(0.005)	0.897(0.005)	0.720(0.006)	0.841(0.010)	0.953(0.018)	0.893(0.009)
Accuracy	0.930(0.002)	0.958(0.002)	0.876(0.003)	0.919(0.005)	0.984(0.006)	0.953(0.004)
F1-score	0.957(0.001)	0.975(0.001)	0.927(0.002)	0.950(0.003)	0.990(0.004)	0.971(0.003)
MCC score	0.757(0.008)	0.859(0.006)	0.547(0.012)	0.725(0.017)	0.939(0.024)	0.848(0.013)
SVM						
AUC	0.867(0.003)	**0.981(0.001)**	**0.946(0.003)**	0.901(0.006)	**0.967(0.014)**	0.927(0.006)
Accuracy	0.939(0.001)	**0.986(0.001)**	**0.976(0.001)**	0.932(0.004)	**0.988(0.005)**	0.969(0.003)
F1-score	0.963(0.001)	**0.991(0.001)**	**0.985(0.001)**	0.957(0.002)	**0.993(0.003)**	0.981(0.002)
MCC score	0.785(0.005)	**0.961(0.002)**	**0.925(0.004)**	0.779(0.012)	**0.958(0.017)**	0.900(0.009)

The number of features is given as mean(standard error)

Bold values indicate the best performances. Since the MKL method was not included in the available packages we implemented in this study, we excluded it for model-based integrated datasets

FS feature selection, *PCA* principal component analysis, *AUC* area under the curve, *MCC* Matthew correlation coefficient, *MKL* multiple kernel learning, *RF* random forest, *SVM* support vector machine

Table 6 The results of MKL, RF, and SVM methods on FS and PCA applied kidney cancer dataset across different integration methods

Performance metrics	FS + PCA applied single omics data			FS + PCA applied concatenate-based integrated data	FS + PCA applied model-based integrated data	PCA applied concatenate-based integrated data, applying FS to each single omics data before the integration
	Methylation	miRNA	RNA-Seq	Methylation + miRNA+ RNA-Seq	Methylation + miRNA+ RNA-Seq	Methylation + miRNA+ RNA-Seq
MKL						
AUC	**0.916(0.004)**	0.909(0.004)	0.752(0.006)	**0.926(0.004)**	–	**0.919(0.004)**
Accuracy	**0.965(0.001)**	0.960(0.002)	0.892(0.003)	**0.967(0.002)**	–	**0.965(0.002)**
F1-score	**0.978(0.001)**	0.975(0.001)	0.937(0.002)	**0.980(0.001)**	–	**0.978(0.001)**
MCC score	**0.884(0.005**	0.868(0.005)	0.627(0.010)	**0.888(0.006)**	–	**0.886(0.005)**
RF						
AUC	0.845(0.006)	0.898(0.006)	0.734(0.005)	0.853(0.006)	0.933(0.019)	0.807(0.007)
Accuracy	0.940(0.002)	0.965(0.002)	0.884(0.003)	0.940(0.002)	0.976(0.007)	0.912(0.003)
F1-score	0.965(0.001)	0.980(0.001)	0.931(0.002)	0.964(0.001)	0.986(0.004)	0.948(0.002)
MCC score	0.775(0.010)	0.857(0.008)	0.584(0.009)	0.788(0.009)	0.914(0.025)	0.683(0.012)
SVM						
AUC	0.856(0.003)	**0.952(0.002)**	**0.834(0.005)**	0.829(0.003)	**0.950(0.015)**	0.911(0.004)
Accuracy	0.894(0.002)	**0.965(0.001)**	**0.930(0.002)**	0.896(0.002)	**0.979(0.006)**	0.947(0.002)
F1-score	0.933(0.001)	**0.978(0.001)**	**0.958(0.001)**	0.936(0.001)	**0.987(0.003)**	0.966(0.001)
MCC score	0.680(0.007)	**0.887(0.005)**	**0.760(0.007)**	0.662(0.007)	**0.928(0.020)**	0.831(0.007)

The number of features is given as mean(standard error)

Bold values indicate the best performance. Since the MKL method was not included in the available packages we implement in this study, we exclude it for model-based integrated datasets

FS feature selection, *PCA* principal component analysis, *AUC* area under the curve, *MCC* Matthew correlation coefficient, *MKL* multiple kernel learning, *RF* random forest, *SVM* support vector machine

integration method, the performance of MKL was found to be higher than that of the RF and SVM methods.

After applying mRMR and PCA for kidney cancer, the results are presented in **Supplementary File, Table S4**. When each omics data is first processed through mRMR feature selection, followed by PCA, and finally integrated, the MKL classification algorithm achieves the highest performance with these integrated data.

3.3 Results for Colon Cancer Dataset

Table S5 illustrates results for the colon cancer dataset when analyzing raw data across different strategies. The NSC method exhibited the lowest performance when raw miRNA was employed, whereas the SVM demonstrated the highest performance when utilizing either raw proteome or raw RNA-Seq data. However, the SVM method performed best in concatenate-based integrated data. In contrast, the RF method was identified as the most efficient approach in the model-based integrated data.

In the case of transformation-based integrated data, the CANetwork method yielded the lowest performance, while the Ada-boost RVM method demonstrated a slightly higher performance than RVM (**Supplementary File, Table S6**).

The results for various scenarios after applying mRMR feature selection are outlined in **Supplementary File, Table S7**. The findings indicated that, following the application of mRMR feature selection, the RF approach exhibited superior performance compared to the MKL and SVM approaches in miRNA data. In contrast, for proteome and RNA-Seq data, the MKL and SVM methods were identified as the most effective approaches, respectively. When integrating omics datasets with the mRMR feature selection method implemented prior to integration, the performance of RF was superior to other approaches.

Table S8 summarizes the results for various scenarios after applying mRMR feature selection and PCA. SVM outperformed other methods when the data was integrated with a model-based approach followed by mRMR feature selection and PCA processes.

3.4 Processing Times and the Results for the Feature Selection Method

We investigated processing (or running) times using various methods across different scenarios. Detailed results are available in **Supplementary File, Table S9-S12**.

In the single omics data of colon, kidney, and thyroid cancers, the NSC method demonstrated superior computational efficiency, making it the most efficient method compared to other methods (**Supplementary File, Table S9**). Conversely, after implementing the feature selection and PCA, SVM emerged as the top-performing method in terms of computational cost. SVM was the most efficient algorithm after integrating the datasets using concatenate-based and model-based integration techniques following feature selection and PCA (**Supplementary File, Table S9**).

For the concatenate-based integrated datasets after applying feature selection to each single omics cancer dataset, the RF method was found to be the fastest algorithm for colon and kidney cancer datasets. In contrast, for the thyroid cancer dataset, SVM was observed to be the most efficient algorithm in terms of computational cost (**Supplementary File, Table S10**). After applying mRMR feature selection to single omics datasets followed by concatenate-based integration, the least costly method for colon, kidney, and thyroid cancer datasets after applying PCA was observed to be the SVM method. See **Supplementary File, Table S10**). For the transformation-based integrated datasets, the least computational cost for colon, kidney and thyroid cancer datasets was achieved by RVM, Ada-boost RVM, and CANetwork, respectively (**Supplementary File, Table S11**).

In the model-based integrated datasets of colon, kidney, and thyroid cancer, NSC surpassed other methods in computational cost efficiency. Nevertheless, after applying feature selection and PCA to the model-based integrated data, SVM emerged as the most efficient algorithm for all cancer datasets. See **Supplementary File, Table S12** for details.

Additionally, we investigated the number of variables determined in the feature selection methods across various strategies, and these findings are documented in **Supplementary File, Table S13-S14**. In RF and SVM algorithms, we did not perform any feature selection process; hence, the number of variables used in these models was the same for all cancer datasets. However, feature selection process is conducted in the NSC algorithm, determining the most appropriate number of variables for each dataset and incorporating them into the model. Several features selected across different strategies are presented in **Supplementary File, Table S13**. Due to the feature selection step in the NSC algorithm, the data subjected to mRMR feature selection and PCA are not included in the analyses conducted by the NSC method. In concatenate-based integrated data, the number of features used in the NSC method was found to be lower than that of the RF and SVM methods.

4 Discussion

Integrating multi-omics data and applying machine-learning techniques are crucial in advancing our understanding of complex biological systems, particularly in cancer diagnosis and precision medicine. In this study, we conducted a comprehensive comparison study of three integration methods in conjunction with powerful machine-learning algorithms on real datasets. Thus, we aimed to provide insights into how omics datasets should be assessed, highlighting the significance of evaluating them separately and in an integrated fashion. We also compared each strategy in terms of computational time. Feldner-Busztin et al. proposed an end-to-end pipeline for machine-learning-based subgroup identification in non-small cell lung cancer (NSCLC) in their study [32]. They also proposed and validated fusion-based classification models to identify subgroups in new samples. Unlike this study, we also demonstrated model-based and graph-based methods. We aimed to demonstrate the effectiveness of various integration methods in subgroup classifications. By comparing the integration and classification methods used in our study and the information obtained from related studies in the literature, each researcher will be able to easily choose the appropriate scenario for their own dataset [33].

Recently, Chierici et al. [34] investigated the performance of RF and SVM methods using concatenate-based integrated data instead of single omics data. Their results indicated similar outcomes for both RF and SVM methods across each strategy. As per their findings, the classification methods employed to predict estrogen receptor status, invasive subtypes of breast carcinoma, and survival in renal clear cell carcinomas demonstrated robust performance when applied to integrated data. However, for myeloid leukemia, they observed that the performance of the classification methods was superior when utilizing single omics data [34]. In our study, we reached similar outcomes. For instance, we observed that the performance of the concatenate-based integrated colon cancer dataset surpassed that of single miRNA and RNA-Seq colon cancer data in the SVM method (**Supplementary File, Table S5**). Similarly, the performance of the NSC method, when omics data were integrated using a concatenate-based approach, outperformed the same method when only the RNA-Seq kidney cancer dataset was preferred (Table 4). This aligns with the observations made by Chierici et al. study [34] and supports the notion that the choice of integration method can impact the performance of classification methods in omics data analysis.

In another study, Ma et al. [35] implemented the "concatenate-based integration" method to integrate omics datasets to predict breast cancer diagnosis across different strategies. They emphasized that the analyses on integrated data were more informative. They followed different strategies: (i) trained the model by integrating the data in its raw form, (ii) trained the model after integrating the data in its raw form and applying variable selection methods, (iii) applied variable selection methods before integrating the data, and then integrated data followed by training the model. They concluded that there was no superiority among these strategies. In our study, we observed that the performances of RF and SVM methods for concatenate-based integrated colon, kidney, and thyroid cancer datasets were close, indicating no significant difference in terms of superiority in applying variable selection before or after integration. The classification performances of concatenate-based data and data with variable selection applied in concatenate-based could be either higher or lower than the classification performances of single data.

Multi-omics integration methods typically rely on statistical and conventional machine-learning techniques, such as iClusterBayes [36], NEMO [37], Multiple Similarity Network Embedding (MSNE) [38], and weight-boosted Multi-Kernel Learning (wMKL) [39]. However, dealing with the high dimensionality of omics datasets and substantial variations in the number of genomic features among different modalities can pose challenges. The use of machine-learning models may encounter the "curse of dimensionality," complicating the analysis of these datasets. Therefore, employing feature selection and/or dimension reduction techniques may be beneficial before the classification process. For instance, Zhang et al. [19] focused on the mRMR feature selection method to predict the diagnosis of glioblastoma multiforme. The authors obtained a dataset comprising a total of 128 variables, including 71 gene expression, 50 gene methylation, 3 miRNAs, and 4 copy number variations. Classification algorithms were applied to the integrated dataset using the MKL method. Their results demonstrated that, compared to other statistical techniques, MKL in the integrated data could enhance the accuracy of glioblastoma multiforme diagnosis. Like Zhang et al. study, we employed the mRMR feature selection method together with integrating the methylation, miRNA, and RNA-Seq data separately for the colon and kidney cancer datasets, and then implemented the MKL classification algorithm. The results showed that the MKL method in integrated data could enhance the accuracy of each colon and kidney cancer diagnosis compared to other methods. However, while the results for miRNA data were consistent with the literature in the thyroid cancer dataset, the results for integrated methylation data were differed. Based on our findings, we conclude that the MKL method for integrated data improves disease classification performance overall. However, it is important to note that the performance of this method may not constantly improve due to potential issues arising from preprocessing steps, as data obtained from innovative technologies can be noisy and require preprocessing stages such as normalization and filtering. Thus, conducting assorted studies with diverse data and evaluating preliminary results while considering these preprocessing steps is critical for future research.

Others have developed "transformation-based integration" techniques to integrate the omics datasets [14]. The kernel-based classification approach was found to be efficient in detecting the nonlinear relationships between samples [14]. For colon and kidney cancer datasets, we found that the kernel-based integration method's performance yielded better results than the graphical-based integration method, which is consistent with results in the literature. However, we observed a slightly higher performance with the graphical-based method for thyroid cancer dataset.

Despite the availability of powerful and sophisticated methodologies, there is still an urgent need for appropriate techniques to harness the potential of large high-throughput datasets [40]. For instance, Cao et al. [39] have introduced a new perspective with their developed method, weight-boosted multi-Kernel learning (wMKL). Recently, there has been a shift toward addressing this issue by incorporating deep learning approaches into multi-omics integration methods [5, 41]. Deep learning techniques may offer a promising solution to overcome the challenges posed by the complex nature of multi-omics data, providing a more effective means of extracting meaningful patterns and insights from such high-dimensional and diverse datasets.

In addition, although many powerful and advanced statistical learning methods have been developed for multi-omics data, class imbalance, commonly seen in these methods, is an inevitable problem. There are resampling approaches such as up-down-smote-rose as a solution to this problem. However, few studies consider the class imbalance situation in multi-omics data. In the study of Yang et al., the class imbalance problem was solved using methods such as synthetic minority oversampling technique and random under-sampling [42]. In the study of Novoloaca et al., the class imbalance problem was addressed using the MCC measure. We also considered this problem by using the MCC measure similarly [43].

In this study, we considered cases where there are only two categories of classes/groups. Nevertheless, this can extend to situations involving multiple classes, increasing the research's applicability and impact. The study included algorithms related to the classification problem and conducted a comprehensive comparison. We believe that a study comparing unsupervised algorithms such as iClusterBayes, NEMO, and MSNE in a similar scope will contribute to the literature.

5 Conclusion

The performances of integration methods along with machine-learning algorithms can exhibit variability across datasets under different scenarios (i.e., raw data, raw data with feature selection applied, etc.). The results showed that the classification models perform relatively better when "concatenate-based" and "model-based integration" methods are used for data integration than when "transformation-based integration" methods are. Furthermore, these two methods yield better results after applying feature selection techniques. On the other hand, considering computational efficiency, the MKL method, which outperforms other classification methods and is relatively faster, can be leveraged after applying feature selection to concatenate-based integrated data.

In situations where the importance of variables is not considered, a "model-based integration" method can be preferred due to its superior classification performance. Nonetheless, it is recommended that more expensive experimentation be conducted to yield findings of broader applicability.

Funding This study was supported by the Research Fund of Erciyes University [TYL-2019-9600]. The funders had no role in study design, data collection and analysis, for decision to publish or prepare the manuscript.

References

1. Shruthi, B.S., Vinodhkumar, P.: Proteomics: a new perspective for cancer. Adv. Biomed. Res. **5**(1), 67 (2016)
2. Manzoni, C., Kia, D.A., Vandrovcova, J., Hardy, J., Wood, N.W., Lewis, P.A., et al.: Genome, transcriptome and proteome: the rise of omics data and their integration in biomedical sciences. Brief. Bioinform. **19**(2), 286–302 (2018)

3. Wörheide, M.A., Krumsiek, J., Kastenmüller, G., Arnold, M.: Multi-omics integration in biomedical research–a metabolomics-centric review. Anal. Chim. Acta. **1141**, 144–162 (2021)
4. Tao, M., Song, T., Du, W., Han, S., Zuo, C., Li, Y., et al.: Classifying breast cancer subtypes using multiple kernel learning based on omics data. Genes (Basel). **10**(3), 200 (2019)
5. Gong, P., Cheng, L., Zhang, Z., Meng, A., Li, E., Chen, J., et al.: Multi-omics integration method based on attention deep learning network for biomedical data classification. Comput. Methods Prog. Biomed. **1**(231), 107377 (2023 Apr)
6. Subramanian, I., Verma, S., Kumar, S., Jere, A., Anamika, K.: Multi-omics data integration, interpretation, and its application. Bioinform Biol. Insights. **14**, 1177932219899051 (2020)
7. Hasin, Y., Seldin, M., Lusis, A.: Multi-omics approaches to disease. Genome Biol. **18**, 1–15 (2017)
8. Lin, E., Lane, H.Y.: Machine learning and systems genomics approaches for multi-omics data. Biomark. Res. **5**, 1–6 (2017)
9. Cantafio, M.E.G., Grillone, K., Caracciolo, D., Scionti, F., Arbitrio, M., Barbieri, V., et al.: From single level analysis to multi-omics integrative approaches: a powerful strategy towards the precision oncology. Road from Nanomedicine to Precis Med. High Throughput, 82969 (2019)
10. Ritchie, M.D., Holzinger, E.R., Li, R., Pendergrass, S.A., Kim, D.: Methods of integrating data to uncover genotype–phenotype interactions. Nat. Rev. Genet. **16**(2), 85–97 (2015)
11. Cavill, R., Jennen, D., Kleinjans, J., Briedé, J.J.: Transcriptomic and metabolomic data integration. Brief. Bioinform. **17**(5), 891–901 (2016)
12. Kim, D., Li, R., Dudek, S.M., Ritchie, M.D.: ATHENA: identifying interactions between different levels of genomic data associated with cancer clinical outcomes using grammatical evolution neural network. BioData Min. **6**(1), 1–14 (2013)
13. Spicker, J.S., Brunak, S., Frederiksen, K.S., Toft, H.: Integration of clinical chemistry, expression, and metabolite data leads to better toxicological class separation. Toxicol. Sci. **102**(2), 444–454 (2008)
14. Yan, K.K., Zhao, H., Pang, H.: A comparison of graph- and kernel-based -omics data integration algorithms for classifying complex traits. BMC Bioinform. **18**(1), 1–13 (2017 Dec)
15. Yang, H., Cao, H., He, T., Wang, T., Cui, Y.: Multilevel heterogeneous omics data integration with kernel fusion. Brief. Bioinform. **21**(1), 156–170 (2020)
16. Alpar, R.: Uygulamalı Çok Değişkenli İstatistiksel Yöntemler [Internet]. Detay (2017)
17. Taskesen, E., Babaei, S., Reinders, M.M.J., de Ridder, J.: Integration of gene expression and DNA-methylation profiles improves molecular subtype classification in acute myeloid leukemia. BMC Bioinform. **16**(4), 1–8 (2015)
18. Vasaikar, S.V., Straub, P., Wang, J., Zhang, B.: LinkedOmics: analyzing multi-omics data within and across 32 cancer types. Nucleic Acids Res. **46**(D1), D956–DD63 (2018)
19. Zhang, Y., Li, A., Peng, C., Wang, M.: Improve glioblastoma multiforme prognosis prediction by using feature selection and multiple kernel learning. IEEE/ACM Trans. Comput. Biol. Bioinforma. **13**(5), 825–835 (2016)
20. El-Manzalawy, Y., Hsieh, T.Y., Shivakumar, M., Kim, D., Honavar, V.: Min-redundancy and max-relevance multi-view feature selection for predicting ovarian cancer survival using multi-omics data 06 Biological Sciences 0604 Genetics. BMC Med. Genet. **11**, 19–31 (2018)
21. Mallik, S., Bhadra, T., Maulik, U.: Identifying epigenetic biomarkers using maximal relevance and minimal redundancy based feature selection for multi-omics data. IEEE Trans. Nanobioscience. **16**(1), 3–10 (2017)
22. Love, M.I., Huber, W., Anders, S.: Moderated estimation of fold change and dispersion for RNA-seq data with DESeq2. Genome Biol. **15**(12), 1–21 (2014)
23. Robinson, M.D., Oshlack, A.: Deseq2论文附录. Genome Biol. **11**(3), 1–9 (2010)
24. Law, C.W., Chen, Y., Shi, W., Smyth, G.K.: Voom: precision weights unlock linear model analysis tools for RNA-seq read counts. Genome Biol. **15**(2), 1–17 (2014)
25. Nadler, S.G., Tritschler, D., Haffar, O.K., Blake, J., Bruce, A.G., Cleaveland, J.S.: Differential expression and sequence-specific interaction of karyopherin α with nuclear localization sequences. J. Biol. Chem. **272**(7), 4310–4315 (1997)

26. Kim, M., Tagkopoulos, I.: Data integration and predictive modeling methods for multi-omics datasets. Molecul. Omics. **14**(1), 8–25 (2018)
27. Cortes, C., Vapnik, V.: Support-vector networks. Mach. Learn. **20**, 273–297 (1995)
28. Gönen, M., Alpaydın, E.: Multiple kernel learning algorithms. J. Machine Learn. Res. **12**, 2211–2268 (2011)
29. Tibshirani, R., Hastie, T., Narasimhan, B., Chu, G.: Diagnosis of multiple cancer types by shrunken centroids of gene expression. PNAS. **99**(10), 6567–6572 (2002)
30. Breiman, L.: Random forests. Mach. Learn. **45**, 5–32 (2001)
31. Chicco, D., Jurman, G.: The advantages of the Matthews correlation coefficient (MCC) over F1 score and accuracy in binary classification evaluation. BMC Genomics. **21**, 1–13 (2020)
32. Feldner-Busztin, D., Nisantzis, P.F., Edmunds, S.J., Boza, G., Racimo, F., Gopalakrishnan, S., et al.: Dealing with dimensionality: the application of machine learning to multi-omics data. Bioinformatics. **39**(2), btad021 (2023)
33. Khadirnaikar, S., Shukla, S., Prasanna, S.R.M.: Machine learning based combination of multi-omics data for subgroup identification in non-small cell lung cancer. Sci. Rep. **13**(1), 4636 (2023)
34. Chierici, M., Bussola, N., Marcolini, A., Francescatto, M., Zandonà, A., Trastulla, L., et al.: Integrative network fusion: a multi-omics approach in molecular profiling. Front. Oncol. **10**, 1065 (2020)
35. Ma, C., Zhang, H.H., Wang, X.: Machine learning for big data analytics in plants. Trends Plant Sci. **19**(12), 798–808 (2014)
36. Mo, Q., Shen, R., Guo, C., Vannucci, M., Chan, K.S., Hilsenbeck, S.G.: A fully Bayesian latent variable model for integrative clustering analysis of multi-type omics data. Biostatistics. **19**(1), 71–86 (2018)
37. Rappoport, N., Shamir, R.: NEMO: cancer subtyping by integration of partial multi-omic data. Bioinformatics. **35**(18), 3348–3356 (2019)
38. Xu, H., Gao, L., Huang, M., Duan, R.: A network embedding based method for partial multi-omics integration in cancer subtyping. Methods. **192**, 67–76 (2021)
39. Cao, H., Jia, C., Li, Z., Yang, H., Fang, R., Zhang, Y., et al.: wMKL: multi-omics data integration enables novel cancer subtype identification via weight-boosted multi-kernel learning. Br. J. Cancer. **130**(6), 1001–1012 (2024)
40. Manochkumar, J., Cherukuri, A.K., Kumar, R.S., Almansour, A.I., Ramamoorthy, S., Efferth, T.: A critical review of machine-learning for "multi-omics" marine metabolite datasets. Comput. Biol. Med. **165**, 107425 (2023)
41. Kang, M., Ko, E., Mersha, T.B.: A roadmap for multi-omics data integration using deep learning. Brief. Bioinform. **23**(1), bbab454 (2022)
42. Yang, Y., Mirzaei, G.: Performance analysis of data resampling on class imbalance and classification techniques on multi-omics data for cancer classification. PLoS One. **19**(2), e0293607 (2024)
43. Novoloaca, A., Broc, C., Beloeil, L., Yu, W.H., Becker, J.: Comparative analysis of integrative classification methods for multi-omics data. Brief. Bioinform. **25**(4), bbae331 (2024)

Sparse Bayesian Clustering of Matrix Data

David Rice, Weining Shen, Chaan Ng, Jiyu Wang, Xiangqi Zhu, and Yuan Wang

Abstract This paper introduces a novel Bayesian framework for probabilistic clustering of matrix-valued data. The proposed approach models the number of clusters as a stochastic partition of the data and introduces a sparsity constraint on the covariance matrices using a beta shrinkage prior for the off-diagonal elements. The effectiveness and superiority of the proposed MCMC algorithm are demonstrated through simulation studies, showing improved estimation of group structures compared to competing methods. It is further tested on two data applications including adrenal lesion clustering and household energy use, aiming to uncover potential disease subtypes and user profile subpopulations.

Keywords Bayesian clustering · Matrix data · Mixture model · Adrenal lesion · Sparsity

1 Introduction

Matrix-structured data is a distinctive type of data where each observation is represented as a rectangular array of values. A feature of this data type is the

D. Rice · Y. Wang (✉)
Washington State University, Pullman, WA, USA
e-mail: yuan.wang@wsu.edu

W. Shen
University of California, Irvine, CA, USA

C. Ng
The University of Texas MD Anderson Cancer Center, Houston, TX, USA

J. Wang
National Renewable Energy Laboratory, Golden, CO, USA

X. Zhu
Oregon State University, Corvallis, OR, USA

Y. Zhao, D.-G. Chen (eds.), *Big Data Analytics in Biostatistics and Bioinformatics*, ICSA Book Series in Statistics,
https://doi.org/10.1007/978-3-032-06649-7_7

preservation of spatial/temporal relationship between entries in the array, making it suitable for various applications. Medical imaging data, such as computerized tomography (CT) scans, electroencephalograms (EEGs), and local field potentials (LFPs) in which the location of irregularities is important, can all be modeled using matrix-structured data. Additionally, it can be applied to model spatiotemporal and multivariate longitudinal data, which are inherently matrix-valued [12, 31–33, 40]. The versatility of this data type has resulted in a large body of literature related to statistical learning of matrices and tensors [3, 30]. For example, matrix regression has been widely used to quantify the association between the predictors and outcomes that involve matrix-valued data [8, 13, 39, 41]. Matrix completion is another popular tool in studying recommender systems and imaging restoration problems [5, 25].

Our focus in this paper is to develop a probabilistic clustering method to model the heterogeneity in the matrix-valued data. Clustering is a well-established problem with many solutions, including classical ones such as K-means and hierarchical clustering [10] and newer ones such as convolutional neural networks (CNNs) [37]. While these methods can be effective, they often disregard the matrix structure in the data. There are some recent works utilizing techniques such as nonnegative matrix factorization [34] and spectral clustering [23]. However, these methods are purely deterministic and hence lack a probabilistic interpretation. One technique that enables us to maintain the matrix structure and follow a probabilistic approach is to represent the data as a finite mixture of matrix distributions, which allows for elegant unsupervised techniques such as expectation-maximization (EM) to be used [7, 11, 21, 28]. However, the EM algorithm assumes a prespecified number of clusters, which is often unknown in real data applications. An intuitive solution to this problem is to consider a Bayesian approach by imposing a prior distribution on the number of clusters [32, 38], which allows estimation of the cluster number based on the data.

For matrix-valued data with large dimensions, sparse covariance (or precision) matrix structures are often utilized to better model the dependence structure in the matrix entries. This is particularly useful to reduce model complexity and improve the interpretation. For example, in brain functional connectivity studies, it is common to impose a sparse covariance or precision matrix structure to help identify important regions of interest in the brain's connectivity network [14, 26]. The sparsity structure, despite its utility, has not been considered in the previous work on matrix clustering (e.g., [32, 38]) to the best of our knowledge. Motivated by these considerations, we propose the sparse Bayesian matrix clustering (SBMC) method, which achieves sparse covariance estimation and infers unknown number of clusters while maintaining a probabilistic interpretation. The main idea is to model the matrix data using a finite mixture of matrix normal distributions within the mixture of finite mixtures (MFM) framework proposed by Miller and Harrison [22]. Then the posterior can be efficiently computed using a Gibbs sampler that iteratively updates the cluster assignments, cluster means, and other parameters using the full conditionals. To induce sparsity on the covariance matrices, we use the beta shrinkage prior in [17]. This prior promotes shrinkage in the off-diagonals of the covariance matrices by imposing a beta and gamma distribution on the off-diagonals and diagonals, respectively. Additionally, the conditional conjugacy nature of this prior allows for analytic full conditionals which integrate nicely within the Gibbs sampler implementation. We showcase the effectiveness of the SBMC method through two real-life data examples. The first dataset comprises 337 CT scans of adrenal lesions, with the objective of uncovering patterns associated with malignancy. The second data application studies the energy usage data from 136 homes in Austin, Texas, focusing on the identification of distinct energy consumption behaviors during the months of November and December.

The rest of this paper is organized as follows. The method section outlines our methodology including a review of the mixture of finite mixtures model and the beta shrinkage prior. The Gibbs sampler section demonstrates how our method can be implemented through presentation of the necessary full conditionals. We conduct simulation studies to compare the effectiveness of SBMC with other algorithms under various settings in Sect. 4. Two data applications are presented in Sect. 5. We conclude with a few remarks about future directions in Sect. 6. Computational code and data used in Sect. 5.2 are available at https://github.com/davidriceciser/SBMC.

2 Method

Let $Y_1, \ldots, Y_n \in R^{p\times q}$ be a random sample of matrix-valued data. Our goal is to model the underlying heterogeneity in $Y_1, \ldots, Y_n$ through a sparse Bayesian matrix clustering (SBMC) approach. Assuming that there are K clusters underneath, each observation is assigned to only one of the K clusters. The mixture of finite mixtures (MFM) model proposed in [22] is used for a probabilistic clustering framework. The MFM model assumes that K is finite and members within the same cluster follow the same distribution. Without knowing the cluster assignment, the marginal distribution of Y_i is a mixture distribution with K components. The choice of K remains an unknown hyperparameter. Learning the probability distribution of K as a function of the observations allows us to reveal the number of clusters presented by the data.

For a given number of K, we denote Z_i the cluster assignment for the ith sample and $f(Y)$ the marginal density for a random matrix Y. The MFM model assumes a finite mixture distribution for $f(Y)$, given K, and a symmetric Dirichlet distribution prior for the cluster assignments. More specifically, given K, we assume

$$
\begin{aligned}
f(Y) &= \sum_{j=1}^{K} \pi_j f_j(Y), \\
\pi &= (\pi_1, \ldots, \pi_k) \sim \mathrm{Dir}_k(\gamma, \ldots, \gamma), \\
P(Z_i = j) &= \pi_j \text{ for } j = 1, \ldots, K.
\end{aligned}
$$

Here $f_j(Y)$ is the conditional density for Y within cluster j, π is the K-dimensional vector of prior probabilities for the assignment clusters $(1, \ldots, K)$, $\gamma > 0$ is a concentration parameter we choose, and $P(Z_i = j)$ is the prior probability that cluster label Z_i for point x_i is equal to j. It is important to note that the choice of γ for the symmetric Dirichlet prior represents our beliefs about the concentration of observations across all clusters. A $\gamma > 1$ concentration assumes the distribution of observations is uniform across clusters, whereas a $\gamma < 1$ concentration assumes that many of the current number of clusters will have 0 observations.

The number of clusters, K, is assigned with a prior distribution on the set of positive integers. The value of K is updated through the Chinese restaurant process where an observation is assigned to an existing group proportional to the number of group members or a new group with probability proportional to the concentration parameter.

While this framework is applicable to a wide class of data types, we focus on matrix-valued data clustering and choose to use the matrix normal distribution for each cluster because of its computational simplicity and convenient interpretation. The matrix normal distribution is a generalization of the multivariate normal distribution for matrix-valued data [9]. A $p \times q$ random matrix Y is normally distributed with matrix mean $M_{p\times q}$, row-wise covariance $U_{p\times p}$, and column-wise covariance $V_{q\times q}$, denoted by $Y \sim N_{p,q}(M, U, V)$, if its column vectorization satisfies

$$\text{vec}(\mathbf{Y}) \sim N_{pq}(\text{vec}(\mathbf{M}), \mathbf{V} \otimes \mathbf{U}). \tag{1}$$

The covariance matrix in (1) satisfies the so-called separable structure and allows the rows and columns of the data have to have different interpretations. This situation arises in our paper when clustering matrix observations where the row and column time scales are different, e.g., in the energy usage example each observation is a 24×7 matrix and the V parameter represents the column-level covariance between days of the week and the U parameter represents the row-level covariance between the hours across the days. The ability to distinguish between the day-to-day and hour-to-hour variance gives insight into what behaviors may be occurring during certain periods of the week.

Now for each observation, we have $Y_i \sim N_{pq}(M_{Z_i}, U, V)$, where $M_1, \ldots, M_K$ are cluster-specific mean parameters. We consider a conjugate matrix normal prior,

$$M_1, \ldots, M_K \overset{\text{i.i.d.}}{\sim} N_{p,q}(M_0, \Sigma_0, \Omega_0), \tag{2}$$

where M_0, Σ_0, and Ω_0 are hyperparameters for the matrix mean, row-wise covariance, and column-wise covariance, respectively. We use a global covariance structure for U and V, i.e., equal covariance parameters across each cluster. Moreover, we consider a sparse prior on them for parsimonious estimation. This is meaningful because the number of free parameters in U and V is as big as $O(p^2 + q^2)$, and by assuming most of the off-diagonal elements are 0, we obtain an interpretable covariance pattern. In general, any sparse priors on covariance matrix can be used in our method (e.g., [36]). We choose the beta shrinkage prior in [17] because of its nice computational and theoretical properties.

To demonstrate how beta shrinkage prior works, let $\Sigma = (\sigma_{jk})$ be a $p \times p$ positive definite matrix. This beta shrinkage prior can be represented as the product of two independent distributions for the diagonal and off-diagonal elements of Σ, respectively:

$$f^u(\Sigma) \propto \prod_{j=1}^{p} f(\sigma_{jj}) \prod_{1 \le j < k \le p} \int f(\sigma_{jk}|\rho_{jk}) f(\rho_{jk}) d\rho_{jk}. \tag{3}$$

The first term assigns independent Gamma priors for the diagonal entries with shape parameter c and rate parameter d, i.e., $f(\sigma_{jj}) \sim \text{Gamma}(\sigma_{jj}|c, d)$ for $j = 1, \ldots, p$. The second term specifies a beta shrinkage prior for the off-diagonal entries through a two-step process as follows:

$$f(\sigma_{jk}|\rho_{jk}) \sim N\left(0, \frac{\rho_{jk}}{1-\rho_{jk}}\tau_1^2\right), \tag{4}$$

$$f(\rho_{jk}) \sim \text{Beta}(\rho_{jk}|a, b), \; 1 \le j < k \le p.$$

Here ρ_{jk} is the shrinkage parameter that controls the variance of the off-diagonal entries. Note that the variance for σ_{jk} depends on a beta distribution with hyperparameters a, b, and global shrinkage constant τ_1^2. Setting $a = b = \frac{1}{2}$ results in the popular half-Cauchy prior, which is what we used in this paper. We assign priors in (3) and (4) on U and V independently.

3 Gibbs Sampler

In this section we outline each step for the implementation of the SBMC Gibbs sampler and describe the full conditional distributions.

3.1 Cluster Assignments

The full conditional for Z_i can be modeled using the Pólya-urn scheme [24]. For an initial number of clusters K_0, each observation X_i is randomly assigned to a cluster label Z_i, where the label corresponds to a particular cluster $C_1, C_2, \ldots, C_{K_0}$.

We then iteratively reassign X_i to a group label Z_i based on the following full conditional:

$$P(Z_i = c|Z_{-i}, \Omega) \propto \begin{cases} (\#c + \gamma) f(Y_i|M_{Z_i}, U, V) \text{ at an existing cluster} \\ \\ \frac{V_n(K_{-i}+1)}{V_n(K_{-i})} \gamma m(Y_i|U, V) \text{ if c is a new cluster,} \end{cases} \tag{5}$$

where $\#c$ is the number of observations in cluster labeled as c, K_{-i} denotes the number of blocks in the partition of the set $\{1, 2, \ldots, n\}/\{i\}$, $f(Y_i|M_{Z_i}, U, V)$ is the matrix normal pdf, and $m(Y_i|U, V)$ is

$$\frac{\exp(-\frac{1}{2}[\text{vec}(Y_i)^T(V^{-1} \otimes U^{-1})\text{vec}(Y_i) + \text{vec}(M_0)^T(\Omega_0^{-1} \otimes \Sigma_0^{-1})\text{vec}(M_0) - \tilde{\mu}^T \tilde{\Sigma} \tilde{\mu}])}{(2\pi)^{pq/2}|V|^{p/2}|U|^{q/2}|\Omega_0|^{p/2}|\Sigma_0|^{q/2}}$$

$$\times |\tilde{\Sigma}^{pq/2}|,$$

where $\tilde{\Sigma}^{-1} = V^{-1} \otimes U^{-1} + \Sigma_0^{-1} \otimes \Sigma_0^{-1}$ and $\tilde{\mu} = \tilde{\Sigma}[(V^{-1} \otimes U^{-1})\text{vec}(Y_i) + (\Omega_0^{-1} \otimes \Sigma_0^{-1})\text{vec}(M_0)]$. Here $V_n(t)$ is defined as

$$V_n(t) = \sum_{k=1}^{\infty} \frac{k_t}{(\gamma k)^{(n)}} p_K(k), \tag{6}$$

where $k_{(t)} = k(k-1)\ldots(k-t+1)$ and $(\gamma k)^{(n)} = \gamma k(\gamma k+1)\ldots(\gamma k+n-1)$.

3.2 Cluster Mean Parameters

The full conditional for the cluster means of cluster j is given by the following formula:

$$\begin{aligned} \text{vec}(M_j)|\cdot &\sim N_{pq}(\zeta_j^{-1}\xi_j, \zeta_j^{-1}), \\ \zeta_j &= (n_j V^{-1} \otimes U^{-1} + \Omega_0^{-1} \otimes \Sigma_0^{-1}), \\ \xi_j &= \text{vec}(U^{-1}(\sum_{i=1}^{n} Y_i I(Z_i = j))V^{-1} + \Sigma_0^{-1} M_0 \Omega_0^{-1}), \end{aligned} \tag{7}$$

where n is the sample size and n_j is the number of observations in cluster j. The closed-form expressions are obtained based on the matrix-normal conjugacy.

3.3 Global Covariance Matrices

To update the covariances matrices $U_{p\times p}$ and $V_{q\times q}$, we use the block Gibbs sampler in [17]. Take U as an example. Consider a partition of U as shown in (8) such that Σ_{11} is a $(p-1)\times(p-1)$ block matrix, σ_{12} is a $(p-1)\times 1$ column vector, and σ_{22} is a scalar.

$$U = \begin{pmatrix} \Sigma_{11} & \sigma_{12} \\ \sigma_{12}^T & \sigma_{22} \end{pmatrix}. \tag{8}$$

Then we define the following matrices of dimension $p\times p$ with similar partitions of S and W:

$$S = \begin{pmatrix} S_{11} & s_{12} \\ s_{12}^T & s_{22} \end{pmatrix}, \quad W = \begin{pmatrix} W_{11} & w_{12} \\ w_{12}^T & 0 \end{pmatrix}, \tag{9}$$

where $S=\sum_{i=1}^n (Y_i - M_j)V^{-1}(Y_i - M_j)^T$ and $W = w_{jk}^2 = \rho_{jk}\tau_1^2/(1-\rho_{jk})$.

We generate samples for σ_{12} and σ_{22} through transformed variables (μ, η) which are defined and sampled as follows:

$$\begin{aligned}
&(\sigma_{12},\sigma_{22}) \to (\mu=\sigma_{12}, \eta=\sigma_{22}-\sigma_{12}^T\Sigma_{11}^{-1}\sigma_{12}) \\
&\mu|\cdot \sim N_{p-1}[\{B+\mathrm{diag}(w_{12}^{-1})\}^{-1}y, \{B+\mathrm{diag}(w_{12}^{-1})\}^{-1}] \\
&B = \Sigma_{11}^{-1}S_{11}\Sigma_{11}^{-1}\eta^{-1}+\lambda\Sigma_{11}^{-1},\ y=\Sigma_{11}^{-1}s_{12}\eta^{-1} \\
&\eta|\cdot \sim GIG(1-nq/2, \lambda, \mu^T\Sigma_{11}^{-1}S_{11}\Sigma_{11}^{-1}\mu - 2s_{12}^T\Sigma_{11}^{-1}\mu + s_{22}),
\end{aligned} \tag{10}$$

where GIG(a,b,c) is the generalized inverse Gaussian with pdf $f(x) \propto x^{a-1}e^{-(bx+c/x)/2}I(x>0)$

$$\begin{aligned}
\rho_{jk} &= 1 - 1/(1+\phi_{jk}), \\
\psi_{jk}|\cdot &\sim \mathrm{Gamma}(a+b, \psi_{jk}+1), \\
\phi_{jk}|\cdot &\sim \mathrm{GIG}(a-1/2, 2\psi_{jk}, \sigma_{jk}^2/\tau_1^2).
\end{aligned} \tag{11}$$

We note that so far, we have simply updated one row and column of U. Permuting a given un-updated column to be the last allows us to repeat our algorithm and systematically update the entire U matrix. This entire process is repeated for the V matrix, where S, W are $q\times q$ matrices, $S=\sum_{i=1}^n (Y_i - M_j)^T U^{-1}(Y_i - M_j)^T$ and np is used instead of nq for the η parameter in (11).

In the implementation, we choose prior cluster mean M_0 to be the element-wise median of all observations, prior covariance Σ_0 a diagonal matrix as $\mathrm{diag}(\sigma_1^2,\ldots,\sigma_p^2)$, and $\Omega_0 = \mathrm{diag}(\omega_1^2,\ldots,\omega_q^2)$ where $\sigma_1,\ldots,\sigma_p$ are the half ranges along rows 1 to p and $\omega_1, \ldots, \omega_q$ are the half ranges along columns 1 to q of the observations, as given in [38].

3.4 Posterior Summary

To summarize the posterior samples, we use Dahl's method [6]. We define L $n \times n$ matrices D_l for $l = 1, .., L$ corresponding to sampler iterations after the burn-in period. In each matrix D_l, the (i, j)th entry is 1 if observations i and j share the same cluster assignment, and 0 otherwise. Define entries for each of the L matrices as $D_l(i, j) = I(Z_i = Z_j)$.

We then define matrix $\bar{D}$ which averages over each of the L observations to give us an element-wise mean in each cell. Denote $\bar{D} = \frac{1}{L}\sum_{l=1} D_l$. Lastly, we choose the observation $\hat{D}$ which has the smallest element-wise Euclidean distance to $\bar{D}$ as follows:

$$\hat{D} = \arg\min_{l} \sum_{i=1}^{n}\sum_{j=1}^{n}((\hat{D}_l)_{ij} - \bar{D}_{ij})^2.$$

The index l of the $\hat{D}_l$ iteration is used to select the representative posterior point estimate iteration sample for cluster assignment, covariance matrices, and mean estimates.

4 Simulations

4.1 The Simulation Setting

To test the effectiveness of our method (SBMC), we compare its performance to the non-sparse Bayesian matrix clustering method (BMC) in [38] as well as two frequentist clustering techniques through a set of simulation studies. A total of four simulation settings are assessed for evaluation, with the sample size $n = 250$, matrix dimension being 10×6 or 20×20, and the signal strength being high or low. Signal strength is defined as a scaling factor that we multiply to the matrix means when generating the data. We choose a high signal strength of 1 and a low signal strength of 0.75. The underlying number of clusters is 6 for each setting. The true cluster sizes are 50, 75, 25, 10, 40, 50 for a total of $n = 250$ observations. The cluster mean patterns for the low-dimensional and high-dimensional settings are displayed in Figs. 1 and 2, respectively. The true covariance matrices U_{true} and V_{true} are generated with diagonals of 1 and off-diagonals determined by a hurdle model. The probability of an off-diagonal entry being nonzero is $\frac{1}{4}$ and the nonzero off-diagonals are generated using a Beta$(1, 5)$ distribution.

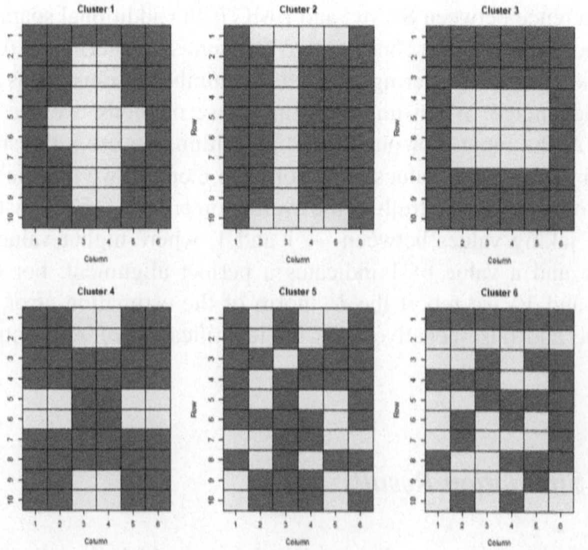

Fig. 1 The six underlying cluster means for the low-dimensional 10×6 simulation setting, where black entries have value 0 and white entries have value 1

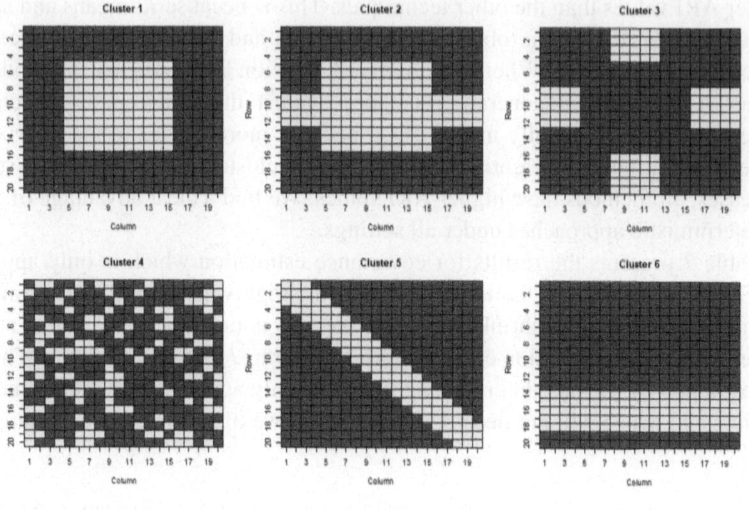

Fig. 2 The six underlying cluster means for the high-dimensional 20×20 simulation setting, where black entries have value 0 and white entries have value 1

In the simulation, each setting is replicated for 50 times. For each replicate, we sample a total of 1000 MCMC iterations after burn-in for inference purpose. For the SBMC and BMC methods, we start the chain with 20 initial clusters. The initial values for U and V are set to the maximum likelihood estimates based on matrix normal distribution, and initial means as the element-wise median M_0. Note that the only difference between SBMC and BMC is the additional sparsity structure in the covariance matrices. We consider two frequentist clustering methods, including K-means and spectral clustering, and set the number of clusters as the true value, 6, to their advantage. When implementing these methods, we use the vectorized matrix data as the input. For our SBMC algorithm, we use a threshold of 0.05 to shrink small off-diagonal values to 0. For each method, we use the adjusted Rand index [29] compared to the truth as the evaluation criteria. The adjusted Rand index is a statistic taking values between -1 and 1, where higher values imply better concordance and a value of 1 indicates a perfect alignment. For the covariance matrices U and V, we report the L_1 norm of the estimation error as well as the false-positive and false-negative rates for identification of zero entries in the off-diagonals.

4.2 The Simulation Results

Table 1 shows the average adjusted Rand index (ARI) for all methods and its standard deviation in the brackets. We find that SBMC and BMC have achieved a high clustering accuracy under all different settings, and both have considerably higher ARI values than the other techniques. This is because K-means and spectral clustering treat the matrix observation as vectors and thus do not take the matrix structure into account. When the matrix dimension increases, all methods have higher ARI values in general. This goes against the intuition of the curse of dimensionality but actually makes sense because more entries in the matrix bring more information to differentiate among different clusters. When the signal strength increases, all methods have higher ARI values. We find a clear advantage of SBMC to deterministic approaches under all settings.

Table 2 presents the results for covariance estimation which is only applicable for SBMC and BMC methods. This finding highlights the benefit of parsimonious estimation by using the shrinkage priors. We also notice that as the signal strength increases, the L_1 estimation error increases for both U and V estimation. This may be explained by the fact that reducing the noise only applies to the matrix means of clusters and hence will not necessarily help improve the covariance estimation.

Table 1 Simulation results: average adjusted Rand index (standard deviation) for SBMC and competing methods

	High dimension		Low dimension	
Method	High sig.	Low sig.	High sig.	Low sig.
SBMC	**0.914**(0.153)	0.708(0.149)	0.834(0.053)	**0.727**(0.032)
BMC	0.842(0.169)	**0.726**(0.148)	**0.843**(0.029)	0.711(0.068)
K-means	0.856(0.119)	0.629(0.092)	0.594(0.058)	0.283(0.067)
Spectral	0.677(0.099)	0.553(0.030)	0.507(0.049)	0.243(0.070)

Table 2 Simulation results: the L_1 estimation error for our method (SBMC) and BMC (in brackets) and the false-positive (F.P.) and false-negative (F.N.) rates for SBMC

		V			U		
		L_1 error	F.P. rate	F.N. rate	L_1 error	F.P. rate	F.N. rate
Low dim.	Low sig.	0.773(0.802)	0.000	0.018	2.132(2.090)	0.290	0.083
	High sig.	0.919(0.902)	0.000	0.025	2.252(2.161)	0.313	0.088
High dim.	Low sig.	4.161(6.926)	0.191	0.019	4.826(4.562)	0.206	0.015
	High sig.	4.161(7.927)	0.204	0.005	6.423(4.805)	0.205	0.037

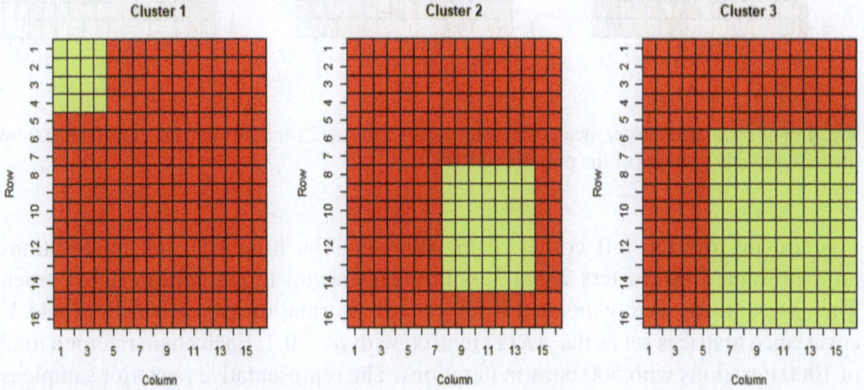

Fig. 3 The cluster means of cluster 1 (left), cluster 2 (middle), and cluster 3 (right) with 1000, 50, and 10 number of observations, respectively

We also report the false-positive and false-negative rates in sparse covariance estimation for our method, where positive corresponds to a zero value in the covariance matrix and negative represents a nonzero value. Our method in general performs well in terms of controlling the false discoveries, in particular, false negatives.

4.3 Additional Simulation Results

To ensure the SBMC clustering algorithm is appropriate for the task of identifying heterogeneity in adrenal lesions, additional simulations are run. These simulations seek to identify whether the algorithm can correctly identify clusters, which have large imbalances in membership, and distribution over the domain we would expect to see in adrenal lesion observations. The cluster mean patterns are displayed in Fig. 3.

The simulation consisted of $n = 160$ observations with true cluster assignments $n_1 = 100$, $n_2 = 50$, and $n_3 = 10$ for clusters 1, 2, and 3, respectively. The cluster means span the regions which we would expect to be populated in adrenal lesion data, with areas associated with low HU unit observations represented by cluster

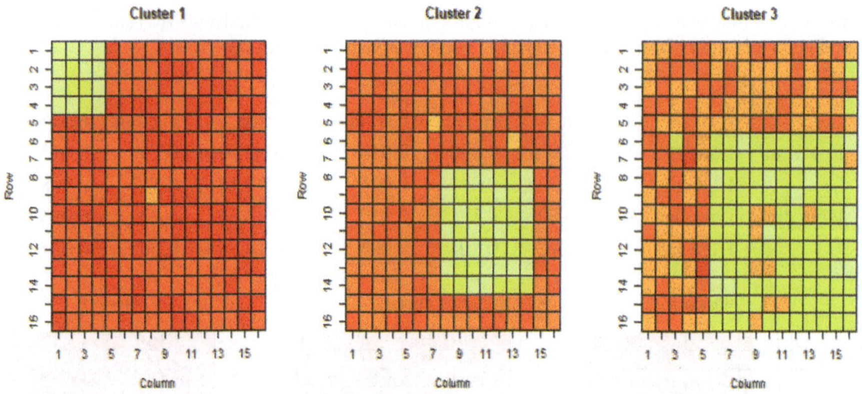

Fig. 4 The estimated cluster means of cluster 1 (left), cluster 2 (middle), and cluster 3 (right) from the representative sample of the posterior distribution

1 occupying the top left corner of the domain. The high HU unit observations are represented by clusters 2 and 3, with means nearer to the bottom right corner. The observations were generated from a matrix-normal distribution with U and V covariance matrices set as the $AR(1)$ matrix, with $\rho = 0.1$. Each chain ran for a total of 1000 iterations with 500 burn-in iterations. The representative posterior sample is chosen using Dahl's method [6], as discussed in Sect. 3.4. Ten replications were run, resulting in an average ARI of 0.980. The true and estimated cluster mean patterns are displayed in Figs. 3 and 4, respectively.

5 Real Data Applications

In this section, we discuss two applications using the proposed SBMC method. The first one is adrenal lesion clustering and its correspondence to the presence of malignant lesions, and the second on detecting clusters in household energy usage.

5.1 Adrenal Lesion Clustering

The adrenal glands are small glands directly above the kidney which are considered functioning if they produce hormones such as cortisol, epinephrine, and norepinephrine [27]. While having nonfunctioning adrenal glands is not considered dangerous, these glands are susceptible to potentially cancerous lesions. The diagnosis of adrenal lesions as malignant or nonmalignant is critical in determining whether a patient has experienced distant migration in the metastatic setting. However, diagnosing adrenal lesions accurately, particularly in the early stages, remains challenging when relying mainly on routine CT imaging [1, 35]. Our research was motivated by an adrenal lesion study that involved patients who had CT imaging available in the MD Anderson Cancer Center's radiology picture archiving and communication system (PACS). Some patients have multiple scans following the injection of contrast medium for enhancement. For our analysis, we exclusively utilized the noncontrast phase scans acquired before contrast injection for all included patients. These patients also underwent pathological diagnoses to establish benignity from malignancy between January 2001 and January 2010. Our dataset comprised a total of 337 nonfunctioning adrenal lesions, where 173 were benign and 164 were malignant. For each lesion, a region of interest (ROI) was carefully drawn freehand, with an electronic cursor and mouse, around the periphery of the adrenal lesion. The size and shape varied among different patients.

The diverse range of sizes and shapes among these lesions pose a significant challenge for analysis, including issues related to rescaling and registration. To address this challenge, we employ the gray-level co-occurrence matrix (GLCM) to summarize the texture features present in the CT imaging data for each lesion's region of interest (ROI). The GLCMs are constructed from the lesion ROIs as follows. First, 16 gray-level bins are constructed from the Hounsfield unit (HU) scale through evaluation of the empirical distribution of all pixels in the 337 lesions. Next, a 16×16 GLCM is constructed for each ROI. In this matrix, the (i, j)th entry represents the count of pixel pairs with gray-level i and j, respectively, that are within a 3×3 spatial neighborhood of each other on the CT scan image. More details of the GLCM interpretation and construction are available in [19].

A nice property of the GLCM matrix is its ability to facilitate the comparison of ROIs with varying sizes and shapes while preserving the spatial heterogeneity within each ROI. As each ROI can be effectively condensed into a 16×16 GLCM matrix, we utilize the SBMC method to cluster the 337 GLCMs after applying a square root transformation. We summarize the posterior inference using Dahl's method on the cluster assignment results based on 3 chains with 1000 MCMC iterations after burn-in and set the concentration parameter γ to be 0.1.

Our method detects eight clusters from the posterior distributions. Their cluster means are shown in Fig. 5. Notably, clusters 2 and 7 exhibit a predominantly bright region that tilts towards the bottom right corner, indicating a higher average number of neighboring pixels with high CT intensity. Clusters 4, 5, and 8, on the other hand, have the peak more towards upper left which is for low-intensity pixels. Based on the pathological diagnosis, we also calculate the proportion of malignant lesions for each cluster. Clusters 2 and 7 are mainly malignant lesions (69.6% and 100%, respectively). Clusters 4, 5, and 8 are mainly benign lesions with 0%, 24.0%, and 11.8% malignancy, respectively. Cluster 5 represents a majority of the observations with 214 samples and has a balanced mix of malignant and benign classifications with 58.4% malignancy. Clusters 1 and 3 have less than 10 members and hence are omitted from the discussion. These findings indicate a strong association between cluster assignments and the cluster mean shape with the distribution of malignant and benign lesions. Furthermore, the disparity between the mean values of the predominantly malignant clusters (clusters 2 and 7) and predominantly benign clusters (clusters 4, 5, and 8) is consistent with current radiology literature in

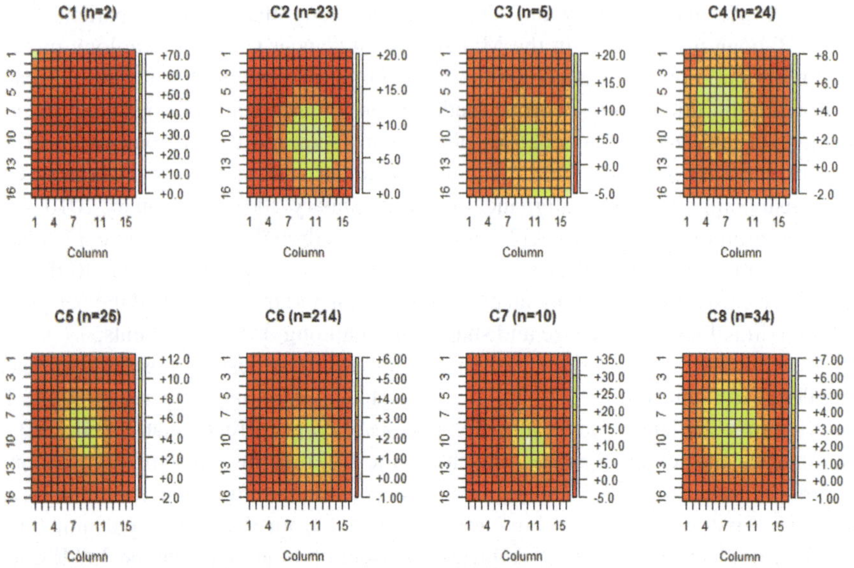

Fig. 5 Adrenal lesion GLCM analysis: each panel shows the posterior mean for the cluster average pattern. Each entry is the square root of the GLCM bin count

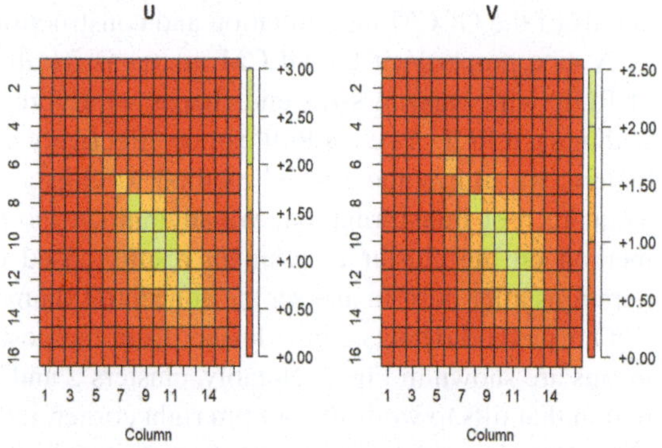

Fig. 6 Adrenal lesion GLCM analysis: the estimated row-wise covariance matrix U and column-wise covariance matrix V

which high HU values in noncontrast scans are used to classify malignancy [16]. Because Hounsfield units are a measure of density, it makes sense that lipid-rich benign lesions which are less than dense than malignant ones have GLCM values concentrated in the upper left.

The row and column covariance matrices U and V are shown in Fig. 6. As expected, the gray levels with large differences in magnitude appear to have sparse covariance entries in the U and V matrices, with 66 and 90 entries being shrunk to 0, respectively, at a 0.15 level (156 entries in total). Most of the non-sparse entries in the covariance matrices appear in gray levels 8–14, where the majority of co-occurrences appear to be located. The U and V matrices overall exhibit a similar pattern as GLCM is a symmetric matrix.

5.2 Energy Usage Clustering

Efficient power allocation through prediction of needs within communities is an important tool to reduce energy expenditure and overall carbon footprint. To maintain the functionality of a power grid, it is important to ensure a sufficient supply of electricity to meet the demands of customers at all times. During periods of historically lower activity, power utilities may opt to reduce electricity production, taking into consideration the decreased demand. The accurate assessment of the appropriate amount of power to inject into the grid relies heavily on various factors, with consumer behavior playing a pivotal role. One approach to gaining insight into consumer behavior is by identifying distinct and diverse patterns in power consumption, particularly during specific times of the year. On the other hand, the flexible energy consumption from building loads provides them great potential to participate in demand response activities in grid operation to solve the problems caused by high-penetration distributed energy resources. The load profiles with similar patterns will have similar characteristics, leading to similar demand response capability. Grid operators can send demand response signals to the building cluster with a higher chance to respond at different time. Our method provides a useful way of modeling the heterogeneity in these patterns, specifically uncovering unique clusters within household energy usage.

Our dataset consists of 136 houses located in Austin, Texas. The power usage for each household was recorded every minute through the year of 2015. To facilitate our analysis, we aggregated the data into hourly intervals and extracted data for the months of November and December (with slight overlap into October due to the uneven division of months into weeks). Each hourly usage curve is then discretized into a 24 hours by 7 days matrix representing the power usage pattern for 1 week. The matrices with zero power usage were removed. At the end, we have 1209 24×7 power usage matrices for the clustering analysis. The overall average weekly power usage is illustrated in Fig. 7. It can be seen that the highest power usage happens between 6 pm and 10 pm. During the weekend (columns 3 and 4), there is a noticeable increase in daytime energy use. For the analysis, we apply a square root transformation to the matrix data entries, followed by normalization of each matrix observation by subtracting the overall average (shown in Fig. 7). Our goal is to detect distinct clusters based on the weekly power usage pattern and to identify clusters of deviations in consumer behaviors from the average energy use.

We apply the SBMC method with 5 initial clusters and a γ value of 0.1. We combine 3 chains each with 4000 MCMC iterations after burn-in and summarize the posterior samples using Dahl's method, which yields 2 clusters. The mean for each cluster is shown in Fig. 8. Cluster 2 (left panel) represents observations that have the highest energy usage on average, particularly concentrated during the evenings. In contrast, cluster 1 (right panel) exhibits a lower average energy usage during the late evening and early morning. This analysis effectively distinguishes three distinct power usage behaviors, providing valuable insights into how power can be allocated during the selected time of year. Furthermore, the average energy used each week

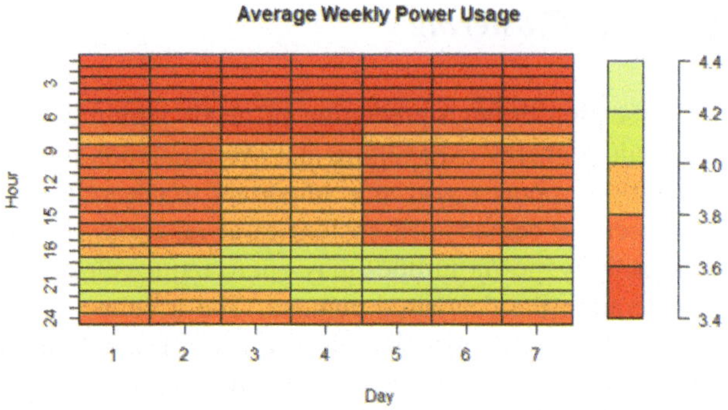

Fig. 7 Average weekly power usage matrix within November and December. Each row represents an hour from 12am to 11:59pm of the day and the columns represent days of the week from Thursday (column 1) to Wednesday (column 7)

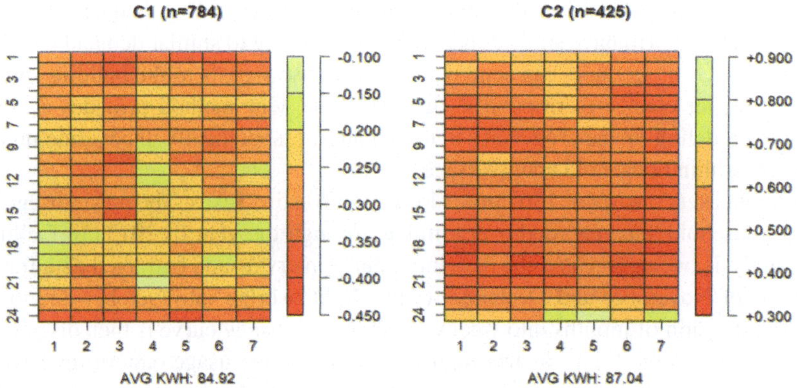

Fig. 8 The average power consumption for the two detected clusters 1 and 2 (left, right), with the average kilowatt hours for each cluster captioned below

for each cluster reinforces the stratification between the two groups, demonstrating that clusters 1 and 2 correspond to low and high energy usage, respectively. The estimated row and column covariance matrices are shown in Fig. 9. The row-wise covariance matrix U shows that the hours 8–17 during a given day exhibit higher covariance with adjacent hours, indicating that if power is being used during this period, it is likely to continue being consumed.

6 Discussion

In this paper, we propose a Bayesian matrix clustering approach that models the heterogeneity in matrix observations under an MFM framework. This approach allows for flexibility in both the number of clusters and the sparsity of the covari-

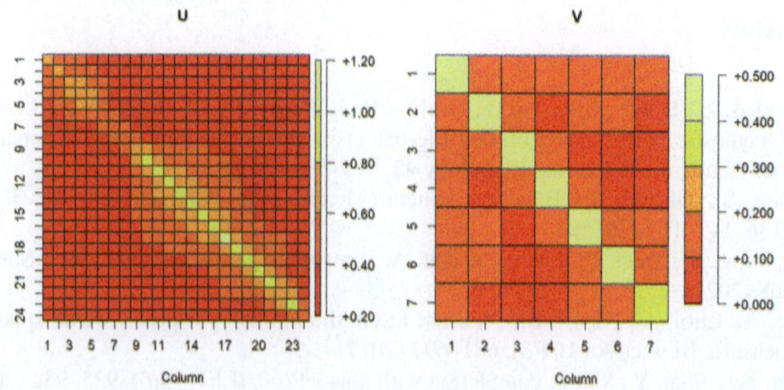

Fig. 9 The estimated row-wise covariance matrix U and column-wise covariance matrix V for power consumption within November and December

ance matrices through modeling the cluster assignment as a Chinese restaurant process and using a beta shrinkage prior for the covariance matrices. Simulations have confirmed the effectiveness of this algorithm under various conditions when compared to Bayesian matrix clustering (without sparsity) and a few frequentist clustering methods. We further demonstrate the utility of our method via two data applications. The application to the adrenal lesion example identifies five substantial clusters that demonstrate patterns in adrenal lesion associated with malignant lesion. These results can help clinicians further detecting lesion subtypes and potentially understanding features and uncertainty for various types of lesions. The application to energy usage allows us to identify three different customer behavior profiles.

Several directions remain open for future research. For example, one may consider the extension to heavy-tailed data by using alternatives to the matrix normal distribution. Our proposed method can be modified to work on higher-dimensional tensor data [15, 18] and sparse precision matrix [2]. On the computational side, more work can be done to improve the computational efficiency of this problem, as the proposed SBMC model currently has a complexity of $O(p^4+q^4+nqp^2+npq^2)$, stemming from matrix multiplication in nested loops within the covariance update. It is also of interest to consider alternative mixture models where the mixture components can be dependent [20] or infinite mixture models such as Dirichlet and Pitman-Yor process mixtures [4].

Acknowledgments Dr. Yuan Wang's work is supported in part by the Simons Foundation Award 713766.

References

1. Altinmakas, E., Hobbs, B.P., Ye, H., Grubbs, E.G., Perrier, N.D., Prieto, V.G., Lee, J.E., Ng, C.S.: Diagnostic performance of 18-f-fdg-pet–ct in adrenal lesions using histopathology as reference standard. Abdominal Radiology **42**, 577–584 (2017)
2. Banerjee, S., Ghosal, S.: Bayesian structure learning in graphical models. J. Multivar. Anal. **136**, 147–162 (2015)
3. Bi, X., Tang, X., Yuan, Y., Zhang, Y., Qu, A.: Tensors in statistics. Annu. Rev. Stat. Appl. **8**, 345–368 (2021)
4. Canale, A., Lijoi, A., Nipoti, B., Prünster, I.: On the pitman–yor process with spike and slab base measure. Biometrika **104**(3), 681–697 (2017)
5. Candes, E.J., Plan, Y.: Matrix completion with noise. Proc. IEEE **98**(6), 925–936 (2010)
6. Dahl, D.B.: Model-based clustering for expression data via a dirichlet process mixture model. Bayesian Inference for Gene Expression and Proteomics **4**, 201–218 (2006)
7. Gao, X., Shen, W., Zhang, L., Hu, J., Fortin, N.J., Frostig, R.D., Ombao, H.: Regularized matrix data clustering and its application to image analysis. Biometrics **77**(3), 890–902 (2021)
8. Guhaniyogi, R., Qamar, S., Dunson, D.B.: Bayesian tensor regression. J. Mach. Learn. Res. **18**(1), 2733–2763 (2017)
9. Gupta, A., Nagar, D.: Matrix Variate Distributions, 1st edn. Chapman and Hall/CRC, New York (1999)
10. Hastie, T., Tibshirani, R., Friedman, J.H., Friedman, J.H.: The Elements of Statistical Learning: Data Mining, Inference, and Prediction, vol. 2. Springer, Berlin
11. Heo, J., Baek, J.: A penalized matrix normal mixture model for clustering matrix data. Entropy **23**(10), 1249 (2021)
12. Hu, W., Pan, T., Kong, D., Shen, W.: Nonparametric matrix response regression with application to brain imaging data analysis. Biometrics **77**(4), 1227–1240 (2021)
13. Hu, W., Shen, W., Zhou, H., Kong, D.: Matrix linear discriminant analysis. Technometrics **62**(2), 196–205 (2020)
14. Huang, S., Li, J., Sun, L., Ye, J., Fleisher, A., Wu, T., Chen, K., Reiman, E., Initiative, A.D.N., et al.: Learning brain connectivity of alzheimer's disease by sparse inverse covariance estimation. NeuroImage **50**(3), 935–949 (2010)
15. Lee, I., Sinha, D., Mai, Q., Zhang, X., Bandyopadhyay, D.: Bayesian regression analysis of skewed tensor responses. Biometrics **79**(3), 1814–1825 (2023)
16. Lee, J.H., Kim, E.K., Hong, A.R., Roh, E., Bae, J.H., Kim, J.H., Shin, C.S., Kim, S.Y., Kim, S.W.: Radiographic characteristics of adrenal masses in oncologic patients. Endocrinol. Metab. **31**(1), 147–152 (2016)
17. Lee, K., Jo, S., Lee, J.: The beta-mixture shrinkage prior for sparse covariances with near-minimax posterior convergence rate. J. Multivar. Anal. **192**, 105067 (2022)
18. Li, J., Mai, Q.: Model-based tensor low-rank clustering. J. Comput. Graph. Stat. **33**(1), 208–218 (2024)
19. Li, X., Guindani, M., Ng, C.S., Hobbs, B.P.: A Bayesian nonparametric model for textural pattern heterogeneity. J. R. Stat. Soc.: Ser. C: Appl. Stat. **70**(2), 459–480 (2021)
20. Lijoi, A., Nipoti, B., Prünster, I.: Dependent mixture models: clustering and borrowing information. Comput. Stat. Data Anal. **71**, 417–433 (2014)
21. Mai, Q., Zhang, X., Pan, Y., Deng, K.: A doubly enhanced em algorithm for model-based tensor clustering. J. Am. Stat. Assoc. **117**(540), 2120–2134 (2022)
22. Miller, J.W., Harrison, M.T.: Mixture models with a prior on the number of components. J. Am. Stat. Assoc. **113**(521), 340–356 (2018)
23. Ng, A., Jordan, M., Weiss, Y.: On spectral clustering: Analysis and an algorithm. Adv. Neural Inf. Proces. Syst. **14**, 849–856 (2001)
24. Pitman, J.: Some developments of the blackwell-macqueen urn scheme. In: Lecture Notes-Monograph Series, pp. 245–267 (1996)

25. Ramlatchan, A., Yang, M., Liu, Q., Li, M., Wang, J., Li, Y.: A survey of matrix completion methods for recommendation systems. Big Data Min. Anal. **1**(4), 308–323 (2018)
26. Rao, N., Cox, C., Nowak, R., Rogers, T.T.: Sparse overlapping sets lasso for multitask learning and its application to fmri analysis. Adv. Neural Inf. Proces. Syst. **26**, 2202–2210 (2013)
27. Rosol, T.J., Yarrington, J.T., Latendresse, J., Capen, C.C.: Adrenal gland: structure, function, and mechanisms of toxicity. Toxicol. Pathol. **29**(1), 41–48 (2001)
28. Ruan, L., Yuan, M., Zou, H.: Regularized parameter estimation in high-dimensional gaussian mixture models. Neural Comput. **23**(6), 1605–1622 (2011)
29. Santos, J.M., Embrechts, M.: On the use of the adjusted rand index as a metric for evaluating supervised classification. In: International Conference on Artificial Neural Networks, pp. 175–184. Springer, Berlin
30. Shi, Y., Shen, W.: Bayesian methods in tensor analysis. *arXiv preprint arXiv:2302.05978* (2023)
31. Sun, W.W., Hao, B., Li, L.: Tensors in modern statistical learning. In: Wiley StatsRef: Statistics Reference Online [Internet], pp. 1–25. Wiley, New York (2021)
32. Viroli, C.: Model Based Clustering for Three-way Data Structures (2011)
33. Viroli, C.: On matrix-variate regression analysis. J. Multivar. Anal. **111**, 296–309 (2012)
34. Wang, Y.-X., Zhang, Y.-J.: Nonnegative matrix factorization: a comprehensive review. IEEE Trans. Knowl. Data Eng. **25**(6), 1336–1353 (2012)
35. Wanis, K.N., Kanthan, R.: Diagnostic and prognostic features in adrenocortical carcinoma: a single institution case series and review of the literature. World J. Surg. Oncol. **13**(1), 1–13 (2015)
36. Xie, F., Cape, J., Priebe, C.E., Xu, Y.: Bayesian sparse spiked covariance model with a continuous matrix shrinkage prior. Bayesian Anal. **17**(4), 1193–1217 (2022)
37. Yamashita, R., Nishio, M., Do, R.K.G., Togashi, K.: Convolutional neural networks: an overview and application in radiology. Insights Imaging **9**, 611–629 (2018)
38. Yin, F., Hu, G., Shen, W.: Analysis of professional basketball field goal attempts via a Bayesian matrix clustering approach. J. Comput. Graph. Stat. **32**(1), 49–60 (2022)
39. Zhang, J., Sun, W.W., Li, L.: Generalized connectivity matrix response regression with applications in brain connectivity studies. J. Comput. Graph. Stat. **32**(1), 252–262 (2023)
40. Zhang, Y., Shen, W., Kong, D.: Covariance estimation for matrix-valued data. J. Am. Stat. Assoc. **118**(544), 2620–2631 (2023)
41. Zhou, H., Li, L.: Regularized matrix regression. J. R. Stat. Soc. Ser. B Stat Methodol. **76**(2), 463–483 (2014)

Bayesian Kernel-Based Modeling and Selection of Genetic Pathways and Genes in Cancer Studies: A Step Toward Targeted Treatment Protocols

Sounak Chakraborty, Zhenyu Wang, and Bimal Ray

Abstract Much attention has been given recently to the development of methods that utilize the large quantity of genetic information available in online databases. Most of the proposed methods look at the entire set of genes and their impact on a disease. Recently a new philosophy emerged which considers using the information available as the genetic pathways, which contain sets of genes and produces a combined effect on a disease. With this newly acquired biological knowledge about pathways the goal is to identify the significant genetic pathways and the corresponding influential genes within a pathway in regard to different diseases. This directly benefits patients by providing targeted treatments based on gene pathway-specific therapies.

In this paper we propose a Bayesian kernel machine model which can incorporate existing information on genetic pathways and gene networks in the analysis of DNA microarray data. The overall effect of each pathway is modeled nonparametrically using a reproducing kernel Hilbert space. Multiple pathways are modeled simultaneously using the additive model structure. The pathway and the gene selection within a pathway is done with the help of mixture priors on the pathway indicator variables and the gene indicator variables, respectively. Our proposed kernel-based method provides a very flexible modeling framework to model both linear and nonlinear pathway effects. It can pinpoint the important pathways along with the active genes within each individual important pathways. An efficient Markov chain Monte Carlo algorithm is developed to fit our proposed model. The effectiveness of our method

---

S. Chakraborty (✉)
Department of Statistics, University of Missouri, Columbia, MO, USA
e-mail: ChakrabortyS@Missouri.edu

Z. Wang
Pfizer Pharmaceuticals, Cambridge, MA, USA

B. Ray
Department of Veterinary Pathobiology, University of Missouri, Columbia, MO, USA
e-mail: RayB@Missouri.edu

Y. Zhao, D.-G. Chen (eds.), *Big Data Analytics in Biostatistics and Bioinformatics*, ICSA Book Series in Statistics,
https://doi.org/10.1007/978-3-032-06649-7_8

is illustrated though several simulation studies and a real data analysis with right-censored survival outcomes.

Keywords Bayesian variable selection · Biological pathways · Survival outcome · Markov chain Monte Carlo · Microarray · Reproducing kernel Hilbert space

1 Introduction

In the last 15 years DNA microarray data have been extensively used for cancer staging, classification, and outcome modeling [10]. A significant part of that effort is to identify or detect a handful of important genes (out of a large number of genes) related to the disease. However, gene selection may not be enough for a complex disease like cancer because often it is noticed that the cancer is not caused by a single gene but a collection of genes and their interactions among themselves. Recent studies showed that cancer is the result of deregulation of one or more signaling pathways which are caused by one or several set(s) of gene mutation [13, 22]. Therefore, focusing just on one pathway or a few pathways might not be enough [7]. Research directed toward identifying pathways related to a disease and detecting relevant genes within an important pathway has generated lots of interest in the last couple of years. Targeting disease relevant pathways will help in reducing trial and error-based treatment decisions when we only consider individual gene sets, and it would eventually reduce the burdens on a patient associated both in terms of health and cost.

A genetic pathway can be described as a set of genes and the map of their specific interactions. These interactions together execute certain biological functions. Biological mechanisms are more related to moderate changes in several genes than dramatic change in a single gene. There are several public and commercial pathway and gene databases, for instance, Gene Ontology (GO) (http://www.geneontology.org/) and Kyoto Encyclopedia of Genes and Genomes (KEGG) (http://www.kegg.jp/), having the information for pathways and their related genes. These databases accumulated the biological gene research knowledge over the years and reveal signaling, metabolic, or regulatory pathways. Figure 1 is steroid hormone biosynthesis pathway from KEGG (http://www.kegg.jp/).

Recent studies show gene expression data are analyzed using pathway information and/or gene-gene network information [25]. Park et al. [21] tried to predict survival time using GO annotation. Telesca et al. [27] attempted to use the prior information about the dependent gene relation in pathways to make inferences about the mean difference in expression data across phenotypes. Liu et al. [19] consider a semiparametric regression model with covariates and a genetic pathway. The covariates are modeled parametrically and the genes in the pathway are modeled using least squares kernel machines (LSKMS). Stingo et al. [25] proposed a Bayesian model to find out relevant pathways and genes related to breast cancer

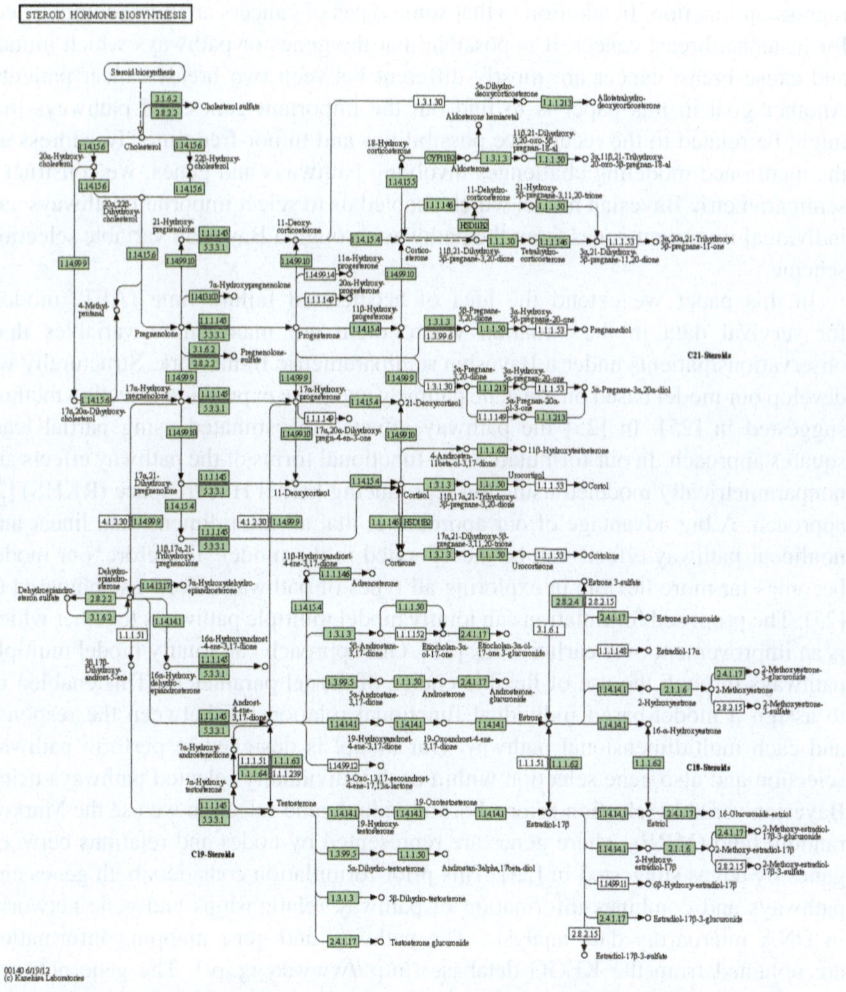

Fig. 1 Steroid hormone biosynthesis pathway from KEGG database

by using the metastasis time and the information of pathway memberships and gene networks in the analysis of DNA microarray data. Their method incorporates both pathway-gene relation and gene-gene relation to find the disease-related pathways and genes simultaneously.

All the abovementioned methods predict the outcome using gene expression data by assuming that they have a certain type of relationship. However, the interactions among the genes in one pathway are very complex and the functional form of the overall pathway effects is not clearly understood. One of our primary goal in this paper is to model the overall pathway effects of a genetic pathway without specifying any restrictive linear or nonlinear structure on the multidimensional regression function. In addition to that some types of cancers are more complicated, for instance, breast cancer. It is possible that the genes or pathways which mutate and cause breast cancer are mostly different between two breast cancer patients. Another goal in this paper is to find out the important genes and pathways that might be related to the recurrence possibilities and tumor-free time. To address all the mentioned modeling challenges involving pathways and genes, we construct a semiparametric Bayesian model which enabled us to select important pathways and individual important genes from the pathway through a Bayesian variable selection scheme.

In this paper we extend the idea of accelerated failure time (AFT) models for survival data in the situation where there are many more variables than observations/patients under a Bayesian semiparametric framework. Structurally we develop our model based on the gene pathway and gene expression selection method suggested in [25]. In [25] the pathway effects are estimated using partial least squares approach. In our formulation the functional forms of the pathway effects are nonparametrically modeled using the reproducing kernel Hilbert space (RKHS) [2] approach. A big advantage of our approach is that all multidimensional linear and nonlinear pathway effects can be incorporated in the model. Therefore, our model becomes far more flexible in exploring all types of pathway effects as compared to [25]. The proposed formulation can jointly model multiple pathways together which is an improvement over earlier work [27]. Our approach can jointly model multiple pathways through the use of flexible choice of kernel parameters. This enabled us to assign a model-based individual functional relationship between the response and each multidimensional pathway. Our model is designed to perform pathway selection and also gene selection within each individually selected pathways using Bayesian variable selection priors. For individual gene selection we use the Markov random field (MRF), where genes are represented by nodes and relations between genes by edges suggested in [25]. This prior formulation considers both genes and pathways and combines information of pathway relationships and gene networks in DNA microarray data analysis. The pathway and gene mapping information are obtained from the KEGG database (http://www.kegg.jp/). The gene network information is used to define Markov random field prior to further explore the gene-gene network/interaction structure within each pathway. We use [29] data set and several simulated data sets to illustrate the effectiveness and utility of our proposed model.

The rest of the paper is organized as follows. In Sect. 2 we have introduced our RKHS-based semiparametric Bayesian model. The step-by-step MCMC algorithm for implementation and model fitting is introduced in Sect. 3. In Sect. 4 we provide two simulation studies and compare the performance of our proposed model against the method proposed by Stingo et al. [25]. The application of the model on the [29] data set is discussed in Sect. 5. Finally, some discussion and concluding remarks are made in Sect. 6.

2 Bayesian Kernel-Based Accelerated Failure Time Model for Simultaneous Pathway and Gene Selection

In modern medical statistics we often have to deal with time-to-event data, otherwise known as survival outcome. Frequently such survival data is hard to analyze with regular regression tools because of the presence of censored observations. Censoring may happen if a patient has not experienced the relevant outcome, such as relapse or death, by the time of the close of the study or a patient is lost to follow-up during the study period. This is also known as right censoring. In survival analysis censoring represents a particular type of missing data and it is an important issue which requires special attention in order to avoid any bias [23].

Accelerated failure time (AFT) models [17] assume multiplicative effect of the covariates on the survival time. It can be used as alternative to the popular Cox proportional hazard model [5]. Cox regression is based on the multiplicative effect on the hazard functions and so it is hard to interpret the regression coefficients in a Cox proportional hazard model, whereas the AFT model is based on the multiplicative effect on the survival times and it can suggest more direct physical interpretation with the regression parameters. For that reason AFT models are often considered more appealing over the Cox proportional hazard model [17]. A simple AFT model can be written as:

$$\log(\boldsymbol{T}_i) = \alpha + \boldsymbol{x}_i'\boldsymbol{\beta} + \epsilon_i, \qquad i = 1, \cdots, n, \tag{1}$$

where $\boldsymbol{T}_i$ is the survival time, α is the intercept, p-vector $\boldsymbol{x}_i$ is the covariates, p-vector $\boldsymbol{\beta}$ is the regression parameters corresponding to the covariates, and ϵ_i's are the error terms which are independent and identically distributed random variables with a common distribution. In (1) the covariates are most commonly modeled using a simple linear predictor.

Let us consider a data set consists of n subjects. For the subject i, we have the survival time t_i and c_i as the censoring time independent of t_i. Then $\delta_i = I\{t_i \le c_i\}$ is the censoring indicator function and $t_i^* = \min(t_i, c_i)$. To fit (1) we can impute the censored data by using the [26] data augmentation approach. Let $\boldsymbol{Y} = (y_1, y_2, \cdots, y_n)'$, and y_i is the augmented data as:

$$\begin{cases} y_i = \log(t_i^*) & \text{if} \quad \delta_i = 1 \\ y_i > \log(t_i^*) & \text{if} \quad \delta_i = 0 \end{cases} \tag{2}$$

Let us consider we have J number of pathways and $\boldsymbol{X}_i^j$, $j = 1, \ldots, J$ is the gene expressions from the genes in the j-th pathway for the i-th individual. In this article we introduce a flexible nonlinear modeling of the pathway-specific covariates in model (1) by introducing functions as $\boldsymbol{f}_i = (f_1(\boldsymbol{X}_i^1), f_2(\boldsymbol{X}_i^2), \cdots, f_J(\boldsymbol{X}_i^J))$, $j = 1, 2, \cdots, J$. Note that $f_j(\boldsymbol{X}_i^j)$ represents the overall effect of the pathway j with gene set $\boldsymbol{X}_i^j$ and J is the total number of the pathways. Therefore, the linear and nonlinear effect of each group of genes in a pathway is modeled via the more general pathway-specific functions/effects $f_j(\boldsymbol{X}_i^j)$. Assuming the error term is *iid* following standard normal distribution, model (1) becomes:

$$Y_i = \alpha + f_1(\boldsymbol{X}_i^1) + \cdots + f_J(\boldsymbol{X}_i^J) + e_i, \quad e_i \overset{\text{iid}}{\sim} N(0, \sigma^2) \tag{3}$$

In the above formulated model 3 we jointly model the effect of J pathways and each pathway effect can have nonlinear flexible structure via nonparametric modeling of the function $f_j()$. Here we adopt reproducing kernel Hilbert space (RKHS) approach to model each pathway-specific function $f_j(\boldsymbol{X}_i^j)$. A Hilbert space is a vector space H with an inner product $\langle g_1, g_2 \rangle$ and the norm $\|g_1\| = \langle g_1, g_1 \rangle^{1/2}$. A RKHS H_K is a Hilbert space of "smooth" functions defined by a kernel $K()$. In a RHKS, there exists a function $K : T \times T \to \mathcal{R}$ with the properties:

- $K(\cdot, \boldsymbol{x}) \in H$.
- For any $g \in H$ and $\boldsymbol{x} \in T$, $\langle K(\cdot, \boldsymbol{x}), g(\cdot) \rangle = g(\boldsymbol{x})$.

Following the representation theorem [16], we have pathway-specific nonlinear function

$$f_j(\boldsymbol{X}_i^j) = \sum_{l=1}^{n} \beta_l^j K(\boldsymbol{X}_i^j, \boldsymbol{X}_l^j | \theta_j), j = 1, \ldots, J, \tag{4}$$

where $K(\boldsymbol{X}_i^j, \boldsymbol{X}_l^j \mid \theta_j)$ is the chosen kernel, $\theta_j > 0$ is the kernel parameter for the j-th pathway, and β_l^j is the kernel coefficients. In our paper, we choose a Gaussian kernel as below:

$$K(\boldsymbol{X}_i^j, \boldsymbol{X}_l^j \mid \theta_j) = \exp\left(-\frac{\|\boldsymbol{X}_i^j - \boldsymbol{X}_l^j\|}{\theta_j} \right) \tag{5}$$

Therefore, inserting (4) in (3) in the kernel representation, we can write our model as:

$$\boldsymbol{Y} = \alpha \mathbf{1}_n + \mathcal{K}\boldsymbol{B} + \boldsymbol{e} \qquad \boldsymbol{e} \sim N(\mathbf{0}, \sigma^2 \boldsymbol{I}_n) \tag{6}$$

where $\boldsymbol{Y} = (y_1, y_2, \cdots, y_n)'$; $\mathcal{K}$ is $n \times n \cdot J$ matrix,

$$\mathcal{K} = \begin{pmatrix} K(\boldsymbol{X}_1^1, \boldsymbol{X}_1^1|\theta_1) & K(\boldsymbol{X}_1^1, \boldsymbol{X}_2^1|\theta_1) & \cdots & K(\boldsymbol{X}_1^1, \boldsymbol{X}_n^1|\theta_1) & \cdots & K(\boldsymbol{X}_1^J, \boldsymbol{X}_n^J|\theta_J) \\ K(\boldsymbol{X}_2^1, \boldsymbol{X}_1^1|\theta_1) & K(\boldsymbol{X}_2^1, \boldsymbol{X}_2^1|\theta_1) & \cdots & K(\boldsymbol{X}_2^1, \boldsymbol{X}_n^1|\theta_1) & \cdots & K(\boldsymbol{X}_2^J, \boldsymbol{X}_n^J|\theta_J) \\ \vdots & \vdots & \ddots & \vdots & \ddots & \vdots \\ K(\boldsymbol{X}_n^1, \boldsymbol{X}_1^1|\theta_1) & K(\boldsymbol{X}_n^1, \boldsymbol{X}_2^1|\theta_1) & \cdots & K(\boldsymbol{X}_n^1, \boldsymbol{X}_n^1|\theta_1) & \cdots & K(\boldsymbol{X}_n^J, \boldsymbol{X}_n^J|\theta_J); \end{pmatrix} \tag{7}$$

and B is $n \cdot J$ vector,

$$\boldsymbol{B}^T = \left(\beta_1^1, \beta_2^1, \cdots, \beta_n^1, \beta_1^2, \beta_2^2, \cdots, \beta_n^2, \cdots \beta_1^J, \beta_2^J, \cdots, \beta_n^J\right) \tag{8}$$

This implies that after the selection of kernels we are transforming the data from the covariate space to kernel space and our model (6) can be viewed as linear in terms of kernel $K()$ but nonlinear in terms of the original covariate $\boldsymbol{x}$. The information from KEGG database (http://www.kegg.jp/)is used to construct two matrices, $\boldsymbol{S}$ and $\boldsymbol{R}$. The $\boldsymbol{S}$ is a $J \times p$ matrix representing the relationship between genes and pathways [25], where the pathway membership of each gene is stored. If gene k belongs to pathway j, in our S matrix we have $s_{jk} = 1$; otherwise, $s_{jk} = 0$, where $k = 1, \ldots, p$ and $j = 1, \ldots, J$. Matrix $\boldsymbol{R}$ is $(p \times p)$ that indicates the relationship between genes. We consider two types of gene-gene relationships in our model. The first one is the genes whose coded proteins combine and form a protein compound. If gene k_1 and k_2 are of that type, we set $r_{k_1,k_2} = 1$ in R [18]. The other relationship between genes is that proteins coded by those genes signal each other and, in this case, $r_{k_1,k_2} = q$, where $q > 0$. And $r_{k_1,k_2} = 0$ otherwise.

2.1 *Priors for Model Parameters*

Suppose the t_i's follow a log-normal distribution, the augmented data y_i's in (6) are normally distributed as:

$$\boldsymbol{Y}|\mathcal{K}, \alpha, \boldsymbol{B}, \sigma^2 \sim \mathcal{N}(\alpha\boldsymbol{1} + \mathcal{K}\boldsymbol{B}, \sigma^2\boldsymbol{I}_n) \tag{9}$$

where $\boldsymbol{I}$ is the identity matrix.

The conjugate priors for the above model are given by

$$\begin{aligned} \alpha|\sigma^2 &\sim \mathcal{N}(\alpha_0, a_\alpha), \\ \boldsymbol{B}|\sigma^2 &\sim \mathcal{N}(\boldsymbol{B}_0, a_B\sigma^2\boldsymbol{I}_{n\times J}), \\ \sigma^2 &\sim \mathcal{IG}(\nu_0/2, \nu_0\sigma_0^2/2), \end{aligned} \tag{10}$$

where the hyperparameters are α_0, a_α, $\boldsymbol{B}_0$, a_B, ν_0, and σ_0. We set $\alpha_0 = 0$ and $\boldsymbol{B}_0 = \boldsymbol{0}$. All other prior parameters are set such that the prior distribution is near-diffuse/weakly informative but proper. More detail description of prior parameter choices are provided in Sect. 4.

2.2 *Marginal Likelihood of the Augmented Data*

To simplify the calculation, we integrate out α, $\boldsymbol{B}$, and σ^2.

- First, we integrate out $\boldsymbol{B}$

$$\begin{aligned}
p(\boldsymbol{Y}|\boldsymbol{X}, \mathcal{K}, \alpha, \sigma^2) &= \int p(\boldsymbol{Y}, \boldsymbol{B}|\boldsymbol{X}, \mathcal{K}, \alpha, \sigma^2) d\boldsymbol{B} \\
&= \int p(\boldsymbol{Y}|\boldsymbol{X}, \mathcal{K}, \boldsymbol{B}, \alpha, \sigma^2) p(\boldsymbol{B}|\sigma^2) d\boldsymbol{B} \\
&\propto \frac{1}{(\sigma^2)^{n/2}} \exp\left[-\frac{(\boldsymbol{Y} - \mathcal{K}\boldsymbol{B})^T(\boldsymbol{Y} - \mathcal{K}\boldsymbol{B})}{2\sigma^2}\right] \\
&\times \frac{1}{(a_B\sigma^2)^{Jn/2}} \exp\left[-\frac{\boldsymbol{B}^T\boldsymbol{B}}{2a_B\sigma^2}\right] d\boldsymbol{B} \\
&\propto \frac{1}{(\sigma^2)^{n/2}} \exp\left(\frac{\boldsymbol{Y}^T(I + a_\beta \mathcal{K}\mathcal{K}^T)^{-1}\boldsymbol{Y}}{2\sigma^2}\right)
\end{aligned} \tag{11}$$

- We integrate out α

$$\begin{aligned}
p(\boldsymbol{Y}|\boldsymbol{X}, \mathcal{K}, \sigma^2) &= \int p(\boldsymbol{Y}, \alpha|\boldsymbol{X}, \mathcal{K}, \sigma^2) d\alpha \\
&= \int p(\boldsymbol{Y}|\boldsymbol{X}, \mathcal{K}\alpha, \sigma^2) p(\alpha|\sigma^2) d\alpha \\
&\propto \int \frac{1}{(\sigma^2)^{n/2}} \exp\left(\frac{\boldsymbol{Y}^T(I + a_{beta}\mathcal{K}\mathcal{K}^T)^{-1}\boldsymbol{Y}}{2\sigma^2}\right) \frac{1}{(a_\alpha\sigma^2)^{1/2}} \\
&\times \exp\left(-\frac{\alpha^2}{2a_\alpha\sigma^2}\right) d\alpha \\
&\propto \frac{1}{(\sigma^2)^{n/2}} \exp\left(-\frac{\boldsymbol{Y}^T(I_n + a_\alpha \boldsymbol{1}^T\boldsymbol{1} + a_\beta \mathcal{K}\mathcal{K}^T)^{-1}\boldsymbol{Y}^T}{2\sigma^2}\right)
\end{aligned} \tag{12}$$

- Finally, we integrate out σ^2

$$\begin{aligned}
p(\boldsymbol{Y}|\boldsymbol{X}, \mathcal{K}) &= \int p(\boldsymbol{Y}, \sigma^2|\boldsymbol{X}, \mathcal{K}) d\sigma^2 \\
&= \int p(\boldsymbol{Y}|\boldsymbol{X}, \mathcal{K}, \sigma^2) p(\sigma^2) d\sigma^2 \\
&\propto \int (\sigma^2)^{-\nu_0/2-1} \exp\left(-\frac{\nu_0\sigma_0^2/2}{\sigma^2}\right) \frac{1}{(\sigma^2)^{n/2}}
\end{aligned} \tag{13}$$

$$\exp\left(-\frac{\boldsymbol{Y}^T(I_n + a_\alpha \boldsymbol{1}^T\boldsymbol{1} + a_\beta \mathcal{K}\mathcal{K}^T)^{-1}\boldsymbol{Y}^T}{2\sigma^2}\right) d\sigma^2$$

$$\propto (\nu_0\sigma_0^2 + \boldsymbol{Y}^T(I_n + a_\alpha \boldsymbol{1}^T\boldsymbol{1} + a_\beta \mathcal{K}\mathcal{K}^T)^{-1}\boldsymbol{Y}^T)^{-\nu_0/2-n/2}$$

2.3 Mixture Priors for Variable Selection

The regression coefficient $\boldsymbol{B}$ in Eq. (6) can be written as:

$$\boldsymbol{B}^T = (\boldsymbol{\beta}_1^T, \boldsymbol{\beta}_2^T, \cdots, \boldsymbol{\beta}_J^T), \tag{14}$$

where $\boldsymbol{\beta}_j$ measures the effect of pathway j and the role of the kernel coefficients in Eq. (4). However, it is to be noted that not all pathways are related to the dependent variable. So in order to identify the important pathways, we assign special Bayesian variable selection priors on $\boldsymbol{\beta}_j$. Our formulation is a direct extension of [9] which arises from a scale mixture of a point mass at 0 and a multivariate normal distribution is described as follows:

$$\boldsymbol{\beta}^j|\phi_j, \sigma^2 \sim \phi_j \mathcal{N}(\boldsymbol{0}, a_\beta\sigma^2\boldsymbol{I}_n) + (1-\phi_j)\mathcal{I}(0) \tag{15}$$

where ϕ_j's are independent Bernoulli random variables. If the pathway j is not related to the dependent variable Y, then all coefficients related to the pathway j, ($\boldsymbol{\beta}_j$), are all set to 0. This in turn makes the entire nonlinear function go to 0 in Eq. (4). This can be interpreted as the overall pathway effect.

2.4 Priors for Pathway and Gene Selection Indicators

From the previous subsection, we know ϕ_j is the pathway selection indicator for j. Let $\boldsymbol{\phi}$ be the pathway selection indicator, and $\boldsymbol{\phi} = (\phi_1, \phi_2, \cdots, \phi_J)$.

$$\begin{cases} \phi_j = 1 & \text{when pathway is } j \text{ selected in the model} \\ \phi_j = 0 & \text{otherwise} \end{cases} \tag{16}$$

We use the independent Bernoulli priors for the pathway selection similarly as done in [25]:

$$p(\boldsymbol{\phi}|\omega_j) = \prod_{j=1}^{J} \omega_j^{\phi_j}(1-\omega_j)^{1-\phi_j} \tag{17}$$

where ω_j is a constant, which represents the a priori probability of pathway j in the model.

Let the gene selection indicator be denoted by $\boldsymbol{\gamma} = (\gamma_1, \gamma_2, \cdots, \gamma_p)^T$, where the i-th gene is selected if $\gamma_i = 1$. We want to construct a prior distribution on γ such that it is able to consider both the pathway membership of each gene (S) and the biological relationships between genes (R). We model these relations using a Markov random field (MRF) suggested in [25]. Our formulation of MRF is an extension of [25], as mentioned before; we consider two types of gene relationships (last paragraph before Sect. 2.1). For the sake of easy understanding of the basic properties and structure of MRF, we include some details about MRF which can also be found in [25]. A MRF is a set of random variables with a Markov property described by an undirected graph. If two genes are not related, they are considered to be conditionally independent given all other genes [3]. The following probability indicates the connections on the MRF of our γ parameter.

$$p(\gamma_k|\eta, \gamma_l, l \in N_k) = \frac{\exp(\gamma_k F(\gamma_k))}{1 + \exp(\gamma_k F(\gamma_k))}, \tag{18}$$

where $F(\gamma_k) = (\mu + \eta \sum_{l \in N_k} \gamma_k)$ and N_k is the set of genes in the same protein compound of gene k and genes that receive/send signal from/to gene k in the MRF given that the pathways of those genes are in the model. The global distribution on the MRF can be expressed as:

$$p(\boldsymbol{\gamma}|\boldsymbol{\phi}) \propto \exp\left(\mu \mathbf{1}_p^T \boldsymbol{\gamma} + \eta \boldsymbol{\gamma}^T \boldsymbol{R} \boldsymbol{\gamma}\right), \tag{19}$$

where matrix $\boldsymbol{R}$ is introduced in the last paragraph before Sect. 2.1, μ is the parameter that relates to the sparsity of the model, and η controls the prior probability of gene selection depending on how many of its related genes are selected. Here η sets the smoothness of the distribution of $\boldsymbol{\gamma}$ over the undirected graph. If a protein from one gene is isolated, then its prior distribution formula (18) becomes a Bernoulli distribution with $p = \exp(\mu)/[1+\exp(\mu)]$. On the other hand, the higher values of η are, the more likely a gene is selected if many of its related genes are already in the model.

Following [25] we impose three restrictions to ensure both interpretability and identifiability of our model. They are as follows:

- No empty pathways, which means no case where a pathway is selected but none of its member genes are in the model.
- No orphan genes, which means no case when a gene is selected in the model but none of the pathways having this gene are in the model.
- No two pathways can have the same set of selected genes in the model.

Given these three restrictions, some of the combination of $\boldsymbol{\phi}$ and $\boldsymbol{\gamma}$ will not be allowed in the model. The joint prior distribution of $(\boldsymbol{\phi}, \boldsymbol{\gamma})$ is:

$$p(\boldsymbol{\phi}, \boldsymbol{\gamma}) \propto \begin{cases} \prod_{j=1}^{J} \omega_j^{\phi_j} (1-\omega_j)^{1-\phi_j} \exp(\mu \mathbf{1}_p^T \boldsymbol{\gamma} + \eta \boldsymbol{\gamma}^T \boldsymbol{R} \boldsymbol{\gamma}) & \text{for valid configurations} \\ 0 & \text{for invalid configurations} \end{cases} \quad (20)$$

2.5 *Prior for the Kernel Parameters*

In our model (4) each pathway has the flexibility of having its own kernel parameter θ_j $(j = 1, \ldots, J)$. The kernel parameter θ_J controls the shape and nonlinearity of each pathway effect. So by this construction we can have different nonlinear structure for each pathway. In this paper we adopted Gaussian kernel (5) and for its θ_j parameter we assign a uniform prior distribution as:

$$p(\theta_j) = \frac{1}{d_{\theta_j} - c_{\theta_j}}, j = 1, \ldots, J \quad (21)$$

We only consider the θ_j's for which the corresponding pathways are in the model, so the overall joint distribution of the kernel parameters is given by:

$$p(\boldsymbol{\theta}) = \begin{cases} \prod_{j \in \mathcal{J}} \frac{1}{d_{\theta_j} - c_{\theta_j}} & \mathcal{J} \text{ is the subset of pathways that are in the model} \\ 0 & \text{otherwise} \end{cases} \quad (22)$$

2.6 *Marginal Posterior Probabilities*

After integrating out $(\alpha, \boldsymbol{\beta}, \sigma^2)$ in Sect. 2.2, our model has the following remaining parameters $(\boldsymbol{\phi}, \boldsymbol{\gamma}, \boldsymbol{\theta})$. Conditioning on $(\boldsymbol{\phi}, \boldsymbol{\gamma}, \boldsymbol{\theta})$, (13) can be written as:

$$f(\boldsymbol{Y}|\boldsymbol{X}, \mathcal{K}, \boldsymbol{\phi}, \boldsymbol{\gamma}, \boldsymbol{\theta}) \propto (\nu_0 \sigma_0^2 + \boldsymbol{Y}^T (I_n + a_\alpha \mathbf{1}^T \mathbf{1} + a_\beta \mathcal{K}\mathcal{K}^T)^{-1} \boldsymbol{Y}^T)^{-\nu_0/2 - n/2} \quad (23)$$

This is a multivariate t-distribution

$$\boldsymbol{Y}|\boldsymbol{X}, \mathcal{K}, \boldsymbol{\phi}, \boldsymbol{\gamma}, \boldsymbol{\theta} \sim \mathcal{T}_{\nu_0}[\mathbf{0}, \sigma_0(I_n + a_\alpha \mathbf{1}^T \mathbf{1} + a_\beta \mathcal{K}\mathcal{K}^T)] \quad (24)$$

with truncation given by censoring indicator in (2). When y_i is censored with $\delta_i = 0$, it follows a univariate truncated t-distribution and can be updated by Gibbs sampling.

The joint posterior probability distribution of the pathway and gene selection indicators is given by:

$$f(\boldsymbol{\phi}, \boldsymbol{\gamma} | \boldsymbol{Y}, \boldsymbol{X}, \mathcal{K}, \boldsymbol{\theta}) \propto f(\boldsymbol{Y} | \boldsymbol{X}, \mathcal{K}, \boldsymbol{\phi}, \boldsymbol{\gamma}, \boldsymbol{\theta}) \cdot p(\boldsymbol{\phi}, \boldsymbol{\gamma}) \tag{25}$$

Similarly, the posterior probability distribution of kernel parameter is

$$f(\boldsymbol{\theta} | \boldsymbol{Y}, \boldsymbol{X}, \mathcal{K}, \boldsymbol{\phi}, \boldsymbol{\gamma}) \propto f(\boldsymbol{Y} | \boldsymbol{X}, \mathcal{K}, \boldsymbol{\phi}, \boldsymbol{\gamma}, \boldsymbol{\theta}) \cdot p(\boldsymbol{\theta}) \tag{26}$$

3 MCMC Algorithm and Posterior Inference Framework

In our model described in Sect. 2 after marginalizing over $(\alpha, \boldsymbol{\beta}, \sigma^2)$, there are only $\boldsymbol{\phi}, \boldsymbol{\gamma}, \boldsymbol{\theta}$ parameters left in the model. We develop a two-step MCMC scheme to sample from the posterior distribution of $\boldsymbol{\phi}, \boldsymbol{\gamma}, \boldsymbol{\theta}$ as follows:

- Step 1: Sample pathway and gene selection indicators from $p(\boldsymbol{\phi}, \boldsymbol{\gamma} | \boldsymbol{Y}, \boldsymbol{X}, \mathcal{K}, \boldsymbol{\theta})$
- Step 2: Sample kernel parameters from $p(\boldsymbol{\theta} | \boldsymbol{Y}, \boldsymbol{X}, \mathcal{K}, \boldsymbol{\phi}, \boldsymbol{\gamma})$

To fit our RKHS model, we will iterate between Step 1 and Step 2. As each step needs detailed attention, Step 1 details are provided in Sect. 3.1 and Step 2 details are provided in Sect. 3.2 separately. It is to be noted here that Sects. 3.1 and 3.2 are both part of the same posterior fitting algorithm. Structurally our MCMC fitting algorithm is similar to [25].

3.1 Step 1: MCMC Algorithm for Pathway and Gene Selection Indicators

We use Metropolis-Hastings algorithm to update the pathway and gene selection indicator parameter $(\boldsymbol{\phi}, \boldsymbol{\gamma})$. In order to select pathways and genes simultaneously and to make sure the selections follow the restrictions we set in Sect. 2.4, at each iteration we make our algorithm to choose one of the following three moves randomly.

3.1.1 Change the Indicator of Gene and Pathway at the Same Time

- Add a pathway and a gene.
  Randomly select a pathway from the subset of pathways that are not in the model and neither are their member genes, so $\phi_j^o = 0$ and $p_j^o = 0$, where p_j^o represents

the number of genes that are included in the model in pathway j. Then randomly select one gene k from the pathway j ($\gamma^o_{j,k} = 0$). Include both the pathway and gene in the model, so that $\phi^p_j = 1$ and $p^p_j = 1$. The proposed (ϕ^p_j, p^p_j) is accepted with probability:

$$\min\left\{1, \frac{f(\boldsymbol{\phi}^p, \boldsymbol{\gamma}^p|\boldsymbol{Y}, \boldsymbol{X}, \mathcal{K})}{f(\boldsymbol{\phi}^o, \boldsymbol{\gamma}^o|\boldsymbol{Y}, \boldsymbol{X}, \mathcal{K})} \cdot \frac{\omega_j \cdot \sum_{j=1}^J I\{\phi^o_j = 0, p^o_j = 0\}}{\sum_{j=1}^J I\{\phi^p_j = 1, p^p_j = 1, \text{C1}\}}\right\} \tag{27}$$

where C1 is clarified below.

- Remove a pathway and a gene.
  Find a subset of the pathways that are in the model and only one of their member genes is selected in the model. Randomly select one of them, so $\phi^o_j = 1$ and $p^o_j = 1$. In addition, the removal of the gene does not create identical subset of genes in different pathways, and this restriction is C1. Remove both the pathway and gene from the model, so that $\phi^p_j = 0$ and $p^p_j = 0$. The proposed (ϕ^p_j, p^p_j) is accepted with probability:

$$\min\left\{1, \frac{f(\boldsymbol{\phi}^p, \boldsymbol{\gamma}^p|\boldsymbol{Y}, \boldsymbol{X}, \mathcal{K})}{f(\boldsymbol{\phi}^o, \boldsymbol{\gamma}^o|\boldsymbol{Y}, \boldsymbol{X}, \mathcal{K})} \cdot \frac{\sum_{j=1}^J I\{\phi^o_j = 1, p^o_j = 1, \text{C1}\}}{\omega_j \cdot \sum_{j=1}^J I\{\phi^p_j = 0, p^p_j = 0\}}\right\} \tag{28}$$

3.1.2 Only Change the Indicator of Gene in an Included Pathway

- Add a gene in an included pathway.
  Find the subset ($\mathcal{J}$) of pathways that have some of their member genes, but not all, in the model. Randomly select one of them j, so $\phi_j = 1$ and $p^o_j < p_j$, where p_j represents the total number of genes in pathway j. And then randomly select one gene k from non-included genes from the pathway $j(\gamma^o_{j,k} = 0)$. Include the gene in the model, so that $\gamma^p_{j,k} = 1$. The proposed move is accepted with probability:

$$\min\left\{1, \frac{f(\boldsymbol{\phi}^o, \boldsymbol{\gamma}^p|\boldsymbol{Y}, \boldsymbol{X}, \mathcal{K})}{f(\boldsymbol{\phi}^o, \boldsymbol{\gamma}^o|\boldsymbol{Y}, \boldsymbol{X}, \mathcal{K})}\right.$$
$$\left.\cdot \frac{\sum_{j=1}^J I\{\phi^o_j = 1, p^o_j < p_j\} \cdot \sum_{j\in\mathcal{J}} \frac{1}{p^p_j(\text{C}2\gamma,\ \text{CI}2\gamma)}}{\sum_{j=1}^J I\{\phi^p_j = 1, p^p_j > 1, \text{C}2\theta,\ \text{CI}2\theta\} \sum_{j\in\mathcal{J}} \frac{1}{p_j - p^o_j}}\right\} \tag{29}$$

  where C2γ, CI2γ, C2θ, and CI2θ are clarified below.

- Remove a gene from an included pathway.

Find the subset ($\mathcal{J}$) of pathways that have more than one of their member genes in the model. And randomly select one of them j, so $\phi_j = 1$ and $p_j^o > 1$. Moreover, at least one of the included genes in the pathway j may not be the sole gene in other included pathways, so that removal of the gene does not create an empty pathway. Then these restrictions are corresponding to C2θ, CI2θ in (29) and (30). After the pathway is selected, the subset of the included member genes is the genes that are not solely representative in other included pathways. And this restrictions are corresponding to C2γ, CI2γ. A gene k is randomly selected from the subset to be removed. C2θ and C2γ ensure the restrictions of the combination of pathways and genes. The proposed move is accepted with probability:

$$\min\left\{1, \frac{f(\boldsymbol{\phi}^o, \boldsymbol{\gamma}^p|\boldsymbol{Y}, \boldsymbol{X}, \mathcal{K})}{f(\boldsymbol{\phi}^o, \boldsymbol{\gamma}^o|\boldsymbol{Y}, \boldsymbol{X}, \mathcal{K})} \cdot \frac{\sum_{j=1}^{J} I\{\phi_j^o = 1, p_j^o > 1, \text{C}2\theta,\ \text{CI}2\theta\} \sum_{j\in\mathcal{J}} \frac{1}{p_j - p_j^p}}{\sum_{j=1}^{J} I\{\phi_j^p = 1, p_j^p < p_j\} \cdot \sum_{j\in\mathcal{J}} \frac{1}{p_j^o(\text{C}2\gamma,\ \text{CI}2\gamma)}}\right\} \tag{30}$$

3.1.3 Only Change the Indicator of the Pathways Not the Genes

- Add a pathway.
  Find the subset of the non-included pathways that have some of the member genes included in the model, and randomly select a pathway j ($\phi_j^o = 0$ and $p_j^o \geq 0$). Change the status of the pathway j, $\phi_j^p = 1$. In addition, avoid selecting a pathway whose included genes are exactly the same as the included genes from an already included pathway. This restriction is corresponding to CI3. Include the pathway j in the model, $p_j^p = 1$. The proposed move is accepted with probability:

$$\min\left\{1, \frac{f(\boldsymbol{\phi}^p, \boldsymbol{\gamma}^o|\boldsymbol{Y}, \boldsymbol{X}, \mathcal{K})}{f(\boldsymbol{\phi}^o, \boldsymbol{\gamma}^o|\boldsymbol{Y}, \boldsymbol{X}, \mathcal{K})} \cdot \frac{\sum_{j=1}^{J} I\{\phi_j^o = 1, p_j^o \geq 1, \text{CI3}\}}{\sum_{j=1}^{J} I\{\phi_j^p = 1, p_j^p \geq 1, \text{C3}\}}\right\} \tag{31}$$

  where C3 is clarified below.
- Remove an included pathway.
  Find the subset of the included pathways that all of the included member genes are associated with other included pathways and randomly select one of them $j(\phi_j^o = 1$ and C3). This guarantees that no orphan gene is in the model. Remove

the pathway j from the model, $p_j^p = 0$. The proposed move is accepted with probability:

$$\min\left\{1, \frac{f(\boldsymbol{\phi}^p, \boldsymbol{\gamma}^o|\boldsymbol{Y}, \boldsymbol{X}, \mathcal{K})}{f(\boldsymbol{\phi}^o, \boldsymbol{\gamma}^o|\boldsymbol{Y}, \boldsymbol{X}, \mathcal{K})} \cdot \frac{\sum_{j=1}^{J} I\{\phi_j^o = 1, p_j^o \geq 1, \text{C3}\}}{\sum_{j=1}^{J} I\{\phi_j^p = 1, p_j^p \geq 1, \text{CI3}\}}\right\} \tag{32}$$

3.2 Step 2: MCMC Algorithm for Kernel Parameters

As $\boldsymbol{\theta}$ (21) have flat priors, we used Metropolis algorithm to update $\boldsymbol{\theta}$. For each included pathway, the proposed θ_j^p is accepted with probability:

$$\min\left\{1, \frac{f(\theta_j^p|\boldsymbol{Y}, \boldsymbol{X}, \mathcal{K}, \boldsymbol{\phi}, \boldsymbol{\gamma})}{f(\theta_j^o|\boldsymbol{Y}, \boldsymbol{X}, \mathcal{K}, \boldsymbol{\phi}, \boldsymbol{\gamma})}\right\} \tag{33}$$

3.3 Posterior Inference

In each iteration, our MCMC algorithm produces one model with included pathways and genes, indicated by $\boldsymbol{\phi}$ and $\boldsymbol{\gamma}$, respectively. The whole procedure produces a list of models. To estimate the marginal posterior probability for pathway j, $p(\phi_j|\boldsymbol{Y}, \boldsymbol{X}, \mathcal{K})$, we count the number of times pathway j appeared in the included pathways for all iterations after a certain burn-in point and then divide the count by the total iteration after the burn-in point. If the posterior probabilities of the pathways pass a user-adopted threshold, they are identified as the important pathways. Similarly, posterior probabilities of gene k in the important pathway j, $p(\gamma_k|\boldsymbol{Y}, \boldsymbol{X}, \mathcal{K}, I\{\phi_j s_j k = 1\})$, can be calculated. To find out overall important genes we can count the number of times gene k appeared in our model, ignoring whether it is in the important pathways. The posterior probabilities of gene k can be calculated as $p(\gamma_k|\boldsymbol{Y}, \boldsymbol{X}, \mathcal{K}\})$.

4 Simulation Study

In this section, we evaluate the proposed model performance using two simulated data sets and compare our model with the one proposed in [25].

To simulate the data, we randomly chose 50 pathways from 243 pathways in the KEGG database (http://www.kegg.jp/), and 1656 genes responding to these 50 pathways. The relationship between the pathways and genes in the simulation data are based on the gene-pathway relations, $\boldsymbol{S}$, and the gene relations, $\boldsymbol{R}$, as provided in the KEGG database (http://www.kegg.jp/). We randomly chose 4 important pathways from the 50 pathways. For each of the 4 important pathways, one important gene is selected randomly and along with the genes near to it to code the same protein compound. Moreover, we selected the genes that send or receive signals from the important protein compound. By this way we have 4 important pathways (out of 50) and 27 important genes. Of them 5 important genes out of 14 genes from the first pathway, 6 out of 11 from the second, 8 out of 43 from the third, and 8 out of 38 from the fourth. This simulation scenario is based on the fact the one gene mutation usually will not form cancer, but several related gene mutations might cause cancer. We also add two fake important genes and two corresponding fake important pathways in the model to check if the proposed model can avoid those two fake important pathways and genes. In reality, it is possible that patients have some mutated genes not related to cancer.

To generate important gene expression microarray data, we first pick a gene which only sends but not receives signal among the important genes in a pathway and let X_{00} represent the value of that gene. Let X_0 be either 2 or -2, and draw X_{00} from $X_{00} \sim U(X_0 - 0.5, X_0 + 0.5)$. For the other genes that are in the same protein compound, select one of them and denote it by X_{01} and $X_{01} \sim \mathcal{N}(\rho X_{00}, 0.5)$, where ρ is a multiplier, and here we let $\rho = 0.95$. For the j-th genes in the same protein compound, its value is generated by $X_{0j} \sim \mathcal{N}(\rho X_{0(j-1)}, 0.5)$. In the neighborhood protein compound, the gene that receives the signal from X_{00} is denoted by X_{10} and $X_{10} \sim \mathcal{N}(\rho X_{00}, 0.5)$, and we can generate other gene values by $X_{1j} \sim \mathcal{N}(\rho X_{1(j-1)}, 0.5)$. If we have other neighborhood protein compounds, their values are generated in similar format. For the fake important gene, we only need to draw X_{00} from $X_{00} \sim U(X_0 - 0.5, X_0 + 0.5)$. The rest of unimportant genes are simulated from a standard normal distribution. We assume nonlinear relationship between the response variable and the important gene variable as follows:

- Let the effect of the first important pathway to be $F1$ and X_k^1 to be the k-th important genes in the first important pathway.

$$F1 = \cos(X_1^1) - 1.5(X_2^1)^2 + \exp(-X_3^1)X_4^1 - 0.8\sin(X_5^1)\cos(X_3^1) + 2X_1^1 * X_5^1 \tag{34}$$

- Let the effect of the second important pathway to be $F2$ and X_k^2 to be the k-th important genes in the first important pathway.

$$F2 = \cos(X_1^2) - 1.5(X_2^2)^2 + \exp(-X_3^2)X_4^2 - 0.8\sin(X_5^2)\cos(X_3^2) + 2X_1^2 * X_5^2 + 0.9X_6^2 \tag{35}$$

- Let the effect of the third important pathway to be $F3$ and X_k^3 to be the k-th important genes in the first important pathway.

$$\begin{aligned} F3 = {} & \cos(X_1^3) - 1.5(X_2^3)^2 + \exp(-X_3^3)X_4^3 - 0.8\sin(X_5^3)\cos(X_3^3) \\ & +2X_1^3 * X_5^3 + 0.9X_6^3\sin(X_7^3) - 0.8\cos(X_6^3)X_7^3 + 2X_8^4 \end{aligned} \tag{36}$$

- Let the effect of the fourth important pathway to be $F4$, and it can be generated similar to the third pathway.
- The response variable t which is the survival time would be generated based on the model below:

$$log(t) = F1 + F2 + F3 + F4 + \epsilon, \qquad \epsilon \sim \mathcal{N}(0, 1) \tag{37}$$

In addition to that, 20% of the observations are randomly censored at time $c \sim Uniform(0, t)$. Therefore, for each sample, we observe $[\boldsymbol{X}, \min(t, c), \delta]$, where δ is the censoring indicator.

In all our model fittings we use weakly informative priors. In Sect. 2.1, we already set $\alpha_0 = 0$ and $\boldsymbol{B}_0 = \boldsymbol{0}$. Moreover, we set $a_\alpha = 100$ and $a_B = 1$. The variance of the inverse gamma distribution exists when the shape parameter is greater than 2, and we set the shape parameter, $\nu_0/2 = 3$, which is the smallest integer that is greater than 2, and the scale parameter, $\nu_0\sigma_0^2/2 = 0.6$, which forms a weakly informative prior. μ decides the sparsity of the model. In our simulation our goal is to select two to six important pathways for each iteration, but different simulation data set require slightly different μ to achieve this goal. We let the model change the μ value based on average pathways in the model in every 2000 iterations. The change of value of μ will initially increase the instability of the pathway selection, but once a suitable μ is selected after first few iterations, it will become more stable. We choose $\eta = 0.08$, which controls the prior probability of gene selection depending on how many its related genes are selected. We set $\omega = 0.1$ as the prior for the probability of important pathway. We denote this set of choice of prior parameters as Prior 1 in Tables 1 and 2. It is to be noted here as our prior parameter choice leads to near-diffuse weak priors, our model is not very sensitive to the choice of the prior parameters as long as we remain in the class of near-diffuse but proper prior. However, to demonstrate the sensitivity of our model, we also include the simulation analysis based on another choice of prior parameter value as Prior 2, where we set $\alpha_0 = 0$, $\boldsymbol{B}_0 = \boldsymbol{0}$, $a_\alpha = 1000$, $a_B = 10$, $\nu_0/2 = 5$, $\nu_0\sigma_0^2/2 = 0.8$, $\eta = 0.05$, $\omega = 0.05$. Prior 2 in Tables 1 and 2 is intended to produce a sparser model, and we want to see that if we force a sparser prior, can the model retrieve some significant pathways and genes without compromising on the false-negative rates?

We have two different simulation scenarios. In Simulation Scenario 1 the important genes are only in the important pathways, and in Simulation Scenario 2 the important genes are not only in the important pathways but a subset of them are also in other pathways. The detail of the scenarios setting is as below:

- Simulation 1:
  We make sure the 27 important genes only appear in the 4 important pathways. The sample size $n = 100$. We replicate the simulation 50 times, generating 50 different data sets. $\mu = -2.8$ is the initial value.

Table 1 Comparison between our model and [25]'s model in terms of pathway and gene selection in Simulation 1. The numbers in the parentheses are related to genes and the numbers outside the parentheses are related to pathways. Detail description of the column headings is provided in the Appendix section

	TP	FP	TN	FN	Run time
True	4 (27)	0 (0)	46 (1629)	0 (0)	
RKHS model (Prior 1)	3.49 (21.67)	0.42 (5.89)	45.58 (1623.11)	0.51 (5.33)	95 mins
RKHS model (Prior 2)	3.35 (21.48)	0.34 (5.77)	45.66 (1623.23)	0.65 (5.52)	95 mins
[25]	2.42 (16.19)	10.23 (44.96)	35.77 (1584.04)	1.58 (10.81)	90 mins

Table 2 Comparison between our model and [25]'s model in terms of pathway and gene selection in Simulation 2. The numbers in the parentheses are related to genes and the numbers outside the parentheses are related to pathways. Detail description of the column headings is provided in the Appendix section

	TP	FP	TN	FN	Run time
True	4 (27)	0 (0)	46 (1629)	0 (0)	
RKHS model (Prior 1)	3.09 (19.19)	1.37 (10.54)	44.63 (1618.46)	0.91 (7.81)	90 mins
RKHS model (Prior 2)	3.02 (19.23)	1.33 (10.41)	44.67 (1618.59)	0.98 (7.77)	90 mins
[25]	1.78 (10.39)	11.12 (78.32)	34.88 (1550.68)	2.22 (16.61)	87 mins

- Simulation 2:
  Similar to Simulation 1, except we add subset of the important genes to three different pathways and $\mu = -5$ is the initial value.

We compare our model with the model introduced in [25] in Tables 1 and 2. In Simulation 1 on average, in our method, we choose 3.49 and 3.35 (respectively, based on our 2 prior parameter settings) out of 4 important pathways, respectively, and that is at least 0.93 more than [25]'s model. Also in Simulation 1 our model has on average only 0.42 and 0.34 false pathway selection, respectively (based on our 2 prior parameter settings), which is much less than [25] approach which is around 10.23. In 50 different replications in Simulation 1, our model selected none of the 2 fake important pathways. For each selected important pathway, at least one of the important genes are selected and none of the unimportant genes are selected, whereas [25]'s model selects one of the fake important pathways frequently. Similarly in Simulation 2 our model selected 3.09 and 3.02, respectively (based on our 2 prior parameter settings), out of 4 important pathways on average, which is lower than Simulation 1, while the false selection becomes 1.37 and 1.33, respectively (based on our 2 prior parameter settings), which is greater than Simulation 1. However, remember that compared to Simulation 1, Simulation 2 is far more challenging as in Simulation 2 some important genes that are in the selected pathways are also present in the unimportant pathways. In Simulation 2 most of the false selections are related to unimportant pathways but with important genes. Even then our RKHS model performs far better compared with [25]'s model. Overall, both simulation studies show a very good advantage of our RKHS model, because our model does not select those mutated genes, when mutation happens during cell reproduction process but not related to the disease or outcome that we are interested in.

Individual significant gene selection is much more difficult for any model. In terms of gene selection also from Tables 1 and 2 we can clearly see that our RKHS model performs consistently well and it is doing far better job in finding important genes and keeping out the unimportant genes from the model than [25]'s model.

Tables 1 and 2 clearly indicate that our RKHS model is not very sensitive to the choice of the prior parameter as long as we remain in the class of near-diffuse but proper prior. In terms of computational speed we can see that our RKHS model is computationally competitive with [25]'s model.

5 Application in Breast Cancer Microarray Data

In this section we apply our RKHS model for [29] breast cancer microarray data. In this data set there are 337 patients with 24481 microarray probes. We focus on 54 lymph-node-negative stage 0 patients. Out of them 21 developed distant metastasis and the rest of them are censored. Our goal is to identify the pathways and genes that do not mutate among all the patients but related to breast cancer distant metastasis.

We first perform a data cleaning and data preparation step. We follow imputation method and we applied a 10-nearest neighbor algorithm to impute missing gene expressions data as suggested in [28]. The pathway and gene mapping information are obtained from Kyoto Encyclopedia of Genes and Genomes (KEGG) database (http://www.kegg.jp/). The gene identifiers are Entrez Gene in KEGG and GenBank accession in breast cancer microarray data. We convert the GenBank accession to Entrez Gene by using Gene ID converter (https://biit.cs.ut.ee/gprofiler/convert). Then we are able to match the gene expression data with the pathway and gene mapping information. A total of 243 pathways and 4363 genes are included in this study after all the initial data cleaning and data preparation step.

In our RKHS model we set $\omega = 0.1$ as the prior for the probability of important pathway, and $\mu = -1.7$ and $\eta = 0.04$ for the gene selection prior. We choose weakly informative priors for all our prior parameters. We set $\alpha_0 = 0$, $\boldsymbol{B}_0 = \mathbf{0}$ (Sect. 2.1), and $a_\alpha = 1000$, $a_\beta = 0.1$. Similar to the simulation study, the variance of the inverse gamma distribution exists when the shape parameter is greater than 2, and we set the shape parameter, $\nu_0/2 = 3$, which is the smallest integer that is greater than 2, and the scale parameter, $\nu_0\sigma_0^2/2 = 0.6$, which forms a weakly informative prior.

In our MCMC we ran 200,000 iterations with the first 150,000 iterations as burn-in. Figure 2 shows the trace plot of the number of selected pathways and genes after the initial burn-in. The number of selected pathways for each iteration mostly ranges between 10 and 20, while the number of selected genes is always between 80 and 110.

In Fig. 3 we report the marginal posterior probability plot for pathway selection. For selection of pathways we adopt a sliding posterior probability-based cutoff

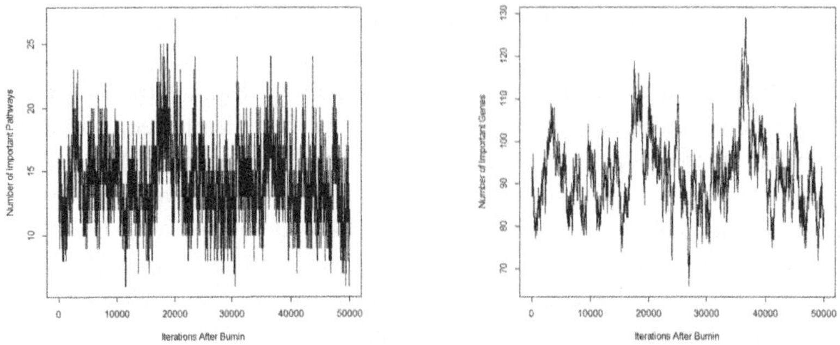

Fig. 2 The trace plots for the number of selected pathways and selected genes. (**a**) The number of selected pathways after burn-in. (**b**) The number of selected genes after burn-in

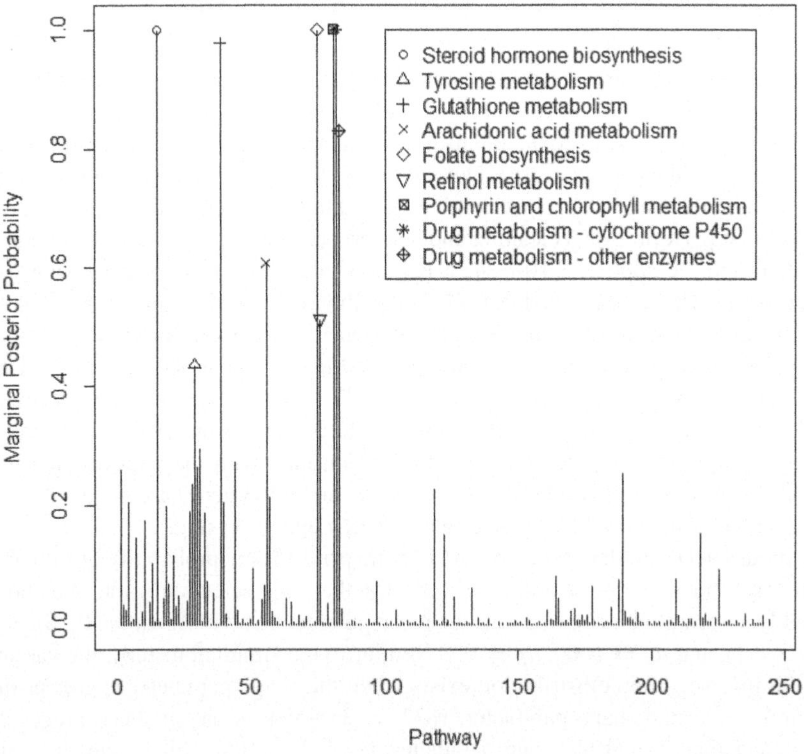

Fig. 3 Marginal posterior probabilities for pathway selection, $p(\phi_j|\boldsymbol{Y}, \boldsymbol{X}, \mathcal{K}) > 0.4$

scheme, where, instead of a preset number for the cutoff, a clinician can have a sliding marginal posterior probability approach. In the sliding marginal posterior probability approach, a clinician can decide if they want to select high- and/or medium-value marginal posterior probability (Fig. 3)-based pathways in their study by moving up or down the posterior probability cutoff number. Figure 3 shows that

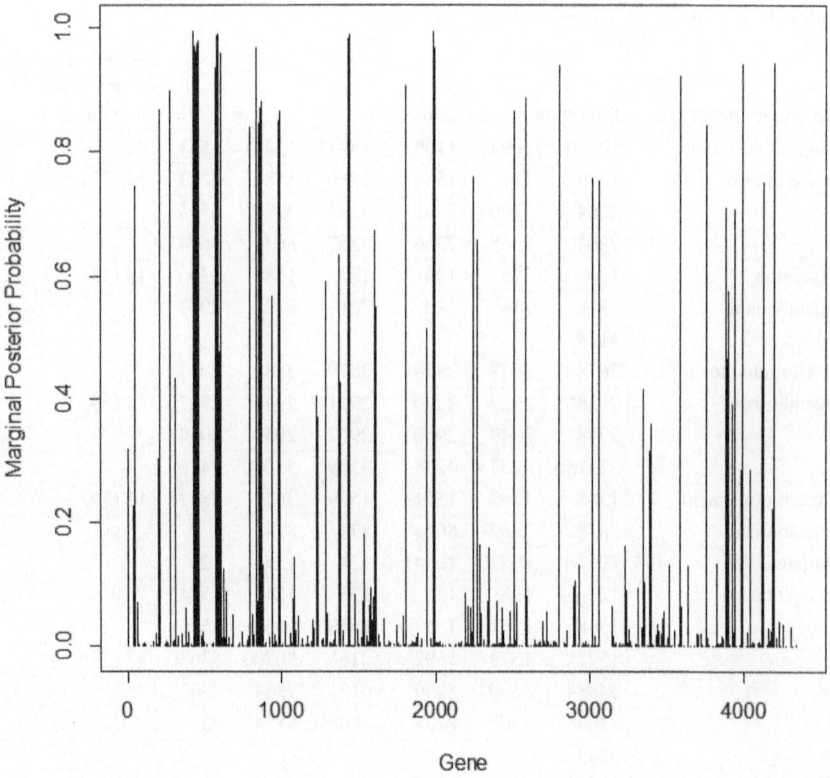

Fig. 4 Marginal posterior probabilities for gene selection, $p(\gamma_j|\boldsymbol{Y}, \boldsymbol{X}, \mathcal{K}) > 0.4$

the nine selected pathways which have the highest posterior probabilities as per a 0.4 threshold (because there is a gap between 0.3 and 0.4 in the figure). Based on the sliding marginal posterior probability principle we notice from Fig. 3 that the cutoff 0.4 can include pathways that have high and medium impacts. In Fig. 4 we report the marginal posterior probability plot for gene selection. Using a similar 0.4 threshold, our RKHS model selected 94 important unique genes. It is to be noted here that the pathway and gene selection thresholds are completely based on user choice and any user based on the full posterior probability plots (Fig. 3) can set their own threshold limits. In Table 3 we list the details of all the nine selected pathways and the Entrez Gene IDs of the selected genes in that pathway. The last column in Table 3 represents the number of genes selected from the total number of genes present in the pathway. Through extensive literature search based on the selected gene ID, we noticed that at least one of the important genes in each selected pathway is related to breast cancer or breast cancer metastasis. It is to be noted that there are several overlapping genes in each of the selected pathways.

Table 3 A summary of selected pathways and genes

Important pathways	Important genes (Entrez ID)						No. of selected genes (total in pathway)
Steroid hormone biosynthesis	10720	10941	1109	1543*	1545*	1551	
	1576	1577*	1584	1586	1588†	3283	24 (37)
	3284	3290	3291	3293	3294*	6715	
	7364*	7365	7366*	7367	8630	8644*	
Tyrosine metabolism	124	125	126	127	128	130	13 (33)
	131	218†	220	221	222	2954	
	4128						
+ Glutathione metabolism	2678	2877	2878	2879	2882	2937	
	2938*	2939	2940	2941	2946*	2947*	24 (39)
	2948	2949	2950	2952	2953	2954	
	373156	4257	4258	4259	51060	9446	
Arachidonic acid metabolism	1558	1562	1571	1579	2678	2877	11 (39)
	2878	2882	8644*	873	874		
Folate biosynthesis	10170	10720	10941	124	125	126	
	127	128	130	131	1543*	1544*	
	1548	1551	1553	1558	1562	1576	
	1577*	1579	1592*	216*	50700	53630	37 (38)
	54884	56603	5959	6121	7364*	7365	
	7366*	7367	8228	8608	8854	9227	
	9249						
Retinol metabolism	10720	10941	7364*	7365	7366*	7367	6 (27)
Porphyrin and chlorophyll metabolism	10720	10941	1109	124	125	126	
	127	128	130	131	1543*	1544*	
	1545*	1548	1551	1553	1558	1562	
	1565*	1571	1572	1576	1577*	2052	
	218†	220	221	222	22977	27294	57 (58)
	2938*	2939	2940	2941	2946	2947	
	2948	2949	2950	2952	2953	2954	
	3290	3291	373156	4257	4258	4259	
	7364*	7365	7366*	7367	8574	8644*	
	873	874	9446				
Drug metabolism: cytochrome P450	10720	10941	124	125	126	127	
	128	130	131	1544*	1548	1551	
	1553	1558	1562	1565*	1571	1576	
	1577*	218†	220	221	222	2326	
	2327	2328	2329	2330	2938*	2939	50 (52)

(continued)

Table 3 (continued)

Important pathways	Important genes (Entrez ID)						No. of selected genes (total in pathway)
	2940	2941	2946*	2947*	2948	2949	
	2950	2952	2953	2954	373156	4128	
	4257	4258	4259	7364*	7365	7366*	
	7367	9446					
Drug metabolism:	10720	10941	1548	1551	1553	1576	11 (32)
other enzymes	1577*	7364*	7365	7366*	7367		

* = genes related to breast cancer; †= genes related to breast cancer metastasis

5.1 *Biological Significance and Pathway-Specific Targeted Treatment*

In this section we investigate the biological importance and the clinical role our RKHS model-based selected pathways can play in breast cancer treatments. Steroid hormone biosynthesis pathway is one such selected pathway, for example, in our RKHS model (Fig. 1 in Sect. 1). Steroid hormones belong to the group of chemical compounds known as steroids. These compounds are biologically synthesized by several organs of humans as well as other animals, and they perform essential functions to maintain homeostasis. These functions include control of metabolism, inflammation, immune functions, and salt and water balance, development of sexual characteristics, and the ability to cope with illness and injury. Such functional activities of steroid hormones require a strict balance of their synthesis to assure appropriate host response. Any abnormal changes in the biosynthetic pathway for steroid hormones can lead to imbalance of the hormonal level in the body. A consequence of such an event will be the abnormality in cellular function and abnormal growth. Postmenopausal women have altered level of steroid hormones and are more susceptible to develop breast cancer. Studies have shown that higher blood levels of testosterone may increase the risk of breast cancer in postmenopausal women. Furthermore, some evidence suggests that higher blood levels of testosterone may also increase breast cancer risk in premenopausal women. Estrogen plays a critical role in hormone-receptor-positive breast cancer growth. These findings underscore the importance of the association of several enzymes and other bioactive molecules in the steroid hormone biosynthetic pathway for analyzing the possibility of the involvement of some of these molecules in breast cancer growth and spread.

Three other notable pathways selected by our RKHS model are :

(1) Tyrosine Metabolism Pathway. Tyrosine is an amino acid that plays an essential role in the metabolism. Tyrosine metabolism is a crucial component to breast cancer and other cancers as well.

(2) Glutathione Metabolism Pathway. Glutathione plays important roles in antioxidant defense, nutrient metabolism, and regulation of cellular events including

gene expression, DNA and protein synthesis, cell proliferation and apoptosis, signal transduction, cytokine production and immune response, and protein glutathionylation. Physiological relevance of glutathione makes the pathway and components of glutathione metabolism a vital part of cancer-associated studies.

(3) Arachidonic Acid Metabolism Pathway. Arachidonic acid and certain other polyunsaturated fatty acids may be transformed into prostaglandins (PG) by the enzyme prostaglandin endoperoxide synthase (PES). Level of prostaglandin E2 is elevated in malignant human breast tissue. An increase of inflammatory component may have a direct consequence in the development of inflammatory breast cancer, the deadliest form of breast cancer.

In Fig. 5 steroid hormone biosynthesis pathway, we recreate where the green boxes represent the protein compound coded by genes. The red number above the boxes are the important genes (Entrez ID) known to be related to breast cancer that our model found. In the lower center of the graph, Entrez gene 1588 is called CYP19A1. CYP19A1 gene codes for an enzyme called aromatase. One of the critical functions of this aromatase is to convert testosterone to estradiol, a form of estrogen [20]. Increased activity of aromatase has been linked to breast cancer due to abundance of estradiol accumulation in the cancer cells [4]. Estradiol increases tumor growth in breast cancer by promoting cell proliferation [8]. In cancer cells it binds to estrogen receptor which subsequently activates a group of hormone-responsive genes that promote DNA synthesis and cell proliferation [6]. Therefore, overactive CYP19A1 gene in breast cancer cells has a poor prognosis for patients due to over-expression of aromatase-driven estradiol synthesis. Consequently, specific aromatase inhibitors have been found to be useful in the treatment of breast cancer [12].

Therefore, through our RKHS model we pinpoint some specific pathways and genes which are medically known to be related to breast cancer and breast cancer metastasis. Our RKHS model-based pathway identification can help in designing a drug to have targeted effect by phenocopying the specific genetic variant. Our method can help drug developers in prioritizing on the number of genetic and pathway associations that are candidates for drug development. Our approach can integrate information from pathway databases and gene expressions and can expand the potential targeted genetic variant list. There are several clinically established cases of fast and effective drug development based on a human genetics-informed approach [11]. The biggest success is the proprotein convertase subtilisin/kexin type 9 (PCSK9) connection to heart disease [1]. Other such cases are missense mutations in the islet-specific zinc transport (SLC30A8) in type 2 diabetes [24], loss-of-function mutations in Niemann-Pick C1-like 1 (NPC1L1) in reducing the risk of coronary heart disease [14], and key mutations in the amyloid precursor protein that protects against Alzheimer's disease and cognitive decline for older patients [15]. We believe our RKHS model can provide similar successful therapeutic hypotheses worthy of more deeper further investigation. It is also to be noted that beyond the known clinically associated genes the model has also selected some new

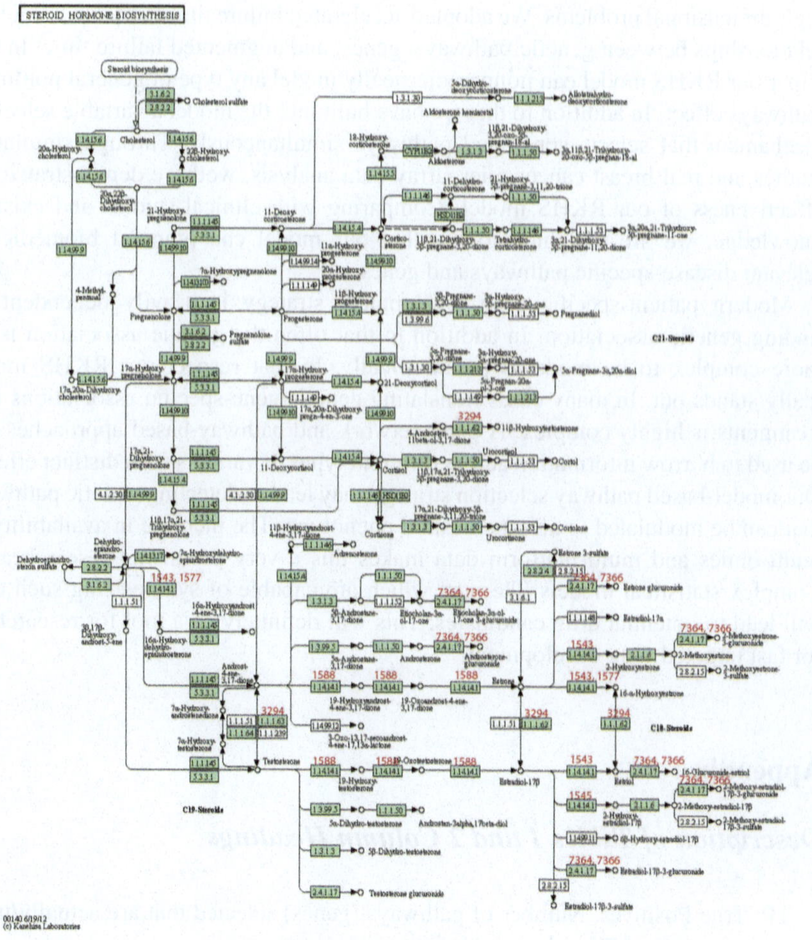

Fig. 5 Steroid hormone biosynthesis pathway with important genes related to breast cancer

candidate genes. From the biology and drug-development research point of view, the information from our posterior probability plots can be used to prioritize the pathways and genes for future new drug design.

6 Discussion

In this paper, we have proposed a Bayesian nonlinear model based on RKHS to model nonlinear genetic pathway and gene selection for right-censored survival outcome data. In our model with prior biological information, pathways and gene-gene relationships are effectively utilized to enhance the gene selection for high-dimensional problems. We adopted accelerated failure time model to model the relationships between genetic pathways, genes, and augmented failure time. In this paper our RKHS model can nonparametrically model any type of general nonlinear pathways effect. In addition to that we have built into the model a variable selection mechanism that selects genes and pathways simultaneously. Through simulation studies and real breast cancer microarray data analysis, we have demonstrated the effectiveness of our RKHS model. Comparing with clinical studies and existing knowledge, we are delighted to see that our model can pinpoint biomedically relevant disease-specific pathways and genes.

Modern patient-specific drug-development strategy is heavily dependent on finding genetic association. In addition to that often the genetic association is far more complex to be modeled parametrically. In that respect our RKHS model really stands out. In many cases translating genetic/gene-specific associations into treatments is highly complex. A gene network and pathway-based approaches can be used to borrow information across different types of variants with distinct effects. Our model-based pathway selection strategy may lead to detecting genetic pathways that can be modulated to affect a desired phenotype. The increase in availability of multi-omics and multi-platform data makes this a very promising research area. Complex statistical models like ours which are capable of synthesizing such data will lead to potential drug candidates. This will definitely be a tool for researchers for fast targeted drug development.

Appendix

Description of Tables 1 and 2 Column Headings

- TP: True Positives. Number of pathways (genes) selected that are actually/truly important out of 50 pathways (1656 genes)
- FP: False Positives. Number of pathways (genes) selected that are not actually/truly important out of 50 pathways (1656 genes)
- TN: True Negatives. Number of pathways (genes) not selected that are actually/truly unimportant out of 50 pathways (1656 genes)
- FN: False Negatives. Number of pathways (genes) not selected that are actually/truly important out of 50 pathways (1656 genes)
- Run Time: Time needed to fit a model in minutes

Simulation Study with One Pathway Having Linear Functional Effect

In this subsection we will do an additional simulation study to understand the effectiveness of our RKHS model when one of the pathway effects is linear. The goal of this study is to demonstrate the ability of our RKHS model to capture simpler linear pathway effect behavior. This simulation study is created using the exact same settings as described in Sect. 4 with only one modification, that is, now the fourth pathway effect is linear. The linear function governing the fourth pathway effect is given by

$$F4 = 0.5 + 1.2X_1^4 - 0.8X_2^4 + 0.2X_3^4 + 1.9X_5^4 - 1.6X_7^4 \quad (38)$$

All other simulation settings including survival time generation, sample size (n=100), number of important genes (=27), and number of important pathways (=4) are kept to be exactly the same as described in Sect. 4. In this simulation we only consider the case when all 27 important genes only appear in the 4 important pathways. We replicate the simulation 50 times, generating 50 different data sets. In this simulation also we chose $\mu = -2.8$ as the initial value. From Table 4 we can see, when the underlying pathway effect function is linear, our RKHS model and [25]'s model work impressively well in terms of TP and FN, although our method gives marginally better results. Considering the FP and TN, we can see our RKHS model is still producing significantly more sparser model than [25]'s model.

Comparison of Our RKHS Model with [25] in Breast Cancer Microarray Data

In this section we provide a comparative analysis of our RKHS method with the approach of [25]. We split the [29] breast cancer microarray data described in Sect. 5 randomly into training set with 80% data and test set with 20% data. We repeat this process ten times, and thus, we have ten separate training and ten corresponding

Table 4 Comparison between our model and [25]'s model in terms of pathway and gene selection in Simulation 3. The numbers in the parentheses are related to genes and the numbers outside the parentheses are related to pathways. Detail description of the column headings is provided in the Appendix section

	TP	FP	TN	FN	Run time
True	4 (27)	0 (0)	46 (1629)	0 (0)	
RKHS model (Prior 1)	3.89 (23.92)	0.46 (5.69)	45.32 (1623.31)	0.11 (3.08)	95 mins
RKHS model (Prior 2)	3.91 (24.17)	0.42 (5.24)	45.38 (1623.76)	0.09 (3.83)	95 mins
[25]	3.61 (21.61)	6.95 (37.22)	39.05 (1591.78)	0.41 (8.39)	90 mins

Table 5 Comparison between our model and [25]'s for the breast cancer microarray data. The numbers in the table are the averages over ten random splits. The numbers in the parentheses are standard deviations

	[25]	RKHS model
Predictive MSE in test set	1.48 (0.26)	1.38 (0.18)
Test set concordance index	0.81 (0.06)	0.87 (0.07)
Number of pathways selected	14 (1.54)	8 (2.05)
Number of genes selected	129 (4.78)	108 (4.69)
Run time	102 mins	120 mins

validation sets. For our RKHS model we adopted the same prior information we used in Sect. 5. For [25]'s model we used the prior parameter setting used in their paper [25]. For both models we ran 200,000 MCMC iterations with the first 150,000 iterations as burn-in. From Table 5 we can see that our RKHS model performs quite favorably in comparison to [25]'s model based on test set predictive MSE and the test set concordance index. Our RKHS model comes out to be more consistent in selecting sparser set of pathways than [25]'s model. Also in terms of the number of genes, our model selects on average 15% less number of genes than [25]'s model. In terms of overlap among pathways found to be important by our RKHS model and [25]'s model, we noticed that on average we have six common pathways that are found to be important by both the models.

Open-Source Software for Model Fitting and Implementation

We have developed all our codes in R and all codes and software are freely available from our GitHub website (https://github.com/sounakchak/BayesianKernelPathway).

References

1. Abifadel, M., Varret, M., Rabès, J.P., Allard, D., Ouguerram, K., Devillers, M., Cruaud, C., Benjannet, S., Wickham, L., Erlich, D., et al.: Mutations in PCSK9 cause autosomal dominant hypercholesterolemia. Nat. Genet. **34**, 154–156 (2003)
2. Aronszajn, N.: Theory of reproducing kernels. Trans. Am. Math. Soc. **68**, 337–404 (1950)
3. Besag, J.: Spatial interaction and the statistical analysis of lattice systems. J. R. Stat. Soc. Ser. B Methodol. **36**, 192–236 (1974)
4. Chen, S.: Aromatase and breast cancer. Front. Biosci. **3**, 922–933 (1998)
5. Cox, D.R.: Regression models and life-tables. J. R. Stat. Soc. Ser. B **34**, 187–220 (1972)
6. DeMayo, F.J., Zhao, B., Takamoto, N., Tsai, S.Y.: Mechanisms of action of estrogen and progesterone. Ann. N. Y. Acad. Sci. **955**, 48–59 (2002)
7. Downward, J.: Cancer biology: Signatures guide drug choice. Nature **439**, 274–275 (2006)
8. Felice, D.L., El-Shennawy, L., Zhao, S., Lantvit, D.L., Shen, Q., Unterman, T.G., Swanson, S.M., Frasor, J.: Growth hormone potentiates 17β-estradiol-dependent breast cancer cell proliferation independently of IGF-I receptor signaling. Endocrinology **154**, 3219–3227 (2013)

9. George, E.I., McCulloch, R.E.: Variable selection via gibbs sampling. J. Am. Stat. Assoc. **88**, 881–889 (2005)
10. Golub, T.R., Slonim, D.K., Tamayo, P., Huard, C., Gaasenbeek, M., Mesirov, J.P., Coller, H., Loh, M.L., Downing, J.R., Caligiuri, M.A., Bloomfield, C.D., Lander, E.S.: Molecular classification of cancer: Class discovery and class prediction by gene expression monitoring. Science **286**, 531–537 (1999)
11. Greene, C.S., Voight, B.F.: Pathway and network-based strategies to translate genetic discoveries into effective therapies. Hum. Mol. Genet. **25**, 94–98 (2016)
12. Gutman, M., Couillard, S., Labrie, F., Candas, B., Labrie, C.: Effects of the antiestrogen em-800 (SCH 57050) and cyclophosphamide alone and in combination on growth of human zr-75-1 breast cancer xenografts in nude mice. Cancer Res. **59**, 5176–5180 (1999)
13. Hanahan, D., Weinberg, R.A.: The hallmarks of cancer. Cell **100**, 57–70 (2000)
14. Myocardial Infarction Genetics Consortium Investigators, Stitziel, N.O., Won, H.H., Morrison, A.C., et al.: Inactivating mutations in npc1l1 and protection from coronary heart disease. N. Engl. J. Med. **371**, 2072–2082 (2014)
15. Jonsson, T., Atwal, J.K., Steinberg, S., Snaedal, J., Jonsson, P.V., Bjornsson, S., Stefansson, H., Sulem, P., Gudbjartsson, D., Maloney, J., et al.: A mutation in app protects against alzheimer's disease and age-related cognitive decline. Nature **488**, 96–99 (2012)
16. Kimeldorf, G., Wahba, G.: Some results on tchebycheffian spline functions. J. Math. Anal. Appl. **33**, 82–95 (1971)
17. Kuo, L., Mallick, B.: Bayesian semiparametric inference for the accelerated failure-time model. Can. J. Stat. **25**, 457–472 (1997)
18. Li, F., Zhang, N.R.: Bayesian variable selection in structured high-dimensional covariate space with application in genomics. J. Am. Stat. Assoc. **105**, 1202–1214 (2010)
19. Liu, D., Lin, X., Ghosh, D.: Semiparametric regression of multidimensional genetic pathway data: least-squares kernel machines and linear mixed models. Biometrics **63**, 1079–1088 (2007)
20. Meinhardt, U., Mullis, P.E.: The aromatase cytochrome p-450 and its clinical impact. Horm. Res. **57**, 145–152 (2002)
21. Park, M.Y., Hastie, T., Tibshirani, R.: Averaged gene expressions for regression. Biostatistics **8**, 212–227 (2007)
22. Sherr, C.J.: Cancer cell cycles. Science **274**, 1672–1677 (1996)
23. Sinha, D., Chen, M.-H., Ghosh, S.K.: Bayesian analysis and model selection for interval-censored survival data. Biometrics **55**, 585–590 (1999)
24. Sladek, R., Rocheleau, G., Rung, J., Dina, C., Shen, L., Serre, D., Boutin, P., Vincent, D., Belisle, A., Hadjadj, S., et al.: A genome-wide association study identifies novel risk loci for type 2 diabetes. Nature **445**, 881–885 (2007)
25. Stingo, F.C., Chen, Y.A., Tadesse, M.G., Vannucci, M.: Incorporating biological information into linear models: a Bayesian approach to the selection of pathways and genes. Ann. Appl. Stat. **5**, 1978–2002 (2011)
26. Tanner, M.A., Wong, W.H.: The calculation of posterior distributions by data augmentation. J. Am. Stat. Assoc. **82**, 528–540 (1987)
27. Telesca, D., Muller, P., Parmigiani, G., Freedman, R.S.: Modeling dependent gene expression. Ann. Appl. Stat. **6**, 542–560 (2012)
28. Troyanskaya, O., Cantor, M., Sherlock, G., Brown, P., Hastie, T., Tibshirani, R., Botstein, D., Altman, R.B.: Missing value estimation methods for DNA microarrays. Bioinformatics **17**, 520–525 (2001)
29. van 't Veer, L.J., et al.: Gene expression profiling predicts clinical outcome of breast cancer. Nature **415**, 530–536 (2002)

Using Guided Regularized Random Forests to Identify Important Biological Pathways and Genes

Tyler Cook, Daniel Brumley, and Sounak Chakraborty

Abstract Microarray data can provide a wealth of knowledge related to predicting a biological outcome. Current research in this area often aims to include information from biological pathways, which can describe gene relationships and interactions, in order to improve understanding of the underlying biological process. Incorporating pathway information is an increasingly attractive option as more knowledge about pathway structure and function becomes available online in publicly accessible databases. Here, a novel method for identifying important biological pathways and genes for classification problems is proposed using guided regularized random forests (GRRF). This approach allows for ranking both pathways and genes, and the regularization of GRRF can help researchers select a compact set of features related to the biological outcome. The proposed methodology is able to successfully identify significant biological pathways and genes and achieve low misclassification rates in both simulation experiments and the analysis of a breast cancer dataset.

Keywords Random forest · Regularization · Gene selection · Pathway selection

1 Introduction

DNA microarrays have provided a valuable tool for medical researchers in recent years, and the analysis of gene expression data has proven to be quite successful in many cases. Researchers are able to identify genes in order to better diagnose and treat a number of diseases. This is an evolving area of study, and much attention has recently been given to advancing beyond investigating individual genes by also incorporating gene relationships and gene dependency structure through genetic

---

T. Cook · D. Brumley
Department of Mathematics & Statistics, University of Central Oklahoma, Edmond, OK, USA

S. Chakraborty (✉)
Department of Statistics, University of Missouri, Columbia, MO, USA
e-mail: chakrabortys@missouri.edu

Y. Zhao, D.-G. Chen (eds.), *Big Data Analytics in Biostatistics and Bioinformatics*, ICSA Book Series in Statistics,
https://doi.org/10.1007/978-3-032-06649-7_9

pathways. It is of interest to determine how to model a biological outcome using genetic data in order to select important pathways and genes for improved medical intervention strategies.

Genetic pathways are groups of genes working together to serve some aggregate function in the cell. Many pathways can be activated or inhibited at several different points along the gene network. This is an important feature to consider in cancer studies since multiple gene mutations are necessary for any cancer tumor growth. Moreover, in recent studies, it has been shown that the interaction of groups of genes in genetic pathways is responsible for metastasis, instead of single genes working alone. For example, a treatment drug targeting a specific gene might be less effective since the pathway could potentially continue to adversely function due to other genes with similar purposes. Vogelstein [35] illustrates several known instances that support a pathway and gene-based analysis. Fortunately, biologists are continually accumulating knowledge concerning genetic pathways. Much of this genetic information is readily available in online databases, such as Gene Ontology (GO), BioCarta, and Kyoto Encyclopedia of Genes and Genomes (KEGG). Utilizing this additional biological information in order to select both important genes and pathways could be one way to improve disease diagnosis and treatment. A more detailed description about genetic pathways and their role in cancer formation is given in Sect. 2, and a schematic display of the data structure can be seen in Fig. 1.

The analysis of gene expression data provides many statistical challenges, and a variety of approaches exist in the literature to handle this type of data.

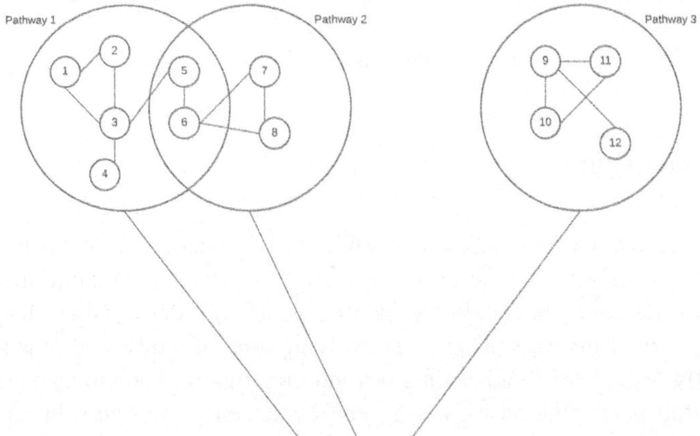

Fig. 1 Diagram outlining the organization of the data as groups of interconnected genes belonging to different pathways where it is possible for genes to belong to multiple pathways. The different pathways then influence the biological response

Identification of differentially expressed genes can be accomplished using a number of different supervised and unsupervised methodologies, and an early review of many commonly used techniques can be found in Butte [3]. Many of these early approaches select genes one at a time. This ignores gene relationships and can often result in multiple testing issues. Much work in has gone into developing appropriate hypothesis tests and methods to address multiple comparisons [10, 28, 30, 34].

Predictive models that simultaneously select genes can also be accomplished using methods such as support vector machines [16], random forests [8], and, more recently, guided regularized random forests (GRRF) [6]. GRRF can model linear and nonlinear relationships since it is based on the random forest methodology. Also, it has the added benefit of selecting a compact feature set, which can be a challenge in genetic studies. In addition, many other statistical learning methods for feature selection exist in the wider variable selection literature, including Bayesian methods [32], gradient boosting [37], support vector machines [1], and neural networks [4].

Recently, several methods focusing on gene set and pathway analysis have also been developed. One of the most popular is gene set enrichment analysis (GSEA) [31]. In GSEA, enrichment scores are calculated to represent whether genes belonging to prespecified sets are overrepresented at the top or bottom of a ranked list of genes, and a hypothesis test is used to evaluate statistical significance. This method has motivated a very large number of similar techniques, and several review and comparison papers exist [20, 21]. Many different predictive, machine learning methods have also been proposed. For example, Park, Hastie, and Tibshirani [24] modeled survival times by creating supergenes from GO groupings and then fitting a Cox model. Additionally, Furey et al. [15] use a support vector machine for classification based on microarray data, and Pang et al. [23] investigated a random forest approach for pathway and gene selection. Bayesian methods are also available, such as Stingo et al. [29], which use a Markov random field to model gene relationships when selecting pathways and genes.

In this chapter, we propose a new method for analyzing gene expression data based on guided regularized random forests that incorporates pathway information. Our aim is to develop a complete procedure that will identify both important pathways and genes when modeling a biological outcome. We will focus on instances where the biological outcome can be treated as a classification problem with an ultimate goal of selecting compact sets of influential pathways and genes. Specifically, we consider pathways and genes to be important or influential if they contribute to the accurate classification of the biological outcome. The method is an adaptation of the random forest approach discussed in Pang et al. [23]. Each pathway is analyzed individually using a GRRF, and the pathways are ranked based on model fit. Important genes can then be identified in the top pathways using variable importance scores from the GRRF. An application of these methods on a breast cancer dataset shows they are able to successfully distinguish a compact set of important pathways and genes. The code used in the analysis is available freely from GitHub at https://github.com/tylerlewiscook/GRRF-Pathways

The remainder of the chapter has the following structure. Section 2 describes the biological background and significance in more detail. Then, in Sect. 3, we describe the specific procedure for the new proposed method. Section 4 contains results from simulation studies of the proposed method. In Sect. 5, we evaluate the performance of the proposed method with an application to a real dataset. Finally, we conclude with a discussion in Sect. 6.

2 Biological Significance

A DNA microarray analysis allows researchers to simultaneously examine the expression levels of thousands of genes. These procedures supply vast amounts of data that can be used to explore various biological questions. One common use of gene expression data is to distinguish groups of genes that are functionally related. Genes in these clusters often work in tandem, and their existence may provide an evolutionary advantage [38]. Another important application of microarray data is identifying differentially expressed genes. This is useful since many diseases, such as cystic fibrosis, are the result of a mutation in a single gene [35]. Determining these genes can therefore improve disease diagnosis.

Methods based on individual gene analysis are an important first step. One logical next step is to utilize genetic pathways to identify both important genes and pathways. This is particularly desirable in cancer research since cancer is a genetic disorder and no individual gene mutation is responsible for cancer development. The p53 signaling pathway, for example, is a well-known example of an important cancer pathway. The p53 protein is a tumor suppressor that has many important roles in preventing cancer, and it has been linked to many different cancers in humans [17]. Figure 2 displays the p53 signaling pathway map from the KEGG database (https://www.genome.jp/kegg-bin/show_pathway?hsa04115) [18]. Deleterious mutations, all having the same effect, can occur at a number of genes along the pathway, so an investigation focusing solely on individual genes could neglect the influence of the pathway [35]. This is a strong argument for a pathway-based analysis. Moreover, many cancer treatments are being developed in order to target specific pathways [9].

Fortunately, knowledge of the gene relationships in pathways is growing, and pathway information is readily available in numerous online databases. These databases are searchable, interactive maps of gene interactions. Many databases cover a variety of areas such as biochemical reactions, cell functions, disease components, drug structure, as well as many others. For example, a researcher interested in learning more about the p53 signaling pathway could access the BioCarta or KEGG database via the Internet and search for this pathway. The search would result in an interactive graphical representation of the pathway that displays related cell functions, pathways, proteins, and genes. One could then select various components in the pathway and be redirected to more detailed information about specific genes, such as a list of other pathways that the gene might belong to. This

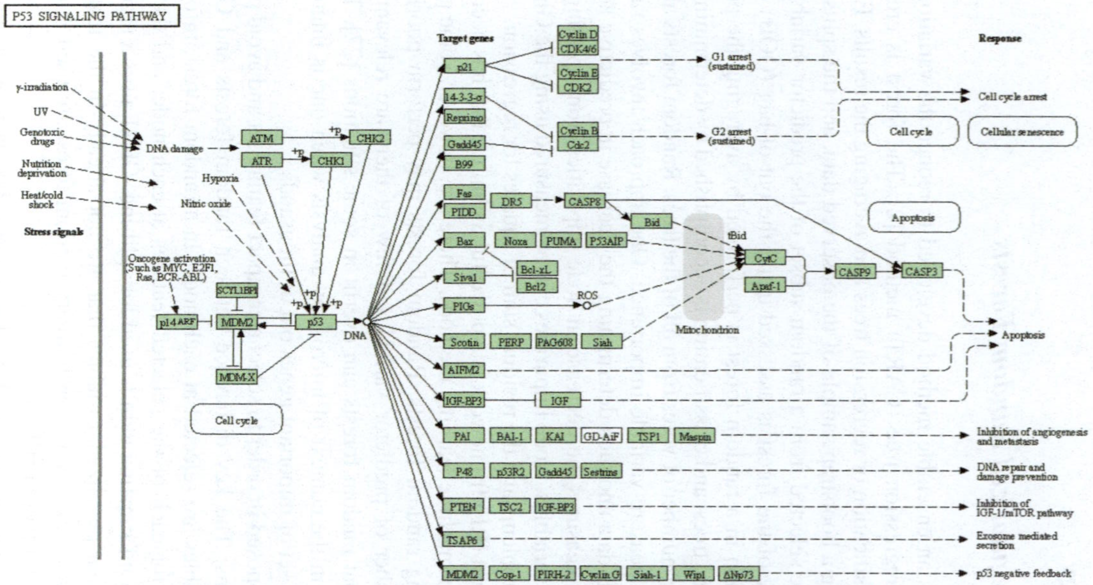

Fig. 2 The p53 signaling pathway map entry from the KEGG database. The diagram displays information such as the genes in the pathway and their relationships. Pathway maps are interactive when viewed on the KEGG website allowing researchers to quickly obtain more information for pathway components

would allow a researcher to use information from pathways that contain sets of overlapping genes. Databases are continually updated, and many include literature references for more detailed information about the different pathways.

3 Methodology

3.1 Guided Regularized Random Forests

A random forest is an ensemble method developed to reduce the variation of the classification and regression tree (CART) method [2]. The forest is created by growing many classification or regression trees and averaging the results. Each tree is constructed using a bootstrap sample of the observed data, and the splits at each node of the tree are selected from a random subset of the predictor variables. The predictive accuracy of the forest is assessed using the out-of-bag (OOB) data for each tree. Regression in a random forest is performed by averaging the predicted values from all of the trees, and classification is accomplished by determining which class had the largest number of votes from all of the trees. Random forests also have a useful ability to measure variable importance. One approach involves randomly permuting the OOB data and then determining the decrease in predictive accuracy. Another approach measures the decrease in node impurities from splitting on the different predictor variables. Node impurities can be measured using the Gini index for classification problems and the residual sum of squares for regression.

The random forest (RF) framework is a powerful technique that has become one of the most popular machine learning methods. There are, however, some potential hazards when using random forests. Random forests may perform poorly when using a large number of predictor variables if few of them are relevant, and it has been shown that random forests can overfit in some situations [27]. This can be a serious issue in the context of microarray analysis when one is interested in identifying a small set of important genes out of thousands.

GRRF were proposed in order to select a compact feature set and avoid potential overfitting problems. The key difference between random forests and GRRF is how splitting variables are selected at each node. In a random forest, information gain is calculated for each of the selected features at each node, and the feature with the maximum information gain is used for splitting. GRRF uses a regularized information gain that penalized variables that are not already in the feature set. Variable importance scores from a preliminary random forest are used in order to "guide" the penalization of GRRF.

To illustrate, consider a study with n observations. For each observation i, let X_i denote the $p \times 1$ vector of features and $Y_i \in \{1, 2, \ldots, C\}$ denote the class membership. One can think of the X_i as representing gene expression levels for the p genes measured in subject i, and Y_i representing a categorical biological outcome such as tumor type.

Classification trees in a RF are grown based on some node impurity criteria. Let $\hat{p}_c^{\nu}$ denote the proportion of observations from class c at node ν. The Gini index at ν is then defined as:

$$Gini(\nu) = \sum_{c=1}^{C} \hat{p}_c^{\nu}(1 - \hat{p}_c^{\nu})$$

From this, one can define the information gain for X_i at node ν as:

$$Gain(X_i, \nu) = Gini(x_i, \nu) - w_L Gini(X_i, \nu^L) - w_R Gini(X_i, \nu^R)$$

where ν^L and ν^R are the two children nodes created by splitting at ν and w_L and w_R are weights corresponding to the proportion of cases in each child node. A random subset of the p features is selected, and the splitting variable at each node is chosen by finding the feature that maximizes $Gain(X_i, \nu)$. Variable importance scores can also be calculated from $Gain(X_i, \nu)$ using:

$$Imp_i = \frac{1}{ntree} \sum_{\nu \in S_{X_i}} Gain(X_i, \nu)$$

where $ntree$ denotes the number of trees and S_{X_i} is the set of nodes split by X_i throughout the forest.

The distinguishing feature of GRRF is how the splitting variable is chosen. In GRRF, a regularized information gain $Gain_R(X_i, \nu)$ is used:

$$Gain_R(X_i, \nu) = \begin{cases} \lambda_i Gain(X_i, \nu) & X_i \notin F \\ Gain(X_i, \nu) & X_i \in F \end{cases}$$

where F is the set of variables used for splitting at previous nodes and $\lambda_i \in (0, 1]$ is the regularization parameter, or penalty coefficient, for X_i. The key idea is that the regularization penalizes features not already in the model, which helps produce a compact feature set.

The penalty coefficient is calculated, or guided, from importance scores from a standard RF using:

$$\lambda_i = (1 - \gamma) * \lambda_0 + \gamma * Imp'_i$$

where Imp'_i is a normalized importance score defined by:

$$Imp'_i = \frac{Imp_i}{max_{j=1}^{p} Imp_j}$$

For the penalty coefficient, λ_0 controls the degree of regularization and γ is a weight for Imp'. Deng and Runger [6] discuss how the size of the feature set can be regulated by changing either parameter, but find that accuracy is improved by focusing on γ. Therefore, they suggest fixing $\lambda_0 = 1$ and consider γ to be the only parameter of interest. Larger penalties for variables that do not have maximum importance scores can be achieved by increasing γ.

3.2 Pathway and Gene Selection with GRRF

Our proposed method is an adaptation of the random forest approach discussed in Pang et al. [23], which analyzed pathways individually. Here, each pathway is analyzed individually with a GRRF using only the genes belonging to that pathway. The pathways are then ranked based on OOB error rate. Important genes can then be identified in the top pathways using variable importance scores from the GRRF. The flowchart in Fig. 3 outlines the procedure.

The first step in this approach, after obtaining gene expression data, is to determine which pathways will be investigated. Pathway information then must be acquired from the relevant databases. This data will be used in order to determine which of the sampled genes belong to each pathway. Once the gene membership for each pathway is known, analysis continues by examining the pathways one at a time.

For each pathway, the subset of genes belonging to that pathway is used as features in GRRF. The results of fitting these series of GRRFs will be used to rank each of the pathways. The GRRF will provide an estimate of the classification error using the OOB data for each of the pathways. The pathways are then ranked according to their OOB errors. It is assumed that important pathways will be better able to predict the response. Therefore, influential pathways are those with the lowest OOB error rates.

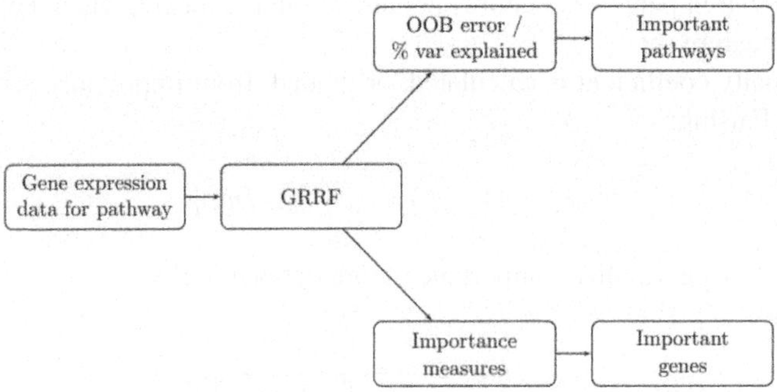

Fig. 3 Flowchart for pathway and gene selection with GRRF

Important genes can also then be identified in the selected pathways using the variable importance results from the GRRF. When performing classification, one can use either the marginal decrease in accuracy or the decrease in the Gini index. The number of genes with nonzero importance scores can be controlled by changing the value of γ. This could be of interest for a researcher desiring a compact set of genes from a pathway with many member genes.

4 Simulation Study

To assess the efficacy of the proposed methodology, we applied GRRF to simulated genetic data and compared its results with two well-known variable selection methods: varSelRF and LASSO logistic regression [8, 33]. The simulations were implemented in *R* using the "RRF", "varSelRF", and "glmnet" packages for the GRRF, varSelRF, and LASSO methods, respectively [5, 7, 12, 26]. In line with [6], we fixed `mtry` $= \sqrt{\text{number of variables in pathway}}$ and `ntree` $= 1000$ for the GRRF and varSelRF methods; we also held $\lambda_0 = 1$ so that γ was the only parameter for GRRF. Beyond this, the default settings for each of the methods were used.

4.1 Pathway Rankings

We simulated a genetic dataset with ten pathways, two of which were significant, and then measured the performance of GRRF, varSelRF, and LASSO in distinguishing significant from nonsignificant pathways.

To accomplish this, we first generate 140 iid random variables sampled from $\mathcal{U}(0, 1)$. Pathways 1–2 are each assigned ten variables: $P_1, \ldots, P_{10}$ and $Q_1, \ldots, Q_{10}$, respectively. The remaining 120 variables are distributed evenly among Pathways 3–10. Within Pathways 1–2, the first five variables are designated significant. Following Deng and Runger [6], we use the significant variables within each pathway to create five redundant variables: $P_{i+10} \leftarrow P_i$ and $Q_{i+10} \leftarrow Q_i$ for $i = 1, \ldots, 5$. Including these redundant features mimics real genetic data and provides an opportunity to showcase the regularization procedure's ability to identify a small set of important variables.

A response Y is then generated via one of the following response models:

RM1: An extension of a model discussed in Friedman [13]. Note $\epsilon \sim \mathcal{N}(0, 1)$.

$$Y = 10\sin(\pi P_1 P_2) + 20(P_3 - 0.5)^2 + 10P_4 + 5P_5 + 15\sin(\pi Q_1 Q_2) + 25(Q_3 - 0.5)^2 + 20Q_4 + 10Q_5 + \epsilon$$

RM2: A variant of RM1 that includes interaction across pathways.

$$Y = 10\sin(\pi P_1 Q_1) + 20(P_2 Q_2 - 0.5)^2 + 10(P_3 + Q_3) + 5(P_4 + Q_5) + 10(P_5 + Q_4) + \epsilon$$

RM3: A simple linear model.

$$Y = \sum_{i=1}^{5} 10(P_i + Q_i) + \epsilon$$

This process is repeated until a sample size of 50 is obtained. The median response $\overline{Y}$ is then computed, and the samples are labeled according to the following rule: If $Y > \overline{Y}$, then the sample is assigned to Class 2; otherwise, the sample belongs to Class 1. In total, 100 datasets were simulated for each of RM1–RM3.

GRRF, varSelRF, and LASSO were then applied to each pathway. The parameter γ of GRRF was selected from $\{0.05, 0.25, 0.5, 0.75, 0.95\}$, resulting in five distinct models: GRRF-0.05, GRRF-0.25, GRRF-0.50, GRRF-0.75, and GRRF-0.95. A fixed grid of values was selected in order to gain insight into how the regularization parameter influences the results. In practice, one could optimize the value of γ using cross-validation. The regularization parameter of LASSO was chosen via 10-fold cross-validation. For each model, the pathways were scored and then ranked using an appropriate metric: minimum OOB error rate for the varSelRF and GRRF models; minimum cross-validated mean for LASSO models. In the event that two or more scores coincided, the ranks at each index set of ties were averaged—for instance, the results $(1, 2, 3, 1, 3, 1)$ would be ranked $(2.0, 4.0, 5.5, 2.0, 5.5, 2.0)$ under this scheme.

The ranks of Pathways 1–2 were recorded, and, in particular, we recorded the rank of the worst-performing pathway. Results are displayed in Tables 1, 2, and 3. Since Pathways 1 and 2 are significant, it would be ideal for those two pathways to achieve high ranks of first and second. Moreover, one would hope that the worst ranking for these two significant pathways would also be high. At first glance, the rankings appear surprisingly high. In particular, we see that the worst performing pathway, on average, never places in the top 3 for any of the models—and it occasionally does not even place in the top 5. However, the results on the individual

Table 1 Average ranking of significant pathways for RM1. Pathways 1 and 2 are significant, so high rankings are desirable

Model	Worst	Pathway 1	Pathway 2
GRRF-0.05	3.865	3.765	1.170
GRRF-0.25	4.205	4.130	1.260
GRRF-0.50	5.330	5.175	1.505
GRRF-0.75	5.920	5.700	2.000
GRRF-0.95	6.170	5.785	2.320
LASSO	4.605	4.545	1.090
varSelRF	6.460	6.190	1.904

Table 2 Average ranking of significant pathways for RM2. Pathways 1 and 2 are significant, so high rankings are desirable

Model	Worst	Pathway 1	Pathway 2
GRRF-0.05	3.375	2.420	2.265
GRRF-0.25	3.585	2.535	2.430
GRRF-0.50	4.515	3.290	3.100
GRRF-0.75	5.255	3.535	3.690
GRRF-0.95	5.440	3.825	3.745
LASSO	3.065	2.050	2.115
varSelRF	5.640	3.945	3.890

Table 3 Average ranking of significant pathways for RM3. Pathways 1 and 2 are significant, so high rankings are desirable

Model	Worst	Pathway 1	Pathway 2
GRRF-0.05	3.265	2.170	2.370
GRRF-0.25	3.640	2.430	2.590
GRRF-0.50	4.895	3.330	3.335
GRRF-0.75	5.480	3.645	3.935
GRRF-0.95	5.470	3.615	4.010
LASSO	3.015	2.090	1.975
varSelRF	5.955	3.810	4.375

pathways are significantly better across the board, which suggests the inflated results are simply an artifact of the ranking procedure.

Comparing performance between models, we see that GRRF outperformed the varSelRF models in all but two cases in RM1 (GRRF-0.75 and GRRF-0.95) but tended not to fare as well against the LASSO models. However, in general, as γ of GRRF decreased—that is, as the GRRF models utilized less regularization—the differences in performance between the GRRF and LASSO models were narrowed as well. In particular, for $\gamma \in \{0.05, 0.25\}$, the GRRF models perform comparably to the LASSO models for each of RM1–RM3, generally differing by no more than half a position in the rankings of the pathways; and, in fact, within RM1, the GRRF models actually edge out the LASSO model with regard to their average rankings of Pathway 1 and the worst performing pathway. This suggests that an appropriately chosen value of γ for GRRF can lead to results that are at least as accurate as the other methods.

4.2 Gene Selection

The next component of our simulation study measured the ability of GRRF, relative to varSelRF and LASSO, to identify the significant genes within predetermined important pathways.

The data generation is the same as in the previous section; however, we ignore Pathways 3–10 as only Pathways 1–2 are significant. We then applied GRRF, varSelRF, and LASSO to each of Pathways 1–2. We allowed γ

of GRRF to range over $\{0.5, 0.55, \ldots, 0.95\} \cup \{0.96, 0.97, 0.98, 0.99\}$; the regularization parameter for LASSO was selected via tenfold cross-validation from $\{0.01, 0.02, 0.03, 0.05, 0.1, 0.2\}$. For each model, we assigned scores for each pathway based on the number of significant genes identified, minus the number of redundancies, as outlined in Deng and Runger [6]—that is, if $(P_1, P_4, P_7, P_{11}, P_{13})$ are identified as significant, we would assign a score of 3, not 4, as P_1 and P_{11} are identical.

As above, this procedure was repeated 100 times for each of RM1–RM3. The results are given in Tables 4, 5, and 6. Within each response model and pathway, the true positive and false positive rates of the GRRF models decreased as γ increased—which is expected, given higher γ values lead to increased regularization. Arguably, the best GRRF models were those for which the true positive and false positive rates were balanced, which roughly occurred for $\gamma \in \{0.85, 0.90, 0.95, 0.96, 0.97\}$. For γ in this range, we see that GRRF outperformed varSelRF across the board in all but a few cases—the most notable exceptions occurring in RM1, where varSelRF achieved a lower false positive rate in Pathway 1 and a higher true positive rate in Pathway 2. We also note that, though LASSO generally outperformed GRRF in terms of significant genes identified, the false positive rates of the LASSO models were typically 2–4 times higher than the GRRF models.

Table 4 Average number of genes selected for RM1. Each pathway contains five genes that are truly significant

Model	P1 true positives	P1 false positives	P2 true positives	P2 false positives
GRRF-0.50	4.25	3.72	3.47	1.77
GRRF-0.55	3.83	3.35	3.23	1.46
GRRF-0.60	3.56	3.25	2.91	1.40
GRRF-0.65	3.39	2.80	2.65	1.19
GRRF-0.70	3.12	2.61	2.68	0.96
GRRF-0.75	2.80	2.35	2.47	1.01
GRRF-0.80	2.78	2.24	2.30	0.87
GRRF-0.85	2.59	2.04	2.23	0.75
GRRF-0.90	2.30	1.78	2.18	0.72
GRRF-0.95	2.26	1.71	2.05	0.68
GRRF-0.96	2.30	1.75	2.04	0.76
GRRF-0.97	2.29	1.73	2.20	0.79
GRRF-0.98	2.26	1.66	2.08	0.76
GRRF-0.99	2.20	1.63	2.00	0.70
LASSO	1.42	1.79	3.74	5.21
varSelRF	1.56	1.42	2.33	1.77

Table 5 Average number of genes selected for RM2. Each pathway contains five genes that are truly significant

Model	P1 true positives	P1 false positives	P2 true positives	P2 false positives
GRRF-0.50	3.97	2.63	3.88	3.07
GRRF-0.55	3.71	2.43	3.65	2.75
GRRF-0.60	3.36	2.07	3.30	2.32
GRRF-0.65	3.25	1.79	3.19	2.21
GRRF-0.70	2.96	1.59	3.07	1.81
GRRF-0.75	2.94	1.45	2.90	1.79
GRRF-0.80	2.75	1.50	2.84	1.60
GRRF-0.85	2.49	1.23	2.57	1.48
GRRF-0.90	2.57	1.10	2.48	1.48
GRRF-0.95	2.45	1.11	2.34	1.33
GRRF-0.96	2.40	1.12	2.39	1.26
GRRF-0.97	2.47	1.02	2.43	1.24
GRRF-0.98	2.40	1.07	2.31	1.26
GRRF-0.99	2.26	1.24	2.39	1.07
LASSO	3.35	4.46	3.13	4.05
varSelRF	1.95	1.49	2.04	1.60

Table 6 Average number of genes selected for RM3. Each pathway contains five genes that are truly significant

Model	P1 true positives	P1 false positives	P2 true positives	P2 false positives
GRRF-0.50	4.20	2.65	4.05	2.60
GRRF-0.55	3.90	2.20	3.85	2.23
GRRF-0.60	3.68	1.88	3.61	1.86
GRRF-0.65	3.45	1.63	3.39	1.76
GRRF-0.70	3.28	1.36	3.23	1.60
GRRF-0.75	3.11	1.22	3.06	1.40
GRRF-0.80	2.94	1.17	2.91	1.35
GRRF-0.85	2.74	1.17	2.81	1.10
GRRF-0.90	2.74	1.10	2.60	1.02
GRRF-0.95	2.62	0.97	2.66	1.02
GRRF-0.96	2.59	1.01	2.58	1.06
GRRF-0.97	2.56	1.01	2.54	0.97
GRRF-0.98	2.51	1.00	2.55	1.13
GRRF-0.99	2.60	0.86	2.59	0.97
LASSO	3.79	4.97	3.77	5.00
varSelRF	2.08	1.34	2.08	1.58

5 Application

The proposed method was further assessed with an application to a publicly available breast cancer dataset consisting of three tumor classes (luminal, basal, and apocrine) for 49 breast cancer patients [11]. A total of 22215 genes and 441 pathways were associated with the dataset. Of the 441 pathways, 129 were taken from the KEGG pathway database and are responsible for metabolism, degradation, biosynthesis, and signal processing; the remaining 312 originate from BioCarta and are mostly related to signal transduction in humans and mice. The data is publicly available from the accompanying website to Pang et al. [23], and we use it here without any additional preprocessing. Computation time using R version 4.3.3 was calculated at 45.77 minutes, and the code used in the analysis is available on GitHub at https://github.com/tylerlewiscook/GRRF-Pathways.

As an initial step, the pathways were separated into two groups according to whether or not the pathway contained less than 10 genes. For the first group, roughly 25% of the pathways, GRRF was ran with $\gamma = 0$ so as to provide minimal regularization; for the second, γ was selected from $\{0.05, 0.10, \ldots, 0.90, 0.95\}$ via tenfold cross-validation. The pathways were then scored and ranked according to minimum OOB.

Table 7 displays the ten most significant pathways along with their corresponding OOB error rates, lengths, and optimal γ values. The results are consistent with recent work in the field. For instance, Palaskas et al. [22] showed that the glycolysis-gluconeogenesis pathway and several glycolysis-related pathways, such as pentose-phosphate and carbon fixation, were linked to the basal subtype of human breast cancer. The KEGG database pathway map for the top pathway, glycolysis-gluconeogenesis (https://www.genome.jp/kegg-bin/show_pathway?map00010), is shown in Fig. 4. Among the aforementioned glycolysis-related pathways, the pentose-phosphate pathway (PPP) has been suggested as a possible target in cancer therapies, as the elevated PPP in cancer cells may help differentiate normal cells

Table 7 Breast cancer dataset results. Pathways labeled with (BC) are from BioCarta, while the others are from KEGG

Pathway	Length	Gamma	Error
Glycolysis-gluconeogenesis	68	0.10	0.022
Downregulated of MTA-3 in ER-negative breast tumors (BC)	19	0.15	0.029
GATA3 participate in activating the Th2 cytokine gene expression (BC)	21	0.05	0.031
Pentose phosphate	22	0.05	0.051
Fructose and mannose metabolism	39	0.05	0.055
Carbon fixation	25	0.05	0.071
CARM1 and regulation of the estrogen receptor (BC)	24	0.70	0.082
Glutathione metabolism	31	0.05	0.088
Valine, leucine, and isoleucine Degradation	46	0.05	0.094
Purine metabolism	112	0.10	0.100

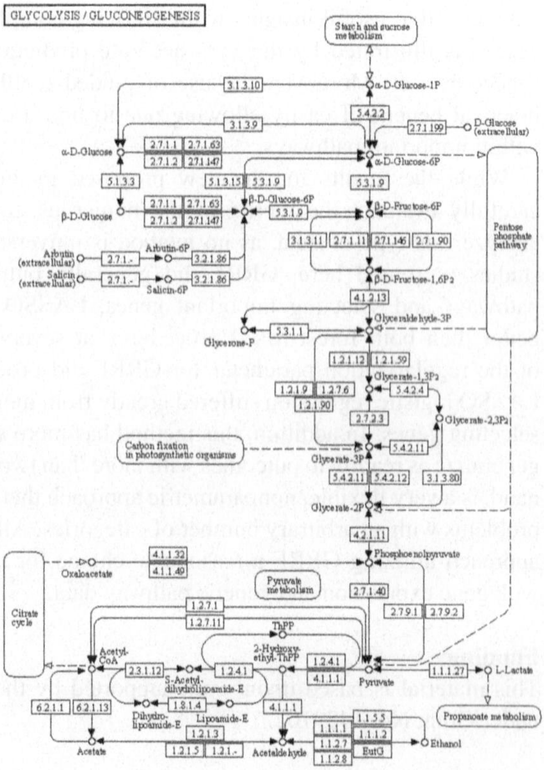

Fig. 4 The structure of the glycolysis-gluconeogenesis pathway taken from the KEGG database

from cancer cells [25]. It is also well known that estrogen plays an important role in breast cancer development and progression, and so it makes sense that three of the top 10 pathways (downregulated of MTA-3 in ER-negative breast tumors, GATA3 participate in activating the Th2 cytokine gene expression, and CARM1 and regulation of the estrogen receptor) are directly linked to activities involving estrogen receptors [14, 19, 36]. Most of the remaining pathways are associated with metabolic processes. The altered metabolisms of cancer cells make the appearance of such pathways in the top 10 plausible [22].

It is also worth noting that none of the pathways in the top 10 have less than 10 genes. In fact, the first pathway with less than 10 genes, sulfur metabolism, only narrowly rounds out the top 25, having placed in the 24th position in the rankings.

6 Discussion

In this chapter, we have developed a novel approach to classify a biological outcome based on gene expression data by taking advantage of known genetic pathways. By utilizing pathway information, our method can help medical researchers and clinicians find useful insights while studying complicated diseases such as cancer. This was illustrated by the very accurate predictions of tumor type for a breast cancer dataset. Moreover, the use of guided regularized random forests has the practical benefit of easily allowing one to find a compact set of important genes within important pathways.

While the results for the new proposed method are promising, one should carefully evaluate the merits of the numerous competing methods available to analyze this type of data, as no method is universally superior. In the simulation studies presented here, GRRF did generally outperform varSelRF for ranking pathways and selecting important genes. LASSO logistic regression performed better than both forest-based procedures in several instances, but certain values of the regularization parameter for GRRF did produce comparable results. Also, LASSO logistic regression suffered greatly from more frequent false positives when selecting genes. In addition, this method has more strict assumptions and does not generalize as readily to outcomes with more than two categories. GRRF, on the other hand, is a very flexible, nonparametric approach that can easily handle classification problems with an arbitrary number of categories. All of these factors make this new approach utilizing GRRF a reasonable choice for modeling a biological outcome with gene expression and genetic pathway data.

Funding
This material is based upon work supported by the National Science Foundation under Grant No. 1429702.

References

1. Bradley, P.S., Mangasarian, O.L.: Feature selection via concave minimization and support vector machines. In: ICML, vol. 98, pp. 82–90 (1998)
2. Breiman, L.: Random forests. Mach. Learn. **45**, 5–32 (2001)
3. Butte, A.: The use and analysis of microarray data. Nat. Rev. Drug. Discov **1**, 951–960 (2002)
4. Castellano, G., Fanelli, A.M.: Variable selection using neural-network models. Neurocomputing **31**, 1–13 (2000)
5. Deng, H.: Guided Random Forest in the RRF Package, arXiv:1306.0237 (2013)
6. Deng, H., Runger, G.: Gene selection with guided regularized random forest. Pattern Recogn. **46**, 3483–3489 (2013)
7. Diaz-Uriarte, R.: Genesrf and varselrf: a web-based tool and r package for gene selection and classification using random forest. BMC Bioinf. **8**, 1–7 (2007)
8. Díaz-Uriarte, R., Alvarez de Andrés, S.: Gene selection and classification of microarray data using random forest. BMC Bioinf. **7**, 1–13 (2006)
9. Downward, J.: Cancer biology: signatures guide drug choice. Nature **439**, 274–275 (2006)
10. Dudoit, S., Shaffer, J.P., Boldrick, J.C.: Multiple hypothesis testing in microarray experiments. Stat. Sci. **18**, 71–103 (2003)
11. Farmer, P., Bonnefoi, H., Becette, V., Tubiana-Hulin, M., Fumoleau, P., Larsimont, D., MacGrogan, G., Bergh, J., Cameron, D., Goldstein, D., et al.: Identification of molecular apocrine breast tumours by microarray analysis. Breast Cancer Res. **7**, 4660–4671 (2005)

12. Friedman, J., Hastie, T., Tibshirani, R.: Regularization paths for generalized linear models via coordinate descent. J. Stat. Softw. **33**, 1–22 (2010). http://www.jstatsoft.org/v33/i01/
13. Friedman, J.H.: Multivariate adaptive regression splines. Ann. Stat. **19**(1), 1–67 (1991)
14. Frietze, S., Lupien, M., Silver, P.A., Brown, M.: Carm1 regulates estrogen-stimulated breast cancer growth through up-regulation of e2f1. Cancer Res. **68**, 301–306 (2008)
15. Furey, T.S., Cristianini, N., Duffy, N., Bednarski, D.W., Schummer, M., Haussler, D.: Support vector machine classification and validation of cancer tissue samples using microarray expression data. Bioinformatics **16**, 906–914 (2000)
16. Guyon, I., Weston, J., Barnhill, S., Vapnik, V.: Gene selection for cancer classification using support vector machines. Mach. Learn. **46**, 389–422 (2002)
17. Hollstein, M., Sidransky, D., Vogelstein, B., Harris, C.C.: p53 mutations in human cancers. Science **253**, 49–53 (1991)
18. Kanehisa, M., Goto, S.: Kegg: Kyoto encyclopedia of genes and genomes. Nucleic Acids Res. **28**, 27–30 (2000)
19. Kumar, R.: Another tie that binds the MTA family to breast cancer. Cell **113**, 142–143 (2003)
20. Maleki, F., Ovens, K., Hogan, D.J., Kusalik, A.J.: Gene set analysis: challenges, opportunities, and future research. Front. Genet. **11**, 654 (2020)
21. Mathur, R., Rotroff, D., Ma, J., Shojaie, A., Motsinger-Reif, A.: Gene set analysis methods: a systematic comparison. BioData Mining **11**, 1–19 (2018)
22. Palaskas, N.J., Larson, S.M., Schultz, N., Komisopoulou, E., Wong, J., Rohle, D., Campos, C., Yannuzzi, N., Osborne, J.R., Linkov, I., et al.: 18f-fluorodeoxy-glucose positron emission tomography marks myc-overexpressing human basal-like breast cancers. Cancer Res. **71**, 5164–5174 (2011)
23. Pang, H., Lin, A., Holford, M., Enerson, B.E., Lu, B., Lawton, M.P., Floyd, E., Zhao, H.: Pathway analysis using random forests classification and regression. Bioinformatics **22**, 2028–2036 (2006)
24. Park, M.Y., Hastie, T., Tibshirani, R.: Averaged gene expressions for regression. Biostatistics **8**, 212–227 (2006)
25. Patra, K.C., Hay, N.: The pentose phosphate pathway and cancer. Trends Biochem. Sci. **39**, 347–354 (2014)
26. R Core Team: R: A Language and Environment for Statistical Computing. R Foundation for Statistical Computing, Vienna (2019). https://www.R-project.org/
27. Segal, M.R.: Machine learning benchmarks and random forest regression. In: UCSF: Center for Bioinformatics and Molecular Biostatistics (2004)
28. Smyth, G.K.: Linear models and empirical bayes methods for assessing differential expression in microarray experiments. Stat. Appl. Genet. Mol. Biol. **3** (2004). https://doi.org/10.2202/1544-6115.1027
29. Stingo, F.C., Chen, Y.A., Tadesse, M.G., Vannucci, M.: Incorporating biological information into linear models: a Bayesian approach to the selection of pathways and genes. Ann. Appl. Stat. **5**, 10–1214 (2011)
30. Storey, J.D., Tibshirani, R.: Statistical significance for genomewide studies. Proc. Natl. Acad. Sci. **100**, 9440–9445 (2003)
31. Subramanian, A., Tamayo, P., Mootha, V.K., Mukherjee, S., Ebert, B.L., Gillette, M.A., Paulovich, A., Pomeroy, S.L., Golub, T.R., Lander, E.S., et al.: Gene set enrichment analysis: a knowledge-based approach for interpreting genome-wide expression profiles. Proc. Natl. Acad. Sci. **102**, 15545–15550 (2005)
32. Tadesse, M.G., Vannucci, M.: Handbook of Bayesian Variable Selection (2021)
33. Tibshirani, R.: Regression shrinkage and selection via the lasso. J. R. Stat. Soc. Ser. B Methodol. **58**, 267–288 (1996)
34. Tusher, V.G., Tibshirani, R., Chu, G.: Significance analysis of microarrays applied to the ionizing radiation response. Proc. Natl. Acad. Sci. **98**, 5116–5121 (2001)
35. Vogelstein, B., Kinzler, K.W.: Cancer genes and the pathways they control. Nat. Med. **10**, 789–799 (2004)

36. Wilson, B.J., Giguère, V.: Meta-analysis of human cancer microarrays reveals GATA3 is integral to the estrogen receptor alpha pathway. Mol. Cancer **7**, 49 (2008)
37. Xu, Z., Huang, G., Weinberger, K.Q., Zheng, A.X.: Gradient boosted feature selection. In: Proceedings of the 20th ACM SIGKDD International Conference on Knowledge Discovery and Data Mining, pp. 522–531 (2014)
38. Yi, G., Sze, S.H., Thon, M.R.: Identifying clusters of functionally related genes in genomes. Bioinformatics **23**, 1053–1060 (2007)

Ultrahigh-Dimensional Discriminant Analysis and Its Application to Gene Expression Data

Li-Pang Chen, Jou-Chin Wu, and Hui-Shan Tsao

Abstract Discriminant analysis has been a commonly used strategy to handle classification with binary or multi-label responses. Under multivariate normal distributions of covariates, a linear or quadratic discriminant function can be derived, which is used as a boundary to classify subjects. In the discriminant function, the estimation of the precision matrix, which is defined as the inverse of the covariance matrix, is a crucial issue because of the sparsity, reflecting that few pairs of variables are informative, which may implicitly affect the accuracy of the classification. While a large body of estimation methods is available to estimate the precision matrix, most methods not only fail to handle ultrahigh-dimensionality in the sense that the dimension of variables is extremely larger than the sample size, but also require longer computational time. In addition, in the presence of nonlinear dependence among variables, existing methods may falsely miss the detection of dependence. To tackle those challenges, we extend the model-free feature screening method to reduce the dimension of variables and detect possibly nonlinear pairwise dependence structure among variables. After that, we adopt several graphical estimation methods to estimate the homogeneous or heterogeneous precision matrices and then implement the estimator to the discriminant function to improve the classification. Numerical studies are conducted to assess the performance of prediction for the proposed method and verify the necessity of taking network structures of variables into account.

Keywords Bioinformatics · Classification · Feature screening · Graphical models · Precision matrix

L.-P. Chen (✉) · J.-C. Wu · H.-S. Tsao
Department of Statistics, National Chengchi University, Taipei, Taiwan
e-mail: lchen723@nccu.edu.tw

Y. Zhao, D.-G. Chen (eds.), *Big Data Analytics in Biostatistics and Bioinformatics*, ICSA Book Series in Statistics,
https://doi.org/10.1007/978-3-032-06649-7_10

1 Introduction

1.1 Background and Literature Review

Classification has been an important topic in supervised learning, whose goal is to use subjects' information to classify them to the desired class. This topic has raised attention in various research fields. A typical classification problem in bioinformatics is to take gene expression variables as the information to identify patients' cancers or tumors. In the literature, [34] applied the support vector machine (SVM) to classify patients to various cancers. Peng et al. [30] proposed a data mining approach with the recursive feature elimination (nRFE) algorithm accommodated to analyze the microRNA data. Yangand Naiman [41] proposed the top scoring set (TSS) method to classify multiple disease states associated with cancer based on gene expression profiles. Saha et al. [36] proposed a two-stage procedure to detect biomarkers and then do classification. Piao et al. [32] proposed a feature subset-based ensemble method to classify multiple cancers. With the number of classes restricted to 2, [8] considered binary classification and examined the causal effect of two different experiments on two types of leukemia (AML and ALL) by incorporating gene expression variables. In addition to those methods, linear discriminant analysis (LDA) and quadratic discriminant analysis (QDA) are also the useful approaches for classification with binary or multi-label classes (e.g., [23]) in recent years due to its convenient implementation and precise classification. The basic idea of LDA and QDA is to derive a linear and quadratic discriminant function, provided that the covariates follow a multivariate normal distribution with positive definite covariance matrices, and use a discriminant function to classify subjects.

While discriminant functions are easy to implement, their natural feature is the estimation of the inverse of covariance matrices, which also refer to precision matrices. According to the theory of graphical models, off-diagonal entries in precision matrices usually reflect the conditional dependence of two variables, and thus, precision matrices characterize the network structure of multivariate (or high-dimensional) variables. Moreover, in biomedical research, some literature (e.g., [16, 25]) found that some gene expressions are usually highly correlated among others, while some of them are not, yielding the network structure. As a result, one can expect that precision matrices are possibly sparse, and the traditional implementation of computing the inverse of empirical estimates of covariance matrices is not an ideal strategy to estimate precision matrices. In contrast, to deal with this concern, some estimation methods have been proposed in the theory of graphical models, including the graphical lasso (glasso, [20]) and the constrained L1-minimization for inverse matrix estimation (clime, [3]). More methods are also summarized in Section 2 of [6]. With the network structures of covariates equipped, various classification methods have been explored, such as [2, 15, 29, 31]. In the applications of discriminant analysis, some methods were proposed to improve the discriminant function with the network structure accommodated. For example, [4] proposed network linear discriminant analysis with binary responses. Chen [11] applied the glasso and neighborhood estimation methods to estimate the precision matrix and implement the estimator on the linear/quadratic discriminant function, where the computational implementation can be found in [9]. Chen [12] considered the nonparametric approach with network structure in variables.

The other challenging feature in gene expression data is the ultrahigh-dimensionality, which reflects that the number of variables is extremely greater than the sample size and only a few gene expressions are informative in classification. In the existing literature, some methods were proposed to address classification with ultrahigh-dimensional data. For example, [1, 37] considered the sparse multinomial logistic regression models. Witten and Tibshirani [39] proposed the penalized linear discriminant method. Mahadi et al. [27] developed the regularized linear discriminant function by modifying the inverse of the covariance matrix. Guo et al. [22] proposed the shrunken centroids regularized discriminant analysis to deal with high-dimensional variables and low sample size in microarray data. Safo and Ahn [35] extended the sparse discrimination methods to handle multi-classification. However, these methods ignore possible network structures in gene expressions. In addition, high-dimensionality usually makes the empirical estimate of the covariance matrix singular or makes it difficult to employ the glasso or clime methods efficiently. To address it, feature screening might be a suitable strategy, whose key idea is to take the correlation between two variables as the signal and then retain the informative variables with higher correlation values, so that the number of retained variables is smaller than the sample size (e.g., [7, 19]). Moreover, together with the target of classification, [10] first reduced the dimension of variables and then used the selected variables to derive the classification models with the network structure in the variables accommodated. However, unlike conventional feature screening methods that are used to determine informative variables associated with a targeted response variable, a rare discussion focuses on capturing informative pairs from ultrahigh-dimensional data and the corresponding implementation for the estimation of the precision matrix.

1.2 Outlined Methods and Contributions

To address those challenges and make discriminant analysis suitable to deal with classification for ultrahigh-dimensional data with network structures in variables, we explore a valid strategy to deal with the estimation of precision matrices. Specifically, we apply a model-free rank-based estimator as a signal to detect informative pairs of gene expressions, so that the "reduced" correlation matrix containing informative pairs of gene expressions can be obtained. After that, we implement the reduced correlation matrix to existing methods, such as the glasso or clime methods, which are different from existing approaches that implement the empirical estimate of the covariance matrix with the ignorance of independent pairs of gene expressions. Moreover, to take classes into account and build quadratic discriminant functions, we also apply the joint graphical lasso (JGL; [18]) method to identify class-dependent network structures of gene expressions. Finally, when estimated precision matrices are obtained, we further derive the linear and quadratic discriminant functions to perform classification and prediction. In general, our estimation procedure is easy to use and can be implemented by some existing packages.

Our proposed method has several contributions and differences from existing literature. First, unlike most feature screening procedures that select main effects depending on the response, our approach aims to retain dependent pairs of variables. This approach enables us to obtain a matrix that contains strong interactions of variables and is convenient for the implementation of the graphical estimation methods. Moreover, due to the reduced dimension, the computation is also faster than the conventional glasso or clime approaches that directly implement the empirical estimate of the covariance matrix. Second, while [40] adopted a similar approach by using the Spearman's ρ, the Chatterjee's measure [5] considered in our development is more sensitive in detecting oscillatory trajectories of variables. Additionally, the sure screening property of pairwise variables detection is ensured, so that one is sufficient to derive the graphical structure based on dependent interactions of variables. Moreover, our study also explores the estimation of heterogeneous network structures among various classes by using the Chatterjee's measure, which is also a main difference from [40]. Finally, provided that the network structure and the precision matrix are estimated, the estimated network structure is adopted to the linear/quadratic discriminant function, which is different from other approaches that select main effects when building discriminant functions (e.g., [17, 22, 27, 39]) or logistic regression models (e.g., [1, 37]).

1.3 Organization of This Article

The remainder is organized as follows. In Sect. 2, we introduce the data structure, the basic idea of discriminant analysis, and network structures in covariates. In Sect. 3, we present our strategy for dealing with precision matrices with ultrahigh-dimensional data and develop a modified linear/quadratic discriminant function for classification and prediction. In Sect. 4, we conduct simulation studies to evaluate the performance of the proposed method, and we apply our method to analyze a gene expression dataset with multiple types of cancer in Sect. 5. Finally, we give a summary and discuss some future research directions in Sect. 6. More information can be found on GitHub: https://github.com/lchen723/UHDClassification.git.

2 Preliminary

2.1 Data Structure and Discriminant Analysis

Let n denote the sample size in a dataset. For a subject $j = 1, \cdots, n$, let $\mathbf{X}_j = (X_{1,j}, \cdots, X_{p,j})^\top$ denote the p-dimensional vector of covariates with the lowercase letter $\mathbf{x}_j$ denoting the realized value, where p can be diverging with n and is denoted as $p \gg n$, i.e., $p = O\{\exp(n^r)\}$ for some $r > 0$ (e.g., [19]). In addition, for $j = 1, \cdots, n$, let Y_j denote a nominal random variable with I different labels for $I \geq 2$. Moreover, let n_i denote the sample size in class i for $i = 1, \cdots, I$, such that $\sum_{i=1}^{I} n_i = n$. Thus, the independent and identically distributed (i.i.d.) dataset is denoted as $\mathcal{D} \triangleq \{\{Y_j, \mathbf{X}_j\} : j = 1, \cdots, n\}$.

The goal is to build a predictive model and classify subjects into their classes. We primarily consider discriminant analysis, which is a commonly used classification method in supervised learning (e.g., [23]). Specifically, given class $Y_j = i$, let $\mathbf{X}_j$ follow the multivariate normal distribution with mean vector $\boldsymbol{\mu}_i$ and a positive definite covariance matrix $\boldsymbol{\Sigma}_i$. Let $\pi_i \triangleq P\left(Y_j = i\right)$ denote the probability that the jth subject is randomly selected from class i, which also satisfies $\sum_{i=1}^{I} \pi_i = 1$. Consequently, the conditional probability of $Y_j = i$ given $\mathbf{X}_j = \mathbf{x}_j$is given by

$$P\left(Y_j = i|\mathbf{X}_j = \mathbf{x}_j\right) = \frac{f_{j|i}(\mathbf{x}_j)\pi_i}{\sum_{l=1}^{I} f_{j|l}(\mathbf{x}_j)\pi_l} \tag{1}$$

for $i = 1, \ldots, I$ and $j = 1, \ldots, n$, where

$$f_{j|i}(\mathbf{x}_j) = \frac{1}{(2\pi)^{p/2}|\boldsymbol{\Sigma}_i|^{1/2}} \exp\left\{-\frac{1}{2}\left(\mathbf{x}_j - \boldsymbol{\mu}_i\right)^\top \boldsymbol{\Sigma}_i^{-1}\left(\mathbf{x}_j - \boldsymbol{\mu}_i\right)\right\} \tag{2}$$

is the density function of $\mathbf{X}_j$ given $Y_j = i$.

For any i and i' with $i \neq i'$, a subject is likely to belong to class i if

$$P\left(Y_j = i|\mathbf{X}_j = \mathbf{x}_j\right) > P\left(Y_j = i'|\mathbf{X}_j = \mathbf{x}_j\right). \tag{3}$$

Then combining (3) with (1) and (2) gives the *quadratic discriminant function*

$$\varphi_i(\mathbf{x}) \triangleq \log(\pi_i) + \frac{1}{2}\log|\boldsymbol{\Theta}_i| - \frac{1}{2}(\mathbf{x} - \boldsymbol{\mu}_i)^\top \boldsymbol{\Theta}_i(\mathbf{x} - \boldsymbol{\mu}_i), \tag{4}$$

where $\boldsymbol{\Theta}_i \triangleq \boldsymbol{\Sigma}_i^{-1}$ is called the *precision matrix* for class i with $i = 1, \cdots, I$. In particular, if $\boldsymbol{\Sigma}_i = \boldsymbol{\Sigma}$ for all $i = 1, \cdots, I$, then (3) yields the *linear discriminant function*

$$\delta_i(\mathbf{x}) \triangleq \log(\pi_i) - \frac{1}{2}\boldsymbol{\mu}_i^\top \boldsymbol{\Theta}\boldsymbol{\mu}_i + \mathbf{x}^\top \boldsymbol{\Theta}\boldsymbol{\mu}_i, \tag{5}$$

where $\boldsymbol{\Theta} \triangleq \boldsymbol{\Sigma}^{-1}$ is the precision matrix by pooling all subjects from all classes. Consequently, a predicted class i^* for a subject is defined as

$$i^* = \underset{i=1,\ldots,I}{\arg\max}\, \delta_i(\widetilde{\mathbf{x}}) \quad \text{or} \quad i^* = \underset{i=1,\ldots,I}{\arg\max}\, \varphi_i(\widetilde{\mathbf{x}}),$$

where $\widetilde{\mathbf{x}}$ represents the covariates from a new subject, provided that $\boldsymbol{\mu}_i$, $\boldsymbol{\Theta}_i$, $\boldsymbol{\Theta}$, and π_i for $i = 1, \cdots, I$ are empirically estimated.

2.2 Network Structures in Covariates

Mathematically, let $\mathbb{V}$ be the set of vertices and let $\mathbb{E} \subset \mathbb{V} \times \mathbb{V}$ denote the set of edges. A *graph* is usually expressed as $\mathbb{G} = (\mathbb{V}, \mathbb{E})$. Given a dataset, vertices represent random variables or gene expressions, and edges connecting two random variables or gene expressions are used to indicate the dependence. Take Fig. 1 as an example, suppose that there are six gene expressions, panel A shows that Gene 2 and Gene 6 are conditionally independent, given other gene expressions, and Gene 1 is conditionally dependent on Gene 3, Gene 4, and Gene 5, given other gene expressions. In the theory of graphical models, the precision matrix can be used to represent the graphical structure: a nonzero value in the (s, t) entry gives an edge between X_s and X_t, and a zero value in the (s, t) entry reflects no edge between X_s and X_t. As a result, panel B in Fig. 1 can represent the network structure in panel A, and it shows that the precision matrix is usually sparse.

Consequently, the goal is to estimate the unknown matrix $\boldsymbol{\Theta}$, so that the network structure can be identified. From the statistical perspective, the first step is to characterize the relationship between random variables and the matrix $\boldsymbol{\Theta}$. Specifically, we first consider the pooled data among I classes, so that the density function of $\mathbf{X}$, which is defined by (2) with the class label i removed, is given by

$$\frac{1}{(2\pi)^{p/2}\,|\boldsymbol{\Sigma}|^{1/2}} \exp\left\{-\frac{1}{2}(\mathbf{x} - \boldsymbol{\mu})^\top \boldsymbol{\Sigma}^{-1}(\mathbf{x} - \boldsymbol{\mu})\right\}. \tag{6}$$

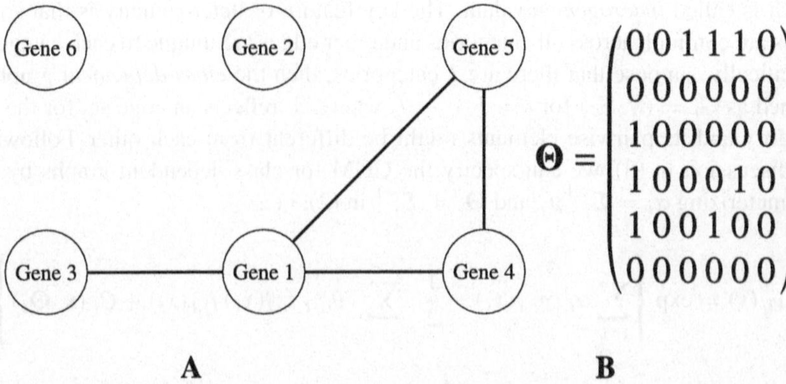

Fig. 1 Illustrative diagrams of the network structure in covariates with $p = 6$. Panel A is the network structure of six gene expressions. Panel B is the precision matrix that reflects the network structure in panel A. Values 1 indicate the existence of edges of variables, such as an entry (1, 3) for a pair of Gene 1 and Gene 3; values 0 reflect the nonexistence of edges of variables, such as an entry (1, 2) for a pair of Gene 1 and Gene 2

Let $\boldsymbol{\alpha} = \boldsymbol{\Sigma}^{-1}\boldsymbol{\mu}$ and $\boldsymbol{\Theta} = \boldsymbol{\Sigma}^{-1}$, then (6) can be re-parameterized as (e.g., [24], p.246)

$$\mathbb{P}_{\boldsymbol{\alpha},\boldsymbol{\Theta}}(\mathbf{x}) = \exp\left\{\sum_{s\in\mathbb{V}} \alpha_s x_s - \frac{1}{2}\sum_{(s,t)\in\mathbb{E}} \theta_{st} x_s x_t + \frac{1}{2}\log\det\left(\frac{\boldsymbol{\Theta}}{2\pi}\right)\right\}, \tag{7}$$

where α_s is the sth component in the vector $\boldsymbol{\alpha}$ and $\boldsymbol{\Theta} = [\theta_{st}]$. The model (7) is called the Gaussian graphical model (GGM). In our study, we further extend (7) to the following complex structure:

$$\mathbb{P}_{\boldsymbol{\alpha},\boldsymbol{\Theta}}(\mathbf{x}) = \exp\left\{\sum_{s\in\mathbb{V}} \alpha_s g_s(x_s) - \frac{1}{2}\sum_{(s,t)\in\mathbb{E}} \theta_{st} f_s(x_s) f_t(x_t) + C(\mathbf{x}, \boldsymbol{\Theta})\right\}, \tag{8}$$

where $C(\mathbf{x}, \boldsymbol{\Theta})$ is a normalizing constant that ensures the integration of (8) is 1, and $f_s(\cdot)$ and $g_s(\cdot)$ are unknown and nonlinear functions. For example, if $p = 2$ with $X_1 \sim N(0, 1)$ and $X_2 = 6\cos(X_1) + \epsilon$ with $\epsilon \sim N(0, 1)$, then (8) with $\mathbf{X} = (X_1, X_2)^\top$ is given by

$$\frac{1}{2\pi}\exp\left\{-\frac{1}{2}\left(x_2^2 - 12x_2\cos(x_1) + 36\cos(x_1)^2 + x_1^2\right)\right\},$$

where $f_1(x_1) = \cos(x_1)$ and $f_2(x_2) = x_2$.

The above discussion for the graphical structure $\mathbb{G}$ implicitly assumes that the variables in a given dataset have a common network. In applications, a general and possible situation is that the same variables are recorded in various categories, which is called *heterogeneous* data. The key feature of heterogeneity is that some edges are common across all categories and other edges are unique to each category. Specifically, suppose that there are I categories, then the *class-dependent* graph is defined as $\mathbb{G}_i = (\mathbb{V}, \mathbb{E}_i)$ for $i = 1, \cdots, I$, where $\mathbb{E}_i$ reflects an edge set for the ith category and its pairwise elements might be different from each other. Following the discussion in (8), we can specify the GGM for class-dependent graphs by re-parameterizing $\boldsymbol{\alpha}_i = \boldsymbol{\Sigma}_i^{-1}\boldsymbol{\mu}_i$ and $\boldsymbol{\Theta}_i = \boldsymbol{\Sigma}_i^{-1}$ in (2), i.e.,

$$\mathbb{P}_{\boldsymbol{\alpha}_i,\boldsymbol{\Theta}_i}(\mathbf{x}) = \exp\left\{\sum_{s\in\mathbb{V}} \alpha_{i,s} g_{i,s}(x_s) - \frac{1}{2}\sum_{(s,t)\in\mathbb{E}_i} \theta_{i,st} f_{i,s}(x_s) f_{i,t}(x_t) + C_i(\mathbf{x}, \boldsymbol{\Theta}_i)\right\}$$

for $i = 1, \cdots, I$, where $\alpha_{i,s}$ is the sth component in the vector $\boldsymbol{\alpha}_i$ and $\boldsymbol{\Theta}_i = [\theta_{i,st}]$ is a $p \times p$ matrix for class i. Then the heterogeneity reflects that $\theta_{i,st} \neq 0$, while $\theta_{j,st} = 0$ for any two categories $i \neq j$ and some fixed pairs (s, t).

Motivated by this, one may realize that directly taking the inverse of the empirical estimation of $\boldsymbol{\Sigma}_i$ or $\boldsymbol{\Sigma}$ may not reflect the estimation of $\boldsymbol{\Theta}_i$ in (4) or $\boldsymbol{\Theta}$ in (5). Furthermore, in the $p \gg n$ setting, the estimators of $\boldsymbol{\Sigma}_i$ and $\boldsymbol{\Sigma}$ are singular, making the matrix non-invertible and failing to construct (4) and (5). Therefore, it is crucial to reasonably estimate the precision matrix by taking the network structure and high-dimensionality into account when implementing the discriminant functions (4) and (5).

3 Methodology

To tackle the estimation of $\boldsymbol{\Theta}_i$ for (4) or $\boldsymbol{\Theta}$ in (5) under the ultrahigh-dimensional data and deal with the classification problem by discriminant functions (4) and (5), we propose the estimation procedure, where the workflow is summarized in Fig. 2. In the following subsections, we will describe the detailed procedures for the steps in Fig. 2.

3.1 Feature Screening for Pairwise Dependence Structure

As shown in panel B of Fig. 1, $\boldsymbol{\Theta}_i$ and $\boldsymbol{\Theta}$ are sparse in the sense that many 0 values are included in off-diagonal entries (k, l) with $k \neq l$, which equivalently reflect the conditional independence between X_k and X_l, given other covariates X_r with $r \in \mathbb{V} \setminus \{k, l\}$. Motivated by this, we first screen out independent or weakly dependent pairs of variables and retain dependent pairs of variables. Specifically, we consider the following active set:

$$\mathcal{S} = \{(k, l) : \text{pairs } (X_k, X_l) \text{ have high dependence for } k, l = 1, \cdots, p; k \neq l\}.$$

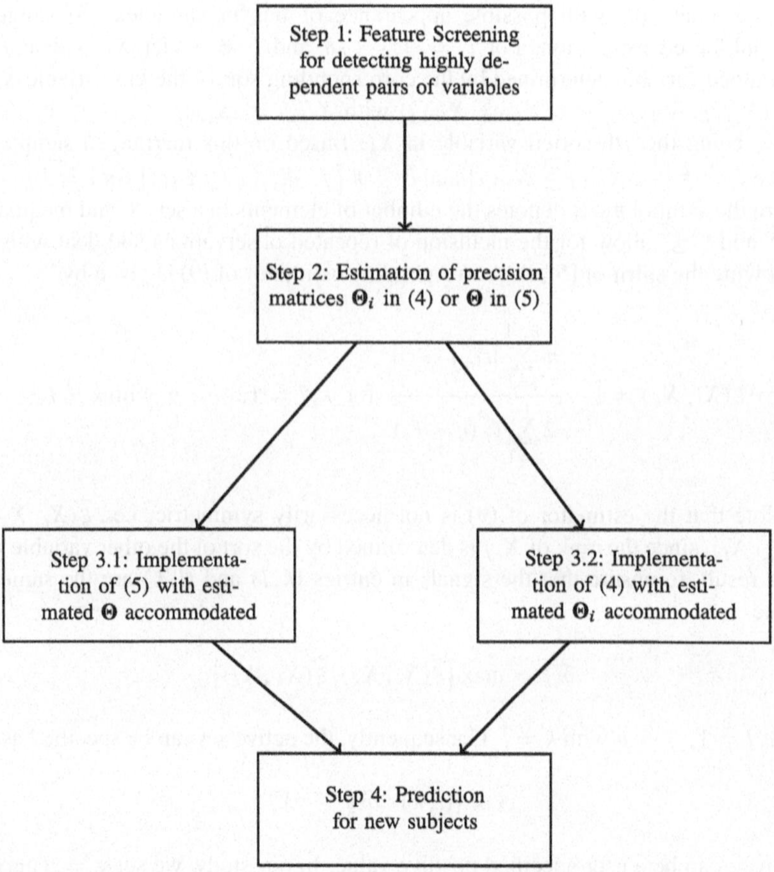

Fig. 2 The workflow of ultrahigh-dimensional discriminant analysis. Step 1 reflects the detection of informative pairs of variable in Sect. 3.1; Step 2 indicates the estimation for precision matrices by using graphical model techniques in Sect. 3.2; Steps 3.1, 3.2, and 4 implement the LDA and QDA methods with the estimators of $\boldsymbol{\Theta}$ and $\boldsymbol{\Theta}_i$ in Sect. 3.3

To detect dependence between (X_k, X_l) for all $k \neq l$, we adopt the following Chatterjee's measure [5]:

$$\xi(X_l, X_k) = \frac{\int \mathrm{var}\left[E\left\{\mathbb{I}(X_l \geq x)|X_k\right\}\right] d\mu_l(x)}{\int \mathrm{var}\left\{\mathbb{I}(X_l \geq x)\right\} d\mu_l(x)}, \tag{9}$$

where $\mathbb{I}(\cdot)$ denotes the indicator function and $\mu_l(\cdot)$ is the law of X_l for $l = 1, \cdots, p$. As commented in [5], (9) is shown to be between 0 and 1 and reflects the correlation coefficient, yielding stronger dependence if the values are higher. As examined in [7], (9) is useful to detect dependence between X_k and X_l in the presence of an oscillatory trajectory or a nonlinear relationship.

To estimate (9) with possible appearance of ties in variables, [5] suggested the rank-based estimation. For $i = 1, \cdots, n$ and $l \neq k$, let $X_{(i),l}$ denote the rearranged variable determined by the corresponding sort of the kth variable $X_{(i),k}$, i.e., $(X_{(1),k}, X_{(1),l}), \cdots, (X_{(n),k}, X_{(n),l})$ with $X_{(1),k} \leq X_{(2),k} \leq \cdots \leq X_{(n),k}$ and $X_{(j),k}$ being the jth sorted variable in X_k. Based on this rearranged sample, we define $\ell_i \triangleq \#\left\{j : X_{(j),l} \geq X_{(i),l}\right\}$ and $r_i \triangleq \#\left\{j : X_{(j),l} \leq X_{(i),l}\right\}$ for $i = 1, \cdots, n$, where the symbol $\#\{\mathcal{A}\}$ denotes the number of elements in a set $\mathcal{A}$, and inequalities "$\geq$" and "$\leq$" allow for the inclusion of repeated observations and deal with ties. Following the spirit of [5], the corresponding estimator of (9) is given by

$$\widehat{\xi}(X_l, X_k) = 1 - \frac{n \sum_{i=1}^{n-1} |r_{i+1} - r_i|}{2 \sum_{i=1}^{n} \ell_i (n - \ell_i)} \quad \text{for } k, l = 1, \cdots, p \text{ with } k \neq l. \tag{10}$$

Note that the estimator of (9) is not necessarily symmetric, i.e., $\widehat{\xi}(X_l, X_k) \neq \widehat{\xi}(X_k, X_l)$, since the rank of $X_{i,l}$ is determined by the sort of the other variable $X_{i,k}$. As a result, to ensure that the signals in entries (k, l) and (l, k) are the same, we define

$$\widehat{\omega}_{lk} = \max\left\{\widehat{\xi}(X_l, X_k), \widehat{\xi}(X_k, X_l)\right\} \tag{11}$$

for $k, l = 1, \cdots, p$ with $k \neq l$. Consequently, the active set can be specified as

$$\widehat{\mathcal{S}} = \{(l, k) : \widehat{\omega}_{lk} > \gamma\}, \tag{12}$$

where γ can be a user-specified positive value. In our study, we set $\gamma = a \max\limits_{s<t} \widehat{\omega}_{st}$ for some constant $a \in (0, 1)$. Finally, we comment that while the strategy of constructing $\widehat{\mathcal{S}}$ follows an idea of feature screening, the main difference is that early feature screening approaches aim to retain variables that are highly associated with the response, but our step is to retain informative pairs of variables.

Alternatively, if we take classes into account, then covariates in different classes reflect heterogeneous data, yielding various precision matrices. To reduce the dimension with the same variables retained for heterogeneous classes at the same time, we consider the following feature screening:

$$\mathcal{I} = \{k : \text{variable } X_k \text{ is informative for cancers in } Y\},$$

which collects all gene expressions that are informative for every class in Y. To estimate $\mathcal{I}$, we adopt the measure (9) with the modification:

$$\xi(Y, X_k) = \frac{\int \text{var}\left[E\left\{\mathbb{I}(Y \geq x) | X_k\right\}\right] d\mu(y)}{\int \text{var}\left\{\mathbb{I}(Y \geq x)\right\} d\mu(y)}, \tag{13}$$

where $\mu(y)$ is the law of Y. Let $\widehat{\tau}_k \triangleq \widehat{\xi}(Y, X_k)$ denote the estimator of (13) derived by the rank-based estimation in (10). Larger values of (13) and their estimates $\widehat{\tau}_k$ reflect stronger dependence between Y and X_k. As a result, the desired informative variables can be determined by

$$\widehat{\mathcal{I}} = \{k : \widehat{\tau}_k > \nu\}, \tag{14}$$

where ν is a prespecified positive constant to ensure that $|\widehat{\mathcal{I}}| < n$. It reflects that variables in $\widehat{\mathcal{I}}$ are informative for every cancer in Y. In our implementation, ν is determined to ensure that the first $\left[\frac{\log n}{n}\right]$ largest $\widehat{\tau}_k$ and the corresponding X_k are selected.

Theoretically, with threshold values γ and ν provided in (12) and (14), one might wonder if $\widehat{\mathcal{S}}$ and $\widehat{\mathcal{I}}$ can retain informative pairs of variables or important variables for the response Y. To answer this question, we state the result in the following theorem, and the proof follows the derivation in [7].

Theorem 1 *Let $\omega_{lk} \triangleq \max\{\xi(X_l, X_k), \xi(X_k, X_l)\}$ and τ_k denote the true values of (9) and (13), respectively. Suppose that the first argument X_l and Y in (9) and (13) are not constants. Then*

(a) Two probabilistic bounds for $\widehat{\omega}_{lk}$ and $\widehat{\tau}_k$:

$$P\left(\max_{1\leq k<l\leq p} |\widehat{\omega}_{lk} - \omega_{lk}| \geq c_1 n^{-\zeta_1}\right) \leq p(p-1)\Big[\exp\Big\{-\log\Big(2c_1 n^{1-\zeta_1} K_1/3\Big)\Big\} + 3\exp\Big(-2n^{1-2\zeta_1} c_1^2 K_1^2/9\Big)\Big]$$

and

$$P\left(\max_{1\leq k\leq p} |\widehat{\tau}_k - \tau_k| \geq c_2 n^{-\zeta_2}\right) \leq p\Big[\exp\Big\{-\log\Big(2c_2 n^{1-\zeta_2} K_2/3\Big)\Big\} + 3\exp\Big(-2n^{1-2\zeta_2} c_2^2 K_2^2/9\Big)\Big],$$

where c_1, c_2, K_1, K_2, ζ_1, and ζ_2 are positive constants with $0 < \zeta_1, \zeta_2 < 1/2$.

(b) The sure screening property:
Assume that $\min_{(k,l)\in\mathcal{S}} \omega_{lk} \geq c_1 n^{-\zeta_1}$ and $\min_{k\in\mathcal{I}} \tau_k \geq c_2 n^{-\zeta_2}$, which reflects that the marginal signal of truly dependent pairs and truly informative variables cannot be small. Then we have that

$$P\left(\widehat{\mathcal{S}} \supseteq \mathcal{S}\right) \geq 1 - q_1\Big[\exp\Big\{-\log\Big(2c_1 n^{1-\zeta_1} K_1/3\Big)\Big\} + 3\exp\Big(-2n^{1-2\zeta_1} c_1^2 K_1^2/9\Big)\Big]$$

and

$$P\left(\widehat{\mathcal{I}} \supseteq \mathcal{I}\right) \geq 1 - q_2\Big[\exp\Big\{-\log\left(2c_2 n^{1-\zeta_2} K_2/3\right)\Big\} \\ +3\exp\left(-2n^{1-2\zeta_2} c_2^2 K_2^2/9\right)\Big],$$

where q_1 and q_2 are the cardinalities of $\mathcal{S}$ and $\mathcal{I}$, respectively.

Under similar conditions as in [7], $\widehat{\omega}_{lk}$ and $\widehat{\tau}_k$ have similar probabilistic bounds that ensure the closeness of the true measure ω_{lk} and τ_k. The probabilistic bounds of $\widehat{\omega}_{lk}$ and $\widehat{\tau}_k$ look similar because they follow the same derivations in [7] with X_l and Y in (9) and (13) treated as the position of the response. In addition, part (a) also yields the sure screening property presented in part (b) with similar probabilistic inequalities. Moreover, the sure screening property in part (b) says that the estimated sets $\widehat{\mathcal{S}}$ and $\widehat{\mathcal{I}}$ are able to include truly dependent pairs of variables and important variables for the response with a large probability. This is due to the fact that the Chatterjee's measure is shown to ensure the sure screening property under the detection of informative variables in ultrahigh-dimensional regression models [7]. While the results and the key strategy of the derivations look similar to [7], the key differences include that the results of $\widehat{\omega}_{lk}$ and $\{\widehat{\mathcal{S}} \supseteq \mathcal{S}\}$ reflect the recruitment of dependent pairs; $\widehat{\tau}_k$ and $\{\widehat{\mathcal{I}} \supseteq \mathcal{I}\}$ indicate the inclusion of informative variables for a nominal response.

3.2 Estimation of Precision Matrices

Given the pairs retained in (12) or variables in (14), we define the matrix $\mathbf{P} \triangleq [\widehat{\omega}_{lk}]_{(l,k)\in\widehat{\mathcal{S}}}$ based on the pooled data, and we define matrices $\mathbf{P}_i \triangleq [\widehat{\omega}_{i,lk}]_{k,l\in\widehat{\mathcal{I}}}$ for heterogeneous class $i = 1, \cdots, I$, where $\widehat{\omega}_{i,lk}$ is defined as (11) with X_k and X_l belonging to class i for $k \neq l$. Note that $\mathbf{P}$ and $\mathbf{P}_i$ are determined by (12) and (14) that may additionally retain independent pairs or non-informative variables because of the user-specified threshold values γ and ν, so that $\mathbf{P}$ and $\mathbf{P}_i$ do not reflect the precision matrices. As a result, as shown in Step 2 of Fig. 2, we use them to estimate the precision matrices $\boldsymbol{\Theta}$ or $\boldsymbol{\Theta}_i$ in the following two subsections.

Before introducing the estimation, we briefly comment on the usage of $\mathbf{P}$ and $\mathbf{P}_i$. Unlike conventional implementations that used conventional covariance matrices in graphical estimation methods, we adopt matrices $\mathbf{P}$ and $\mathbf{P}_i$. The main reason is that the Chatterjee's measure is also used to detect dependent/independent pairs of variables and reflects the correlation of two variables. In addition, the Chatterjee's measure is more sensitive in detecting dependent pairs of variables. For example, if two variables are independent, the Chatterjee's measure gives a value close to zero and is smaller than the empirical covariance. With penalty functions equipped in graphical estimation methods, zero-valued entries in precision matrices can also be identified. On the other hand, note that [40] also adopted a similar approach by using the Spearman's rho correlation in graphical estimation methods. The main difference between [40] and our approach is that the Chatterjee's measure is able to detect non-monotone and oscillatory trajectory between variables in high-dimensional settings. Moreover, as discussed in Sect. 3.2.2, we also make extensions to the estimation of heterogeneous network structure, which is also the main difference from [40].

3.2.1 Estimation with Pooled Samples

Due to the sparsity, we can rewrite $\boldsymbol{\Theta} \triangleq \text{Diag}(\boldsymbol{\Phi}, \mathbf{I})$, where $\boldsymbol{\Phi}$ is a submatrix of the precision matrix $\boldsymbol{\Theta}$ and reflects the network structure of variables, i.e., all entries with nonzero values in $\boldsymbol{\Phi}$ are pairs in $\mathbb{E}$, $\mathbf{I}$ is an identity matrix, and "Diag" represents the block diagonal matrix with diagonal entries being submatrices. Therefore, with dependent pairs selected in $\mathbf{P}$, it is sufficient to adopt $\mathbf{P}$ to estimate $\boldsymbol{\Phi}$.

When $\mathbf{P}$ is derived based on the pooled samples, we primarily adopt the glasso and clime methods to derive the estimator of $\boldsymbol{\Phi}$ because of the availability of the R packages `glasso` and `clime`, respectively. For the glasso method, we estimate $\boldsymbol{\Phi}$ by maximizing the following penalized function:

$$\log\{\det(\boldsymbol{\Phi})\} - \text{trace}(\mathbf{P}\boldsymbol{\Phi}) - \lambda \sum_{s \neq t} |\phi_{st}|, \tag{15}$$

where λ is a tuning parameter and ϕ_{st} is the parameter in the entry (s, t) of $\boldsymbol{\Phi}$. Equivalently, the maximization of (15) can be written as solving the *subgradient equation*

$$\boldsymbol{\Phi}^{-1} - \mathbf{P} - \lambda \boldsymbol{\Psi} = \mathbf{0}, \tag{16}$$

where $\boldsymbol{\Psi}$ is the symmetric matrix with diagonal elements being zero. For off-diagonal elements $s \neq t$, $\psi_{st} = \text{sign}(\phi_{st})$ if $\phi_{st} \neq 0$, and $\psi_{st} \in [-1, 1]$ if $\phi_{st} = 0$.

In contrast, motivated by the optimization of (15), [3] developed the clime method, whose key spirit is to solve the following optimization problem:

$$\min_{\boldsymbol{\Phi}} \|\boldsymbol{\Phi}\|_1$$

$$\text{s.t.} \|\boldsymbol{\Phi}^{-1} - \mathbf{P}\|_\infty \leq \lambda, \tag{17}$$

where $\|\mathbf{A}\|_\infty$ is the infinity norm of a matrix $\mathbf{A}$. We denote $\widetilde{\boldsymbol{\Phi}} \triangleq [\widetilde{\phi}_{st}]$ as the estimator of $\boldsymbol{\Phi}$ derived from (16) or (17). The detailed computational implementation can be found in [3, 20], respectively. Finally, we note that there exists a tuning parameter λ in (16) and (17), which is used to control the selection of variables. In applications, it can be determined by Bayesian information criterion (BIC) or cross-validation (CV); detailed discussion can be referred to [3, 13, 20]. Consequently, the resulting estimator of the precision matrix $\boldsymbol{\Theta}$ is given by $\widetilde{\boldsymbol{\Theta}} = \text{Diag}(\widetilde{\boldsymbol{\Phi}}, \mathbf{I})$.

We comment on the difference between the proposed and existing approaches. The conventional glasso or clime methods directly estimate $\boldsymbol{\Theta}$ by implementing the empirical estimate of the covariance matrix in place of $\mathbf{P}$ in (16) and (17), which may falsely include non-informative pairs of variables or falsely exclude informative pairs with the oscillatory trajectories between two variables. In addition, those conventional implementations may incur longer and unstable computation if one simply uses the $p \times p$ covariance matrix with $p \gg n$, which is also found in [3] and verified by the order $\sqrt{\log p/n}$ derived by Cai et al. [3]. In contrast, our strategy is valid for reducing the matrix by removing independent pairs of variables. Under the reduced matrix $\mathbf{P}$, we further adopt the glasso and clime methods to derive the estimator of the precision matrix under a reasonably fast computation time.

Moreover, following a similar discussion in [40], we have that the reduced matrix $\widetilde{\boldsymbol{\Phi}}$ has the sparsity consistency regardless of estimation methods (15) and (17), i.e., $\text{sign}(\widetilde{\phi}_{st}) = \text{sign}(\phi_{st})$ for all $(s, t) \in \mathbb{E}$ and $\text{sign}(\widetilde{\phi}_{st}) = 0$ for all $(s, t) \in \mathbb{E}^c$. Furthermore, accompanied by the result of the feature screening in Sect. 3.1, truly independent pairs of variables have been screened out in $\widetilde{\boldsymbol{\Theta}}$, so that the estimator $\widetilde{\boldsymbol{\Theta}}$ still enjoys the sparsity consistency in the $p \gg n$ setting. It indicates that our estimated graph $\widetilde{\boldsymbol{\Theta}}$ can fully reflect the true graph in the ultrahigh-dimensional environment and is valid for identifying the gene network accurately to improve classification. Our simulation studies also reveal this property from a numerical perspective.

3.2.2 Estimation with Heterogeneous Samples

In the quadratic discriminant function (4), there exist I precision matrices $\boldsymbol{\Theta}_1, \cdots, \boldsymbol{\Theta}_I$ that share the same variables, which can be regarded as multiple graphical models since some edges are common across all categories and other edges are unique to each category (e.g., [6], Section 3.3; [18]). In this way, we follow Sect. 3.2.1 to consider the decomposition of $\boldsymbol{\Theta}_i \triangleq \text{Diag}(\boldsymbol{\Phi}_i, \mathbf{I})$ for class $i = 1, \cdots, I$, where $\boldsymbol{\Phi}_i \triangleq [\phi_{i,kl}]$ is the submatrix of the precision matrix $\boldsymbol{\Theta}_i$ and $\phi_{i,kl}$ is a value of the entry (k, l) in $\mathbb{E}_i$. In the end, it is sufficient to estimate $\boldsymbol{\Phi}_i$.

We primarily implement $\mathbf{P}_i$ defined in the beginning of Sect. 3.2 to the JGL method and jointly estimate $\boldsymbol{\Phi}_i$ with homogeneous/heterogeneous dependence taken into account, where the penalized likelihood function is given by

$$\mathcal{L}(\boldsymbol{\Phi}_1, \cdots, \boldsymbol{\Phi}_I) = \sum_{i=1}^{I} \left[\log\{\det(\boldsymbol{\Phi}_i)\} - \text{trace}(\mathbf{P}_i \boldsymbol{\Phi}_i) - \Gamma(\boldsymbol{\Phi}_i)\right], \tag{18}$$

where $\Gamma(\boldsymbol{\Phi}_i)$ is the penalty function and can be specified as the group graphical lasso

$$\Gamma(\boldsymbol{\Phi}_i) = \lambda_1 \sum_{i=1}^{I} \sum_{s \neq t} |\phi_{i,st}| + \lambda_2 \sum_{i=1}^{I} \left(\sum_{s \neq t} \phi_{i,st}^2 \right)^{1/2}$$

with two tuning parameters λ_1 and λ_2 accommodated. The optimization algorithm for (18) can be found in [18], and the computational implementation can be achieved by the package JGL with $\mathbf{P}_i$ equipped. Let $\widehat{\mathbf{\Phi}}_1, \cdots, \widehat{\mathbf{\Phi}}_I$ denote the estimators derived by maximizing (18). Therefore, the resulting estimator of $\mathbf{\Theta}_i$ is given by $\widehat{\mathbf{\Theta}}_i = \text{Diag}(\widehat{\mathbf{\Phi}}_i, \mathbf{I})$ for $i = 1, \cdots, I$.

Theoretically, since the objective function (18) is based on the glasso method, by a similar discussion in Sect. 3.2.1, it is expected that each reduced matrix $\widetilde{\mathbf{\Phi}}_i$ has the sparsity consistency in the sense that $\text{sign}(\widetilde{\phi}_{i,st}) = \text{sign}(\phi_{i,st})$ for all $(s, t) \in \mathbb{E}_i$ and $i = 1, \cdots, I$, suggesting that the JGL method based on the Chatterjee's measure is valid for detecting the same/differential edges among various classes, which is similar to the numerical finding in [18] and is reflected in our simulation studies. Consequently, one may expect that "unique" and class-dependent edges can be used to reflect the corresponding network structures in each class and improve classification.

3.3 Classification and Prediction via Discriminant Functions

When the estimators of $\mathbf{\Theta}$ and $\mathbf{\Theta}_i$ for $i = 1, \cdots, I$ are ready, we now implement them to discriminant functions. Specifically, we implement $\mathbf{\Theta}$ to (5) with the training set $\mathcal{T}$

$$\widehat{\delta}_i(\mathbf{x}) = \log(\widehat{\pi}_i) - \frac{1}{2}\widehat{\boldsymbol{\mu}}_i^\top \widehat{\mathbf{\Theta}} \widehat{\boldsymbol{\mu}}_i + \mathbf{x}^\top \widehat{\mathbf{\Theta}} \widehat{\boldsymbol{\mu}}_i, \tag{19}$$

where $\widehat{\boldsymbol{\mu}}_i$ and $\widehat{\pi}_i$ are empirical estimators of $\boldsymbol{\mu}_i$ and π_i, respectively. In addition, under the training set $\mathcal{T}$, replacing $\mathbf{\Theta}_i$ in (4) by $\widehat{\mathbf{\Theta}}_i$ gives

$$\widehat{\varphi}_i(\mathbf{x}) = \log(\widehat{\pi}_i) + \frac{1}{2}\log\left|\widehat{\mathbf{\Theta}}_i\right| - \frac{1}{2}(\mathbf{x} - \widehat{\boldsymbol{\mu}}_i)^\top \widehat{\mathbf{\Theta}}_i (\mathbf{x} - \widehat{\boldsymbol{\mu}}_i). \tag{20}$$

In fact, (19) and (20) follow NetLDA and NetQDA in [11] due to the implementation of estimated precision matrices and network structures. The key difference comes from the estimation of precision matrices. Specifically, our approach is able to handle ultrahigh-dimensionality by retaining highly dependent pairs of variables and removing weakly dependent ones. Regarding the implementation of the quadratic discriminant function, we take heterogeneity into account and consider the joint estimation for $\mathbf{\Theta}_i$ instead of estimating $\mathbf{\Theta}_i$ separately (e.g., [9, 11]).

Finally, given a new subject in the validation set $\mathcal{V}$ with a covariate $\mathbf{x}_{\text{new}}$, we compute $\widehat{\delta}_i(\mathbf{x}_{\text{new}})$ and $\widehat{\varphi}_i(\mathbf{x}_{\text{new}})$ for $i = 1, \cdots, I$, and the predicted class for such a new subject, denoted i^*, is determined by

$$i^* = \underset{i \in \{1,2,\cdots,I\}}{\arg\max}\ \widehat{\delta}_i(\mathbf{x}_{\text{new}}) \text{ and } i^* = \underset{i \in \{1,2,\cdots,I\}}{\arg\max}\ \widehat{\varphi}_i(\mathbf{x}_{\text{new}}).$$

3.4 Assessment of Performance and Prediction

For a subject $j \in \mathcal{V}$, let $\widehat{Y}_j$ denote the predicted class label and define Y_{0j} as the true class label. For class $i = 1, \ldots, I$, we first calculate the number of true positives (TP), the number of false positives (FP), and the number of false negatives (FN):

$$\mathrm{TP}_i = \sum_{j \in \mathcal{V}} \mathbb{I}\left(Y_{0j} = i, \widehat{Y}_j = i\right), \quad \mathrm{FP}_i = \sum_{j \in \mathcal{V}} \mathbb{I}\left(Y_{0j} \neq i, \widehat{Y}_j = i\right),$$

and

$$\mathrm{FN}_i = \sum_{j \in \mathcal{V}} \mathbb{I}\left(Y_{0j} = i, \widehat{Y}_j \neq i\right).$$

Given TP, FP, and FN, precision (PRE) and recall (REC) are defined as follows:

$$\mathrm{PRE} = \frac{\sum_{i=1}^{I} \mathrm{TP}_i}{\sum_{i=1}^{I} \mathrm{TP}_i + \sum_{i=1}^{I} \mathrm{FP}_i} \text{ and } \mathrm{REC} = \frac{\sum_{i=1}^{I} \mathrm{TP}_i}{\sum_{i=1}^{I} \mathrm{TP}_i + \sum_{i=1}^{I} \mathrm{FN}_i}. \tag{21}$$

Moreover, the F-score is defined as

$$\mathrm{F} = 2 \times \frac{\mathrm{PRE} \times \mathrm{REC}}{\mathrm{PRE} + \mathrm{REC}}. \tag{22}$$

As commented in [11, 15], it is obvious to see that PRE and REC are equal to 1 if all subjects are correctly classified, i.e., FP and FN are equal to 0; PRE and REC are equal to 0 if subjects are all misclassified. Thus, values of PRE, REC, and F-score are between 0 and 1. It also indicates that higher values of PRE, REC, and F-score reflect more accurate classification and satisfactory performance of prediction.

4 Numerical Studies

4.1 Simulation Setup

In this section, we use simulation studies to assess the performance of the proposed method. Let $p = 3000, 5000, 10000$ denote the dimension of covariates and denote $n = 200$ or 500 as sample sizes. We consider the following two scenarios to generate the data $\mathcal{D} = \{\{Y_j, \mathbf{X}_j\} : j = 1, \cdots, n\}$:

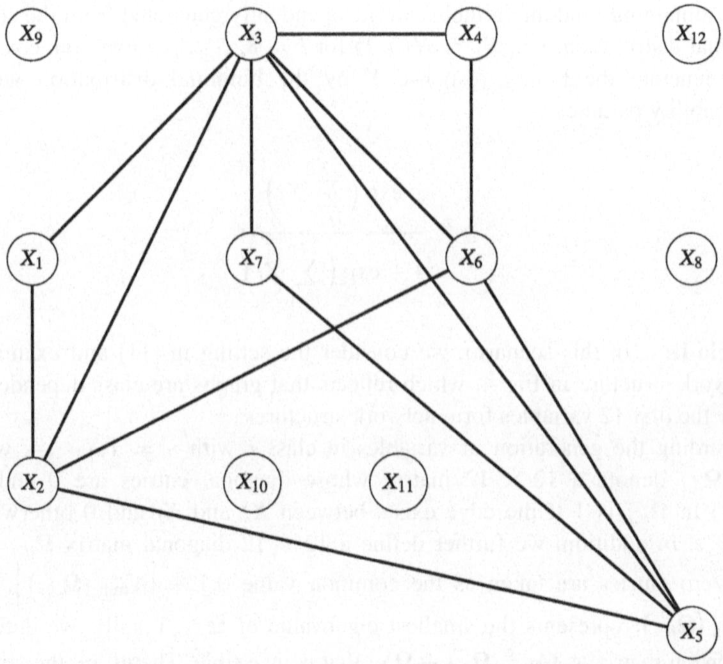

Fig. 3 The graphical structure in Scenario I. It implies that seven variables X_1–X_7 form a network structure and the remaining variables are independent of each other

Scenario I: In this scenario, we consider the setting in Section 8.4.1 of [26] and examine the graphical structure in Fig. 3, which reveals that the variables share the same graph regardless of classes.

Following [26], we consider the nonlinear relationship among variables based on this graph. We first generate the random variable X_1 from the standard normal distribution, i.e., $X_1 \sim N(0, 1)$. After that, some of variables are generated sequentially. Specifically,

$$X_2 = 6\cos(X_1) + \epsilon_2 \text{ with } \epsilon_2 \sim N(0, 1);$$

$$X_3 = 5\sin(X_1) + X_2 + \epsilon_3 \text{ with } \epsilon_3 \sim N(0, 1);$$

$$X_4 = 5\cos(X_3X_6) + 3X_3 + 3X_6 + \epsilon_4 \text{ with } \epsilon_4 \sim N(0, 1);$$

$$X_5 = 0.05(X_2 + X_6)^3 + \epsilon_5 \text{ with } \epsilon_5 \sim N(0, 1);$$

$$X_6 \sim N(0, 1);$$

$$X_7 = 6\cos(0.2[X_3 + \log\{|5X_5 + 1|\}]) + \epsilon_7 \text{ with } \epsilon_7 \sim N(0, 1).$$

The remaining random variables are independently generated from the standard normal distribution, i.e., $X_i \sim N(0, 1)$ for $i = 8, \cdots, p$. Given the covariates, we generate the binary response Y by the binomial distribution with the probability parameter

$$\varrho \triangleq \frac{\exp\left(\sum_{i=1}^{7} X_i\right)}{1+\exp\left(\sum_{i=1}^{7} X_i\right)}.$$

Scenario II: In this scenario, we consider the setting in [11] and examine the network structure in Fig. 4, which reflects that graphs are class-dependent and only the first 12 variables form network structures.
Regarding the generation of variables in class i with $i = 1, \cdots, 4$, we first let $\mathbf{\Omega}_{o,i}$ denote a 12×12 matrix whose diagonal entries are 0 and entry (s, t) in $\mathbf{\Omega}_{o,i}$ is 1 if the edge exists between X_s and X_t and 0 otherwise for $s \neq t$. In addition, we further define a 12×12 diagonal matrix $\mathbf{\Omega}_{d,i}$ whose nonzero entries are taken as the common value $0.1 + \left|\Lambda_{\min}\left(\mathbf{\Omega}_{o,i}\right)\right|$, where $\Lambda_{\min}\left(\mathbf{\Omega}_{o,i}\right)$ represents the smallest eigenvalue of $\mathbf{\Omega}_{o,i}$. Finally, we define the precision matrix as $\mathbf{\Theta}_i \triangleq \mathbf{\Omega}_{o,i} + \mathbf{\Omega}_{d,i}$ that is invertible. Therefore, the covariate vectors $(X_1, X_2, \cdots, X_{12})^\top$ in class i are generated from a multivariate normal distribution with mean zero and the covariance matrix $\mathbf{\Sigma}_i = \mathbf{\Theta}_i^{-1}$ for $i = 1, \ldots, 4$. The remaining $p - 12$ covariates are independently generated from the standard normal distribution, i.e., $X_i \sim N(0, 1)$ for $i = 13, 14, \cdots, p$.

4.2 Simulation Results

Given the dataset generated in Sect. 4.1, we implement the methods in Sect. 3 to do classification. To compare the performance with the proposed method, we examine the conventional glasso, clime, and JGL methods in lieu of the inverse of the empirical estimate of the covariance matrix in the linear or quadratic discriminant function due to the singularity of the matrix $\mathbf{\Sigma}$ or $\mathbf{\Sigma}_i$ in ultrahigh-dimensional data. In addition, we also examine some state-of-the-art methods that do not take the network structure into account, including naive Bayes (naiveBayes; [28]), support vector machine (SVM; [28]), sparse multinomial logistic regression models (Tian-logistic; [37]), regularized logistic regression (glmnet; [21]), shrunken centroids regularized discriminant analysis (rda; [22]), and regularized linear discriminant analysis with nonlinear covariance matrix (RLDA; [27]).

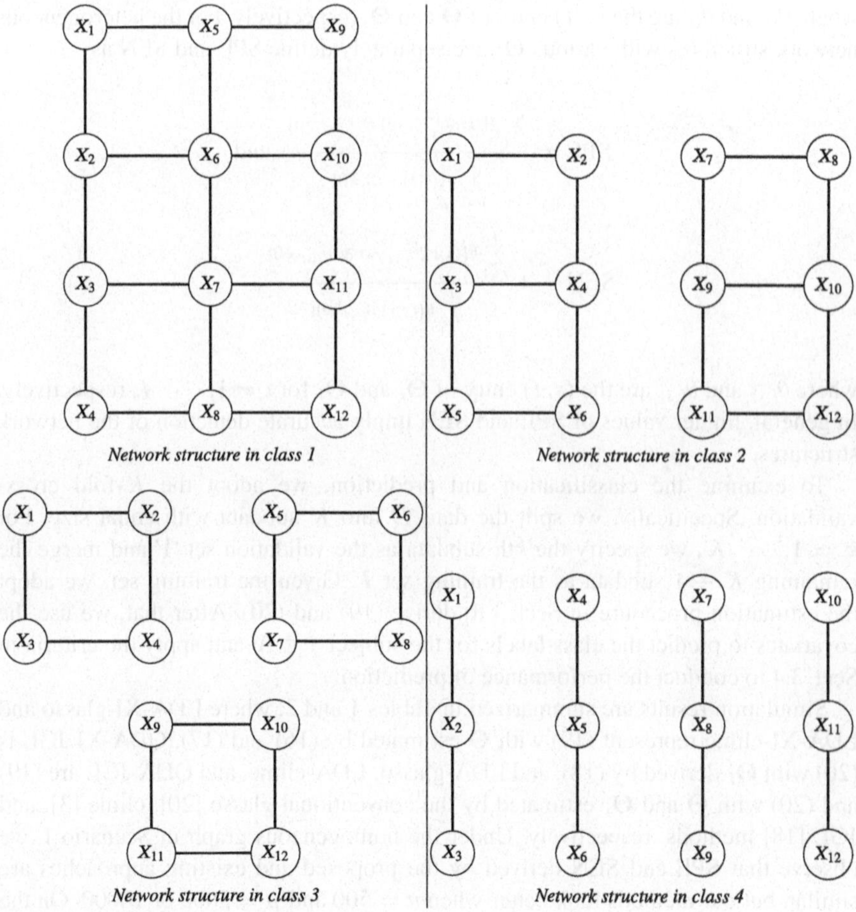

Fig. 4 The graphical structure in Scenario II. It indicates that four different classes contain variables with various network structures, yielding the heterogeneous precision matrices among different classes

To see the performance of estimating precision matrices, we record specificity (SPE) and sensitivity (SEN), where the former reflects the proportion of zero coefficients that were correctly estimated to be zero and the latter indicates the proportion of nonzero coefficients that were correctly estimated to be nonzero. That is, under the homogeneous network structure with $\mathbf{\Theta}$, SPE and SEN are, respectively, defined as

$$\text{SPE} = \frac{\#\{(s,t) : \widehat{\theta}_{st} = 0 \,\&\, \theta_{st} = 0\}}{\#\{(s,t) : \theta_{st} = 0\}} \quad \text{and} \quad \text{SEN} = \frac{\#\{(s,t) : \widehat{\theta}_{st} \neq 0 \,\&\, \theta_{st} \neq 0\}}{\#\{(s,t) : \theta_{st} \neq 0\}},$$

where $\widehat{\theta}_{st}$ and θ_{st} are the (s,t) entry of $\widehat{\boldsymbol{\Theta}}$ and $\boldsymbol{\Theta}$, respectively. For the heterogeneous network structures with various $\boldsymbol{\Theta}_i$, we separately define SPE and SEN as

$$\text{SPE} = \frac{\sum_{i=1}^{I} \#\{(s,t):\widehat{\theta}_{i,st}=0 \ \& \ \theta_{i,st}=0\}}{\sum_{i=1}^{I} \#\{(s,t):\theta_{i,st}=0\}} \quad \text{and}$$

$$\text{SEN} = \frac{\sum_{i=1}^{I} \#\{(s,t):\widehat{\theta}_{i,st}\neq 0 \ \& \ \theta_{i,st}\neq 0\}}{\sum_{i=1}^{I} \#\{(s,t):\theta_{i,st}\neq 0\}},$$

where $\widehat{\theta}_{i,st}$ and $\theta_{i,st}$ are the (s,t) entry of $\widehat{\boldsymbol{\Theta}}_i$ and $\boldsymbol{\Theta}_i$ for $i = 1, \cdots, I$, respectively. In general, higher values of SPE and SEN imply accurate detection of the network structures.

To examine the classification and prediction, we adopt the K-fold cross-validation. Specifically, we split the data $\mathcal{D}$ into K subdata with equal size. For $k = 1, \cdots, K$, we specify the kth subdata as the validation set $\mathcal{V}$ and merge the remaining $K - 1$ subdata as the training set $\mathcal{T}$. Given the training set, we adopt the estimation procedure in Sect. 3 to derive (19) and (20). After that, we use the covariates to predict the class labels for the subject $j \in \mathcal{V}$ and apply the criteria in Sect. 3.4 to conduct the performance of prediction.

Simulation results are summarized in Tables 1 and 2, where LDA-XI-glasso and LDA-XI-clime represent (19) with $\boldsymbol{\Theta}$ estimated by (16) and (17), QDA-XI-JGL is (20) with $\boldsymbol{\Theta}_i$ derived by (18), and LDA-glasso, LDA-clime, and QDA-JGL are (19) and (20) with $\boldsymbol{\Theta}$ and $\boldsymbol{\Theta}_i$ estimated by the conventional glasso [20], clime [3], and JGL [18] methods, respectively. Under the homogeneous graph in Scenario I, we observe that SPE and SEN derived by the proposed and existing approaches are similar, but our methods look better when $n = 500$ and $p = 5000$ or 10000. On the other hand, when graphs are heterogeneous, as shown in Scenario II, the proposed QDA-XI-JGL method has higher SPE and SEN than the existing methods.

With the estimated network structures equipped, we find that LDA-XI-glasso, LDA-XI-clime, QDA-XI-JGL, LDA-glasso, LDA-clime, and QDA-JGL have relatively higher values of PRE, REC, and F-score, suggesting that they are generally better than other existing methods that ignore the effects of network structures regardless of Scenarios I or II. It indicates that the classification performance might be affected by the pairwise interactions of variables and the estimation of $\boldsymbol{\Theta}$ or $\boldsymbol{\Theta}_i$. Compared with the LDA and QDA methods with $\boldsymbol{\Theta}$ or $\boldsymbol{\Theta}_i$ estimated by the proposed or existing methods, we find that the proposed methods have better classification performance. It indicates that the implementation of the empirical estimates of $p \times p$ covariance matrices in the glasso, clime, and JGL methods may lead to an inaccurate estimator of precision matrices. In contrast, the results verify the validity of our proposed method with the implementation of $\mathbf{P}$ and $\mathbf{P}_i$.

The other interesting phenomenon in the numerical results is that the increase in sample size does not necessarily provide higher values of PRE, REC, or F-

Table 1 Simulation result for Scenario I. Methods contain the proposed methods in Sects. 3.2 and 3.3 and some state-of-the-art methods. Under various dimensions p and sample sizes n, SPE and SEN are used to examine the accuracy of network structure detection; PRE, REC, and F-score are used to conduct the accuracy of classification

		$n = 200$					$n = 500$				
p	Methods	SPE	SEN	PRE	REC	F-score	SPE	SEN	PRE	REC	F-score
3000	LDA-XI-glasso	0.849	0.998	0.831	0.947	0.885	0.849	1.000	0.819	0.994	0.898
	LDA-XI-clime	0.849	1.000	0.784	0.929	0.851	0.849	1.000	0.762	0.975	0.855
	QDA-XI-JGL	–	–	0.965	0.965	0.965	–	–	0.960	0.960	0.960
	LDA-glasso	0.829	1.000	0.799	0.824	0.811	0.838	0.996	0.797	0.986	0.882
	LDA-clime	0.843	1.000	0.798	0.775	0.786	0.862	0.999	0.788	0.812	0.800
	QDA-JGL	–	–	0.793	0.793	0.793	–	–	0.808	0.808	0.808
	naiveBayes	–	–	0.725	0.998	0.838	–	–	0.728	0.981	0.835
	SVM	–	–	0.726	1.000	0.841	–	–	0.724	1.000	0.839
	Tian-logistic	–	–	0.739	1.000	0.848	–	–	0.736	1.000	0.847
	glmnet	–	–	0.742	1.000	0.850	–	–	0.743	1.000	0.851
	rda	–	–	0.723	1.000	0.839	–	–	0.718	1.000	0.835
	RLDA	–	–	0.650	0.650	0.650	–	–	0.324	0.324	0.324
5000	LDA-XI-glasso	0.849	0.998	0.810	0.901	0.853	0.849	1.000	0.817	0.948	0.878
	LDA-XI-clime	0.849	0.998	0.810	0.901	0.853	0.849	1.000	0.816	0.883	0.848
	QDA-XI-JGL	–	–	0.975	0.975	0.975	–	–	0.953	0.953	0.953
	LDA-glasso	0.852	0.999	0.799	0.722	0.759	0.626	1.000	0.755	0.897	0.820
	LDA-clime	0.834	0.996	0.799	0.799	0.799	0.691	0.999	0.757	0.896	0.821
	QDA-JGL	–	–	0.781	0.781	0.781	–	–	0.783	0.761	0.772
	naiveBayes	–	–	0.674	0.995	0.801	–	–	0.688	0.980	0.808
	SVM	–	–	0.674	1.000	0.803	–	–	0.668	1.000	0.800
	Tian-logistic	–	–	0.699	1.000	0.821	–	–	0.684	1.000	0.812
	glmnet	–	–	0.719	1.000	0.834	–	–	0.687	1.000	0.813
	rda	–	–	0.676	1.000	0.806	–	–	0.678	1.000	0.808
	RLDA	–	–	0.636	0.636	0.636	–	–	0.426	0.426	0.426
10000	LDA-XI-glasso	0.849	0.998	0.806	0.892	0.847	0.849	1.000	0.830	0.939	0.881
	LDA-XI-clime	0.849	0.998	0.806	0.892	0.847	0.849	1.000	0.817	0.926	0.868
	QDA-XI-JGL	–	–	0.940	0.940	0.940	–	–	0.918	0.918	0.918
	LDA-glasso	0.869	0.999	0.798	0.705	0.748	0.325	1.000	0.808	0.908	0.855
	LDA-clime	0.841	0.996	0.798	0.709	0.751	0.641	0.999	0.823	0.828	0.825
	QDA-JGL	–	–	0.771	0.771	0.771	–	–	0.832	0.809	0.820
	naiveBayes	–	–	0.628	0.992	0.765	–	–	0.631	0.971	0.763
	SVM	–	–	0.633	1.000	0.773	–	–	0.631	1.000	0.773
	Tian-logistic	–	–	0.670	0.998	0.799	–	–	0.645	0.999	0.783
	glmnet	–	–	0.672	0.997	0.799	–	–	0.652	0.999	0.787
	rda	–	–	0.594	0.953	0.731	–	–	0.629	1.000	0.772
	RLDA	–	–	0.570	0.570	0.570	–	–	0.531	0.531	0.531

Table 2 Simulation result for Scenario II. Methods contain the proposed methods in Sects. 3.2 and 3.3 and some state-of-the-art methods. Under various dimensions p and sample sizes n, SPE and SEN are used to examine the accuracy of network structure detection; PRE, REC, and F-score are used to conduct the accuracy of classification

		$n = 200$					$n = 500$				
p	Methods	SPE	SEN	PRE	REC	F-score	SPE	SEN	PRE	REC	F-score
3000	LDA-XI-glasso	–	–	0.745	0.745	0.745	–	–	0.741	0.741	0.741
	LDA-XI-clime	–	–	0.750	0.750	0.750	–	–	0.741	0.741	0.741
	QDA-XI-JGL	0.993	1.000	0.995	0.995	0.995	0.988	1.000	0.948	0.948	0.948
	LDA-glasso	–	–	0.735	0.735	0.735	–	–	0.694	0.694	0.694
	LDA-clime	–	–	0.510	0.510	0.510	–	–	0.670	0.670	0.670
	QDA-JGL	0.292	0.980	0.766	0.782	0.774	0.230	1.000	0.759	0.753	0.756
	naiveBayes	–	–	0.272	0.272	0.272	–	–	0.259	0.259	0.259
	SVM	–	–	0.181	0.181	0.181	–	–	0.206	0.206	0.206
	Tian-logistic	–	–	0.335	0.335	0.335	–	–	0.200	0.200	0.200
	glmnet	–	–	0.379	0.379	0.379	–	–	0.335	0.335	0.335
	rda	–	–	0.244	0.244	0.244	–	–	0.250	0.250	0.250
	RLDA	–	–	0.255	0.255	0.255	–	–	0.217	0.217	0.217
5000	LDA-XI-glasso	–	–	0.720	0.720	0.720	–	–	0.714	0.714	0.714
	LDA-XI-clime	–	–	0.750	0.750	0.750	–	–	0.714	0.714	0.714
	QDA-XI-JGL	0.986	1.000	0.995	0.995	0.995	0.975	1.000	0.882	0.882	0.882
	LDA-glasso	–	–	0.700	0.700	0.700	–	–	0.554	0.554	0.554
	LDA-clime	–	–	0.700	0.700	0.700	–	–	0.656	0.656	0.656
	QDA-JGL	0.407	0.961	0.753	0.769	0.761	0.279	1.000	0.733	0.733	0.733
	naiveBayes	–	–	0.264	0.264	0.264	–	–	0.260	0.260	0.260
	SVM	–	–	0.177	0.177	0.177	–	–	0.206	0.206	0.206
	Tian-logistic	–	–	0.300	0.300	0.300	–	–	0.233	0.233	0.233
	glmnet	–	–	0.415	0.415	0.415	–	–	0.342	0.342	0.342
	rda	–	–	0.243	0.243	0.243	–	–	0.246	0.246	0.246
	RLDA	–	–	0.250	0.250	0.250	–	–	0.225	0.225	0.225
10000	LDA-XI-glasso	–	–	0.695	0.695	0.695	–	–	0.743	0.743	0.743
	LDA-XI-clime	–	–	0.750	0.750	0.750	–	–	0.743	0.743	0.743
	QDA-XI-JGL	0.980	0.994	0.990	0.991	0.990	0.960	1.000	0.882	0.882	0.882
	LDA-glasso	–	–	0.649	0.649	0.649	–	–	0.717	0.717	0.717
	LDA-clime	–	–	0.680	0.680	0.680	–	–	0.612	0.612	0.612
	QDA-JGL	0.565	0.941	0.755	0.755	0.755	0.374	1.000	0.725	0.725	0.725
	naiveBayes	–	–	0.255	0.255	0.255	–	–	0.257	0.257	0.257
	SVM	–	–	0.177	0.177	0.177	–	–	0.202	0.202	0.202
	Tian-logistic	–	–	0.225	0.225	0.225	–	–	0.225	0.225	0.225
	glmnet	–	–	0.425	0.425	0.425	–	–	0.329	0.329	0.329
	rda	–	–	0.244	0.244	0.244	–	–	0.238	0.238	0.238
	RLDA	–	–	0.200	0.200	0.200	–	–	0.300	0.300	0.300

score under Scenarios I and II. As noted in [38], small sample sizes resulted in higher accuracy. In particular, the results of Tian-logistic, glmnet, and SVM in Tables 1 and 2 are consistent with the finding in [33] who examined the logistic regression and SVM and concluded a negative relationship between sample size and the classification accuracy. In addition, other methods considered in Tables 1 and 2 also show the similar pattern. According to the discussion in [33], this issue might be caused by K-fold cross-validation or possible overfitting/overoptimistic.

For the comparisons between LDA and QDA, as expected, we observe that LDA-glasso, LDA-clime, and QDA-JGL have comparable results under Scenario I and the LDA-based methods are generally better than the QDA-based methods; the results are opposite under Scenario II. In contrast, while it is expected to see that QDA-XI-JGL has the satisfactory performance under Scenario II, it is interesting to see that QDA-XI-JGL is still better than LDA-XI-glasso and LDA-XI-clime under Scenario I. The main reason might be the construction of discriminant function: the LDA-XI-glasso and LDA-XI-clime methods adopt (12) to reduce the size of the matrices, and then implement $\mathbf{P}$ to the glasso or clime methods, while the QDA-XI-JGL method first employs (13) to retain the covariates that are informative for the response, which ensures that the same variables are collected for the implementation of the JGL method. In addition, Scenario I reflects that two different classes have the same network structure, which can be treated as a special case of heterogeneous network structure, and the JGL method is still valid for addressing class-dependent network structure with the common edges in each class.

Finally, for the computational time, while it is not recorded in our report, the experiments reveal that the proposed methods spend less time in obtaining the results, whereas other existing methods require longer computational times, especially when p becomes larger.

5 Analysis of Gene Expression Data

In this section, we apply the proposed and some state-of-the-art methods in Sect. 4.2 to analyze the GCM dataset, which contains 16,063 gene expression values and 14 human cancers, including breast (BR), prostate (PR), leukemia (LE), colorectal (CO), lung (LU), bladder (BL), CNS, uterus (UT), lymphoma (LY), renal (RE), pancreas (PA), ovary (OV), melanoma (ME), and mesothelioma (ML). This dataset contains 198 tumor samples, which are automatically separated as the training set $\mathcal{T}$ with size 144 and the validation set $\mathcal{V}$ with size 54 in record. The sample sizes in each class are summarized in Table 3.

Following the strategy in Fig. 2, we first implement (11) to determine the matrix $\mathbf{P}$ and class-dependent matrices $\mathbf{P}_i$ for $i = 1, \cdots, 14$ under the training data $\mathcal{T}$. After that, we apply (16), (17), and (18) to derive the estimators of $\boldsymbol{\Theta}$ and $\boldsymbol{\Theta}_i$ for $i = 1, \cdots, 14$. To ease the visualization, we display the resulting graphs for the first 35 gene expressions obtained by the glasso, clime, and JGL methods in Figs. 5 and 6, respectively. We observe that gene expressions in Fig. 5 are different from

Table 3 Sample sizes for each cancer. The first row with $\mathcal{T}$ contains sample sizes of the training data in cancer labels, the second row with $\mathcal{V}$ contains sample sizes of the validation set in cancer labels, and the last row with "Total" contains sample sizes of the whole data in cancer labels

	BR	PR	LE	CO	LU	BL	CNS	UT	LY	RE	PA	OV	ME	ML
$\mathcal{T}$	8	8	8	8	16	8	8	8	24	8	8	8	8	16
$\mathcal{V}$	3	4	2	4	4	4	2	3	6	4	3	6	3	6
Total	11	12	10	12	20	12	10	11	30	12	11	14	11	22

those in Fig. 6. It might be due to various strategies for the estimation of precision matrices. From Fig. 5, we can see that the glasso method tends to retain more pairs of gene expressions, which seems to be consistent with the finding in [3]. On the other hand, with different class labels accommodated, Fig. 6 reveals that graphs G2, G5, G9, and G14 contain class-dependent edges, yielding that network structures of common gene expressions are different from each other. For example, according to the genes' accession numbers from the dataset, RC_AA262655_s_at (`X13173`) has the connections with other gene expressions under the cancers PR, LU, and ML, but pairs with H19570_s_at (`X9487`), X52008_at (`X4228`), and X58298_s_at (`X6221`) uniquely exist for those cancers. In particular, graphs G9 and G14 contain more complex heterogeneous edges than graphs G2 and G5.

Given the estimated precision matrices, we use the training data $\mathcal{T}$ to construct linear and quadratic discriminant functions (19) and (20), respectively. The confusion matrices of classification results under the training data $\mathcal{T}$ are displayed as heatmaps in Fig. 7. In general, Fig. 7 shows that some diagonal entries have ratios 1 that reflect perfect classification; meanwhile, there are some misclassifications. For comparison, we can see that QDA has better fit than LDA because class-dependent precision matrices are taken into account.

Finally, we input the gene expressions $\mathbf{X}$ in the validation set $\mathcal{V}$ into the estimated discriminant functions (19) and (20) to predict the subjects' cancer. The resulting confusion matrices based on different methods are displayed in Fig. 8, which shows comparable results among methods, and some of the classes are accurately predicted, while others contain misclassifications. Moreover, to closely assess the performance of prediction numerically, we compute measures (21) and (22) for the predicted and true classes in $\mathcal{V}$ and summarize those values in Table 4. Consistent with the findings in simulation studies, we observe that QDA-XI-JGL has the highest values of PRE, REC, and F-score, reflecting the best prediction performance among all approaches. With the accompaniment of the findings in Fig. 6, the classification results might be affected by some pairs of gene expressions for a specific cancer tumor, such as pairs (RC_AA262655_s_at, H19570_s_at), (RC_AA262655_s_at, X52008_at), and (RC_AA262655_s_at, X58298_s_at) for the cancers PR, LU, and ML, respectively.

In contrast, with $\boldsymbol{\Theta}$ or $\boldsymbol{\Theta}_i$ estimated using the conventional glasso, clime or JGL methods, the LDA and QDA methods have unsatisfactory performance for classification and are generally worse than the proposed methods, which might be caused by ultrahigh-dimensionality or the possible ignorance of nonlinear

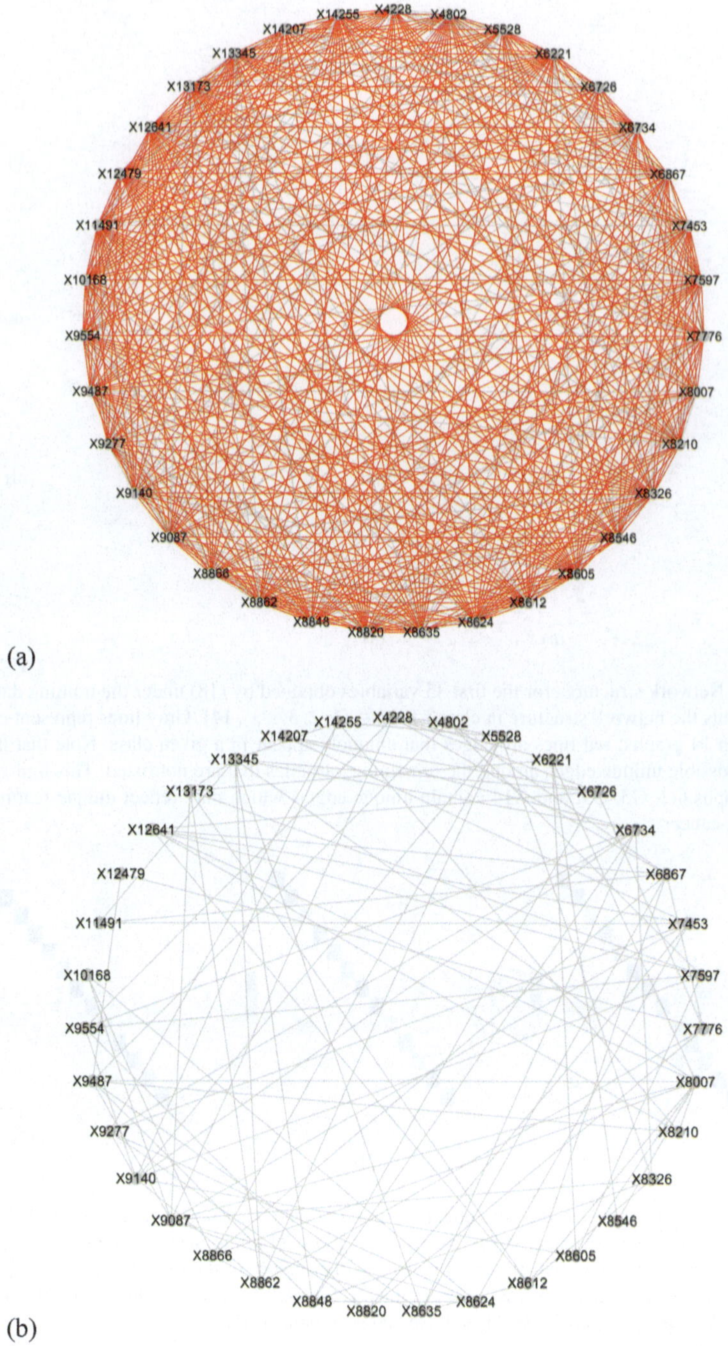

Fig. 5 Network structures for the first 35 variables obtained by the (**a**) glasso (15) and (**b**) clime (17) methods under the training data $\mathcal{T}$. Red lines in the panel A indicate additional edges selected by the glasso method, compared with the panel (**b**). The comparison between (**a**) and (**b**) reveals that the glasso method tends to retain more edges than the clime method

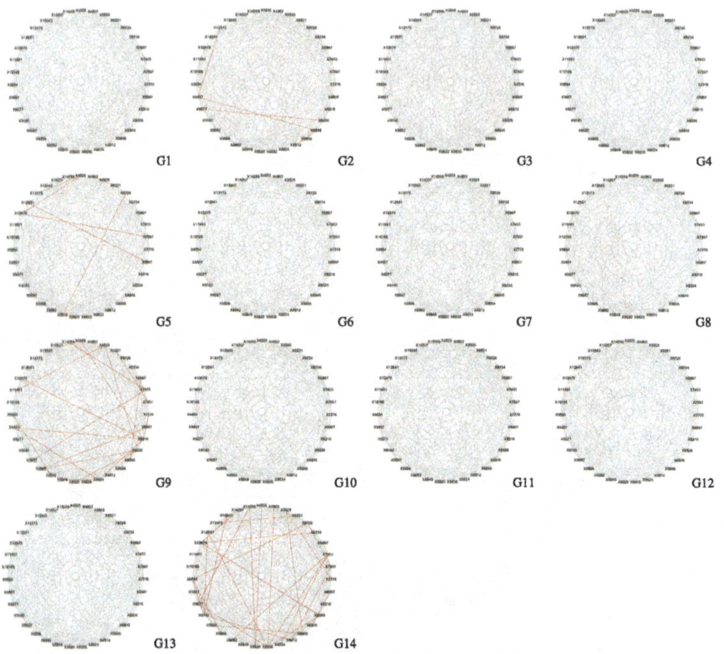

Fig. 6 Network structures for the first 35 variables obtained by (18) under the training data $\mathcal{T}$. Gi represents the network structure in class i for $i \in \{1, 2, 3, \cdots, 14\}$. Gray lines represent common edges in 14 graphs; red lines are edges that uniquely appear in a given class. Note that there are some possible unique edges among the remaining variables that are not listed. This figure reveals that graphs G2, G5, G9, and G14 contain unique edges, which may reflect unique features for a specific cancer

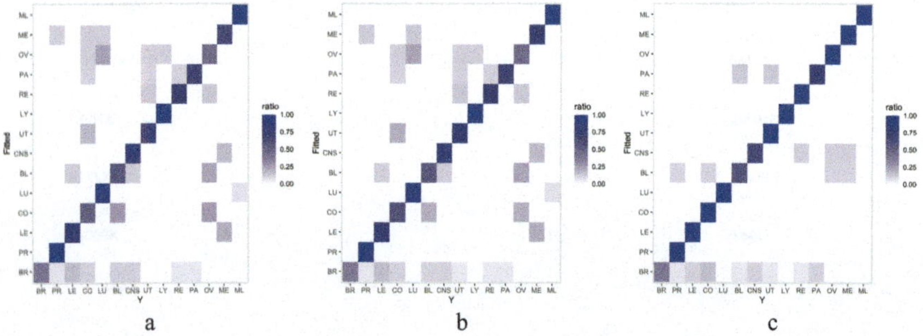

Fig. 7 Heatmaps for classification under the training data $\mathcal{T}$. Panel (**a**) is the result of LDA-XI-glasso derived by (15), panel (**b**) is the result of LDA-XI-clime derived by (17), and panel (**c**) is the result of QDA-XI-JGL derived by (18). Darker colors in the diagonal entries imply more accurate classification, and lighter colors in the off-diagonal entries indicate less misclassification. The QDA method (panel (**c**)) seems to have better classification

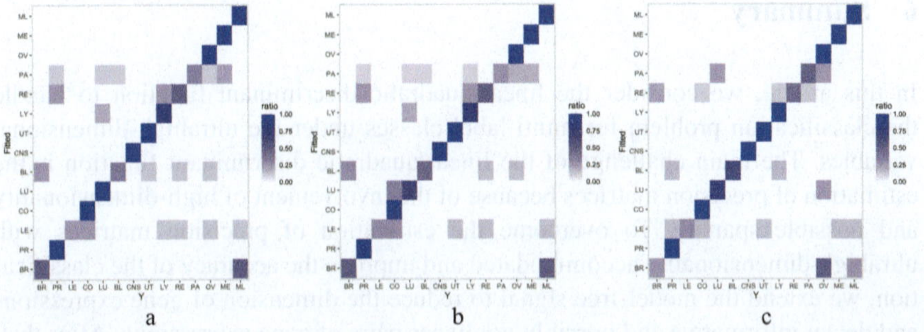

Fig. 8 Heatmaps for prediction under the validation set $\mathcal{V}$. Panel (**a**) is the result of LDA-XI-glasso derived by (15), panel (**b**) is the result of LDA-XI-clime derived by (17), and panel (**c**) is the result of QDA-XI-JGL derived by (18). Darker colors in the diagonal entries imply more accurate classification, and lighter colors in the off-diagonal entries indicate less misclassification. The QDA method (panel (**c**)) seems to have better prediction

Table 4 Numerical results: prediction for the GCM data. Methods contain the proposed methods in Sects. 3.2 and 3.3 and some state-of-the-art methods. PRE, REC, and F-score are used to conduct the accuracy of classification

Method	PRE	REC	F-score
LDA-XI-glasso	0.764	0.764	0.764
LDA-XI-clime	0.757	0.757	0.757
QDA-XI-JGL	0.847	0.847	0.847
LDA-glasso	0.500	0.500	0.500
LDA-clime	0.751	0.705	0.728
QDA-JGL	0.771	0.771	0.771
naiveBayes	0.111	0.111	0.111
SVM	0.713	0.713	0.713
Tian-logistic	0.148	0.148	0.148
glmnet	0.240	0.250	0.245
rda	0.563	0.563	0.563
RLDA	0.074	0.074	0.074

relationship between two gene expressions. Finally, among the comparisons of state-of-the-art methods that ignore the effects of network structure, we find that the SVM method performs better than other existing approaches but does not outperform network-based methods. Moreover, there are two notable situations on the dimensions and network structure of gene expressions. First, in the same line of handling variable selection and regularization, the performance of the Tian-logistic [37] and glmnet [21] methods is not better than the rda [22] method. Second, while the RLDA [27] method is based on the regularized inverse covariance matrix, which is different from the conventional implementation of the covariance matrix, it is surprising to see that its performance is not satisfactory. It might be due to the fact that this method does not take network structure into account as well.

6 Summary

In this article, we consider the linear/quadratic discriminant function to handle the classification problem for multi-label classes under the ultrahigh-dimensional variables. The main challenge of the linear/quadratic discriminant function is the estimation of precision matrices because of the involvement of high-dimensionality and possible sparsity. To overcome the estimation of precision matrices with ultrahigh-dimensionality accommodated and improve the accuracy of the classification, we extend the model-free signal to reduce the dimension of gene expressions and detect informative and possibly nonlinear pairs of gene expressions. After that, reduced correlation matrices $\mathbf{P}$ enable us to employ the glasso and clime methods to obtain the estimator of precision matrices. Moreover, with class-dependency accommodated, we first use the model-free signal to define matrices $\mathbf{P}_i$, and use them to compute the class-dependent precision matrices $\boldsymbol{\Theta}_i$ by using the JGL method. Numerical results reveal that our strategy provides accurate prediction and outperforms other existing methods that may not be valid for handling ultrahigh-dimensional data.

The current estimation procedure has several possible extensions. First, the discriminant function is basically derived based on the normal distributions of $\mathbf{X}$. It is important to develop new flexible classification models, such as nonparametric approaches, with ultrahigh-dimensionality and network structures accommodated. The second concern is about the data. In the current development, we implicitly assume that variables are precisely measured and free of noise, such as measurement errors or missing values. In the presence of noisy data, it is interesting to propose new strategies (e.g., [13]) to improve (9) and (10) and derive the estimators of precision matrices. Finally, as shown in numerical studies, there is an issue related to sample sizes and the accuracy of classification based on machine learning methods. To improve the classification, extending the sample size determination (e.g., [38]) or the cross-validation strategy (e.g., [33]) based on the current development could be possible solutions, which deserve careful exploration in the near future.

References

1. Abramovich, F., Grinshtein, V., Levy, T.: Multiclass classification by sparse multinomial logistic regression. IEEE Trans. Inf. Theory **67**, 4637–4646 (2021)
2. Bielza, C., Li, G., Larrañaga, P.: Multi-dimensional classification with Bayesian networks. Int. J. Approx. Reason. **52**, 705–727 (2011)
3. Cai, T., Liu, W., Luo, X.: A constrained ℓ_1 minimization approach to sparse precision matrix estimation. J. Am. Stat. Assoc. **106**, 594–607 (2011)
4. Cai, W., Guan, G., Pan, R., Zhu, X., Wang, H.: Network linear discriminant analysis. Comput. Stat. Data Anal. **117**, 32–44 (2018)
5. Chatterjee, S.: A new coefficient of correlation. J. Am. Stat. Assoc. **116**, 2009–2022 (2021)
6. Chen, L.-P.: Estimation of graphical models: an overview of selected topics. Int. Stat. Rev. **92**, 194–245 (2024)

7. Chen, L.-P.: A note of feature screening via rank-based coefficient of correlation. Biom. J. **65**, 2100373 (2023)
8. Chen, L.-P., Hsu, W.-H.: CHEMIST: an R package for causal inference with high-dimensional error-prone covariates and misclassified treatments. Jpn. J. Stat. Data Sci. **8**, 349–365 (2025)
9. Chen, L.-P.: NetDA: an R package for network-based discriminant analysis subject to multi-label classes. J. Probab. Stat. **2022**, Article ID 1041752, 1–14 (2022a)
10. Chen, L.-P.: Classification and prediction for multi-cancer data with ultrahigh-dimensional gene expressions. PLOS One **17**, e0274440 (2022b)
11. Chen, L.-P.: Network-based discriminant analysis for multiclassification. J. Classif. **39**, 410–431 (2022c)
12. Chen, L.-P.: Nonparametric discriminant analysis with network structures in predictor. J. Stat. Comput. Simul. **92**, 3836–3861 (2022d)
13. Chen, L.-P., Yi, G.Y.: De-noising analysis of noisy data with graphical models. Electron. J. Stat. **16**, 3861–3909 (2022)
14. Chen, L.-P., Yi, G.Y.: Analysis of noisy survival data with graphical proportional hazards measurement error models. Biometrics **77**, 956–969 (2021)
15. Chen, L.-P., Yi, G.Y., Zhang, Q., He, W.: Multiclass analysis and prediction with network structured covariates. J. Stat. Distrib. Appl. **6**, 6 (2019)
16. Chen, L.-P.: Multiclassification to gene expression data with some complex features. Biostatistics and Biometrics Open Access J. **9**, 555751 (2018)
17. Clemmensen, L., Kuhn, M.: Package sparseLDA: sparse discriminant analysis (2016). https://cran.r-project.org/package=sparseLDA
18. Danaher, P., Wang, P., Witten, D.M.: The joint graphical lasso for inverse covariance estimation across multiple classes. J. R. Stat. Soc. Ser. B Stat Methodol. **76**, 373–397 (2014)
19. Fan, J., Lv, J.: Sure independence screening for ultrahigh dimensional feature space. J. R. Stat. Soc. Ser. B **70**, 849–911 (2008)
20. Friedman, J., Hastie, T., Tibshirani, R.: Sparse inverse covariance estimation with the graphical lasso. Biostatistics **9**, 432–441 (2008)
21. Friedman, J., Hastie, T., Tibshirani, R., Narasimhan, B., Tay, K., Simon, N., Qian, J., Yang, J.: Package glmnet: lasso and elastic-net regularized generalized linear models (2023). https://CRAN.R-project.org/package=glmnet
22. Guo, Y., Hastie, T., Tibshirani, R.: Regularized linear discriminant analysis and its application in microarrays. Biostatistics **8**, 86–100 (2007)
23. Hastie, T., Tibshirani, R., Friedman, J.: The Elements of Statistical Learning: Data Mining, Inference, and Prediction. Springer, New York (2008)
24. Hastie, T., Tibshirani, R., Wainwright, M.: Statistical Learning with Sparsity: The Lasso and Generalizations. Chapman and Hall/CRC, New York (2015)
25. Herrgård, M.J., Covert, M.W., Palsson, B.Ø.: Reconciling gene expression data with known genome-scale regulatory network structures. Genome Res. **13**, 2423–2434 (2003)
26. Liang, F., Jia, B.: Sparse Graphical Modeling for High Dimensional Data: A Paradigm of Conditional Independence Tests. CRC Press, Boca Raton, FL (2023)
27. Mahadi, M., Ballal, T., Moinuddin, M., Al-Naffouri, T.Y., Al-Saggaf, U.M.: Regularized linear discriminant analysis using a nonlinear covariance matrix estimator. IEEE Trans. Signal Process. **72**, 1049–1064 (2024)
28. Meyer, D., Dimitriadou, E., Hornik, K., Weingessel, A., Leisch, F., Chang, C.-C., Lin, C.-C.: Package e1071: Misc Functions of the Department of Statistics, Probability Theory Group (Formerly: E1071), TU Wien (2024). https://CRAN.R-project.org/package=e1071
29. Miguel Hernández-Lobato, J., Hernández-Lobato, D., Suárez, A.: Network-based sparse Bayesian classification. Pattern Recogn. **44**, 886–900 (2011)
30. Peng, S., Zeng, X., Li, X., Peng, X., Chen, L.: Multi-class cancer classification through gene expression profiles: microRNA versus mRNA. J. Genet. Genomics **36**, 409–416 (2009)
31. Peterson, C.B., Stingo, F.C., Vannucci, M.: Joint Bayesian variable and graph selection for regression models with network-structured predictors. Stat. Med. **35**, 1017–1031 (2016)

32. Piao, Y., Piao, M., Ryu, K.H.: Multiclass cancer classification using a feature subset-based ensemble from microRNA expression profiles. Comput. Biol. Med. **80**, 39–44 (2017)
33. Rajput, D., Wang, W.-J., Chen, C.-C.: Evaluation of a decided sample size in machine learning applications. BMC Bioinf. **24**, 48 (2023)
34. Ramaswamy, S., Tamayo, P., Rifkin, R., et al.: Multiclass cancer diagnosis using tumor gene expression signatures. Proc. Natl. Acad. Sci. USA **98**, 15149–15154 (2001)
35. Safo, S.E., Ahn, J.: General sparse multi-class linear discriminant analysis. Comput. Stat. Data Anal. **99**, 81–90 (2016)
36. Saha, S., Mitra, S., Yadav, R.K.: A stack-based ensemble framework for detecting cancer microRNA biomarkers. Genom. Proteom. Bioinform. **15**, 381–388 (2017)
37. Tian, Y., Rusinek, H., Masurkar, A.V., Feng, Y.: ℓ_1-penalized multinomial regression: estimation, inference, and prediction, with an application to risk factor identification for different dementia subtypes. Stat. Med. **43**, 5711–5747 (2024)
38. Vabalas, A., Gowen, E., Poliakoff, E., Casson, A.J.: Machine learning algorithm validation with a limited sample size. PLOS One **14**, e0224365 (2019)
39. Witten, D.M., Tibshirani, R.: Penalized classification using Fisher's linear discriminant. J. R. Stat. Soc. Ser. B **73**, 753–772 (2011)
40. Xue, L., Zou, H.: Regularized rank-based estimation of high-dimensional nonparanormal graphical models. Ann. Stat. **40**, 2541–2571 (2012)
41. Yang, S., Naiman, D.Q.: Multiclass cancer classification based on gene expression comparison. Stat. Appl. Genet. Mol. Biol. **13**, 477–496 (2014)

Part III
Deep Learning and Neural Network

Deep Image-on-Scalar Regression Model with Hidden Confounders

Xiaohe Chen, Rongjie Liu, and Chao Huang

Abstract The application of integrative regression analysis using neuroimaging data from diverse sources has been crucial in investigating the relationship between clinical factors and brain structures, thereby aiding in the comprehension of the mechanisms underlying neurological diseases such as Alzheimer's disease (AD). However, it usually suffers from imaging heterogeneities caused by differences in study design, protocol, environment, population, or other hidden confounders. To address this challenge, this paper introduces a novel model known as the deep image-on-scalar regression model with hidden confounders (DISRM-HC), which can simultaneously detect hidden confounders and learn primary effects from variables of interest by employing the functional surrogate variable analysis and deep neural networks. Compared to existing solutions, our DISRM-HC can successfully handle imaging heterogeneities and capture complex patterns of primary effects. In our model, we establish estimation procedures for both unknown varying coefficients and hidden confounders. The asymptotic properties of the estimation procedures are systematically investigated as well. Subsequently, the finite-sample performance of our proposed DISRM-HC is assessed using synthetic datasets generated from Monte Carlo simulations and a real data example on diffusion MRI images from the Alzheimer's Disease Neuroimaging Initiative (ADNI) study.

Keywords Alzheimer's disease · Deep learning · Hidden confounder · Imaging heterogeneity · Neuroimaging

X. Chen
Department of Statistics, Florida State University, Tallahassee, FL, USA
e-mail: xc20j@fsu.edu

R. Liu
Department of Statistics, University of Georgia, Athens, GA, USA
e-mail: rjliu@uga.edu

C. Huang (✉)
Department of Epidemiology & Biostatistics, University of Georgia, Athens, GA, USA
e-mail: chaohuang@uga.edu

Y. Zhao, D.-G. Chen (eds.), *Big Data Analytics in Biostatistics and Bioinformatics*, ICSA Book Series in Statistics,
https://doi.org/10.1007/978-3-032-06649-7_11

1 Introduction

With the advancements in modern imaging technology, numerous extensive medical imaging databases have been established, supporting studies like the Osteoarthritis Initiative (OAI) [20] and the Alzheimer's Disease Neuroimaging Initiative (ADNI) [18]. These studies often seek to determine the association between imaging responses and several covariates of interest, such as age and gender. The image-on-scalar regression models are commonly adopted to establish this association. However, existing image-on-scalar regression models face three significant challenges: (i) the high-dimensional nature of images, (ii) complex association patterns between imaging responses and covariates of interest, and (iii) imaging heterogeneity resulting from variations in data collection procedures, such as diverse study environments, protocols, designs, and other unknown factors in multiple centers or phases. Consequently, it's crucial to detect the complex association patterns with high-dimensional imaging responses while properly accounting for imaging heterogeneity.

A widely used method for handling high-dimensional imaging data is the mass univariate analysis (MUA) [4]; the MUA involves statistical regression analysis at each voxel and generates a statistical parametric map [16]. The application of smoothing techniques further reduces the noise component of image measures and enhances the precision of primary effect estimates under MUA [23]. Nevertheless, spatial correlations are not considered in MUA. Many spatially varying coefficient models (or function-on-scalar models) [2, 14, 17, 29] are proposed to address this limitation, where the regression coefficients are modeled using spatially varying functions across voxels and the within-image variability are characterized via some stochastic processes [17]. Most existing statistical estimation procedures represent the spatially varying functions through pre-specified basis functions, such as kernels or splines [17]. While these approaches offer computational convenience and interpretability, they may lack the flexibility needed to accurately model the complex and heterogeneous spatial association patterns often observed between imaging responses and covariates across voxels. As a result, important features of the underlying spatially varying functions may be inadequately captured, potentially leading to biased or oversimplified estimates. As a powerful tool in computer vision [10], deep neural networks have been considered in approximating the mean function (or coefficient functions) on a compact set by the universal approximation theorem [25–27]. However, the estimation performance is affected when imaging heterogeneity exists [6]. Currently, there are two approaches to tackling the heterogeneity in imaging studies. The first one is the image-based meta-analysis technique, in which study-specific statistical analyses are performed first and the results are combined afterward [21]. The second one is to apply either fixed-effect or mixed-effect models to capture the imaging heterogeneity. These methods estimate primary effects while adjusting study (site or phase) related known covariates and (unknown) hidden factors. To identify those unknown factors, surrogate variable analysis has been developed in various genomic studies [12, 24]. The ideas in

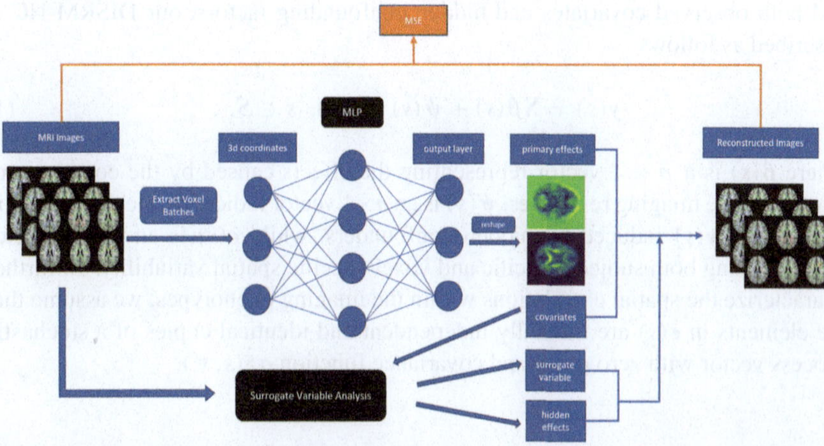

Fig. 1 Workflow of DISRM-HC architecture

surrogate variable analysis can also be adapted to imaging data analysis. However, imaging data presents three additional characteristics, spatial smoothness, spatial correlation, and low-dimensional representation [29], which are not considered in the direct surrogate variable analysis.

To address these challenges, we propose a novel model known as the deep image-on-scalar regression model with hidden confounders (DISRM-HC), which can simultaneously detect hidden confounders and learn primary effects from variables of interest by employing the functional surrogate variable analysis and deep neural networks. The workflow of our DISRM-HC is presented in Fig. 1. In particular, estimation procedures for unknown association patterns and hidden confounders are established through deep neural networks. The asymptotic properties of the estimation procedures are systematically investigated as well. Subsequently, the finite-sample performance of our proposed DISRM-HC is assessed using synthetic datasets generated from Monte Carlo simulations and a real data example on diffusion MRI images from the ADNI study. The code and validation datasets for our DISRM-HC can be found in https://github.com/xhech/DISRM-HC.

2 Method

Suppose we have collected the medical image scans and covariates of interest from n uncorrelated subjects. All the image scans have been registered to a common spatial domain $\mathcal{S} \in \mathbb{R}^D$ ($D = 2$ for 2D slice and $D = 3$ for 3D volume), where the imaging signals are observed across m voxels $\{s_k\}_{k=1}^m$. Let $\boldsymbol{y}(\boldsymbol{s})$ be an $n \times 1$ vector, including the imaging signals at voxel $\boldsymbol{s} \in \mathcal{S}$, while $\mathbf{X}$ be an $n \times p$ matrix, including all p covariates of interest. To investigate the relationship between imaging responses and both observed covariates and hidden confounding factors, our DISRM-HC is described as follows:

$$y(s) = \mathbf{X}\boldsymbol{\beta}(s) + \boldsymbol{\psi}(s) + \boldsymbol{\epsilon}(s),\ s \in \mathcal{S}, \tag{1}$$

where $\boldsymbol{\beta}(s)$ is a $p \times 1$ vector representing the effects caused by the covariates of interest on the imaging responses. $\boldsymbol{\psi}(s)$ is an $n \times 1$ vector indicating the deterministic changes on $\boldsymbol{y}(s)$ induced by hidden confounders, while $\boldsymbol{\epsilon}(s)$ is an $n \times 1$ vector characterizing both subject-specific and voxel-specific spatial variability. To further characterize the spatial correlations within the imaging phenotypes, we assume that the elements in $\boldsymbol{\epsilon}(s)$ are mutually independent and identical copies of a stochastic process vector with zero mean and covariance function $\sigma^2(s, s')$.

2.1 Estimation Procedure

In this paper, we propose an integrative approach consisting of two steps: (i) functional surrogate variable analysis to detect $\boldsymbol{\psi}(s)$ induced by hidden confounders and (ii) deep learning framework to discover the patterns in primary effects $\boldsymbol{\beta}(s)$.

Functional Surrogate Variable Analysis We apply the orthogonal decomposition of $\boldsymbol{\psi}(s)$ onto the column space of $\mathbf{X}$ and re-parametrize model (1) as

$$y(s) = \mathbf{X}\boldsymbol{\beta}^*(s) + \boldsymbol{\psi}^*(s) + \boldsymbol{\epsilon}(s),\ s \in \mathcal{S}, \tag{2}$$

where $\boldsymbol{\beta}^*(s) = \boldsymbol{\beta}(s) + \mathbf{P}_X\boldsymbol{\psi}(s)$, and $\boldsymbol{\psi}^*(s) = (\mathbf{I}_n - \mathbf{X}\mathbf{P}_X)\boldsymbol{\psi}(s)$, and $\mathbf{P}_X = (\mathbf{X}^\top\mathbf{X})^{-1}\mathbf{X}^\top$. For the coefficient $\boldsymbol{\beta}^*(s)$, we can derive an asymptotically unbiased estimator through the local linear kernel smoothing method. Specifically, some notations are introduced as follows. Let $\boldsymbol{e}^{\otimes 2} = \boldsymbol{e}\boldsymbol{e}^\top$ for any vector $\boldsymbol{e}$ and $\mathbf{C} \otimes \mathbf{D}$ be the Kronecker product of two matrices $\mathbf{C}$ and $\mathbf{D}$. In addition, we denote $K_{H_\beta}(s) = |\mathbf{H}_\beta|^{-1}K(\mathbf{H}_\beta^{-1}s)$ and $\boldsymbol{w}_{H_\beta}(s_k - s) = (1, (s_k - s)^\top\mathbf{H}_\beta^{-1})^\top$, where $K(\cdot)$ is the kernel function, and $\mathbf{H}_\beta$ is the positive definite bandwidth matrix and $|\mathbf{H}_\beta|$ is its determinant. For fixed $\mathbf{H}_\beta$, the estimator of $\boldsymbol{\beta}^*(s)$ is derived as

$$\widehat{\boldsymbol{\beta}}^*(s) = \mathbf{P}_X \sum_{k=1}^{m} \varrho_k(\mathbf{H}_\beta, s)\boldsymbol{y}(s_k), \tag{3}$$

where $\varrho_k(\mathbf{H}_\beta, s) = (1, \mathbf{0}_{1\times d})\{\sum_{k=1}^m K_{H_\beta}(s_k - s)\boldsymbol{w}_{H_\beta}^{\otimes 2}(s_k - s)\}^{-1}K_{H_\beta}(s_k - s)\boldsymbol{w}_{H_\beta}(s_k - s)$. Since there is no linearity assumption on the coefficient function $\boldsymbol{\beta}^*(s)$, the local linear smoother in (3) is a biased estimator [3]. To overcome this issue, a standard technique considered here is bias correction. Following the pre-asymptotic substitution method in [3], the bias term can be obtained by using local cubic fit with a pilot bandwidth selected in (3). denoted as $\widehat{\boldsymbol{\beta}}^*(s)$. Then, we consider a rank-q representation of the hidden confounders in $\boldsymbol{\psi}^*(s)$, i.e., $\mathbf{Z}\boldsymbol{\alpha}(s)$, where $\mathbf{Z}$ is an $n \times q$ (full column rank) loading matrix characterizing the potential hidden confounders and $\boldsymbol{\alpha}(s)$ is a $q \times 1$ vector representing the corresponding effect. To estimate the loading matrix $\mathbf{Z}$, we first construct the extended residual matrix denoted by $\bar{\mathbf{R}} = (\boldsymbol{R}(s_1), \ldots, \boldsymbol{R}(s_m))$ with $\boldsymbol{R}(s_k) = \boldsymbol{y}(s_k) - \mathbf{X}\widehat{\boldsymbol{\beta}}^*(s_k), k = 1, \ldots, m$. Given $\mathbf{X}$ and $\boldsymbol{\psi}(s)$, the conditional expectation of $\bar{\mathbf{R}}$ can be approximated by $\mathbf{Z}\bar{\mathbf{A}}$, where $\bar{\mathbf{A}} = (\boldsymbol{\alpha}(s_1), \ldots, \boldsymbol{\alpha}(s_m))$ [29]. Therefore, the loading matrix $\mathbf{Z}$ can be estimated through the singular value decomposition (SVD) on the extended residual matrix $\bar{\mathbf{R}}$, i.e., $\bar{\mathbf{R}} = \mathbf{U}\boldsymbol{\Delta}\mathbf{V}^\top$, where $\mathbf{U}$ and $\mathbf{V}$ represent the left and right singular vectors and $\boldsymbol{\Delta}$ represents the diagonal matrix containing ordered singular values of $\bar{\mathbf{R}}$. Then, the first q columns of $\mathbf{U}$, represented as $\mathbf{U}_{1:q}$, are the estimators of linear combinations of columns of $\mathbf{Z}$, i.e., $\mathbf{U}_{1:q} = \widehat{\mathbf{ZQ}}$, where $\mathbf{Q}$ is a $q \times q$ orthonormal matrix [6], which leads to an approximation form of model (2):

$$\boldsymbol{y}(s) = \mathbf{X}\boldsymbol{\beta}^*(s) + \mathbf{U}_{1:q}\boldsymbol{\gamma}(s) + \boldsymbol{\epsilon}(s), \ s \in \mathcal{S},$$

where $\boldsymbol{\gamma}(s) = \mathbf{Q}^\top\boldsymbol{\alpha}(s)$. Similar to $\widehat{\boldsymbol{\beta}}^*(s)$, we can also derive a local linear kernel estimator for $\boldsymbol{\gamma}(s)$, denoted by $\widehat{\boldsymbol{\gamma}}(s)$. Then, let $\mathbf{G} = (\mathbf{I}_n - \mathbf{X}\mathbf{P}_X)^{-1}\mathbf{ZQ}$, we can construct the estimating equation:

$$\mathbf{X}\widehat{\boldsymbol{\beta}}^*(s) + \mathbf{U}_{1:q}\widehat{\boldsymbol{\gamma}}(s) = \mathbf{X}\boldsymbol{\beta}(s) + \mathbf{G}\widehat{\boldsymbol{\gamma}}(s).$$

By assuming that $\boldsymbol{\beta}(s)$ and $\boldsymbol{\gamma}(s)$ are orthogonal after mean centering, we can derive the estimator of $\mathbf{G}$ as

$$\widehat{\mathbf{G}} = \mathbf{U}_{1:q} + \mathbf{X}\int_{\mathcal{S}} (\widehat{\boldsymbol{\beta}}^*(s) - \bar{\boldsymbol{\beta}}^*)(\widehat{\boldsymbol{\gamma}}(s) - \bar{\boldsymbol{\gamma}})^\top ds \boldsymbol{\Omega}^{-1}, \tag{4}$$

where $\bar{\boldsymbol{\beta}}^* = \int_{\mathcal{S}} \widehat{\boldsymbol{\beta}}^*(s)ds$, $\bar{\boldsymbol{\gamma}} = \int_{\mathcal{S}} \widehat{\boldsymbol{\gamma}}(s)ds$, and $\boldsymbol{\Omega} = \int_{\mathcal{S}} (\widehat{\boldsymbol{\gamma}}(s) - \bar{\boldsymbol{\gamma}})(\widehat{\boldsymbol{\gamma}}(s) - \bar{\boldsymbol{\gamma}})^\top ds$.

Thus, a statistically consistent estimator of $\boldsymbol{\psi}(s)$ can be derived as $\widehat{\mathbf{G}}\widehat{\boldsymbol{\gamma}}(s)$, and model (1) can be further written as

$$\widetilde{\boldsymbol{y}}(s) = \mathbf{X}\boldsymbol{\beta}(s) + \boldsymbol{\epsilon}(s), \ s \in \mathcal{S}, \tag{5}$$

where $\widetilde{\boldsymbol{y}}(s) = \boldsymbol{y}(s) - \widehat{\mathbf{G}}\widehat{\boldsymbol{\gamma}}(s)$ indicate the confounder-adjusted imaging responses.

Learning Coefficients Through MLP Neural Networks In this paper, we consider using MLP neural networks to estimate all the varying coefficients in $\boldsymbol{\beta}(s)$ concurrently. Specifically, we define a L-layer fully connected neural network $\mathcal{N}(s|\sigma, \boldsymbol{\Theta}) \doteq \mathcal{N}(s|\sigma, \{\mathbf{W}_l, \boldsymbol{b}_l\}_{l=0}^L)$ as follows:

$$\mathbf{W}_L\sigma(\cdots \mathbf{W}_1\sigma(\mathbf{W}_0 s + \boldsymbol{b}_0) + \boldsymbol{b}_1 \cdots) + \boldsymbol{b}_L, \tag{6}$$

where the input vector is the coordinate information $s \in \mathcal{S}$, $\sigma(\cdot)$ is the activation function (we choose the logistic activation function in this paper, i.e., $\sigma(u) =$

$\{1+\exp(u)^{-1}\}^{-1}$), and $\mathbf{W}_l \in \mathbb{R}^{h_{l+1}\times h_l}$ and $\boldsymbol{b}_l \in \mathbb{R}^{h_{l+1}}$ are the weight and bias parameters from the l-th hidden layer to the $(l+1)$-th hidden layer, $l = 0, \ldots, L$. Then, to approximate the varying coefficients in $\boldsymbol{\beta}(\boldsymbol{s})$, we build up p distinct $(L+1)$-layer fully connected neural networks. Specifically, the first L layers are commonly shared across all neural networks and parameterized by $\boldsymbol{\Theta}$, while the output layer is distinct, i.e., for the j-th varying coefficient in $\boldsymbol{\beta}(\boldsymbol{s})$, denoted as $\beta_j(\boldsymbol{s})$, the $(L+1)$-th layer in the corresponding neural network is parameterized by $\{\mathbf{W}_{L+1,j}, \boldsymbol{b}_{L+1,j}\}$, $j = 1, \ldots, p$. Furthermore, to improve the interpretability of detected primary effect $\boldsymbol{\beta}(\boldsymbol{s})$, we impose the sparsity assumption on the patterns of each varying coefficient in $\boldsymbol{\beta}(\boldsymbol{s})$ by utilizing the hard thresholding techniques. Specifically, a thresholding function is applied to $\beta_j(\boldsymbol{s})$, i.e., $T_{\beta_j(\boldsymbol{s})}(t_j, B) = \mathbf{1}\{|\beta_j(\boldsymbol{s})| > t_j\} \cdot \min(|\beta_j(\boldsymbol{s})|, B) \cdot \operatorname{sign}(\beta_j(\boldsymbol{s}))$, $j = 1, \ldots, p$, where $\mathbf{1}\{\cdot\}$ the indicator function and t_j is the threshold to be learned from the data. In practice, we set the upper truncation bound $B = 10^{10}$ so it has no impact on the output. To compute the threshold, we can randomly permute images across subjects multiple times to obtain a null distribution of the estimated coefficients and set the threshold as desired quantiles of the absolute values of the estimates. Consequently, the MLP neural network-based representation of the varying coefficient $\beta_j(\boldsymbol{s})$ can be written as

$$\mathcal{N}(\boldsymbol{s}|\sigma, \boldsymbol{\Theta}, \boldsymbol{\Theta}_j) = T_{\beta_j(\boldsymbol{s})}(\mathbf{W}_{L+1,j}\mathcal{N}(\boldsymbol{s}|\sigma, \boldsymbol{\Theta}) + \boldsymbol{b}_{L+1,j}, t_j, B),$$

where $\boldsymbol{\Theta}_j = \{\mathbf{W}_{L+1,j}, \boldsymbol{b}_{L+1,j}, t_j\}$, $1 \le j \le p$. In particular, the network parameters, $\boldsymbol{\Theta}$ and $\{\boldsymbol{\Theta}_j\}_{j=1}^p$, can be learned by minimizing the mean squared error (MSE) loss as follows:

$$\frac{1}{m}\sum_{k=1}^{m}\left\|\tilde{\boldsymbol{y}}(\boldsymbol{s}_k) - \mathbf{X}\overline{\mathcal{N}}(\boldsymbol{s}_k|\sigma, \boldsymbol{\Theta}, \{\boldsymbol{\Theta}_j\}_{j=1}^p)\right\|^2, \tag{7}$$

where $\overline{\mathcal{N}}(\boldsymbol{s}_k|\sigma, \boldsymbol{\Theta}, \{\boldsymbol{\Theta}_j\}_{j=1}^p)$ is a $p \times 1$ vector with the j-th element $\mathcal{N}(\boldsymbol{s}|\sigma, \boldsymbol{\Theta}, \boldsymbol{\Theta}_k)$. We also illustrate the overall estimation procedure in Algorithm 1.

Remark 1 In our estimation procedure, we consider the spatial correlation in constructing both the estimator of varying coefficient $\boldsymbol{\gamma}(\boldsymbol{s})$ and the neural network-based estimation of $\boldsymbol{\beta}(\boldsymbol{s})$. For the coefficient $\boldsymbol{\gamma}(\boldsymbol{s})$, compared to the voxel-wise regression analysis, we adopt the local linear kernel estimator to borrow information from the neighborhood voxels. For the refined MLP-based estimator of $\boldsymbol{\beta}(\boldsymbol{s})$, the spatial correlation is taken into account as the weight and bias parameters in the first L layers are commonly shared across all neural networks and learned using imaging intensities from all pixels $\boldsymbol{s} \in \mathcal{S}$. Although we vectorized the voxel-wise residuals in identifying the unobserved confounders $\mathbf{G}$, it does not destroy the spatial correlation as the unobserved confounders $\mathbf{G}$ are invariant across voxels.

Algorithm 1 Estimation procedure of parameters in model (1)

Normalize d-dimensional coordinates $\boldsymbol{s}$ for each image voxel.
Perform functional surrogate variable analysis to get the estimates for surrogate variable $\mathbf{G}$ and hidden effects $\boldsymbol{\gamma}(\boldsymbol{s})$, i.e., $\widehat{\mathbf{G}}$ and $\widehat{\boldsymbol{\gamma}}(\boldsymbol{s})$.
Train a neural network to estimate $\boldsymbol{\beta}(\boldsymbol{s})$:
for epoch < max_epochs **do**
  Divide voxels into multiple batches of size b, $\{\mathcal{S}_b\}$.
  for each batch **do**
    Feed $\boldsymbol{s} \in \mathcal{S}_b$ into MLPs $\{\mathcal{N}(\boldsymbol{s}|\sigma, \boldsymbol{\Theta}, \boldsymbol{\Theta}_j)\}_{j=1}^{p}$.
    Optimize MSE loss function

$$\frac{1}{b}\sum_{\boldsymbol{s}\in\mathcal{S}_b} \|\boldsymbol{y}(\boldsymbol{s}) - \widehat{\mathbf{G}}\widehat{\boldsymbol{\gamma}}(\boldsymbol{s}) - \mathbf{X}\overline{\mathcal{N}}(\boldsymbol{s}|\sigma, \boldsymbol{\Theta}, \{\boldsymbol{\Theta}_k\}_{k=1}^{p})\|^2$$

  end for
end for
Input coordinates to the trained model to estimate $\boldsymbol{\beta}(\boldsymbol{s})$.

2.2 *Theoretical Analysis*

In this section, we establish the theoretical properties of our proposed method. First, some function classes for the nonparametric functions are defined. Similar definitions also can be found in existing literature [27].

Definition 1 (Smooth Functions) For $D \in \mathbb{N}_+$, $C \in \mathbb{R}_+$ and $P = P' + P''$, where $P' = \lceil P - 1 \rceil$, i.e., the largest integer no greater than $P - 1$, a function $f : \mathbb{R}^D \to \mathbb{R}$ is said to be P-smooth, if for every $(p_1, \cdots, p_D) \in \mathbb{N}_0^D$ with $\sum_{d=1}^{D} p_d = P'$, we have:

- the partial derivative $\left\{\partial^{P'}/(\partial u_1^{p_1} \cdots \partial u_D^{p_D})\right\} f$ exists;
- for any $\boldsymbol{u} \in \mathbb{R}^D$,

$$\left|\left\{\frac{\partial^{P'}}{\partial u_1^{p_1} \cdots \partial u_D^{p_D}}\right\} f(\boldsymbol{u})\right| < C;$$

- for all $\boldsymbol{u}, \boldsymbol{u}' \in \mathbb{R}^D$,

$$\left|\left\{\frac{\partial^{P'}}{\partial u_1^{p_1} \cdots \partial u_D^{p_D}}\right\} f(\boldsymbol{u}) - \left\{\frac{\partial^{P'}}{\partial u_1^{p_1} \cdots \partial u_D^{p_D}}\right\} f(\boldsymbol{u}')\right| \le C\|\boldsymbol{u} - \boldsymbol{u}'\|_2^{P''}.$$

Definition 2 (Piecewise Smooth Functions) For K', $Q \in \mathbb{N}_+$ and $P \in \mathbb{R}_+$, a function $f : \mathbb{R}^D \to \mathbb{R}$ is said to be K'-component Q-sided piecewise P-smooth if there exist $g_k : \mathbb{R}^D \to \mathbb{R}$ and $\Omega_k \subset \mathbb{R}^D$ for $k = 1, \ldots, K'$, such that $f(\boldsymbol{u}) =$

$\sum_{k=1}^{K'} g_k(\boldsymbol{u}) \cdot \mathbf{1}(\boldsymbol{u} \in \Omega_k)$, where g_k is P-smooth, and $\Omega_k \subset \mathbb{R}^D$ is a Q-sided D-dimensional polytope.

Definition 3 (Candidate Neural Network Function) For $D, L', K', Q, H \in \mathbb{N}_+$ and $\kappa \in \mathbb{R}_+$, define $\mathcal{G}_{D,L',K',Q}^{H,\kappa}$ to be the collection of all functions $g : \mathbb{R}^D \to \mathbb{R}$ that satisfy:

- When $L' = 0$, there exist $\xi_{h,b,d}^{[1]}, \xi_{h,b}^{[2]}, \xi_h^{[3]} \in (-\kappa, \kappa)$, $h = 0, \ldots, H, b = 0, \ldots, 4D + Q, d = 0, \ldots, D$, such that

$$g(\boldsymbol{u}) = \sum_{h=1}^{H} \xi_h^{[3]} \sigma \left(\sum_{b=1}^{4D+Q} \xi_{h,b}^{[2]} \sigma \left(\sum_{d=1}^{D} \xi_{h,b,d}^{[1]} u_d + \xi_{h,b,0}^{[1]} \right) + \xi_{h,0}^{[2]} \right) + \xi_0^{[3]}.$$

- When $L' > 0$, there exist $g_k \in \mathcal{G}_{D,0,K',Q}^{H,\kappa}$ and $h_{k,b} \in \mathcal{G}_{D,L'-1,K',Q}^{M,\kappa}$, $k = 1, \ldots, K', b = 1, \ldots, D$, such that $g(\boldsymbol{u}) = \sum_{k=1}^{K'} g_k \left(h_{k,1}(\boldsymbol{u}), \ldots, h_{k,D}(\boldsymbol{u})\right)$.

Definition 1 provides a general characterization of function smoothness by imposing bounds on derivatives up to a specified order, i.e., P, which reflects the smoothness level of the functions we study. Definition 2 introduces a class of piecewise smooth functions, where each piece is supported on a multidimensional polytope, where Q is the number of sides of the polytope that characterizes the boundary of the piecewise functions and K' is the number of components in the recursive construction of the true functions and the candidate functions. This structural assumption is well-suited for medical imaging applications, as activation regions typically exhibit moderate geometric complexity, reflecting the spatial organization of underlying biological structures and functions [27]. Definition 3 characterizes a family of neural network functions constructed by recursively composing and summing two-layer fully connected feed-forward networks, where the constant κ s the bound of absolute values of the weight parameters in the neural network functions and L' and H correspond to the number of layers and the number of hidden nodes in the recursive construction of the two-layer feed-forward neural networks. While the logistic activation function is used in this paper, analogous results can be achieved with the ReLU activation function. In the theoretical analysis, we study the family of piecewise smooth functions described in Definition 2, to which $\boldsymbol{\beta}(s)$ is assumed to belong, and then employ the candidate neural network function described in Definition 3 to approximate the true $\boldsymbol{\beta}(s)$ function.

Throughout the paper, the following assumptions are used to facilitate the technical details. Some of the assumptions might be weakened, but the current version simplifies the proof.

Assumption 1 *The rows in* $\mathbf{X}$, *denoted as,* $\boldsymbol{x}_1, \ldots, \boldsymbol{x}_n$, *are i.i.d with* $\mathbb{E}[\boldsymbol{x}_i] = \mathbf{0}$, $\mathbb{E}[\|\boldsymbol{x}_i\|_2^4] < c_1$, *and* $\|Cov(\boldsymbol{x}_i)\|_F^2 < c_2$, *where* $\|\cdot\|_F$ *is the Frobenius norm. In addition, there exist constants* $c_3, c_4 \in \mathbb{R}_+$, *such that* $\mathbb{E}(\exp[c_3\{\boldsymbol{x}_i^T \boldsymbol{\beta}(s) + \boldsymbol{\epsilon}(s)\}^2]) < c_4$, *for all* $s \in \mathcal{S}$.

Assumption 2 *The true spatially varying functions* $\{\beta_j(\cdot)\}_{j=1}^{p}$ *are* K'*-component* Q*-sided piecewise* P*-smooth functions. In addition, for the corresponding spatial domain* $\mathcal{S}$*, there exists a constant* $c_5 \in \mathbb{R}_+$ *such that* $\mathcal{S} \subset [-c_5, c_5]^D$*.*

Assumption 3 *There exist a constant* $c_6 \in \mathbb{R}+$ *such that* $\inf_{\beta_j(s)\neq 0} |\beta_j(s)| > c_6$ *and* $\mu(\{s \in \mathcal{S} : \beta_j(s) \neq 0\})/\mu(\mathcal{S}) \ll 1$*, for* $j = 1, \ldots, p$*, where* μ *is the Lebesgue measure in* $\mathcal{S} \subset \mathbb{R}^D$*.*

Assumption 4 *The neural network approximation functions belong to the class specified in Definition 3, i.e.,* $\mathcal{N}(s|\sigma, \boldsymbol{\Theta}, \boldsymbol{\Theta}_k) \in \mathcal{G}_{D,L',K',Q}^{H,\kappa}$ *for* $k = 1, \ldots, p$*, where* $\kappa = (nm)^{c_7}$ *for some constant* $c_7 \in \mathbb{R}_+$*.*

Assumption 5 *The hard threshold parameters satisfy that* $\max(t_1, \ldots, t_p) \to 0$ *as* $n \to 0$*, and* $\min(t_1, \ldots, t_p) > c_8 \log(n)^{-1}$ *for some* $c_8 \in \mathbb{R}+$*.*

Assumption 1 imposes mild moment conditions on the covariates. Assumption 2 requires the true spatially varying functions to exhibit a certain degree of smoothness, a standard condition in the literature on varying coefficient models [6, 29]. Additionally, it is assumed that the domain of these functions lies within a compact set—a reasonable assumption in imaging studies, where spatial domains are inherently bounded. Assumption 3 introduces a sparsity condition on the main effects, along with a minimum signal strength requirement, ensuring a separation between zero and the weakest nonzero effect. This reflects common characteristics of activation patterns observed in medical imaging data [27]. Assumption 4 defines the class of candidate neural network functions used to approximate the true coefficient functions in the varying coefficient model. Assumption 5 requires that the hard thresholding values converge to zero at a controlled rate, imposing a lower bound on this rate of convergence. This condition is analogous to the penalty weight assumptions commonly seen in regularization frameworks [27, 28].

Assumption 6 *Both* n *and* m *converge to* ∞ *with* $m/n \to \infty$*. Let* $|\cdot|_d$ *be the determinant of some given matrix. Then* $|\mathbf{H}_\beta|_d = o(1)$*,* $m|\mathbf{H}_\beta|_d \to \infty$*, and* $|\mathbf{H}_\beta|_d^{-1}|\log(|\mathbf{H}_\beta|_d)|^{1-2/l} \leq m^{1-2/l}$ *for* $l \in (2, 4)$*.*

Assumption 7 *Let* λ_i, λ_j *be the* i*-th and* j*-th largest singular value of* $\boldsymbol{\psi}^*(s) = (\mathbf{I}_n - \mathbf{X}\mathbf{P}_X)\boldsymbol{\psi}(s)$*, then* $\lambda_i = O(\lambda_j)$*,* $\lambda_j = O(\lambda_i)$*, and* $m^{-1/2}\lambda_i \to \infty$ *hold for all* $1 \leq i, j \leq q$*.*

Assumption 8 *The kernel function* $K(\cdot)$ *is Lipschitz continuous and a symmetric density function with bounded support* $\mathcal{S}$*. Moreover,*

$$\inf_{|\mathbf{H}|<h_0, s\in S} |\Omega_K(\mathbf{H}, s)|_D$$

is above 0 for some small scalar h_0*, where* $\Omega_K(\mathbf{H}, s) = \int_S K_H(t-s) z_H^{\otimes 2}(t-s)dt$*.*

Assumption 9 *$\boldsymbol{\beta}(s)$ and $\boldsymbol{\gamma}(s)$ are orthogonal after mean centering:*

$$\int_{\mathcal{S}} (\boldsymbol{\beta}(s) - \bar{\boldsymbol{\beta}})(\boldsymbol{\gamma}(s) - \bar{\boldsymbol{\gamma}})^\top ds = 0,$$

where $\bar{\boldsymbol{\beta}} = \int_{\mathcal{S}} \boldsymbol{\beta}(s)ds$ and $\bar{\boldsymbol{\gamma}} = \int_{\mathcal{S}} \boldsymbol{\gamma}(s)ds$.

Assumption 10 *Suppose $\boldsymbol{\epsilon}(s) = \boldsymbol{\zeta}(s)+\boldsymbol{e}(s)$ consists of a component $\boldsymbol{\zeta}(s)$ capturing individual variability and a random error component $\boldsymbol{e}(s)$. For all the elements in $\boldsymbol{e}(s)$, $\mathbb{E}[\sup_s |e_i(s)|^l] < \infty$ for some $l > 4$.*

Assumption 11 *Each component of $\{\boldsymbol{\zeta}(s) : s \in \mathcal{S}\}$, $\{\boldsymbol{\zeta}(s)\boldsymbol{\zeta}^\top(s') : (s, s') \in \mathcal{S}\}$, and $\{\boldsymbol{\omega}^\top \boldsymbol{\zeta}(s) : s \in \mathcal{S}\}$ are Donsker classes.*

Assumption 6 concerns the choice of smoothing bandwidths and aligns with standard practices in the literature [6, 29]. Assumption 7 adopts the spiked eigenvalue model, which ensures that the effects of latent factors are sufficiently strong to be identified via singular value decomposition. Assumption 8 is a common condition in the context of kernel smoothing methods [6]. Assumption 9 is the central assumption underlying surrogate variable analysis. Assumption 10 imposes a uniform bound on the higher-order moments of the error term $\epsilon_{ij}(s)$ for all $s \in \mathcal{S}$. Assumption 11 avoids smoothness conditions on the sample path $\zeta(s)$; see [29] for further discussion.

Finally, we present the estimation consistency of detected unobserved confounders $\widehat{\boldsymbol{G}}$ and the error bound of estimated coefficients $\widehat{\boldsymbol{\beta}}(s)$. The detailed proof can be found in the Appendix.

Theorem 1 *Under Assumptions 1–11, we have the following results: (i) The columns of $\widehat{\mathbf{G}}$ span the same column space as the columns of $(\mathbf{I}_n - \mathbf{X}\mathbf{P}_X)^{-1}\mathbf{Z}$ in probability.*
(ii) The L_2 estimation error satisfies

$$\mathbb{E}\left\{\frac{1}{m}\sum_{k=1}^{m} \|\boldsymbol{\beta}(s_k) - \widehat{\boldsymbol{\beta}}(s_k)\|^2\right\} \le c_{100}\left\{\log(nm)^3\left(\frac{H}{nm} + H^{-\frac{2P}{D}}\right) + \frac{1}{n}\right\}$$

for some constant $c_{100} \in \mathbb{R}_+$ and sufficiently large n and m.

3 Simulation Studies

We used the following image-on-scalar regression model to generate the simulated 3d imaging response for each voxel $s_k \in \mathcal{S}$ for each subject i:

$$y_i(s_k) = \sum_{j=1}^{p} x_{ij}\beta_j(s_k) + \sum_{j=1}^{q} z_{ij}\gamma_j(s_k) + \psi_i(s_k) + \epsilon_i(s_k),$$

for $k = 1, \ldots, m, i = 1, \ldots, n$. We set the number of subjects $n = 100$, and the dimension of the 3d imaging response to be $64 \times 64 \times 8$, which means $m = 32768$. We set the number of covariates $p = 3$, where $x_{i1}, x_{i2} \sim N(1, 1)$, and $x_{i3} \sim \text{Ber}(0.5)$. We set the number of hidden factors $q = 2$, where

$$z_{i1} \sim \begin{cases} N(0.5, 0.25), & i \leq 50 \\ N(-0.5, 0.25), & i > 50 \end{cases},$$

indicating the potential batch effect, while $z_{i2} = \sum_{j=1}^{3} x_{ij}\phi_j + \omega_i$ with $\omega_i \sim N(0, 0.25)$, $\phi_t = u_t(2b_t - 1), t = 1, 2, 3$, and $b \sim \text{Ber}(0.5)$, which characterizes other unknown observed confounders. We considered four scenarios when simulating u_t. (1) z_{i2} is independent of $\{x_{ij}\}_{j=1}^{3}$: $u_t = 0$, (2) z_{i2} is weakly correlated with $\{x_{ij}\}_{j=1}^{3}$: $u_t \sim U(0, 0.2)$, and (3) z_{i2} is moderately correlated with $\{x_{ij}\}_{j=1}^{3}$: $u_t \sim U(0.2, 0.5)$. The individual stochastic function $\psi_i(s)$ was simulated in the form of Karhunen-Loeve expansion as $\psi_i(s) = \xi_{i1}\eta_1(s) + \xi_{i2}\eta_2(s)$, where $\xi_{il} \sim N(0, 0.01)$ for $l = 1, 2$, and $\{\eta_l(s)\}_{l=1}^{2}$ are the eigen functions: $\psi_1(s) = 2s/m - 1$, and $\psi_2(s) = s/m - 0.5$. The noise term ϵ_{im} was generated from $N(0, \sigma_i^2/\delta)$ with $\sigma_i^2 \sim \text{IG}(10, 9)$ and δ is a term controlling the scale of the noise or equivalently the signal-noise ratio (SNR). We consider four scenarios to simulate ϵ_{im}: (1) very low SNR, $\delta = 0.5$; (2) low SNR, $\delta = 1$; (3) medium SNR, $\delta = 5$; and (4) high SNR, $\delta = 10$. We specified primary effects $\{\beta_j(s)\}_{j=1}^{3}$ and hidden effects $\{\gamma_j(s)\}_{j=1}^{2}$ with the sparse patterns illustrated in Figs. 2 and 3, respectively. In addition, three image responses randomly generated under high SNR and weak correlation scenarios are presented in Fig. 4.

We constructed a fully connected neural network with 64 hidden units for each layer with ReLU activation function to estimate primary effects. We set the batch

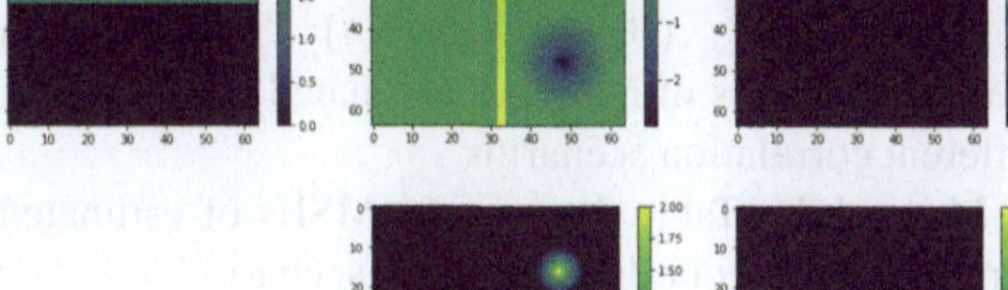

Fig. 2 Sparse patterns of primary effects: $\beta_1(s)$ (left), $\beta_2(s)$ (middle), and $\beta_3(s)$ (right)

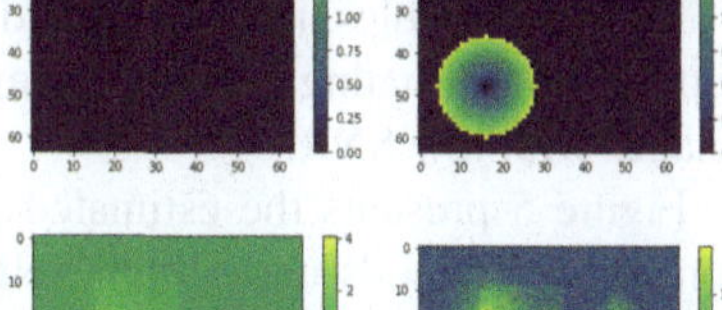

Fig. 3 Sparse patterns of hidden effects: $\gamma_1(s)$ (left) and $\gamma_2(s)$ (right)

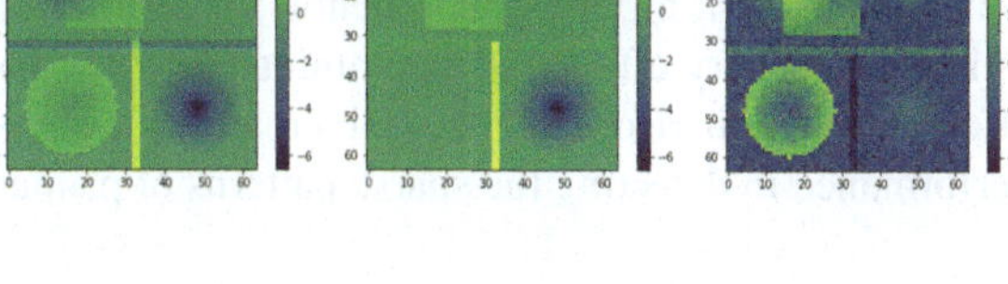

Fig. 4 Visualization of three randomly simulated image responses

Table 1 Mean and standard deviation of MSEs of estimated primary effects under high SNR and three different correlation scenarios

Correlation	Independent	Weak	Moderate
DISRM-HC	**0.00077 (0.00018)**	**0.00125 (0.00085)**	**0.00185 (0.00061)**
MUA	0.00574 (0.00432)	0.00752 (0.00388)	0.00670 (0.00442)
DSVA	0.00705 (0.00877)	0.00261 (0.00047)	0.00335 (0.00085)
FHFRM	0.01165 (0.00358)	0.01027 (0.00585)	0.01252 (0.00367)
IRRNN	0.03495 (0.00425)	0.04347 (0.01998)	0.04162 (0.01559)

Table 2 Mean and standard deviation of MSEs of estimated primary effects under weak correlation and four different SNR scenarios

SNR	Very low	Low	Medium	High
DISRM-HC	**0.00121 (0.00033)**	**0.00096 (0.00038)**	**0.00083 (0.00027)**	**0.00126 (0.00085)**
MUA	0.12545 (0.00845)	0.03550 (0.00464)	0.00675 (0.00437)	0.00587 (0.00437)
DSVA	0.12237 (0.00749)	0.03178 (0.00181)	0.00348 (0.00040)	0.00267 (0.00047)
FHFRM	0.01605 (0.00339)	0.01285 (0.00350)	0.01186 (0.00363)	0.01184 (0.00359)
IRRNN	0.03908 (0.00237)	0.03320 (0.00254)	0.03595 (0.00375)	0.04347 (0.01998)

size of input coordinates as 64 with an adjustable learning rate starting from 0.002, and trained using Adam [11] optimizer for 250 epochs. Note that we didn't apply fine-tuning for every simulation scenario; instead, we used the same set of hyper-parameters, which may not demonstrate the optimal performance, but it's sufficient to demonstrate that DISRM outperforms other existing methods according to the results we will present below.

We compared our model with other four competing methods, including massive univariate analysis (MUA) [4], direct surrogate variable analysis (dSVA) [12], functional hybrid factor regression model (FHFRM) [6], and image response regression via deep neural networks (IRRNN) [27]), and assessed the estimation performance in terms of primary effects by evaluating the average and standard deviation of the mean squared error (MSE) per each simulation, which is defined as $\frac{1}{mp}\sum_{k=1}^{m}\sum_{j=1}^{p}(\beta_j(s_k) - \widehat{\beta}_j(s_k))^2$. Table 1 presents the comparison of all five methods in terms of MSEs of estimated primary effects under high SNR and three different correlation scenarios.

Meanwhile, Table 2 gives the MSEs of estimated primary effects under weak correlation and four different SNR scenarios.

From both tables, it can be found that, compared to other methods, our model is superior in estimating the primary effects in all simulation scenarios, especially for images with low SNR.

Figure 5 presents the estimated primary effects by DISRM and the other four competing methods under high SNR and weak correlation scenarios. From Fig. 5 we can observe a mixing phenomenon for all four competing methods, where the estimated primary effects are contaminated by the patterns in hidden confounding effects. In comparison, our model greatly alleviates this issue and shows great performance in detecting the sparse patterns of primary effects.

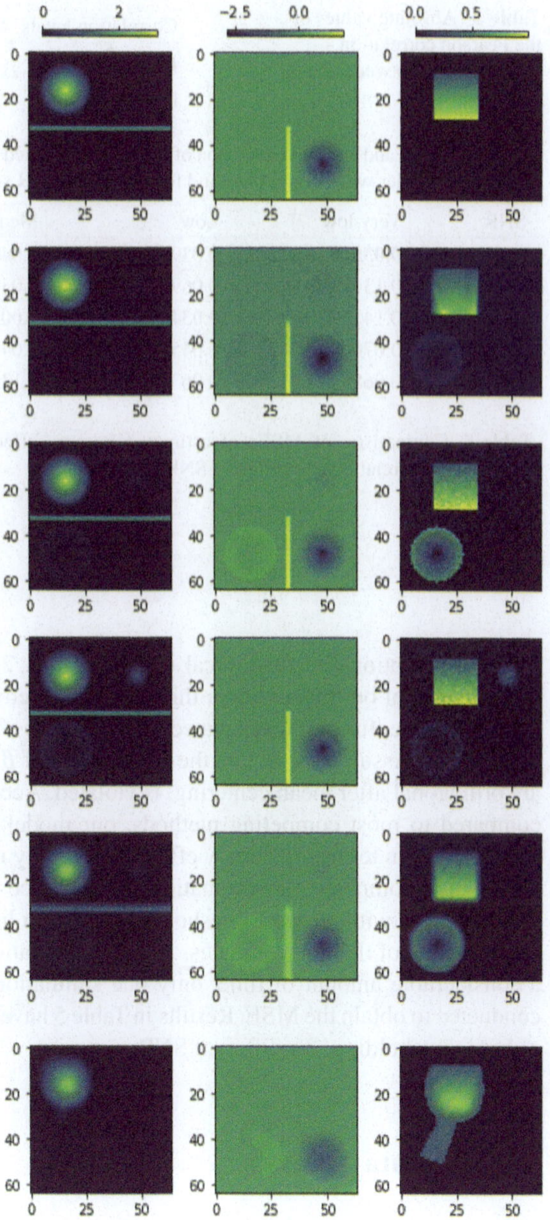

Fig. 5 Ground truth of primary effects (Row 1) and the estimation performance for five methods: DISRM (Row 2), MUA (Row 3), DSVA (Row 4), FHFRM (Row 5), and IRRNN (Row 6)

Next, we set $q = 1$ by only keeping one hidden confounder, z_{i2}, in the generative model, and calculated the absolute value of the Pearson correlation coefficient between $\mathbf{Z}$ and detected confounding factor $\widehat{\mathbf{G}}$ under high SNR and four different correlation scenarios between z_{i2} and $\{x_{ij}\}_{j=1}^{3}$. It can be found from Table 3 that $\mathbf{Z}$ and $\widehat{\mathbf{G}}$ span the same column space, which corresponds to both our

Table 3 Absolute values of the Pearson correlation coefficients ρ between Z and $\widehat{G}$ when $q = 1$

Correlation levels	Independent	Weak	Moderate
$\lvert\widehat{\rho}(Z, \widehat{G})\rvert$	0.9999	0.9995	0.9986
p-value	<0.0001	<0.0001	<0.0001

Table 4 Mean and standard deviation of MSEs of estimated primary effects with violated model assumption under weak correlation and four different SNR scenarios

SNR	Very low	Low	Medium	High
DISRM-HC	**0.03520 (0.02202)**	0.03994 (0.02737)	0.04040 (0.02882)	0.03180 (0.02034)
MUA	0.13421 (0.06720)	0.06903 (0.02489)	0.03990 (0.02493)	0.03898 (0.02490)
DSVA	0.14197 (0.00746)	**0.03496 (0.00267)**	**0.00149 (0.00015)**	**0.00053 (0.00013)**
FHFRM	0.07009 (0.04320)	0.04509 (0.02414)	0.04383 (0.02381)	0.04377 (0.02377)
IRRNN	0.06896 (0.01564)	0.06312 (0.02485)	0.13612 (0.11059)	0.08584 (0.02004)

Table 5 Comparison of MSEs of estimated primary effects with/without hard thresholding under weak correlation and different SNR scenarios

SNR	Very low	Low	Medium	High
With threshold	0.00302	0.00225	0.00212	0.00117
No threshold	0.00306	0.00473	0.00906	0.00262

model assumption and theoretical results in Sect. 2, and further ensures the good performance of our model under this simulation setting.

Finally, we further investigated the robustness of our model when the key assumption, Assumption 9, i.e., the row vectors of $\boldsymbol{\beta}(s)$ and the row vectors of $\boldsymbol{\gamma}(s)$ are orthogonal after mean centering, is violated. According to the results in Table 4, compared to most competing methods, our model can provide robust estimation performance in terms of primary effects, especially in low SNR scenarios.

We also compared the estimation performance of the primary effects in two different both without hard thresholding and with hard thresholding applied at the 0.95 quantile of the null estimates. As the permutation of neural networks will take a considerable amount of time, only one simulation run under each scenario was conducted to obtain the MSE. Results in Table 5 have demonstrated the effectiveness of hard thresholding, for different SNR scenarios.

4 Real Data Analysis

4.1 Data Description

Data used in the preparation of this article were obtained from the ADNI database (adni.loni.usc.edu). The ADNI was launched in 2003 by the National Institute on Aging, National Institute of Biomedical Imaging and Bioengineering, Food and Drug Administration, private pharmaceutical companies, and nonprofit organizations as a $60 million, 5-year public-private partnership. The primary goal of ADNI has been to test whether serial magnetic resonance imaging (MRI), positron-emission tomography, other biological markers, and clinical and neuropsychological assessment can be combined to measure the progression of mild cognitive impairment (MCI) and early Alzheimer's disease (AD). Determination of sensitive and specific markers of very early AD progression is intended to aid researchers and clinicians in developing new treatments and monitoring their effectiveness, as well as lessening the time and cost of clinical trials. The principal investigator of this initiative is Michael W. Weiner, MD, at the VA Medical Center and University of California, San Francisco. ADNI is the result of efforts of many coinvestigators from a broad range of academic institutions and private corporations, and subjects have been recruited from over 50 sites across the USA and Canada. The goal was to recruit 800 subjects, but the initial study (ADNI-1) has been followed by ADNI-GO and ADNI-2. To date, these 3 protocols have recruited over 1,500 adults, ages 55–90, to participate in the research, consisting of cognitively normal older individuals, people with early or late MCI, and people with early AD. The follow-up duration of each group is specified in the protocols for ADNI-1, ADNI-2, and ADNI-GO. Subjects originally recruited for ADNI-1 and ADNI-GO had the option to be followed in ADNI-2. For up-to-date information, see www.adni-info.org.

4.2 Data Processing

In this data analysis, we consider the baseline DTI dataset with $n = 213$ subjects from 16 sites in the ADNI study. Detailed information about the ADNI study can be found in the Web Appendix. As described in [13] and [15], the diffusion-weighted image data was processed by two key steps including using the FMRIB software library (FSL) FDT [1] and TBSS [22] pipelines to construct the diffusion tensor images and register them to create a mean image and a mean skeleton. Specifically, the DTIs were constructed from the diffusion-weighted image data for all subjects, and the FA maps were computed from the DTIs after eddy current correction and automatic brain extraction using the FSL FDT pipeline. Then, through the FSL TBSS pipeline, we aligned the FA maps into a common space by using nonlinear registration and created and thinned the mean FA image to obtain a mean FA skeleton, which represents the centers of all white-matter tracts common to the group. Subsequently, we projected each subject's aligned FA maps onto this skeleton. To improve computing efficiency, we downsampled the original images from (182,218,182) to (73,87,73) and applied a mask to filter redundant voxels near the image edges. Three axial slices of one randomly selected preprocessed FA map are illustrated in Fig. 6.

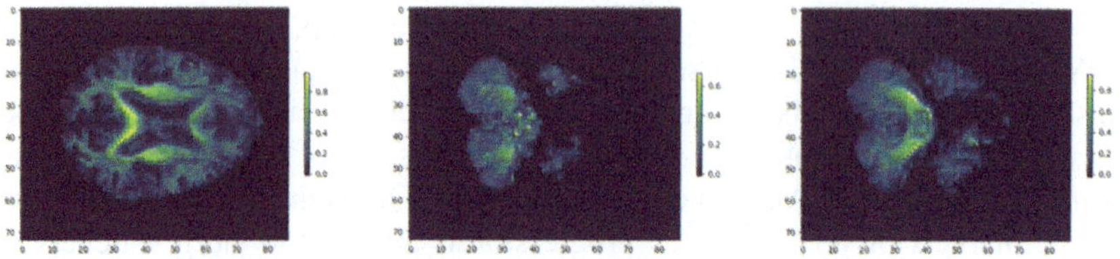

Fig. 6 Three axial slices of one randomly selected preprocessed FA maps

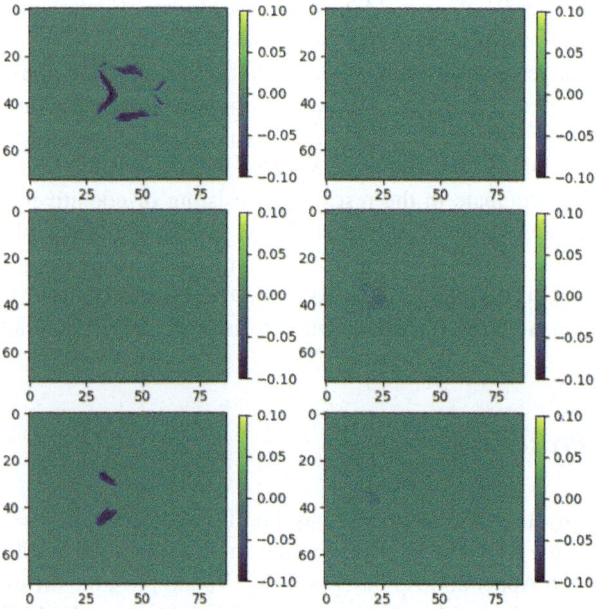

Fig. 7 Some axial slices of the estimated age effect (left) and gender effect (right)

4.3 Data Analysis

This real data analysis aims to investigate the relationship between FA maps and some covariates of interest, i.e., age and gender, while handling the potential hidden confounders. We first applied our functional surrogate variable analysis and identified one hidden factor through the factor analysis tool in [19]. Then, we trained the neural network for 400 epochs with a voxel batch size of 128 on masked baseline FA maps to estimate the primary effects of age and gender, while adjusting for the identified hidden factor. Figure 7 shows three axial slices of the estimated age and gender effects on FA maps. By utilizing the JHU DTI-based white-matter atlas [5], which segmented the brain into 48 regions of interest (ROIs), we identified some important ROIs where age and gender may have impacts. For example, according to DISRM estimated varying coefficients, the age effect can be

Table 6 p-values for testing the association between the hidden factor and covariates

	Age	Gender	EDU	CN	MCI	AD
p-value	0.994	0.992	0.587	0.184	0.160	0.001

found on the corpus callosum and the hippocampus, while the gender effect can be found on the longitudinal fasciculus and the inferior fronto-occipital fasciculus. All these detected ROIs are highly related to brain aging and consistent with the findings in existing literature [7–9, 15].

We further explored the correlation between identified hidden factors and variables including age, gender, education years (EDU), as well as diagnostic status including normal control (CN), mild cognitive impairment (MCI), and Alzheimer's disease (AD). We tested if there is no association pattern between the identified hidden factor and these covariates. Table 6 shows the p-values of the hypothesis tests. From the table, we can see this identified hidden confounder has a significant association with AD status, which indicates that AD could be a potential confounder to be included in the analysis.

5 Discussion and Conclusion

Image-on-scaler regression has been challenged by the high dimensionality nature of images, complex spatial association patterns, and heterogeneity from diverse data sources. In this paper, we introduce surrogate variable analysis from genomic studies to imaging data analysis to alleviate image heterogeneity and employ neural networks to capture complex spatial association patterns, and by utilizing voxels as samples for neural network inputs, we can reverse the dimension of subjects and voxels to avoid the high-dimensional image vs limited sample size issue in medical image data analysis. By addressing these problems, our model provides insight into integrating traditional statistical models with modern deep-learning tools to handle complex data.

However, there also exist limitations to our proposed model. Assumption 9 in Sect. 2.2 should be satisfied to be able to derive the surrogate variable. However, simulation studies have shown that our model can offer robust estimates of primary effects compared to competing methods even if the assumption is violated. Also, statistical inference for estimated primary effects is not provided. Due to the inclusion of neural networks, the asymptotic distribution of the test statistic under null hypothesis would be quite complicated to derive, wild bootstrap could be considered to compute the p-value, but this could be extremely time-consuming as the neural network needs to be retrained numerous times. In addition, we assume images to be single-channel in this model, but an extension to multiple image measurements can also be possible.

Funding The research of Dr. Huang was partially supported by the National Institutes of Health (NIH) under Award Number UL1TR002378. The content is solely the responsibility of the authors and does not necessarily represent the official views of the NIH.

Appendix

First, some definitions are provided here, which will be used in the following lemmas and the proof of Theorem 1.

Definition 4 (Piecewise Smooth Generalized Hierarchical Interaction Model) For $D, D', L', K', Q \in \mathbb{N}_+$ and $P \in \mathbb{R}_+$, a function $f : \mathbb{R}^D \to \mathbb{R}$ is called a K'-component Q-sided piecewise P-smooth generalized hierarchical interaction model of depth L' and order D', if it satisfies:

- When $L' = 0$, there exist $\boldsymbol{a}_d \in \mathbb{R}^D, d = 1, \ldots, D', g : \mathbb{R}^{D'} \to \mathbb{R}$, and $\Omega \subset \mathbb{R}^D$, such that $f(\boldsymbol{u}) = g(\boldsymbol{a}_1^\top \boldsymbol{u}, \ldots, \boldsymbol{a}_{D'}^\top \boldsymbol{u}) \times \mathbf{1}_\Omega(\boldsymbol{u})$, where g is P-smooth, Ω is a Q-sided D-dimensional polytope, and $K' = 1$.
- When $L' > 0$, there exist $g_k : \mathbb{R}^{D'} \to \mathbb{R}$, $h_{k,d} : \mathbb{R}^D \to \mathbb{R}$, and $\Omega_k \subset \mathbb{R}^D$, such that

$$f(\boldsymbol{u}) = \sum_{k=1}^{K'} g_k(h_{k,1}(\boldsymbol{u}), \ldots, h_{k,D'}(\boldsymbol{u})) \times \mathbf{1}_{\Omega_k}(\boldsymbol{u}),$$

  where g_k is P-smooth and $h_{k,d}$ is a K'-component P-smooth generalized hierarchical interaction model of depth $L' - 1$ and order D', and $\Omega_k \subset \mathbb{R}^D$ is a Q-sided D-dimensional polytope, $k = 1, \ldots, K', d = 1, \ldots, D'$.

Definition 5 (Covering Number) Let $\mathcal{F}$ be a collection of functions $f : \mathbb{R}^p \to \mathbb{R}$. Moreover, let $A \subset \mathbb{R}^p$ and $\delta > 0$. A finite collection $f_1, \ldots, f_L : \mathbb{R}^p \to \mathbb{R}$ is called a $(\delta, \|\cdot\|_{\infty,A})$-cover of $\mathcal{F}$ if for any $f \in \mathcal{F}$, there exists an $l \in \{1, \ldots, L\}$ such that $\sup_{x \in A} |f(x) - f_l(x)| < \delta$. Furthermore, the $(\delta, \|\cdot\|_{\infty,A})$-covering number of $\mathcal{F}$ is the cardinality of the smallest $(\delta, \|\cdot\|_{\infty,A})$-cover of $\mathcal{F}$, denoted as $\mathfrak{N}(\mathcal{F}, \delta, \|\cdot\|_{\infty,A})$, abbreviated as $\mathfrak{N}(\mathcal{F}, \delta)$.

Definition 4 describes a family of piecewise smooth functions, which covers a wide range of functions. For instance, when $D = 2$, the nonzero regions of $\boldsymbol{\beta}$ can be partitioned into a finite number of hexagons, and $\boldsymbol{\beta}$ is Lipschitz continuous inside each partition, $\boldsymbol{\beta}$ is a 6-sided-piecewise 1-smooth generalized hierarchical interaction model of depth 1 and order 2. When $K = 1$ and $\mathcal{S} \subset \Omega_1$, the function is smooth over the entire spatial domain.

Second, we present two lemmas that will be used in the proof of Theorem 1. Since these lemmas have already been stated and proved in [27], we include them here without reproducing the proofs.

Lemma 1 *Suppose $\mathcal{F}_{n,m}$ is an arbitrary collection of functions with domain $\mathcal{S}$ and range $\mathbb{R}^p$. Let $\bar{\boldsymbol{\beta}}'_{n,m}$ be the least square estimator based on the corresponding threshold function class $T(t_{n,m}, \infty) \circ \mathcal{F}_{n,m}$, that is,*

$$\bar{\boldsymbol{\beta}}'_{n,m} = \arg \min_{\boldsymbol{\beta} \in T(t_{n,m}, \infty) \circ \mathcal{F}_{n,m}} \frac{1}{nm} \sum_{k=1}^{m} \sum_{i=1}^{n} \left[y_i(s_k) - \psi(s_k) - \boldsymbol{x}_i^\top \boldsymbol{\beta}(s_k) \right]^2,$$

where $t_{n,m} = c_{20} \log(nm)^{-1}$ for some $c_{20} \in \mathbb{R}_+$. Moreover, let $B_{n,m} = c_{21} \log(nm)$ for some $c_{21} \in \mathbb{R}_+$, and let $\bar{\boldsymbol{\beta}}_{n,m} = T(0, B_{n,m}) \circ \bar{\boldsymbol{\beta}}'_{n,m}$. Define

$$\Delta_{n,m}^2 = m^{-1} \sum_{k=1}^{m} [\boldsymbol{\beta}(s_k) - \bar{\boldsymbol{\beta}}_{n,m}(s_s)]^2$$

Then there exists a constant $c_{30} > 0$ such that

$$\begin{aligned}\mathbb{E}\left[\Delta_{n,m}^2\right] \leq\, & c_{30}\left\{1 + \log \mathfrak{N}[\mathcal{G}_{D,L',K',Q}^{H,\kappa} \circ \mathcal{F}_{n,m}, (nm)^{-1} B_{n,m}^{-1}]\right\} \log(nm)^2 (nm)^{-1} \\ & + c_{30} \log(nm) H^{-2P/D} \\ & + c_{30} \inf_{\boldsymbol{\beta}_{n,m} \in T(t_{n,m}, \infty) \circ \mathcal{F}_{n,m}} m^{-1} \sum_{k=1}^{m} \|\boldsymbol{\beta}(s_k) - \boldsymbol{\beta}_{n,m}(s_k)\|_2^2 + c_{30} n^{-1}\end{aligned}$$

Lemma 2 *Let $k \in \mathbb{N}_+$. Suppose random vector $(\boldsymbol{X}_k, Y_k) \in \mathbb{R}^D \times \mathbb{R}$ satisfies $\mathbb{E}[Y_k^2] \leq \infty$ and has conditional mean function $f(\boldsymbol{x}) = \mathbb{E}[Y_k \mid \boldsymbol{X}_k = \boldsymbol{x}]$ for all k. Moreover, suppose f is a K'-component Q-sided piecewise P-smooth generalized hierarchical interaction model of depth L' and order D' with $P > 1$. Let $\kappa = k^{c_{40}}$ for some $c_{40} \in \mathbb{R}_+$. Then for sufficiently large H and for all k,*

$$\inf_{f \in \mathcal{G}_{D',L',K',Q}^{H,\kappa}} \int \left|f(x) - \widehat{f}_k(x)\right|^2 \mathrm{Pr}_{\boldsymbol{X}_k}(dx) \leq c_{50} \log(k)^3 H^{-\frac{2P}{D}},$$

where $c_{50} \in \mathbb{R}_+$ is a constant.

Proof of Theorem 1

(i) Since $\mathbf{G} = (\mathbf{I}_n - \mathbf{X}\mathbf{P}_X)^{-1}\mathbf{Z}\mathbf{Q}$, $\mathbf{G}$ can be seen as the linear combination of columns in $(\mathbf{I}_n - \mathbf{X}\mathbf{P}_X)^{-1}\mathbf{Z}$, indicating that they share the same column space, so we only need to show $\widehat{\mathbf{G}} = \mathbf{G} + o_p(1)$ to prove Theorem 1. According to Eq. (4) and Lemma 1 in [6], we have $\widehat{\mathbf{G}} = (\mathbf{I}_n - \mathbf{X}\mathbf{P}_X)\mathbf{G} + \mathbf{X} \int_{\mathcal{S}} (\boldsymbol{\beta}^*(s) - \bar{\boldsymbol{\beta}}^*)(\boldsymbol{\gamma}(s) - \bar{\boldsymbol{\gamma}})^\top ds \boldsymbol{\Omega}^{-1} + o_p(1)$. Plugging in $\boldsymbol{\beta}^*(s) = \boldsymbol{\beta}(s) + \mathbf{P}_X \boldsymbol{\psi}(s)$, we have: $\widehat{\mathbf{G}} = \mathbf{G} + \mathbf{X} \int_{\mathcal{S}} (\boldsymbol{\beta}(s) - \bar{\boldsymbol{\beta}})(\boldsymbol{\gamma}(s) - \bar{\boldsymbol{\gamma}})^\top ds \boldsymbol{\Omega}^{-1} + o_p(1)$. Under Assumption 9, $\widehat{\mathbf{G}} = \mathbf{G} + o_p(1)$, which completes the proof.

(ii) Let

$$\Delta_{n,m}^2 = m^{-1}\sum_{k=1}^{m}[\boldsymbol{\beta}(s_k) - \bar{\boldsymbol{\beta}}_{n,m}(s_k)]^2$$

By Lemma 1, $\Delta_{n,m}^2 \leq c_{30}\sum_{k=1}^{3}\Delta_{k,n,m}^2$, where

$$\Delta_{1,n,m}^2 = \{1 + \log \mathfrak{N}[\mathcal{G}_{D,L',K',Q}^{H,\kappa} \circ \mathcal{G}_{D,L',K',Q}^{H,\kappa}, (nm)^{-1}B_{n,m}^{-1}]\}\log(nm)^2(nm)^{-1}$$

$$\Delta_{2,n,m}^2 = \inf_{\boldsymbol{\beta}_{n,m}\in T(t_{n,m},\infty)\circ\mathcal{G}_{D,L',K',Q}^{H,\kappa}} m^{-1}\sum_{k=1}^{m}\|\boldsymbol{\beta}(s_k) - \boldsymbol{\beta}_{n,m}(s_k)\|_2^2$$

$$\Delta_{3,n,m}^2 = \log(nm)H^{-\frac{2P}{D}} + n^{-1}$$

For $\Delta_{1,N,V}^2$, we have $\mathcal{G}_{D,L',K',Q}^{H,\kappa} \circ \mathcal{G}_{D,L',K',Q}^{H,\kappa} \subset \mathcal{G}_{D,2L',K',Q}^{H,\kappa}$ by Definition 4. Moreover,

$$1 + \log \mathfrak{N}[\mathcal{G}_{D,2L',K',Q}^{H,\kappa}, (nm)^{-1}B_{n,m}^{-1}] \leq c_{60}\log(nm)H$$

for some $c_{60} \in \mathbb{R}_+$ [27]. Then

$$\Delta_{1,n,m}^2 \leq c_{60}\log(nm)^3(nm)^{-1}H$$

For $\Delta_{2,n,m}^2$. Since β_j is assumed to be a K'-component Q-sided piecewise P-smooth function, it is also a K'-component Q-sided piecewise P-smooth generalized hierarchical interaction model of depth L' and order D for any $L' \geq 0$. Then by Lemma 2, we have

$$\Delta_{2,n,m}^2 \leq c_{70}\log(nm)^3 H^{-\frac{2P}{D}}$$

for some $c_{70} \in \mathbb{R}_+$.

Finally, we have:

$$\begin{aligned}\Delta_{n,m}^2 &\leq c_{80}\log(nm)^3(nm)^{-1}H + c_{80}\log(nm)^3 H^{-\frac{2P}{D}} \\ &\quad + c_{80}\log(nm)H^{-\frac{2P}{D}} + c_{80}n^{-1} \\ &\leq c_{100}\left(\log(nm)^3[(nm)^{-1}H + H^{-\frac{2P}{D}}] + N^{-1}\right)\end{aligned}$$

for some $c_{80}, c_{100} \in \mathbb{R}_+$.

References

1. Behrens, T.E.J., et al.: Characterization and propagation of uncertainty in diffusion-weighted MR imaging. In: Magn. Reson. Med. Official J. Int. Soc. Magn. Reson. Med. **50**(5), 1077–1088 (2003)
2. Chen, Y., et al.: Local region sparse learning for image-on-scalar regression. Stat **1050**, 27 (2016)
3. Fan, J., Gijbels, I.: Local Polynomial Modelling and Its Applications. Chapman and Hall, London (1996)
4. Friston, K.J.: Statistical parametric mapping. In: Kötter, R. (ed.) Neuroscience Databases: A Practical Guide, pp. 237–250. Springer US, Boston, MA (2003)
5. Hua, K., et al.: Tract probability maps in stereotaxic spaces: analyses of white matter anatomy and tract-specific quantification. Neuroimage **39**(1), 336–347 (2008)
6. Huang, C., Zhu, H.: Functional hybrid factor regression model for handling heterogeneity in imaging studies. Biometrika **109**(4), 1133–1148 (2022)
7. Huang, C., Srivastava, A., Liu, R.: Geo-FARM: geodesic factor regression model for misaligned pre-shape responses in statistical shape analysis. In: Proceedings of the IEEE/CVF Conference on Computer Vision and Pattern Recognition, pp. 11496–11505 (2021)
8. Huang, C., et al.: FGWAS: functional genome wide association analysis. Neuroimage **159**, 107–121 (2017)
9. Jin, Y., et al.: 3D tract-specific local and global analysis of white matter integrity in Alzheimer's disease. Hum. Brain Mapp. **38**(3), 1191–1207 (2017)
10. Khan, S., et al.: A Guide to Convolutional Neural Networks for Computer Vision. Morgan & Claypool Publishers, California (2018)
11. Kingma, D., Ba, J.: Adam: A Method for Stochastic Optimization. arXiv preprint arXiv:1412.6980 (2014)
12. Lee, S., et al.: An improved and explicit surrogate variable analysis procedure by coefficient adjustment. Biometrika **104**(2), 303–316 (2017)
13. Li, J., Huang, C., Zhu, H.: A functional varying-coefficient single-index model for functional response data. J. Am. Stat. Assoc. **112**(519), 1169–1181 (2017)
14. Li, X., Wang, L., Wang, H.J.: Sparse learning and structure identification for ultrahigh-dimensional image-on-scalar re-gression. J. Am. Stat. Assoc. **116**(536), 1994–2008 (2021)
15. Luo, X., Zhu, L., Zhu, H.: Single-index varying co-efficient model for functional responses. Biometrics **72**(4), 1275–1284 (2016)
16. Mechelli, A., et al.: Voxel-based morphometry of the human brain: methods and applications. Curr. Med. Imaging **1**(2), 105–113 (2005)
17. Morris, J.S.: Functional regression. Annu. Rev. Stat. Appl. **2**, 321–359 (2015)
18. Mueller, S.G., et al.: The Alzheimer's disease neuroimaging initiative. Neuroimaging Clin. **15**(4), 869–877 (2005)
19. Onatski, A.: Determining the number of factors from empirical distribution of eigenvalues. Rev. Econ. Stat. **92**(4), 1004–1016 (2010)
20. Peterfy, C.G., Schneider, E., Nevitt, M.: The osteoarthritis initiative: report on the design rationale for the magnetic resonance imaging protocol for the knee. Osteoarthr. Cartil. **16**(12), 1433–1441 (2008)
21. Salimi-Khorshidi, G., et al.: Meta-analysis of neuroimaging data: a comparison of image-based and coordinate-based pooling of studies. NeuroImage **45**, 810–823 (2009)
22. Smith, S.M., et al.: Tract-based spatial statistics: voxelwise analysis of multi-subject diffusion data. Neuroimage **31**(4), 1487–1505 (2006)
23. Wang, J.-L., Chiou, J.-M., Müller, H.-G.: Functional data analysis. Annu. Rev. Stat. Appl. **3**(1), 257–295 (2016)
24. Wang, J., et al.: Confounder adjustment in multiple hypothesis testing. Ann. Stat. **45**, 1863–1894 (2017)

25. Wang, S., Cao, G., Shang, Z.: Estimation of the mean function of functional data via deep neural networks. Stat **10**(1), e393 (2021)
26. Wu, S., Beaulac, C., Cao, J.: Neural networks for scalar input and functional output. Stat. Comput. **33**(5), 118 (2023)
27. Zhang, D., et al.: Image response regression via deep neural networks. J. R. Stat. Soc. Series B Stat. Methodol. **85**(5), 1589–1614 (2023)
28. Zhao, P., Yu, B.: On model selection consistency of Lasso. J. Mach. Learn. Res. **7**(Nov), 2541–2563 (2006)
29. Zhu, H., Li, R., Kong, L.: Multivariate varying co-efficient model for functional responses. Ann. Stat. **40**(5), 2634–2666 (2012)

Transfer Learning for Causal Effect Estimation

Song Wei, Hanyu Zhang, Ronald Moore, Rishikesan Kamaleswaran, and Yao Xie

Abstract We present a Transfer Causal Learning (TCL) framework when target and source domains share the same covariate/feature spaces whereas the treatment assignment mechanisms might differ, aiming to improve causal/treatment effect estimation accuracy in limited data. Limited data is very common in medical applications, where some rare medical conditions, such as sepsis, are of interest. Our proposed method, named ℓ_1-TCL, incorporates ℓ_1 regularized transfer learning (TL) for nuisance models (e.g., propensity score model); the TL estimator of the nuisance parameters is plugged into downstream average treatment effect estimators (e.g., inverse probability-weighted estimator). We establish non-asymptotic recovery guarantees for the ℓ_1-TCL with generalized linear model (GLM) under the sparsity assumption in the high-dimensional setting and demonstrate the empirical benefits of ℓ_1-TCL through extensive numerical simulation for GLM and recent neural network nuisance models. Our method is subsequently extended to real data and generates meaningful insights consistent with medical literature, a case where all baseline methods fail.

This work is partially supported by an NSF CAREER CCF-1650913, NSF DMS-2134037, CMMI-2015787, CMMI-2112533, DMS-1938106, DMS-1830210, R01GM139967-02S1, the Coca-Cola Foundation, and an Emory Hospital grant. The implementation using benchmark dataset is available online at https://github.com/SongWei-GT/L1-TCL.

S. Wei · H. Zhang · Y. Xie (✉)
Georgia Institute of Technology, Atlanta, GA, USA
e-mail: yao.xie@isye.gatech.edu

R. Moore
Duke University, Durham, NC, USA

R. Kamaleswaran
Georgia Institute of Technology, Atlanta, GA, USA

Duke University, Durham, NC, USA

Y. Zhao, D.-G. Chen (eds.), *Big Data Analytics in Biostatistics and Bioinformatics*, ICSA Book Series in Statistics,
https://doi.org/10.1007/978-3-032-06649-7_12

Keywords Causal effect estimation · Electronic medical record · Generalized linear model · Lasso · Transfer learning

1 Introduction

Causal effect estimation from observational data has attracted much attention in many fields since it is crucial for informed decision-making and effective intervention design. Several unbiased estimators for the average treatment effect (ATE) have been proposed, e.g., the inverse probability-weighted (IPW) estimator, outcome regression (OR) estimator, and doubly robust (DR) estimator, which have shown good empirical performances and strong theoretical guarantees; see, e.g., [70], for a survey of those estimators. However, there is less study for the situations with limited data present in the target study. In modern applications, advanced data acquisition techniques make it possible to collect datasets from other domains, referred to as the source domains, which are related to (but different from) that of the target study. Transfer learning (TL), aiming to boost performance in the target domain with knowledge gained from the source domain, has shown promise in practice [55].

1.1 Motivating Application and Dataset

Our work is motivated by a real study, where the goal is to estimate the causal/treatment effect of vasopressor therapy among septic patients who are admitted to the intensive care unit (ICU) at an academic level 1 trauma center. The corresponding dataset (i.e., the target domain dataset) contains in-hospital electronic medical records (EMRs) derived from this facility in the year 2018, and we report the summary statistics of the patient demographics in Table 1.

Table 1 Summary statistics of the patient demographics in the selected cohort in the real-data example. Q1 and Q3 stand for the 25% and 75% quantiles (also gives the interquartile range)

	Source		Target	
	Treatment	Control	Treatment	Control
Number of patients	207	1249	58	700
Age, median and [Q1,Q3]	63.0 [51.0,70.5]	64.0 [53.0,74.0]	55.5 [37.25,67.5]	58.0 [41.0,68.0]
Male, number and percentage	131 (63.3%)	652 (52.2%)	38 (65.5%)	449 (64.1%)
28-D Mortality, number and percentage	43 (20.8%)	117 (9.4%)	20 (34.5%)	71 (10.1%)
Total hospital days, median and [Q1,Q3]	22.0 [12.5,33.5]	13.0 [8.0,21.0]	25.5 [13.0,45.5]	18.0 [10.0,31.0]

Due to *limited* data availability, IPW estimation on target domain dataset shows that vasopressor therapy increases the risk of 28-day mortality (see Table 5 for evidence), and such a "finding" contradicts the established medical literature [2]. In this work, we aim to correct this using the available source domain dataset derived from one geographically adjacent medical facility.

In other words, our goal is to estimate the treatment effect from a limited observational dataset with the help of another observational dataset, which *shares the same covariate space but can have different treatment assignment mechanism*; we will call it *Transfer Causal Learning* (TCL) problem in the following. Given that both domains may differ not only in treatment assignment mechanisms (see Fig. 2 for evidence) but also in the patients' responses to treatment, a naive integration of both datasets can be impractical and lead to biased estimates due to the disproportionate amount of source domain data. Thus, developing a principled data-integrative approach to effectively utilize the abundant source domain data to enhance the estimation accuracy of the target domain treatment effect is of significant interest.

1.2 Literature

TL has been applied to causal inference in a distinct yet more straightforward manner, owing to the unique treatment-and-control structure. For instance, [46, 47] proposed a novel neural network (NN) architecture tailored to causal effect estimation by considering shared and group-specific layers in the potential outcome models for treatment and control groups. However, adapting TL techniques from the supervised learning setting to handle data integration for causal effect estimation is nontrivial, as it requires counterfactual information. In causal inference, this problem is solved by the aforementioned plug-in estimators (e.g., IPW, OR, and DR estimators), which involve preliminary stage nuisance parameter estimation for the propensity score (PS) and/or OR models. Hence, a natural solution is to apply data-integrative TL to the supervised nuisance parameter estimation problem and subsequently evaluate the plug-in estimators for ATE using target domain data, where the hope is to improve ATE estimation accuracy by enhancing the quality of estimated nuisance parameters, regardless of whether the ground truth ATEs are the same across both domains.

Recently, there has been increased interest in applying data-integrative TL techniques to causal inference. One notable line of research [17, 67] has focused on combining observational and experimental/randomized datasets to address the limited amount of randomized data, thereby leveraging the benefits of both types of datasets. Similarly, [68] explored the use of multiple observational datasets, including a limited target domain dataset with additional potential confounders. However, the above methods are not suitable for our TCL problem since obtaining randomized datasets can be especially challenging and unethical in life-threatening conditions (e.g., sepsis), and methods designed for heterogeneous covariate spaces

[5, 68] typically rely on domain-specific covariate spaces for their algorithmic designs. To the best of our knowledge, [24] is the only work that has developed a data-integrative heuristic for the TCL problem, which used the neural network weights estimated from the source domain as the warm start of the subsequent target domain NN training. Despite its improved empirical performance, the theoretically grounded approach for the TCL problem is still largely missing. For other related works on applying TL in causal inference, we refer readers to an extended literature review in Appendix A and a survey study by [70].

1.3 Contribution

In this work, we present a generic framework for the Transfer Causal Learning problem, called ℓ_1-TCL framework. It entails data-integrative transfer learning of the nuisance parameter and plug-in estimation for causal effect in the target domain. The transfer learning stage comprises two steps: (i) rough estimation using abundant source domain data and (ii) bias correction step via ℓ_1 regularized estimation of the difference between the target and source domain nuisance parameters using target domain data. Subsequently, the estimated nuisance parameters are plugged into the unbiased causal effect estimators, including IPW, OR, and DR estimators. Most importantly, as shown in [4], with the help of Lasso in the high-dimensional setting, we can establish non-asymptotic recovery guarantees for the causal effect estimators when the nuisance models (i.e., PS and OR models) are parameterized as generalized linear models (GLMs) and under the sparsity assumption on the target and source nuisance parameters' difference. Furthermore, we incorporate recently developed nonparametric PS and OR models in ℓ_1-TCL to improve robustness to model misspecification, and we show improved performance of our ℓ_1-TCL framework using NN-based approaches [46, 47] by comparing with existing TL approaches [24] for ATE estimation on a benchmark pseudo-real-dataset [7]. The ℓ_1-TCL framework is subsequently applied to a real study and reveals that vasopressor therapy could prevent mortality within septic patients [2], which all baseline approaches fail to show.

1.4 Notations

Superscript ^{T} denotes vector or matrix transpose, and $\|\cdot\|_p$ denotes the vector ℓ_p norm. We use upper case letters (e.g., $\boldsymbol{X}$) to denote random variables (r.v.s) and the corresponding lowercase letters with additional subscripts (e.g., $\boldsymbol{x}_1, \boldsymbol{x}_2, \ldots$) to denote their realizations. For asymptotic notations, $f(n) = o(g(n))$ or $g(n) \gg f(n)$ means for all $c > 0$, there exists $k > 0$ such that $0 \leq f(n) < cg(n)$ for all $n \geq k$; $f(n) = \mathcal{O}(g(n))$ means there exist positive constants c and k, such that $0 \leq f(n) \leq cg(n)$ for all $n \geq k$.

2 Methodology

We study the causal inference problem under Neyman–Rubin potential outcome framework [43, 50]. In this section, we will review the IPW estimator, introduce the formal TCL problem setup, and present our ℓ_1-TCL with a generalized linear propensity score model. Additionally, we will extend these contents to OR and DR estimators.

2.1 Background

Potential Outcome Framework Consider the tuple (X, Z, Y) in the target domain, where random vector $X \in \mathcal{X} \subset \mathbb{R}^d$ represents covariates measured before receipt of treatment, r.v. $Z \in \{0, 1\}$ is treatment indicator ($Z = 1$ if treated) and r.v. Y is the *observed outcome*:

$$Y = Y_1 Z + (1 - Z)Y_0.$$

Here, Y_0 and Y_1, referred to as *potential outcomes*, are the values of the outcome that would be seen if the subject were to receive control or treatment. Throughout this work, we are interested in estimating the ATE (or average causal effect), which is formally defined as

$$\tau = \mathbb{E}[Y_1] - \mathbb{E}[Y_0].$$

In an observational study, the treatment Z is typically not statistically independent from (Y_0, Y_1) since the characteristics that determine the treatment assignment may also be correlated, or "confounded," with the potential outcome. To handle this problem, a common practice is to assume there are "no unmeasured confounders" (also known as the ignorability assumption):

$$(Y_0, Y_1) \perp\!\!\!\perp Z \mid X.$$

In the following, we shall continue our study under the above assumption.

Inverse Probability Weighting The propensity score $e(X) = \mathbb{P}(Z = 1|X)$ is the probability of treatment given covariates and specifies the treatment assignment mechanism. Rosenbaum and Rubin [41] showed:

$$(Y_0, Y_1) \perp\!\!\!\perp Z \mid e(X),$$

which leads to an unbiased estimator for ATE through inverse probability weighting. Consider n samples from the target domain:

$$\mathcal{D}_i = (\boldsymbol{x}_i, z_i, y_i), \quad i = 1, \ldots, n, \tag{1}$$

and let $\widehat{e}(\boldsymbol{x}_i)$ be the estimated propensity score for i-th subject, the IPW estimator for ATE is

$$\widehat{\tau}_{\mathrm{IPW}} = \frac{1}{n}\sum_{i=1}^{n} \frac{z_i y_i}{\widehat{e}(\boldsymbol{x}_i)} - \frac{(1-z_i)y_i}{1-\widehat{e}(\boldsymbol{x}_i)}. \tag{2}$$

Due to space consideration, we defer the introduction of OR and DR estimators to Appendix "Additional Details on the Potential Outcome Framework". We refer readers to the survey studies by Lunceford and Davidian [28], Bang and Robins [3], Yao et al. [70] for further background knowledge.

2.2 Problem Setup

Inductive Multitask Transfer Learning Our TCL problem studies the causal effect estimation in the inductive multitask TL setup [34], where the feature spaces across both domains are the same, but the feature distribution, treatment assignment rule, and underlying causal effect can be different. From now on, we will refer to (1) as samples from the target domain. Assume we additionally observe n_{s} samples of the covariates, treatment, and outcome tuple $(\boldsymbol{X}_{\mathrm{s}}, Z_{\mathrm{s}}, Y_{\mathrm{s}})$ from the source domain:

$$\mathcal{D}_{i,\mathrm{s}} = (\boldsymbol{x}_{i,\mathrm{s}}, z_{i,\mathrm{s}}, y_{i,\mathrm{s}}), \quad i = 1, \ldots, n_{\mathrm{s}}.$$

In our motivating real example, $n \ll n_{\mathrm{s}}$, rendering it difficult to get an accurate ATE estimate by solely using target domain data and necessitating the use of source domain data. The challenge is that neither the nuisance models (e.g., the PS model) nor the ground truth ATEs are the same between both domains, making naively merging two datasets impractical. To be precise, consider that the PS models take the following forms:

$$\mathbb{P}(Z=1|\boldsymbol{X}) = e(\boldsymbol{X};\beta_{\mathrm{t}}), \quad \mathbb{P}(Z_{\mathrm{s}}=1|\boldsymbol{X}_{\mathrm{s}}) = e_{\mathrm{s}}(\boldsymbol{X}_{\mathrm{s}};\beta_{\mathrm{s}}), \tag{3}$$

where functions $e(\cdot)$, $e_{\mathrm{s}}(\cdot)$ have known form with unknown nuisance parameters $\beta_{\mathrm{t}}, \beta_{\mathrm{s}} \in \mathbb{R}^{d_1}$. Our TCL aims to integrate both domains' data to accurately estimate the target domain ATE.

An Illustrative Example To help readers understand this TCL setup and elucidate why the TCL problem is nontrivial, we present a toy example as follows:

$$\underline{\text{Treatment assignment}}: \quad \mathbb{P}(Z = 1|X_1, X_2) = g(\beta_1 X_1 + \beta_2 X_2),$$

$$\underline{\text{Causal relationship}}: \quad Y = \tau Z + \alpha X_2 + \epsilon,$$

where $g(x) = 1/(1 + e^x)$ is the sigmoid function. The goal is to infer the causal effect from treatment Z to outcome Y, given potential confounding variables X_1 and X_2; the additive noise ϵ is independent of the aforementioned r.v.s. The treatment assignment and the causal relationship are visualized in Fig. 1; further experimental details can be found in Appendix "Motivating Toy Example".

Although IPW is consistent, it is still empirically challenging to obtain a reliable estimate from limited amount of data, as verified by the estimate using target-only causal learning (`TO-CL`) in Table 2, and this necessitates the use of source domain data. One naive way is to integrate (or merge) both datasets in the PS model nuisance parameter estimation stage for causal learning, i.e., `Merge-CL`. However, due to different treatment assignments, `Merge-CL` may not help improve estimation accuracy. To make things worse, since $n_s \gg n$ ($n_s = 1000$ and $n = 100$ in this toy example), the `Merge-CL` estimate will bias toward the source domain causal effect, leading to a potentially worse downstream plug-in IPW estimator, as verified in Table 2.

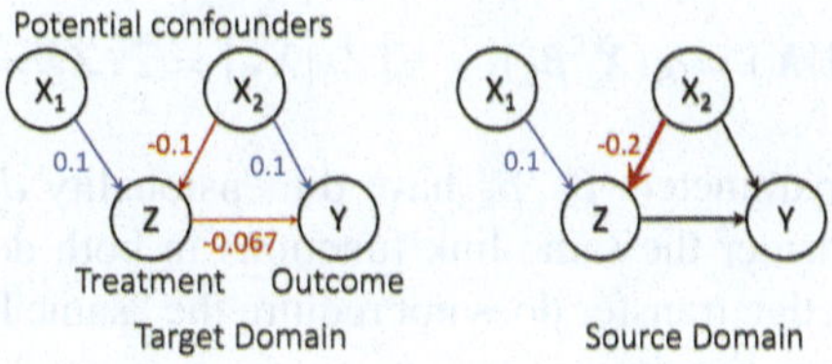

Fig. 1 The treatment assignments differ between target and source domains (highlighted by the bold red arrow). We do not assume that the ATEs are the same for both domains

Table 2 Comparison of ATE estimation accuracy: the truth is $\tau = -0.067$. Our proposed ℓ_1-TCL yields the most accurate one, which correctly recovers the *inhibiting* effect

Data used	Target only	Both domains	
Learning framework	`TO-CL`	`Merge-CL`	ℓ_1-TCL
IPW estimate	0.0002	0.0441	−0.0013

2.3 Proposed Method

We begin with a simple yet popular generalized linear model (GLM) [33] parameterization of the *nuisance models* (i.e., PS (3) and OR (9) models). A GLM for r.v. $\widetilde{Z}$ with parameter β and predictor $\widetilde{\boldsymbol{X}}$ is

$$\widetilde{Z} \mid \widetilde{\boldsymbol{X}} \sim \mathbb{P}(\widetilde{Z}|\widetilde{\boldsymbol{X}}) = F(\widetilde{Z}) \exp\{\widetilde{Z}\widetilde{\boldsymbol{X}}^{\mathrm{T}}\beta - G(\widetilde{\boldsymbol{X}}^{\mathrm{T}}\beta)\}, \text{ which satisfies } \mathbb{E}[\widetilde{Z}|\widetilde{\boldsymbol{X}}] = G'(\widetilde{\boldsymbol{X}}^{\mathrm{T}}\beta).$$

Here, $G'(\cdot)$, known as the (inverse) link function, is the derivative of $G(\cdot)$; common nonlinear choices include sigmoid link function $G'(x) = 1/(1 + e^{-x})$ on a domain $x \in \mathbb{R}$ and exponential link function $G'(x) = 1 - e^{-x}$ on a domain $x \in [0, \infty)$. The function $F(\cdot)$ normalizes, ensuring a valid probability distribution. Given samples $(\widetilde{\boldsymbol{x}}_i, \widetilde{z}_i)$, $i = 1, \ldots, n$, the maximum likelihood estimation (MLE) of the GLM model parameter is given by

$$\widehat{\beta}_{\mathrm{MLE}} = \arg\min_b \sum_{i=1}^{n} -\widetilde{z}_i \widetilde{\boldsymbol{x}}_i{}^{\mathrm{T}} b + G\left(\widetilde{\boldsymbol{x}}_i{}^{\mathrm{T}} b\right).$$

As the treatment indicator is binary, the GLM parameterization with link function $G'(\cdot) = g(\cdot)$ can be expressed as follows:

$$\mathbb{E}[Z|\boldsymbol{X}] = \mathbb{P}(Z = 1|\boldsymbol{X}) = g(\boldsymbol{X}^{\mathrm{T}}\beta_{\mathrm{t}}), \quad \mathbb{E}[Z_{\mathrm{s}}|\boldsymbol{X}_{\mathrm{s}}] = \mathbb{P}(Z_{\mathrm{s}} = 1|\boldsymbol{X}_{\mathrm{s}}) = g(\boldsymbol{X}_{\mathrm{s}}^{\mathrm{T}}\beta_{\mathrm{s}}), \tag{4}$$

where the nuisance parameters $\beta_{\mathrm{t}}, \beta_{\mathrm{s}}$ have dimensionality $d_1 = d$. Without loss of generality, we consider the same link functions in both domains; however, the success of the knowledge transfer does not require the "same link function" as long as the link functions are known.

Assumption to Guarantee Knowledge Transferability The key assumption guaranteeing the success of the knowledge transfer is the sparsity of the nuisance parameter difference Δ_β, which is defined as

$$\Delta_\beta = \beta_{\mathrm{t}} - \beta_{\mathrm{s}}. \tag{5}$$

Definition 1 (s-Sparse Vector) A vector $v \in \mathbb{R}^d$ is said to be s-sparse (with $0 \le s \le d$) if this vector has at most s nonzero elements, i.e., $\|v\|_0 \le s$.

We posit that the mechanisms guiding treatment assignments should exhibit substantial similarity across both domains, a concept encapsulated by the *s-sparse Δ_β assumption*. This assumption is supported by the fact that the two trauma centers involved in our study are geographically adjacent and share a common set of clinicians. These shared clinicians likely apply consistent decision-making

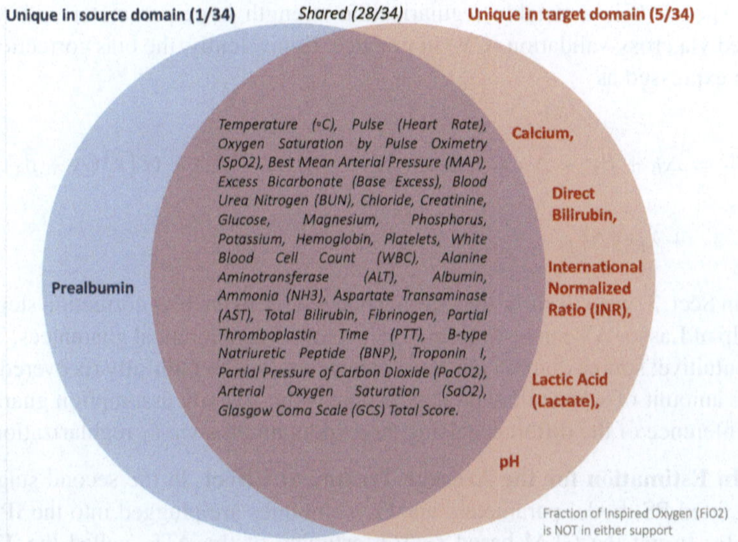

Fig. 2 Support of the PS model parameters via ℓ_1 regularized logistic regression in both domains in the real example. This figure shows that the supports of β_{t} and β_{s} only differ on 6 out of 34 covariates (listed in Table 4). Since the PS model parameter essentially shows how the clinicians assign treatment based on collected EMR data, the "similar support" observation could be evidence that Δ_β in our real example is sparse

criteria when treating patients, as inferred from the supports of the fitted PS model parameters shown in Fig. 2.

ℓ_1 Regularized Data-Integrative TL for PS Model The first stage involves two steps: (i) leveraging source domain data to estimate β_{s}, which serves as a rough estimator of β_{t} due to their sparse difference, and (ii) using ℓ_1 regularization to learn the difference Δ_β from target domain data, which corrects the bias of the first-step rough estimator, i.e.,

$$\begin{aligned}
&\underline{\text{Rough estimation for PS model}} : \widehat{\beta}_{\text{s}} = \arg\min_b \frac{1}{n_{\text{s}}} \sum_{i=1}^{n_{\text{s}}} -z_{i,\text{s}} \boldsymbol{x}_{i,\text{s}}^{\text{T}} b + G\left(\boldsymbol{x}_{i,\text{s}}^{\text{T}} b\right), \\
&\underline{\text{Bias correction for PS model}} : \widehat{\beta}_{\text{t}} = \arg\min_b \frac{1}{n} \sum_{i=1}^{n} -z_i \boldsymbol{x}_i^{\text{T}} b \\
&\qquad + G\left(\boldsymbol{x}_i^{\text{T}} b\right) + \lambda_{\text{PS}} \|b - \widehat{\beta}_{\text{s}}\|_1.
\end{aligned} \tag{6}$$

Here, $\lambda_{\text{PS}} > 0$ is a tunable regularization strength hyperparameter and will be selected via cross-validation (CV) in practice. Equivalently, the bias correction step can be expressed as

$$\widehat{\beta}_{\text{t}} = \widehat{\Delta}_{\beta} + \widehat{\beta}_{\text{s}}, \quad \widehat{\Delta}_{\beta} = \arg\min_{\Delta} \sum_{i=1}^{n} -z_i \boldsymbol{x}_i^{\text{T}}(\Delta + \widehat{\beta}_{\text{s}}) + G\left(\boldsymbol{x}_i^{\text{T}}(\Delta + \widehat{\beta}_{\text{s}})\right)$$
$$+ \lambda_{\text{PS}} \|\Delta\|_1. \tag{7}$$

Later in Sect. 3, we will show that, even when $n \ll d$ in the bias correction step, with the help of Lasso, Δ_{β} can be faithfully recovered with theoretical guarantees. This is quite intuitive: source domain nuisance parameters can be faithfully recovered using a large amount of source domain data, whereas the sparsity assumption guarantees valid inference of the difference using target domain data via ℓ_1 regularization.

Plug-In Estimation for the Average Treatment Effect In the second stage, the above fitted PS model parameters via TL techniques are plugged into the IPW (2) estimator to get the GLM-based ℓ_1-TCL estimate of the ATE, called the TLIPW estimate, as follows:

$$\widehat{\tau}_{\text{TLIPW}} = \frac{1}{n} \sum_{i=1}^{n} \frac{z_i y_i}{g(\boldsymbol{x}_i^{\text{T}} \widehat{\beta}_{\text{t}})} - \frac{(1 - z_i) y_i}{1 - g(\boldsymbol{x}_i^{\text{T}} \widehat{\beta}_{\text{t}})}. \tag{8}$$

2.4 Extension to OR and DR Estimators

Depending on the confidence in the PS and/or OR model specification, one can also apply TL techniques to OR or DR estimators (defined in (19) and (20) in Appendix "Additional Details on the Potential Outcome Framework") similarly to get the GLM-based ℓ_1-TCL estimate of the ATE, which we will call TLOR and TLDR estimators.

In our TCL, the generalized linear OR model has the following form, for $z \in \{0, 1\}$:

$$\mathbb{E}[Y_z|\boldsymbol{X}] = m_z(\boldsymbol{X}; \alpha_{z,\text{t}}), \quad \mathbb{E}[Y_{z,\text{s}}|\boldsymbol{X}_{\text{s}}] = m_{z,\text{s}}(\boldsymbol{X}_{\text{s}}; \alpha_{z,\text{s}}), \tag{9}$$

where functions $m_z(\cdot), m_{z,\text{s}}(\cdot)$ have known form with unknown nuisance parameters $\alpha_{z,\text{t}}, \alpha_{z,\text{s}} \in \mathbb{R}^{d_2}$. For simplicity, we parameterize the OR model via linear regression; however, our method and theory can be extended to handle GLM parameterization for the OR model. Specifically, for $z \in \{0, 1\}$, let

$$\mathbb{E}[Y_z|\boldsymbol{X}] = \boldsymbol{X}^{\text{T}} \alpha_{z,\text{t}}, \quad \mathbb{E}[Y_{z,\text{s}}|\boldsymbol{X}_{\text{s}}] = \boldsymbol{X}_{\text{s}}^{\text{T}} \alpha_{z,\text{s}}, \tag{10}$$

where the OR model nuisance parameters have dimensionality $d_2 = d$.

Similarly, the transferability guarantee comes from the assumption of the following differences:

$$\Delta_{\alpha,z} = \alpha_{z,\mathrm{t}} - \alpha_{z,\mathrm{s}}, \quad z \in \{0, 1\}, \tag{11}$$

are s-sparse, i.e., $\|\Delta_{\alpha,0}\|_0, \|\Delta_{\alpha,1}\|_0 \le s$. This enables us to apply those above ℓ_1 regularized TL techniques to estimate the OR model parameters in the target domain with the help of source domain data: for $z \in \{0, 1\}$, denote $n_{z,\mathrm{s}} = \#\{i : z_{i,\mathrm{s}} = z\}$ (# represents the cardinality of a set), and let $\lambda_{\mathrm{OR}} > 0$ be the tunable regularization strength hyperparameter:

$$\underline{\text{Rough estimation for OR model}} : \widehat{\alpha}_{z,\mathrm{s}} = \arg\min_{\alpha} \frac{1}{n_{z,\mathrm{s}}} \sum_{z_{i,\mathrm{s}}=z} \left(y_{i,\mathrm{s}} - \boldsymbol{x}_{i,\mathrm{s}}^{\mathrm{T}}\alpha\right)^2,$$

$$\begin{aligned}\underline{\text{Bias correction for OR model}} : \widehat{\alpha}_{z,\mathrm{t}} = \arg\min_{\alpha} & \frac{1}{n_z} \sum_{z_i=z} \left(y_i - \boldsymbol{x}_i^{\mathrm{T}}\alpha\right)^2 \\ & + \lambda_{\mathrm{OR}} \|\alpha - \widehat{\alpha}_{z,\mathrm{s}}\|_1.\end{aligned} \tag{12}$$

Finally, we plug the TL estimates of the nuisance model parameters to get the ℓ_1-TCL estimates of the ATE:

$$\widehat{\tau}_{\mathrm{TLOR}} = \frac{1}{n_1} \sum_{z_i=1} \boldsymbol{x}_i^{\mathrm{T}} \widehat{\alpha}_{1,\mathrm{t}} - \frac{1}{n_0} \sum_{z_i=0} \boldsymbol{x}_i^{\mathrm{T}} \widehat{\alpha}_{0,\mathrm{t}}, \tag{13}$$

$$\begin{aligned}\widehat{\tau}_{\mathrm{TLDR}} = \frac{1}{n} \sum_{i=1}^{n} & \frac{z_i y_i - \boldsymbol{x}_i^{\mathrm{T}} \widehat{\alpha}_{1,\mathrm{t}} (z_i - g(\boldsymbol{x}_i^{\mathrm{T}} \widehat{\beta}_{\mathrm{t}}))}{g(\boldsymbol{x}_i^{\mathrm{T}} \widehat{\beta}_{\mathrm{t}})} \\ & - \frac{(1 - z_i) y_i + \boldsymbol{x}_i^{\mathrm{T}} \widehat{\alpha}_{0,\mathrm{t}} (z_i - g(\boldsymbol{x}_i^{\mathrm{T}} \widehat{\beta}_{\mathrm{t}}))}{1 - g(\boldsymbol{x}_i^{\mathrm{T}} \widehat{\beta}_{\mathrm{t}})}.\end{aligned} \tag{14}$$

3 Theoretical Analysis

Typically, to make valid inferences by solely using target domain data, we need a sufficiently large amount of target domain data such that $n \gg d$. However, in our setting, such an assumption does not hold; to make things even worse, we may encounter $n < d$ case. Fortunately, with the help of Lasso for high-dimensional regression, recovery guarantees can still be established when we have abundant source domain data, which only require target domain sample size n to be on the order of $\log d$. In this section, we present the main results and their interpretations; complete details, including the technical assumptions and proofs, can be found in Appendices "Non-asymptotic Recovery Guarantee for TLIPW", "Non-asymptotic

Table 3 Locations of all theoretical results in the Appendix

	Nuisance parameter estimation	Plug-in ATE estimation
TLIPW	Lemma 1 (Appendix "Non-asymptotic Recovery Guarantee for TLIPW")	Theorem 1 (Appendix "Non-asymptotic Recovery Guarantee for TLIPW")
TLOR	Lemma 3 (Appendix "Non-asymptotic Recovery Guarantee for TLOR")	Theorem 2 (Appendix "Non-asymptotic Recovery Guarantee for TLOR")
TLDR	Lemma 1, Lemma 3	Theorem 3 (Appendix "Non-asymptotic Recovery Guarantee for TLDR")

Recovery Guarantee for TLOR", and "Non-asymptotic Recovery Guarantee for TLDR". Furthermore, the superior empirical performance of the GLM parametric approach is verified via numerical simulation in Appendix "Additional Details of the GLM-Based Experiments".

Main Theoretical Results When the PS model is correctly specified, and the difference is s-sparse, i.e., $\|\Delta_\beta\|_0 \leq s$, in the large sample limit $n, n_s \to \infty$, consider the following *regime*:

$$n \gg s^2 \log d, \quad n_s \gg nd^2, \tag{15}$$

By taking

$$\lambda_{PS} = \mathcal{O}\left(\sqrt{\log d}\left(\frac{1}{\sqrt{n}} + \frac{d}{\sqrt{n_s}}\right)\right),$$

we can show that, under standard technical assumptions, with probability at least $1 - 1/n$, the absolute estimation error is upper bounded as

$$|\widehat{\tau}_{TL} - \tau| = \mathcal{O}\left(\underbrace{s\sqrt{\frac{\log d}{n}}}_{\text{bias correction error}} + \underbrace{sd\sqrt{\frac{\log d}{n_s}}}_{\text{rough estimation error}}\right),$$

where $\widehat{\tau}_{TL}$ can be either the TLIPW estimator $\widehat{\tau}_{TLIPW}$ (8) or the TLDR estimator $\widehat{\tau}_{TLDR}$ (14).

Complete details are deferred to the appendix, including the assumptions, lemmas, formal statements of the non-asymptotic theoretical guarantees, and all proofs. To help readers find these results, in Table 3, we provide a summary of our results.

Interpretations Similar to the two-stage estimation, the proofs are done by plugging the non-asymptotic upper bound on the vector ℓ_1-norm of the nuisance parameter to the absolute error bound of the downstream plug-in estimators, resulting in *the error bound decomposition as above*. In particular, the bias correction term is $\mathcal{O}(s\sqrt{\log d/n})$ (which aligns with that of the classic Lasso estimator, cf. Theorem 7.1 [6]) and dominates the rough estimation error term due to $n_s \gg nd^2$ (15); however, according to the above error upper bound, the condition on source domain sample size can be relaxed to $n_s \gg s^2d^2 \log d$ to achieve consistency. Without the help of the source domain, the overall error rate will be similar to that of the rough estimation, which requires $n \gg d^2$ target domain samples to achieve a satisfying error bound (cf. Theorem 1 [4]). In contrast, the abundant source domain data, characterized by $n_s \gg nd^2$ in the considered regime (15), relaxes the requirement on target domain sample size to $n \gg s^2 \log d$ to achieve the same satisfying error bound.

In our proof, we invoke the compatibility condition [9] for the sample covariance matrix, which is standard in high-dimensional Lasso literature. Alternatively, if we consider the classic restricted eigenvalue condition [6, 32, 58], we can prove ℓ_2 error bound that scales as $\sqrt{s}$ instead of s; see Remark 2 in Appendix 6 on why we consider ℓ_1 error bound for nuisance parameter estimation over the ℓ_2 bound. Lastly, our non-asymptotic analysis shows that the error upper bound with probability at least $1 - \varepsilon$ (for any $\varepsilon \in (0, 1)$) will have a $\mathcal{O}(s\sqrt{\log(1/\epsilon)/n})$ term. When we consider the probability converging to one at a polynomial rate, i.e., $\varepsilon = 1/n^\kappa$ for positive integer κ, this term will be $\mathcal{O}(s\sqrt{\log n^\kappa/n})$ and dominated by the $\mathcal{O}(s\sqrt{\log d/n})$ term in the above bound under our considered regime (15). The above result corresponds to the $\kappa = 1$ case.

Additional Theoretical Results Our theory can be extended to TLOR and TLDR estimators when the OR model specification is correct with s-sparse differences $\|\Delta_{\alpha,z}\|_0 \le s$ ($z \in \{0, 1\}$). One additional notable assumption is the "balanced" samples in the treatment and control groups, i.e., we assume there exists a constant $r \in (0, 1)$ such that, for $z \in \{0, 1\}$:

$$\liminf_{n\to\infty} \frac{n_z}{n} \ge r, \quad \liminf_{n_s\to\infty} \frac{n_{z,s}}{n_s} \ge r, \tag{16}$$

where $n_z = \#\{i : z_i = z\}$ and $n_{z,s} = \#\{i : z_{i,s} = z\}$, then, by taking

$$\lambda_{\mathrm{OR}} = \mathcal{O}\left(\sqrt{\log d}\left(\frac{1}{\sqrt{rn}} + \frac{d}{\sqrt{rn_s}}\right)\right),$$

for $\widehat{\tau}_{\mathrm{TL}} = \widehat{\tau}_{\mathrm{TLOR}}$ or $\widehat{\tau}_{\mathrm{TLDR}}$, we can show that, under standard technical assumptions, with probability at least $1-1/n$, the absolute estimation error can be upper bounded as follows:

$$|\widehat{\tau}_{\mathrm{TL}} - \tau| = \mathcal{O}\left(s\sqrt{\log d}\left(\frac{1}{\sqrt{rn}} + \frac{d}{\sqrt{rn_s}}\right)\right).$$

Remark We acknowledge that the theoretical results can be strengthened, and we refer readers to Appendix "Developments of ℓ_1 Regularized Transfer Learning Approaches" for a survey on recent theoretical developments of ℓ_1 regularized transfer learning. Notably, [26] showed that, for extremely sparse difference, the ℓ_1 regularization hyperparameter can be chosen as large as $\mathcal{O}(\sqrt{n_s \log d})$, and the ℓ_1 error upper bound can be improved as $\mathcal{O}(\sqrt{s \log d/n}$ (cf. Theorem 1 therein), which is faster than our rate $\mathcal{O}(s\sqrt{\log d/n})$. Nevertheless, we want to emphasize that our main contribution is the adaption of ℓ_1 regularized transfer learning to causal inference and its application in healthcare. In contrast, the theoretical results here are mainly for completeness purposes.

4 Real-Data Example

In this real experiment, we aim to investigate whether vasopressor therapy can *prevent* mortality within sepsis patients. Vasopressor therapy for septic patients has been shown to decrease the risk of 28-day mortality [2]. Therefore, it is worth observing the underlying *inhibiting* causal effect of this treatment. Indeed, [61] showed that vasopressor therapy could have an inhibiting effect on sepsis via a Granger causal graph approach, suggesting its inhibiting effect on mortality as well.

Data Description We created a retrospective cohort using EMR data from two adjacent academic level 1 trauma centers in the Southeastern USA in 2018 (see Table 1 for patient demographics). The data were analyzed in accordance with an institutional review board, and relevant ethics approval information will be provided upon acceptance.

The primary outcome is 28-day mortality (i.e., the patient's death within 28 days or less after the time of admission) is a common metric for sepsis observational studies [52], and it defines the binary outcome variable in our causal effect estimation problem. Patients are considered to be treated if they received any vasopressor therapy (norepinephrine, epinephrine, dobutamine, dopamine, phenylephrine, or vasopressin) within 12 hours before sepsis onset. Patient data is organized into hourly bins from admission to discharge, averaging multiple measurements per hour if needed. To ensure comparable data lengths for causal effect estimation, patients must meet Sepsis-3 criteria, and we examine at most 12 hours of data before and after sepsis onset, resulting in a 25-hour subset of the full patient encounter.

Our study analyzes 34 covariates from EMR data, including 4 vital signs and 30 laboratory (lab) results (see Table 4). Since covariate names are self-explanatory, we do not provide additional descriptions. To address missing data issue—common due to irregular recording—we use the fill-forward method to replace missing hourly values with the most recent preceding value. Remaining missing values are imputed using the population median.

Table 4 List of covariates in the real-data example. In the ICU environment, vital signs are usually recorded at hourly intervals; however, patients on the floor may only have measurements for every 8 hours. The lab tests are most commonly ordered on a daily basis, but this can change based on the patient's status and the clinician's request

Type	Name
Vital sign	Temperature (°C), Pulse (Heart Rate), Oxygen Saturation by Pulse Oximetry (SpO2), Best Mean Arterial Pressure (MAP)
Lab result	Excess Bicarbonate (Base Excess), Blood Urea Nitrogen (BUN), Calcium, Chloride, Creatinine, Glucose, Magnesium, Phosphorus, Potassium, Hemoglobin, Platelets, White Blood Cell Count (WBC), Alanine Aminotransferase (ALT), Albumin, Ammonia (NH3), Aspartate Transaminase (AST), Direct Bilirubin, Total Bilirubin, Fibrinogen, International Normalized Ratio (INR), Lactic Acid (Lactate), pH, Partial Thromboplastin Time (PTT), Prealbumin, B-type Natriuretic Peptide (BNP), Troponin I, Fraction of Inspired Oxygen (FiO2), Arterial Oxygen Saturation (SaO2), Partial Pressure of Carbon Dioxide (PaCO2), Glasgow Coma Scale (GCS) Total Score

Baseline Approaches Fail to Capture the Inhibiting Causal Effect Here, we consider the PS model parameterized by GLM (4) with sigmoid link and IPW estimator for ATE; later in Sect. 5.3, we will extend this experiment using NN-based ATE estimator. We begin with solely using target domain data to estimate ATE, i.e., the `TO-CL` mentioned in our toy example. By considering both datasets as the target domain dataset, `TO-CL` yields ATEs 0.12 in the target domain and 0.057 in the source domain. Those results are counterintuitive and contradict established results in the medical literature [2, 61]. Indeed, the estimate in the source domain is almost zero, which is closer to the established inhibiting treatment effect [2] than that of the target domain, potentially due to its larger sample size. Naively merging two domains' data, which we call `Merge-CL` framework, is a tempting choice, given that two studied trauma centers sometimes share clinicians; it leads to a point estimate of 0.082, which aligns with the intuition that `Merge-CL` "drags" the `TO-CL` estimate of the target domain toward that of the source domain, as the source domain has more samples. Due to space limitations, complete details, such as training details, are deferred to Appendix "Additional Details of the Real-Data Example".

The Proposed ℓ_1-TCL Could Yield the Correct Treatment Effect Estimate Now, we apply the TLIPW estimator (8) in our ℓ_1-TCL, yielding a point estimate of -0.011; this gives a more reasonable conclusion that vasopressor therapy has an inhibiting causal effect on mortality in sepsis patients, agreeing with existing medical literature. Additionally, we perform bootstrap uncertainty quantification (UQ) with 200 bootstrap trials, each with 700 random samples (with replacement)

Table 5 Comparison of estimated ATEs in the real-data example: the only reasonable result is given by our proposed ℓ_1-TCL, which indicates *inhibiting* causal effect from the vasopressor therapy to 28-day mortality in sepsis patients

Data used	Target domain only	Both domains	
framework	`TO-CL`	`Merge-CL`	ℓ_1-TCL
Point estimate	0.120	0.082	−0.011
Bootstrap mean	0.072	0.130	−0.85
Bootstrap median	0.072	0.120	−0.067
Bootstrap 90% CI	[0.015, 0.134]	[0.016, 0.275]	[−7.257, 1.951]

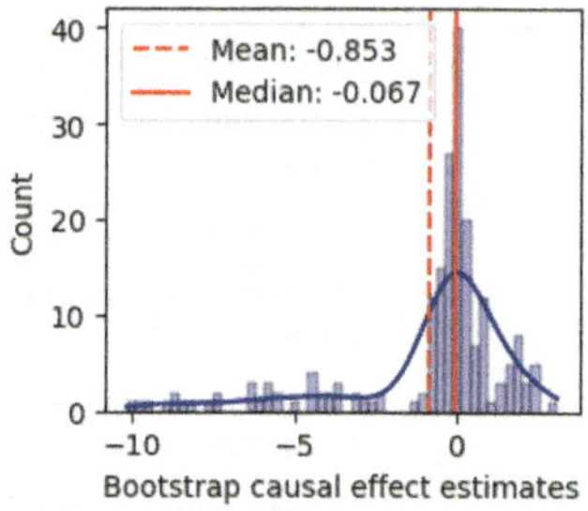

Fig. 3 Histogram of the 200 ℓ_1-TCL estimates on the bootstrap samples

from the target domain. The baseline frameworks (i.e., `TO-CL` and `Merge-CL`) all show statistically significant promoting causal effects, verified by the 90% bootstrap CI, which again violates established medical findings. In contrast, despite the 90% CI containing zero, the mean and median of bootstrap ℓ_1-TCL causal effect estimates suggest that vasopressor therapy can prevent 28-day mortality within sepsis patients (Table 5).

Limitation Reliable decision-making is essential in healthcare, a major application of our ℓ_1-TCL. One common approach is UQ; however, as reflected by the bootstrap distribution of our ℓ_1-TCL estimates in Fig. 3, the long tail (the tail to the left leads to overly small estimates) and large variance (which results in wider bootstrap CI) suggest that bootstrap could be less effective for constructing CI. In the experiments to obtain the point estimate, we find our ℓ_1-TCL extremely sensitive to the choice of hyperparameters. Therefore, we iteratively refine grids of hyperparameters (by putting finer grids around the selected hyperparameter) to get a reliable point estimate. Unfortunately, such a practice incurs very high computational costs when we construct bootstrap CIs, and we use a fixed grid of hyperparameters for all 200 repeats. This leads to unreasonably large or small ℓ_1-TCL estimates for "extreme" bootstrap samples since the preselected grid does not cover the empirical optimal choice. As a result, we would claim that the most reliable estimate(s) for drawing causal conclusions in our ℓ_1-TCL framework would be the bootstrap median and the point estimate with hyperparameter selected from iteratively refined grids, which both suggest inhibiting causal effects from the treatment. Developing a principled approach for UQ in the TCL problem can be a meaningful future direction, which is outside the scope of this work and left for future study.

5 A Generic Framework for Transfer Causal Learning

Inspired by the superior performance of the GLM-based parametric approach, we now extend our method into a generic framework for the TCL problem by considering arbitrary parameterization of the *nuisance model* (i.e., PS (3) and/or OR (9) models), which is called ℓ_1-TCL framework. This extension can benefit from improved robustness to model misspecification, and it can be applied to the Conditional Average Treatment Effect estimation in the presence of a heterogeneous causal effect.

5.1 ℓ_1-TCL Framework

Consider arbitrary parameterization of the nuisance model with finite-dimensional nuisance parameter $\theta \in \Theta$. Given dataset $\mathcal{D}$, suppose the estimator for nuisance parameter can be obtained as $\widehat{\theta} = \arg\min_{\theta\in\Theta} \mathcal{L}(\theta; \mathcal{D})$, where $\mathcal{L}$ is the loss function. In our setup, the ground truth nuisance parameters differ across both domains, i.e., $\theta_{\mathrm{t}} \neq \theta_{\mathrm{s}}$. We assume their difference $\theta_{\mathrm{t}} - \theta_{\mathrm{s}}$ is sparse such that this difference can be estimated from the target domain using ℓ_1 regularization to correct the bias of the rough estimator obtained from the source domain. Formally, the *nuisance parameter estimation stage* of our proposed ℓ_1-TCL is given by

$$\underline{\text{Rough estimation}}: \widehat{\theta}_{\mathrm{s}} = \arg\min_{\theta\in\Theta} \mathcal{L}(\theta; \mathcal{D}_{\mathrm{s}}),$$

$$\underline{\text{Bias correction}}: \widehat{\theta}_{\mathrm{t}} = \arg\min_{\theta\in\Theta} \mathcal{L}(\theta; \mathcal{D}_{\mathrm{t}}) + \lambda\|\theta - \widehat{\theta}_{\mathrm{s}}\|_1,$$

where $\mathcal{D}_{\mathrm{s}} = \{\mathcal{D}_{i,\mathrm{s}}, i = 1, \ldots, n_{\mathrm{s}}\}$ and $\mathcal{D}_{\mathrm{t}} = \{\mathcal{D}_i, i = 1, \ldots, n\}$ are the collections of source and target domain samples, respectively, and $\lambda > 0$ is a tunable hyperparameter. In the subsequent *plug-in estimation stage*, the IPW estimator (2), OR estimator (19), and DR estimator (20) are evaluated using the estimated nuisance parameters above to get the ℓ_1-TCL estimate of the ATE. Please see a graphical illustration in Fig. 4.

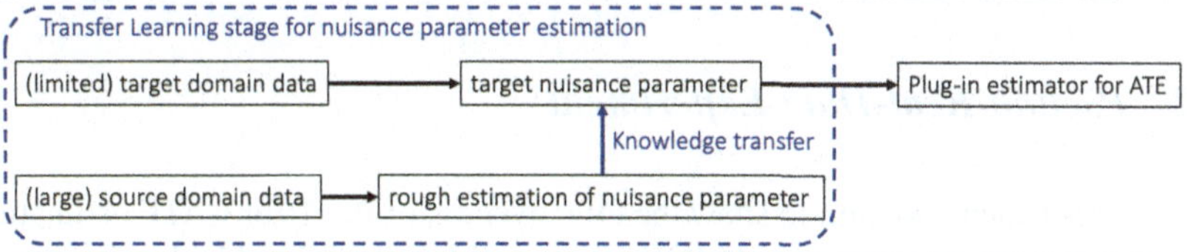

Fig. 4 Illustration of the general approach for TCL problem. In our ℓ_1-TCL framework, the nuisance parameter estimation stage leverages ℓ_1 regularized TL, and the plug-in estimation stage can be IPW, OR, and DR estimators

Nonparametric Approach Based on Neural Networks While there exist many recent efforts on improving robustness in causal inference, such as meta-learning [63] and super learning [37], using NN to parameterize the nuisance models [23] remains to be the most straightforward and effective. In next subsection, we adapt two recent NN architectures to our ℓ_1-TCL: Treatment-Agnostic Representation Network (TARNet) [46] and Dragonnet [47]. Details on their loss functions are provided in Appendix "Neural Network-Based Nuisance Models for Causal Effect Estimation". For our NN-based ℓ_1-TCL, the nuisance parameter estimation involves standard NN training with source domain data, followed by bias correction. Specifically, we estimate the sparse difference between target and source NN weights with zero initialization, as detailed in (7) for GLM. Full details of our NN-based ℓ_1-TCL approach are available in Appendix "Experimental Configurations and Training Details".

Application Heterogeneous causal effect has recently drawn increasing attention in causal inference, and there have been many popular machine learning approaches, such as meta-learning [12] and heterogeneous transfer learning (i.e., TL under the heterogeneous covariate space setting) [5], applied to this problem. Typically, this problem is approached via the Conditional Average Treatment Effect (CATE) instead of ATE, i.e.,

$$\tau_S = \mathbb{E}[Y_1|\boldsymbol{X} \in S] - \mathbb{E}[Y_0|\boldsymbol{X} \in S],$$

which studies the causal effect within a sub-cohort of patients whose covariates lie in a targeted subset of the covariate space, i.e., $S \subset \mathcal{X}$. Built on our ℓ_1-TCL, we introduce a *Partition-then-Transfer* (ParT) approach for CATE estimation.

Consider samples from a single dataset as in (1), let $S_t \subset \mathcal{X}$ be the target subset, and the goal is to estimate τ_{S_t}. ParT first partitions the covariate space into $\mathcal{X} = S_s \cup S_t$, resulting in a source-target domain partition: $\mathcal{D}_s = \{\mathcal{D}_i : \boldsymbol{x}_i \in S_s\}$ and $\mathcal{D}_t = \{\mathcal{D}_i : \boldsymbol{x}_i \in S_t\}$. Then, ℓ_1-TCL can be readily applied to leverage knowledge gained from $\mathcal{D}_s$ to help estimate the CATE (or target domain ATE) τ_{S_t}. In practice, the target subset S_t is usually defined by a binary or categorical covariate, naturally partitioning the covariate space based on the labels. Given that these partitions originate from the same dataset, it's reasonable to assume similar treatment assignment mechanisms across domains, making our ℓ_1-TCL applicable.

5.2 *Pseudo-Real-Data Experiment*

In this experiment, we aim to show the effectiveness of ParT for CATE estimation, which also demonstrates the good performance of its building block, i.e., our ℓ_1-TCL framework, by comparing with baseline frameworks. As ground truth causal effects are inaccessible in most real studies, we consider a commonly used pseudo-real-dataset, i.e., the Infant Health and Development Program (IHDP) dataset [7,

18]. It includes 747 subjects (139 treated and 608 control), with 6 continuous and 19 categorical covariates (of which 18 are binary). We arbitrarily pick one binary covariate (denoted by X_{par}) and assign subjects with labels 0 and 1 to source and target domains, respectively, resulting in $n_s = 546, n = 201$. The goal is to study the ATE in the target domain, or the CATE for the subjects with $X_{\text{par}} = 1$. Due to space consideration, additional details for the dataset, configurations, training, and results are deferred to Appendix "Additional Details of NN-Based Experiments".

Comparison with Baselines We compare ℓ_1-TCL framework with two baseline learning frameworks: TO-CL introduced above and the "warm-start" TCL baseline (WS-TCL) by Künzel et al. [24], which used the estimated NN weights in the source domain as the warm-start of the subsequent target domain NN training. For each framework, the nuisance model for PS and OR is either Dragonnet or TARNet with hyperparameters selected based on minimum average NN regression loss on a randomly selected validation target domain dataset; the estimated nuisance parameters are subsequently plugged into IPW, OR, and DR estimators to get the estimated ATEs.

We report both in-sample (i.e., training and validation target datasets) and out-of-sample (i.e., testing target dataset) absolute estimation errors over 1000 trials in Table 6, from which we can observe the following: (i) transfer learning helps improve estimation accuracy for all *ATE estimators* (we will call a specific nuisance model coupled with a specific plug-in estimator as an ATE estimator); (ii) in almost all cases, our proposed ℓ_1-TCL outperforms the existing WS-TCL approach; (iii) most importantly, the best results (highlighted in bold fonts) are given by our proposed ℓ_1-TCL framework.

Table 6 Mean and standard deviation of absolute errors of estimated ATEs over 1000 trials using IHDP dataset. The primary goal is to compare three learning frameworks: we can observe that TL can help improve ATE estimation accuracy for all ATE estimators (highlighted in green for each column), and our proposed ℓ_1-TCL yields the best in-sample and out-of-sample results (highlighted in bold font)

	Dragonnet			3-Headed Variant of TARNet		
In-sample	IPW	OR	DR	IPW	OR	DR
TO-CL	$6.668_{(11.234)}$	$0.573_{(0.579)}$	$0.612_{(0.711)}$	$4.307_{(4.408)}$	$0.5_{(0.437)}$	$0.415_{(0.349)}$
WS-TCL	$5.28_{(12.068)}$	$0.49_{(0.445)}$	$0.503_{(0.7)}$	$2.815_{(3.203)}$	$0.41_{(0.373)}$	$0.337_{(0.273)}$
ℓ_1-TCL	$4.724_{(11.038)}$	$0.386_{(0.406)}$	$0.404_{(0.443)}$	$2.804_{(3.149)}$	$0.394_{(0.434)}$	$\mathbf{0.289}_{(0.238)}$
	Dragonnet			3-Headed Variant of TARNet		
Out-of-sample	IPW	OR	DR	IPW	OR	DR
TO-CL	$28.568_{(43.776)}$	$0.639_{(0.713)}$	$2.095_{(3.909)}$	$4.873_{(5.842)}$	$0.603_{(0.594)}$	$0.36_{(0.301)}$
WS-TCL	$16.416_{(28.332)}$	$0.54_{(0.533)}$	$1.203_{(2.063)}$	$4.182_{(5.588)}$	$0.469_{(0.447)}$	$0.324_{(0.282)}$
ℓ_1-TCL	$13.872_{(24.138)}$	$0.425_{(0.454)}$	$0.747_{(0.94)}$	$4.193_{(5.502)}$	$0.42_{(0.439)}$	$\mathbf{0.301}_{(0.259)}$

Hyperparameter Selection Criteria In Table 9, the hyperparameters are chosen based on minimizing average NN *regression* loss. For completeness, we also report results using NN *classification* cross-entropy (CE) loss and mean squared error (MSE) in Table 9 of Appendix 6. These results reaffirm that ℓ_1-TCL outperforms baselines, though the overall best performance is worse than that in Table 6. This suggests that the selection criterion based on *OR* model is better suited to our application. Such a finding aligns with the poor performance of the IPW estimator observed in Table 6, which could be a result of severe *PS* model misspecification. These findings are consistent with [47], who focused only on the OR estimator.

Furthermore, a recent study by Machlanski et al. [29] indicates that proper hyperparameter tuning can reduce performance gaps among causal effect estimators. Thus, we employ another commonly used criterion in causal inference [72]—the Standard Mean Difference (SMD)—and present the results in Table 12 of Appendix "An Alternative Hyperparameter Selection Criterion". The results reveal that the three-headed variant of TARNet with the DR estimator for ATE estimation, using hyperparameters selected by SMD, achieves the best results for the IHDP dataset in our setting. Therefore, we will use this configuration for subsequent experiments.

5.3 ℓ_1-TCL with NN-Based Nuisance Model on Real Data

Given the superior performance of SMD as the hyperparameter selection criterion, we report the SMDs of the GLM-based real-data experimental results in Table 7, which reaffirms that our ℓ_1-TCL can output the most reliable causal effect estimate. Additionally, we apply the NN-based methods to real data and report the point estimates of the ATE and the SMD in the right-hand side of Table 7. As shown in this table, the results selected by SMD support inhibiting treatment effect, i.e., vasopressor therapy does decrease the risk of 28-day mortality in sepsis patients, agreeing with established results in medical literature [2].

Table 7 SMDs of the point estimates in Table 5 (left), and the results using the NN-based method (right). In the first row, we specify nuisance model parameterization (with additional details such as link function and hyperparameter selection criterion) and the plug-in estimator. The results selected by SMD indicate an inhibiting effect from treatment to mortality, agreeing with both common sense and existing medical literature

Model specification	GLM-Sigmoid-IPW			3 Headed-TARNet-SMD-DR		
Data-integrative method	TO-CL	Merge-CL	ℓ_1-TCL	TO-CL	WS-TCL	ℓ_1-TCL
Point estimate	0.12	0.082	− 0.011	− 12.612	− 11.851	− 9.676
SMD	0.242	0.268	**0.225**	0.1731	0.1721	**0.1720**

The bold fonts denote best performed method in that setting

6 Conclusion

This work proposes a framework to adapt transfer learning to causal inference, which can address the limited data issue in many real applications. Our ℓ_1-TCL not only enjoys theoretical guarantees but also can be used along with recently developed nonparametric ATE estimators. Importantly, it shows promise in estimating the causal effect in real applications, especially in the medical setting, as evidenced by our experimental results. We outline several promising follow-up directions in Appendix 6. With our open-source implementation, we hope our ℓ_1-TCL can be applied in more real applications that face the limited data issue.

Appendix of Transfer Learning for Causal Effect Estimation

Appendix A: Extended Literature Survey

Background on Transfer Learning

Transfer learning [55] has received increasing attention due to its empirical success in various fields, ranging from machine learning problems, such as natural language processing [14], recommendation system [35], and computer vision [57], to science problems, such as predictions of protein localization [31], biological imaging diagnosis [48], integrative analysis of "multi-omics" (e.g., genomics) data [21, 53, 59], cancer image classification [20, 45], drug sensitivity prediction [56] and discovery [4], and so on. Based on whether or not the target and source domains, as well as the target and source tasks, are the same, transfer learning problems can be categorized into several subproblems [34]; in this study, we focus on "Inductive Multi-Task Transfer Learning" and our ℓ_1 regularization-based approach can be categorized as "Transferring Knowledge of Parameters." Our work only leverages a particular transfer learning technique, and we refer readers to [34, 62, 73] for comprehensive surveys on transfer learning.

Developments of ℓ_1 Regularized Transfer Learning Approaches

The idea of using ℓ_1 regularization to develop a theoretically grounded TL approach could date back to [15], who considered a support vector machine with parameter decomposed as a summation of a shared term and a task-specific term and proposed a learning algorithm by imposing ℓ_1 regularization on the task-specific terms in all domains. Recently, this idea was applied to GLM by Bastani [4], and this seminal work has motivated several follow-up studies: [54] extended this work to multisource TL problems, [25] proved minimax optimality under liner regression setting and later on showed minimax rate of convergence for high-dimensional GLM estimation [26], and so on. Our work follows this line of study and adapts the ℓ_1 regularized TL approach proposed by Bastani [4] to develop a theoretically grounded method for TCL. However, the theoretical results may be strengthened using those aforementioned recent developments. Most importantly, it is important to recognize that our work points out a new direction on leveraging recently developed principled TL methods to contribute to the TCL problem, which we will discuss in detail in Appendix E.

Connections Between Transfer Learning and Causal Inference

There have been works leveraging causal inference to help with TL problems, such as domain adaption, by exploring the invariant causal relationships between both domains, which is referred to as the causal transfer learning problem [40]. While the causal transfer learning problem has been studied from both empirical [30, 69, 71] and theoretical [10, 40] perspectives, the reverse study on adapting TL techniques to causal inference (i.e., our proposed TCL problem) only starts to attract some attention recently.

In fact, although there have been efforts trying to harvest the benefits of unconfounded experimental/randomized data [11, 16], there is limited work in developing data-integrative methods to combine observational data with the randomized data (or observational data with additional covariates) until the recent line of research [17, 67, 68]. However, such experimental data is not always available in reality, and the fundamental problem of estimating causal effects from two sets of observational data lying in the same space but (possibly) with different treatment mechanism and covariate distribution receives little attention.

Existing works on this direction include the aforementioned "warm-start" knowledge transfer approach under our TCL setting [24] and a special neural network architecture designed based on the shared covariate space and the domain-specific covariate spaces [5]. Here, we not only provide a theoretically grounded approach for the TCL problem but also use numerical evidence to show our proposed ℓ_1-TCL outperforms the existing warm-start method.

Appendix B: Additional Background Knowledge

Additional Details on the Potential Outcome Framework

The gold-standard approach to estimating the causal effect is randomized controlled trials (RCT), where subjects are randomized to receive treatment or placebo (i.e., the control group). However, RCT is unethical in most studies, such as the medical study. Therefore, the main question is how to estimate causal effect from observational data.

In this work, we approach this problem under the potential outcome framework [43]. Let us recall the notations we used: random vector $\boldsymbol{X} \in \mathbb{R}^d$ represents covariates measured prior to receipt of treatment, r.v. $Z \in \{0, 1\}$ is treatment indicator, and r.v. Y is the observed outcome, which is defined using potential outcomes Y_0 and Y_1: $Y = Y_1 Z + (1 - Z)Y_0$. The ATE (or average treatment effect) is the estimand in this study and is defined as $\tau = \mathbb{E}[Y_1] - \mathbb{E}[Y_0]$.

Apparently, observing Y_0 and Y_1 simultaneously is impossible, making it a tempting choice to estimate $\mathbb{E}[Y_0]$ and $\mathbb{E}[Y_1]$ using the sample average outcome in the control and treatment group and take their difference as an estimate of the ATE. Unfortunately, the problem is $\mathbb{E}[Y|Z = 0] = \mathbb{E}[Y_0|Z = 0] \neq \mathbb{E}[Y_0]$ and $\mathbb{E}[Y|Z = 1] = \mathbb{E}[Y_1|Z = 1] \neq \mathbb{E}[Y_1]$, as the treatment Z is typically not statistically independent from (Y_0, Y_1) due to some pretreatment covariates in $\boldsymbol{X}$. Such a problem is also referred to as "selection bias."

In observational study, although $(Y_0, Y_1) \perp\!\!\!\perp Z$ is unlikely to hold, it may be possible to identify those pretreatment covariates that related to (or can affect) both potential outcome and treatment, referred to as "confounders." If we assume the covariate vector $\boldsymbol{X}$ contains all such confounders, we would have $(Y_0, Y_1) \perp\!\!\!\perp Z \mid \boldsymbol{X}$, which is referred to as "no unmeasured confounders" or ignorability assumption [39]. Under this assumption, we shall have:

$$\begin{aligned} \mathbb{E}[Y|Z = 1] &= \mathbb{E}\{\mathbb{E}[Y|Z = 1, \boldsymbol{X}]\} = \mathbb{E}\{\mathbb{E}[Y_1|Z = 1, \boldsymbol{X}]\} \\ &= \mathbb{E}\{\mathbb{E}[Y_1|\boldsymbol{X}]\} = \mathbb{E}[Y_1]. \end{aligned} \tag{17}$$

Similarly,

$$\mathbb{E}[Y|Z = 0] = \mathbb{E}\{\mathbb{E}[Y|Z = 0, \boldsymbol{X}]\} = \mathbb{E}[Y_0].$$

The above observations actually motivate the unbiased estimator using the outcome regression model, i.e., the OR estimator (19). Under the no unmeasured confounding assumption, the ATE τ is identifiable from observational data.

The propensity score $e(\boldsymbol{X}) = \mathbb{P}(Z = 1|\boldsymbol{X})$ is the probability of treatment given covariates, which specifies the treatment assignment mechanism. Rosenbaum and Rubin [41] showed that $(Y_0, Y_1) \perp\!\!\!\perp Z \mid e(\boldsymbol{X})$, which implies that $\mathbb{E}[I(Z = 1)|Y_1, \boldsymbol{X}] = e(\boldsymbol{X})$ (here, $I(A) = 1$ if event A is true and 0 otherwise). Therefore, we will have:

$$\begin{aligned} \mathbb{E}\left[\frac{ZY}{e(\boldsymbol{X})}\right] &= \mathbb{E}\left\{\mathbb{E}\left[\frac{I(Z = 1)Y_1}{e(\boldsymbol{X})} \,\middle|\, Y_1, \boldsymbol{X}\right]\right\} \\ &= \mathbb{E}\left\{\frac{Y_1}{e(\boldsymbol{X})}\mathbb{E}[I(Z = 1)|Y_1, \boldsymbol{X}]\right\} = \mathbb{E}[Y_1]. \end{aligned} \tag{18}$$

Similarly,

$$\mathbb{E}\left[\frac{(1-Z)Y}{1-e(\boldsymbol{X})}\right]=\mathbb{E}[Y_0].$$

The above observations actually motivate the application of IPW [19] for ATE estimation and show that IPW estimator (2) is unbiased under correct PS model specification.

An alternative unbiased estimator uses the (potential) outcome regression model:

$$m_z(\boldsymbol{X})=\mathbb{E}[Y_z|\boldsymbol{X}], \quad z\in\{0,1\}.$$

Given samples (1), for $z\in\{0,1\}$, let $n_z=\#\{i : z_i=z\}$ and $\widehat{m}_z(\boldsymbol{x}_i)$ be the fitted potential outcome for i-th subject, the OR estimator for ATE is given by

$$\widehat{\tau}_{\mathrm{OR}}=\frac{1}{n_1}\sum_{z_i=1}\widehat{m}_1(\boldsymbol{x}_i)-\frac{1}{n_0}\sum_{z_i=0}\widehat{m}_0(\boldsymbol{x}_i). \tag{19}$$

One common drawback of both IPW and OR estimators is that they require correct specification of the PS and OR models, respectively, which is challenging in practice. To fix this issue, an augmented IPW estimator (also known as DR estimator) is proposed [38, 42, 44]—the main idea is that by incorporating an augmented term (which is related to the OR model) in IPW, the estimator will be doubly robust. To be precise, given samples (1), the DR estimator for ATE is defined as

$$\begin{aligned}\widehat{\tau}_{\mathrm{DR}}&=\frac{1}{n}\sum_{i=1}^{n}\left[\frac{z_i y_i}{\widehat{e}(\boldsymbol{x}_i)}-\frac{z_i-\widehat{e}(\boldsymbol{x}_i)}{\widehat{e}(\boldsymbol{x}_i)}\widehat{m}_1(\boldsymbol{x}_i)\right] \\ &\quad-\frac{1}{n}\sum_{i=1}^{n}\left[\frac{(1-z_i)y_i}{1-\widehat{e}(\boldsymbol{x}_i)}+\frac{z_i-\widehat{e}(\boldsymbol{x}_i)}{1-\widehat{e}(\boldsymbol{x}_i)}\widehat{m}_0(\boldsymbol{x}_i)\right] \\ &=\frac{1}{n}\sum_{i=1}^{n}\left[\widehat{m}_1(\boldsymbol{x}_i)+\frac{z_i(y_i-\widehat{m}_1(\boldsymbol{x}_i))}{\widehat{e}(\boldsymbol{x}_i)}\right] \\ &\quad-\frac{1}{n}\sum_{i=1}^{n}\left[\widehat{m}_0(\boldsymbol{x}_i)+\frac{(1-z_i)(y_i-\widehat{m}_0(\boldsymbol{x}_i))}{1-\widehat{e}(\boldsymbol{x}_i)}\right].\end{aligned} \tag{20}$$

Notice that

$$\mathbb{E}[Y_1] = \mathbb{E}\left[\frac{ZY}{e(X)} - \frac{Z - e(X)}{e(X)} m_1(X)\right] = \mathbb{E}\left[m_1(X) + \frac{Z(Y - m_1(X)\}}{e(X)}\right],$$

$$\mathbb{E}[Y_0] = \mathbb{E}\left[\frac{(1-Z)Y}{1-e(X)} + \frac{Z - e(X)}{1-e(X)} m_0(X)\right]$$

$$= \mathbb{E}\left[m_0(X) + \frac{(1-Z)(Y - m_0(X))}{1-e(X)}\right].$$

Therefore, the DR estimator is unbiased when either the PS model or the OR model is correctly specified, i.e., it is doubly robust.

Lastly, those aforementioned estimators for ATE all have nice theoretical properties; see, e.g., [65, 66] for the theory of IPW estimator and [3, 38] for the theory of DR estimator. There are also other approaches to estimate causal effects using propensity score, such as matching; see [28] for a nice survey on the use of propensity scores in causal inference and [70] for a recent comprehensive survey on causal inference.

Neural Network-Based Nuisance Models for Causal Effect Estimation

In this part, we briefly review the aforementioned NN-based approaches for ATE estimation: TARNet [46] and Dragonnet [47], which can both be categorized as representation learning methods according to [70].

TARNet Consider covariate vector, treatment, and observed outcome tuple (X, Z, Y) tuple with realizations $\mathcal{D} = \{(\boldsymbol{x}_i, z_i, y_i),\ i = 1, \ldots, n\}$. TARNet finds a representation of the covariates, denoted by $\Phi(\boldsymbol{x}_i)$, which maps the covariate vector onto a representation space, and hypothesis of the potential outcome variable, denoted by $m_{z_i}(\Phi(\boldsymbol{x}_i))$, simultaneously by minimizing the following regularized objective function:

$$\min_{m_0, m_1, \Phi} \mathcal{L}_{\text{TAR}}(m_0, m_1, \Phi;\ \mathcal{D}) = \frac{1}{n}\sum_{i=1}^{n} w_i \widetilde{L}\left(m_{z_i}(\Phi(\boldsymbol{x}_i));\ y_i\right)$$
$$+ \lambda_{\text{CPLX}} \mathrm{R}(m_0, m_1)$$
$$+ \lambda_{\text{BAL}}\, \text{IPM}\left(\{\Phi(\boldsymbol{x}_i)\}_{i:z_i=0}, \{\Phi(\boldsymbol{x}_i)\}_{i:z_i=1}\right),$$

where $\mathrm{R}(\cdot,\cdot)$ represents the model complexity, $\text{IPM}(\cdot,\cdot)$ represents the Integral Probability Metric (IPM) [51], such as the Maximum Mean Discrepancy and the Wasserstein Distance, evaluated on two empirical distributions defined by two collections of data points on the representation space, and weights w_i's compensate for the difference in treatment group size and are defined as follows:

$$w_i = \frac{z_i}{2u} + \frac{1 - z_i}{2(1 - u)}, \quad i = 1, \ldots, n, \quad u = \frac{1}{n}\sum_{i=1}^{n} z_i.$$

The loss function $\widetilde{L}$ for the network training is decomposed into two terms, i.e., $\widetilde{L}\left(m_z(\Phi(\cdot)); \cdot\right), z \in \{0, 1\}$, which correspond to the control and treatment groups, respectively. The weights for the treatment and control functions are updated only if the sample belongs to that group. Either the MSE or log-loss can be used as $\widetilde{L}$, depending on whether the outcome variable is continuous or binary. Most importantly, to handle the problem of variance arising from treatment imbalance, the TARNet objective includes the empirical IPM to upper bound this variance. Hyperparameter $\lambda_{\text{BAL}} > 0$ controls the trade-off between outcome regression model fitting and the treatment-and-control distribution balances. When $\lambda_{\text{BAL}} = 0$, it corresponds to the TARNet; otherwise, it corresponds to the counterfactual regression.

Dragonnet Similarly, Dragonnet creates a shared representation of the covariates that can be used to predict the treatment and potential outcomes. It uses an NN for the shared representation followed by two NNs used for predicting potential outcomes of the treatment and control groups, respectively. However, instead of using an IPM layer, [47] incorporated a mapping layer for the propensity score, which is named the "propensity score head" and denoted by $e(\cdot)$, to connect the shared representation of the covariates with the estimated propensity scores. To be precise, the objective function is

$$\min_{\theta} \mathcal{L}_{\text{Dragon}}(\theta; \mathcal{D}) = \frac{1}{n}\sum_{i=1}^{n} \underbrace{\left(m_{z_i}(\theta; \boldsymbol{x}_i) - y_i\right)^2}_{\text{NN regression loss}} + \lambda_{\text{BAL}} \underbrace{\text{CE}\left(e(\theta; \boldsymbol{x}_i), z_i\right)}_{\text{NN classification CE loss}}, \tag{21}$$

where $\text{CE}(\cdot, \cdot)$ is the binary classification cross-entropy loss and $\lambda_{\text{BAL}} > 0$ is a tunable hyperparameter controlling the trade-off between outcome regression model fitting and the treatment-and-control distribution balances.

For further details of TARNet and Dragonnet, we refer readers to the original papers. In our numerical experiments, we use the open-source implementation[1] of TARNet and Dragonnet on the IHDP dataset, and readers can find further implementation details therein.

[1] The are two implementations on GitHub, one is from the Dragonnet paper author, https://github.com/claudiashi57/dragonnet, and the other is a reproduction of the results using PyTorch: https://github.com/alecmn/dragonnet-reproduced.

Appendix C: Theory

Non-asymptotic Recovery Guarantee for TLIPW

We begin our theoretical analysis with the TLIPW estimator. We will first prove the non-asymptotic upper bound on the ℓ_1 regularized TL estimator for PS model (6) and then plug it into the error bound for unbiased IPW estimator (2) to get the final recovery guarantee for the TLIPW estimator.

Guarantee for PS Model Estimation with Knowledge Transfer

Let us begin with the necessary assumptions.

Assumption 1 The covariates in both target and source domains are uniformly bounded, i.e., there exists $M_X > 0$ such that $\|\boldsymbol{x}_i\|_\infty \leq M_X, i = 1, \ldots, n$, and $\|\boldsymbol{x}_{i,\mathrm{s}}\|_\infty \leq M_X, i = 1, \ldots, n_\mathrm{s}$.

The above assumption is a slightly different from the "standardized design matrix" assumption in [4], which requires the squared matrix F-norms of design matrices $(\boldsymbol{x}_1, \ldots, \boldsymbol{x}_n)^\mathrm{T}$ and $(\boldsymbol{x}_{1,\mathrm{s}}, \ldots, \boldsymbol{x}_{n_\mathrm{s},\mathrm{s}})^\mathrm{T}$ to be n and n_s, respectively. However, we will see they serve the same purpose when proving Lemma 1 (to be presented). Denote the sample covariance matrices as follows:

$$\Sigma = \frac{1}{n}\sum_{i=1}^{n} \boldsymbol{x}_i\boldsymbol{x}_i^\mathrm{T} \in \mathbb{R}^{n\times n}, \quad \Sigma_\mathrm{s} = \frac{1}{n_\mathrm{s}}\sum_{i=1}^{n_\mathrm{s}} \boldsymbol{x}_{i,\mathrm{s}}\boldsymbol{x}_{i,\mathrm{s}}^\mathrm{T} \in \mathbb{R}^{n_\mathrm{s}\times n_\mathrm{s}}. \tag{22}$$

Assumption 2 The source domain sample covariance matrix Σ_s is positive-definite (PD); in particular, we assume that Σ_s has minimum eigenvalue $\psi > 0$.

Here, Assumption 2 ensures we can faithfully recover β_s using MLE from the source domain data, and this assumption is mild when $n_\mathrm{s} > d$, which is satisfied under our considered regime (15).

Definition 2 (Compatibility Condition) The compatibility condition with constant $\phi > 0$ is met for the index set $\mathcal{I} \subset \{1, \ldots, d\}$ and the matrix $\Sigma \in \mathbb{R}^{d\times d}$, if for all $u \in \mathbb{R}^d$ satisfying $\|u_{\mathcal{I}^c}\|_1 \leq 3\|u_{\mathcal{I}}\|_1$, the following condition holds:

$$u^\mathrm{T}\Sigma u \geq \frac{\phi^2}{\#\mathcal{I}}\|u_{\mathcal{I}}\|_1^2,$$

where (recall that) # represents the cardinality of a set, and $u_{\mathcal{I}}$ is a vector with j-th elements being u_j, i.e., j-th element in vector u, if j belongs to index set $\mathcal{I}$ and zero otherwise.

A standard assumption in high-dimensional Lasso literature is as follows.

Assumption 3 The index set $\mathcal{I} = \mathrm{supp}(\Delta_\beta)$ (5) and target domain sample covariance matrix Σ (22) meet the above compatibility condition with constant $\phi > 0$.

This assumption guarantees the identifiability of Δ_β, and it holds automatically when the target domain sample covariance is PD. However, when $n < d$, the target domain sample covariance is rank-deficient, and Assumption 3 is crucial for the identifiability of Δ_β.

Assumption 4 The function $G(\cdot)$ is strongly convex with $\gamma > 0$, i.e., for all w_1, w_2 in its domain, the following holds:

$$G(w_1) - G(w_2) \geq G'(w_2)(w_1 - w_2) + \gamma \frac{(w_1 - w_2)^2}{2}.$$

Assumption 4 is standard in GLM literature, and it is automatically satisfied when the link function $G'(\cdot) = g(\cdot)$ (4) is linear, i.e., $g(x) = x$ with domain $x \in [0, 1]$. Now, we are ready to present the recovery guarantee for the ℓ_1 regularized TL for the PS model nuisance parameters.

Lemma 1 (Transferable Guarantee for PS Model) *Under Assumptions 1, 2, 3, and 4, when the PS model* (4) *is correctly specified and the difference* Δ_β (5) *is s-sparse, the following holds for the estimator* $\widehat{\beta}_{\mathrm{t}}$ (6) *with regularization strength parameter* $\lambda_{\mathrm{PS}} > 0$*:*

$$\mathbb{P}\left(\left\| \widehat{\beta}_{\mathrm{t}} - \beta_{\mathrm{t}} \right\|_1 \geq \frac{5\lambda_{\mathrm{PS}}}{\gamma} \left(\frac{1}{8\psi^2} + \frac{1}{\psi} + \frac{s}{\phi^2} \right) \right)$$
$$\leq 2d \exp\left(-\frac{2\lambda_{\mathrm{PS}}^2 n}{125 M_X^2} \right) + 2d \exp\left(-\frac{2\lambda_{\mathrm{PS}}^2 n_{\mathrm{s}}}{5d^2 M_X^2} \right). \tag{23}$$

Remark 2 As one will see later in the next subsection, the above error bound is invoked when we upper bound the error for the estimated propensity scores, i.e., $|g(x_i^{\mathrm{T}}\beta_{\mathrm{t}}) - g(x_i^{\mathrm{T}}\widehat{\beta}_{\mathrm{t}})|$, which involves applying Hölder's inequality to get

$$x_i^{\mathrm{T}}(\beta_{\mathrm{t}} - \widehat{\beta}_{\mathrm{t}}) \leq |x_i^{\mathrm{T}}(\beta_{\mathrm{t}} - \widehat{\beta}_{\mathrm{t}})| \leq \|x_i\|_{p_1} \|\beta_{\mathrm{t}} - \widehat{\beta}_{\mathrm{t}}\|_{p_2},$$

with $1/p_1 + 1/p_2 = 1$, $p_1, p_2 \geq 1$. Notice that common choices include $(p_1, p_2) = (2, 2)$ and $(\infty, 1)$. As mentioned earlier, we can invoke restricted eigenvalue condition [6, 32, 58] to upper bound $\|\beta_{\mathrm{t}} - \widehat{\beta}_{\mathrm{t}}\|_2$, which scales as $\sqrt{s}$ instead of s; however $\|x_i\|_2$ will scale as $\sqrt{n}$ under Assumption 1, which typically dominates the sparsity term in our regime (15). Therefore, the overall error upper bound on ATE estimate will deteriorate to $\mathcal{O}(\sqrt{sn \log d/n})$, compared with $\mathcal{O}(s\sqrt{\log d/n})$ (to be presented below). This explains why we use the compatibility condition to obtain the ℓ_1 error bound for the estimated nuisance parameters instead of using the restricted eigenvalue condition to get the ℓ_2 error bound.

Guarantee for Plug-In TLIPW Estimator

To bound the absolute estimation error $|\widehat{\tau}_{\mathrm{TLIPW}} - \tau|$, we additionally need some (mild) technical assumptions.

Assumption 5 The target domain outcomes are uniformly bounded, i.e., there exists $M_Y > 0$ such that $|y_i| \le M_Y, i = 1, \ldots, n$.

This technical assumption helps simplify the analysis; however, our following theoretical analysis will also hold for sub-Gaussian (see Definition 3) outcome random variables as shown by the techniques used in the proof of Theorem 3, case (I).

Assumption 6 The propensity scores evaluated on the target domain data are bounded away from zero and one, i.e., there exists $0 < m_g < 1/2$ such that

$$m_g \le e(\boldsymbol{x}_i) = g(\boldsymbol{x}_i^{\mathrm{T}} \beta_{\mathrm{t}}) \le 1 - m_g, \quad i = 1, \ldots, n.$$

Assumption 6 is standard for proving the theoretical guarantee of IPW estimator; see [65, 66] for classic asymptotic analysis for the IPW estimator's $\sqrt{n}$-consistency and asymptotic normality (cf. Theorems 1 and 4.1 [66] respectively). Now, by leveraging Hoeffding's inequality, we can establish the following concentration result.

Lemma 2 *Under Assumptions 5 and 6, for any $t > 0$, we have:*

$$\mathbb{P}\left(\left|\frac{1}{n}\sum_{i=1}^{n} \frac{z_i y_i}{g(\boldsymbol{x}_i^T \beta_{\mathrm{t}})} - \frac{(1 - z_i) y_i}{1 - g(\boldsymbol{x}_i^T \beta_{\mathrm{t}})} - \tau\right| \ge t\right) \le 4 \exp\left(-\frac{m_g^2 t^2 n}{8 M_Y^2}\right). \tag{24}$$

Before presenting the non-asymptotic guarantee for the TLIPW estimator, we additionally impose the following technical assumption for simplicity.

Assumption 7 The link function $g(\cdot)$ is L-Lipschitz with constant $L > 0$, i.e., for x_1, x_2 in its domain, we have $|g(x_1) - g(x_2)| \le L|x_1 - x_2|$.

Finally, with the help of the above lemmas, we can establish the non-asymptotic upper bound on the absolute estimation error of $\widehat{\tau}_{\mathrm{TLIPW}}$ as follows.

Theorem 1 (Non-asymptotic Recovery Guarantee for $\widehat{\tau}_{\mathrm{TLIPW}}$ (8)) *Under Assumptions 1, 2, 3, 4, 5, 6, and 7, for any constant $\delta > 0$, if the PS model* (4) *is correctly specified and the difference Δ_β* (5) *is s-sparse, as $n, n_{\mathrm{s}} \to \infty$, suppose* (15) *holds, i.e.,*

$$s\sqrt{\frac{\log d}{n}} = o(1), \quad d\sqrt{\frac{n}{n_{\mathrm{s}}}} = \mathcal{O}(1),$$

we take ℓ_1 regularization strength parameter to be

$$\lambda_{\text{PS}} = \sqrt{\frac{5M_X^2 \log(6nd)}{2n} \max\left\{25, \frac{nd^2}{n_{\text{s}}}\right\}}, \tag{25}$$

and we will have

$$\mathbb{P}\left(|\widehat{\tau}_{\text{TLIPW}} - \tau| \le (1+\delta)\left(C_1 s \sqrt{\frac{\log n + \log d}{n} \max\left\{1, \frac{nd^2}{25n_{\text{s}}}\right\}} + \frac{2M_Y}{m_g}\sqrt{\frac{\log n}{n}}\right)\right) \ge 1 - \frac{1}{n}, \tag{26}$$

where constant $C_1 = C_1(M_X, M_Y, \psi, \phi; \gamma, m_g, L)$ is defined as

$$C_1 = \frac{100\sqrt{5}M_X^2 M_Y L}{\sqrt{2}m_g^2 \gamma}\left(\frac{1}{8\psi^2} + \frac{1}{\psi} + \frac{1}{\phi^2}\right).$$

Proofs

Proof Outline of Lemma 1 This proof mostly follows the proof of Theorem 6 in [4]. The differences in our setting come from *(i)* The Bernoulli r.v.s are sub-Gaussian with variance bounded by $1/4$, which implies

$$\mathbb{E}[Z - g(X^{\text{T}}\beta_{\text{t}})] = 0, \quad \text{Var}(Z - g(X^{\text{T}}\beta_{\text{t}})) \le 1/4 + 1 = 5/4.$$

We need to substitute the variance terms with this upper bound (i.e., $5/4$).

(ii) By Assumption 1, we have:

$$\sum_{i=1}^{n} (\boldsymbol{x}_i)_j^2 \le n M_X^2,$$

where $(\boldsymbol{x}_i)_j$ denotes the j-th element in the vector $\boldsymbol{x}_i$. This implies that $\sum_{i=1}^{n}(z_i - g(\boldsymbol{x}_i^{\text{T}}\beta_{\text{t}}))(\boldsymbol{x}_i)_j$ is $(\sqrt{5n}M_X/2)$-sub-Gaussian (cf. Lemma 16 in [4]). Notice that this is different from "$\sum_{i=1}^{n}(\boldsymbol{x}_i)_j^2 = n$" due to the "normalized feature assumption" in the proof of Lemma 4 [4]. Therefore, in addition to substituting the variance terms as mentioned in (i), we need to include the additional M_X term due to different model assumptions. Lastly, we perform the same modification to Lemma 5 and its proof in [4], and these lead to (23). For complete details of the proof, we refer readers to Appendix C in [4].

Proof of Lemma 2 For correctly specified propensity score model (4), the IPW estimator is unbiased as shown in (18). Notice that Assumptions 5 and 6 ensures

$$\left|\frac{z_i y_i}{g(\boldsymbol{x}_i^{\mathrm{T}}\beta_{\mathrm{t}})}\right| \leq \frac{M_Y}{m_g}.$$

By Hoeffding's inequality, we have:

$$\mathbb{P}\left(\left|\frac{1}{n}\sum_{i=1}^{n}\frac{z_i y_i}{g(\boldsymbol{x}_i^{\mathrm{T}}\beta_{\mathrm{t}})} - \mathbb{E}[Y_1]\right| \geq t\right) \leq 2\exp\left(-\frac{m_g^2 t^2 n}{2M_Y^2}\right).$$

Similarly, we have $\mathbb{E}\left[\frac{(1-Z)Y}{1-e(X)}\right] = E[Y_0]$, and we can show:

$$\mathbb{P}\left(\left|\frac{1}{n}\sum_{i=1}^{n}\frac{(1-z_i)y_i}{1-g(\boldsymbol{x}_i^{\mathrm{T}}\beta_{\mathrm{t}})} - \mathbb{E}[Y_0]\right| \geq t\right) \leq 2\exp\left(-\frac{m_g^2 t^2 n}{2M_Y^2}\right).$$

Recall that $\tau = \mathbb{E}[Y_1] - \mathbb{E}[Y_0]$, we have:

$$\begin{aligned}
&\mathbb{P}\left(\left|\frac{1}{n}\sum_{i=1}^{n}\frac{z_i y_i}{g(\boldsymbol{x}_i^{\mathrm{T}}\beta_{\mathrm{t}})} - \frac{(1-z_i)y_i}{1-g(\boldsymbol{x}_i^{\mathrm{T}}\beta_{\mathrm{t}})} - \tau\right| \geq t\right) \\
&\leq \mathbb{P}\left(\left|\frac{1}{n}\sum_{i=1}^{n}\frac{z_i y_i}{g(\boldsymbol{x}_i^{\mathrm{T}}\beta_{\mathrm{t}})} - \mathbb{E}[Y_1]\right| \geq t/2\right) \\
&+ \mathbb{P}\left(\left|\frac{1}{n}\sum_{i=1}^{n}\frac{(1-z_i)y_i}{1-g(\boldsymbol{x}_i^{\mathrm{T}}\beta_{\mathrm{t}})} - \mathbb{E}[Y_0]\right| \geq t/2\right) \\
&\leq 4\exp\left(-\frac{m_g^2 t^2 n}{8M_Y^2}\right).
\end{aligned}$$

We complete the proof. □

Proof of Theorem 1 On one hand, plugging the regularization parameter choice (25) into (23) yields:

$$\mathbb{P}\left(\|\widehat{\beta}_{\mathrm{t}} - \beta_{\mathrm{t}}\|_1 \geq \frac{5\lambda_{\mathrm{PS}}}{\gamma}\left(\frac{1}{8\psi^2} + \frac{1}{\psi} + \frac{s}{\phi^2}\right)\right) \leq \frac{2}{3n}. \tag{27}$$

On the other hand, by setting $t = \frac{2M_Y}{m_g}\sqrt{\frac{\log(12n)}{n}}$ in (24), we have:

$$\mathbb{P}\left(\left|\frac{1}{n}\sum_{i=1}^{n}\frac{z_i y_i}{g(\boldsymbol{x}_i^{\mathrm{T}}\beta_{\mathrm{t}})} - \frac{(1-z_i)y_i}{1-g(\boldsymbol{x}_i^{\mathrm{T}}\beta_{\mathrm{t}})} - \tau\right| \geq \frac{2M_Y}{m_g}\sqrt{\frac{\log(12n)}{n}}\right) \leq \frac{1}{3n}. \tag{28}$$

Due to Assumptions 5 and 6, we have:

$$\left|\frac{1}{n}\sum_{i=1}^{n}\frac{z_i y_i}{g(\boldsymbol{x}_i^{\mathrm{T}}\beta_{\mathrm{t}})}-\frac{z_i y_i}{g(\boldsymbol{x}_i^{\mathrm{T}}\widehat{\beta_{\mathrm{t}}})}\right|\leq\frac{1}{n}\sum_{i=1}^{n}\frac{M_Y|g(\boldsymbol{x}_i^{\mathrm{T}}\beta_{\mathrm{t}})-g(\boldsymbol{x}_i^{\mathrm{T}}\widehat{\beta_{\mathrm{t}}})|}{m_g\left(m_g-|g(\boldsymbol{x}_i^{\mathrm{T}}\beta_{\mathrm{t}})-g(\boldsymbol{x}_i^{\mathrm{T}}\widehat{\beta_{\mathrm{t}}})|\right)}. \tag{29}$$

Since $g(\cdot)$ is L-Lipschitz, we have:

$$|g(\boldsymbol{x}_i^{\mathrm{T}}\beta_{\mathrm{t}})-g(\boldsymbol{x}_i^{\mathrm{T}}\widehat{\beta_{\mathrm{t}}})|\leq L|\boldsymbol{x}_i^{\mathrm{T}}(\beta_{\mathrm{t}}-\widehat{\beta_{\mathrm{t}}})|\leq L\|\boldsymbol{x}_i\|_\infty\left\|\widehat{\beta_{\mathrm{t}}}-\beta_{\mathrm{t}}\right\|_1,$$

where the last inequality comes from Hölder's inequality. Due to Assumption 5 and the fact that $f(x)=x/(m_g-x)$ monotonically increase on a domain $0\leq x<m_g$, we can further bound the right-hand side (RHS) of (29) as follows:

$$\begin{aligned}\left|\frac{1}{n}\sum_{i=1}^{n}\frac{z_i y_i}{g(\boldsymbol{x}_i^{\mathrm{T}}\beta_{\mathrm{t}})}-\frac{z_i y_i}{g(\boldsymbol{x}_i^{\mathrm{T}}\widehat{\beta_{\mathrm{t}}})}\right|&\leq\frac{1}{n}\sum_{i=1}^{n}\frac{M_X M_Y L\left\|\widehat{\beta_{\mathrm{t}}}-\beta_{\mathrm{t}}\right\|_1}{m_g\left(m_g-M_X L\left\|\widehat{\beta_{\mathrm{t}}}-\beta_{\mathrm{t}}\right\|_1\right)}\\&\leq\frac{1}{n}\sum_{i=1}^{n}\frac{M_X M_Y L\left\|\widehat{\beta_{\mathrm{t}}}-\beta_{\mathrm{t}}\right\|_1}{m_g^2/2}.\end{aligned}\tag{30}$$

The above inequality will hold since, for large enough n, n_{s} and in the regime (15), Lemma 1 guarantees $M_X L\left\|\widehat{\beta_{\mathrm{t}}}-\beta_{\mathrm{t}}\right\|_1\to 0$, and therefore we will have $M_X L\left\|\widehat{\beta_{\mathrm{t}}}-\beta_{\mathrm{t}}\right\|_1\leq m_g/2$. Similarly, we can obtain

$$\left|\frac{1}{n}\sum_{i=1}^{n}\frac{(1-z_i)y_i}{1-g(\boldsymbol{x}_i^{\mathrm{T}}\beta_{\mathrm{t}})}-\frac{(1-z_i)y_i}{1-g(\boldsymbol{x}_i^{\mathrm{T}}\widehat{\beta_{\mathrm{t}}})}\right|\leq\frac{1}{n}\sum_{i=1}^{n}\frac{M_X M_Y L\left\|\widehat{\beta_{\mathrm{t}}}-\beta_{\mathrm{t}}\right\|_1}{m_g^2/2}. \tag{31}$$

Now, (27) and (28) tell us that, with probability as least $1-1/n$,

$$\begin{aligned}&|\widehat{\tau}_{\mathrm{TLIPW}}-\tau|\\&\leq\left|\widehat{\tau}_{\mathrm{TLIPW}}-\frac{1}{n}\sum_{i=1}^{n}\frac{z_i y_i}{g(\boldsymbol{x}_i^{\mathrm{T}}\beta_{\mathrm{t}})}-\frac{(1-z_i)y_i}{1-g(\boldsymbol{x}_i^{\mathrm{T}}\beta_{\mathrm{t}})}\right|\\&\quad+\left|\frac{1}{n}\sum_{i=1}^{n}\frac{z_i y_i}{g(\boldsymbol{x}_i^{\mathrm{T}}\beta_{\mathrm{t}})}-\frac{(1-z_i)y_i}{1-g(\boldsymbol{x}_i^{\mathrm{T}}\beta_{\mathrm{t}})}-\tau\right|\\&<\frac{20M_X M_Y L\lambda_{\mathrm{PS}}}{m_g^2\gamma}\left(\frac{1}{8\psi^2}+\frac{1}{\psi}+\frac{s}{\phi^2}\right)+\frac{2M_Y}{m_g}\sqrt{\frac{\log(12n)}{n}}\\&\leq\frac{20M_X M_Y L\lambda_{\mathrm{PS}}}{m_g^2\gamma}\left(\frac{1}{8\psi^2}+\frac{1}{\psi}+\frac{1}{\phi^2}\right)s+\frac{2M_Y}{m_g}\sqrt{\frac{\log(12n)}{n}}.\end{aligned}$$

Here, the last inequity above assumes $s \geq 1$; however, this inequality is merely to make the result look more concise, and we can handle the $s = 0$ case in a similar manner. Plugging the λ_{PS} choice (25) into the above equation, and notice that, for any constant $\delta > 0$, for large enough n the following holds:

$$\sqrt{\log(12n)} = \sqrt{\log 12 + \log n} \leq (1+\delta)\sqrt{\log n}, \quad \sqrt{\log(6nd)} \leq (1+\delta)\sqrt{\log(nd)}.$$

We can obtain the non-asymptotic result in (26). Now we complete the proof.

Non-asymptotic Recovery Guarantee for TLOR

Guarantee for OR Model Estimation with Knowledge Transfer

Now we prove the non-asymptotic guarantee for our proposed TLOR estimator.

Definition 3 A random variable $Z \in \mathbb{R}$ is σ-sub-Gaussian if $\mathbb{E}\left[e^{tz}\right] \leq e^{\sigma^2 t^2/2}$ for all $t \in \mathbb{R}$.

Many classical distributions are sub-Gaussian; typical examples include any bounded, centered distribution, or the normal distribution. For $z \in \{0, 1\}$, we denote the "noise terms" in the OR models (10) as follows:

$$\epsilon_z = Y_z - \mathbb{E}[Y_z|X] = Y_z - X^{\mathrm{T}}\alpha_{z,\mathrm{t}},$$

$$\epsilon_{z,\mathrm{s}} = Y_{z,\mathrm{s}} - \mathbb{E}[Y_{z,\mathrm{s}}|X_{\mathrm{s}}] = Y_{z,\mathrm{s}} - X_{\mathrm{s}}^{\mathrm{T}}\alpha_{z,\mathrm{s}}.$$

Assumption 8 The noise terms are sub-Gaussian, i.e., for $z \in \{0, 1\}$, there exist constants $\sigma, \sigma_{\mathrm{s}} > 0$ such that ϵ_z is σ-sub-Gaussian, and $\epsilon_{z,\mathrm{s}}$ is σ_{s}-sub-Gaussian.

Assumption 9 For $z \in \{0, 1\}$, the index set $\mathcal{I} = \mathrm{supp}(\Delta_{\alpha,z})$ (11) and target domain sample covariance matrix Σ (22) meet the compatibility condition with $\phi_z > 0$.

Lemma 3 (Transferable Guarantee for OR Model, cf. Theorem 5 [4]) *Under Assumptions 1, 2, (8), and 9, assume the sample balanceness condition* (16) *holds, for $z \in \{0, 1\}$, when the OR model* (10) *is correctly specified and the difference $\Delta_{\alpha,z}$* (11) *is s_z-sparse, i.e.,*

$$\|\Delta_{\alpha,0}\|_0 \leq s_0, \quad \|\Delta_{\alpha,1}\|_0 \leq s_1,$$

the following holds for the estimator $\widehat{\alpha}_{z,\mathrm{t}}$ (12) *with regularization strength parameter* $\lambda_{\mathrm{OR}} > 0$*:*

$$\mathbb{P}\left(\left\|\widehat{\alpha}_{z,\mathrm{t}} - \alpha_{z,\mathrm{t}}\right\|_1 \geq 5\lambda_{\mathrm{OR}}\left(\frac{1}{4\psi^2} + \frac{1}{\psi} + \frac{s_z}{2\phi_z^2}\right)\right)$$
$$\leq 2d \exp\left(-\frac{rn\lambda_{\mathrm{OR}}^2}{200\sigma^2 M_X^2}\right) + 2d \exp\left(-\frac{rn_{\mathrm{s}}\lambda_{\mathrm{OR}}^2}{2d^2\sigma_{\mathrm{s}}^2 M_X^2}\right). \tag{32}$$

Guarantee for Plug-In TLOR Estimator

Here, we impose an additional technical assumption that the covariates in the target domain are sub-Gaussian such that there exists constant $\sigma_X > 0$:

$$\mathbb{P}\left(\left|\frac{1}{n}\sum_{i=1}^{n} \boldsymbol{x}_i^{\mathrm{T}}\alpha_{z,\mathrm{t}} - \mathbb{E}[Y_z]\right| > t\right) \leq 2\exp\left(-\frac{nt^2}{2\sigma_X^2}\right), \quad z \in \{0, 1\}. \tag{33}$$

Theorem 2 (Non-asymptotic Recovery Guarantee for $\widehat{\tau}_{\mathrm{TLDR}}$ **(14))** *Under Assumptions 1, 2, 8, and 9, suppose the sample balances condition* (16) *holds and the covariates in target domain follow a sub-Gaussian distribution* (33)*, as* $n, n_{\mathrm{s}} \to \infty$*, suppose* (15) *holds, for any constant* $\delta > 0$*, when the OR model* (10) *is correctly specified with* s_z*-sparse* $\Delta_{z,\alpha}$ (11) *(for* $z \in \{0, 1\}$*), i.e.,*

$$\|\Delta_{\alpha,0}\|_0 \leq s_0, \quad \|\Delta_{\alpha,1}\|_0 \leq s_1,$$

then by taking

$$\lambda_{\mathrm{OR}} = \sqrt{2M_X^2 \log(12nd) \max\left\{\frac{100\sigma^2}{rn}, \frac{d^2\sigma_{\mathrm{s}}^2}{rn_{\mathrm{s}}}\right\}}, \tag{34}$$

we will have:

$$\mathbb{P}\Bigg(|\widehat{\tau}_{\mathrm{TLOR}} - \tau| \leq (1+\delta)\Bigg(C_2\sigma(s_0 + s_1)\sqrt{\frac{\log n + \log d}{rn}\max\left\{100, \frac{n\sigma_{\mathrm{s}}^2 d^2}{n_{\mathrm{s}}\sigma^2}\right\}}$$
$$+ 2\sigma_X\sqrt{\frac{2\log n}{rn}}\Bigg)\Bigg) \geq 1 - \frac{1}{n}. \tag{35}$$

where constant $C_2 = C_2(M_X, \psi, \phi_0, \phi_1; m_g)$ is defined as follows:

$$C_2 = 5\sqrt{2}M_X^2\left(\frac{1}{m_g} - 1\right)\left(\frac{1}{2\psi^2} + \frac{2}{\psi} + \frac{1}{2\phi_0^2} + \frac{1}{2\phi_1^2}\right). \tag{36}$$

Proof

The proof of Lemma 3 mostly follows that of Theorem 5 in [4] and we omit it here. We only give detailed proof of the main theorem.

Proof of Theorem 2 The absolute error of the TLOR estimator (13) can be decomposed as follows:

$$\begin{aligned}
|\widehat{\tau}_{\mathrm{TLOR}} - \tau| &\le \left|\frac{1}{n_1}\sum_{z_i=1} \boldsymbol{x}_i^{\mathrm{T}}(\widehat{\alpha}_{1,\mathrm{t}} - \alpha_{1,\mathrm{t}})\right| + \left|\frac{1}{n_0}\sum_{z_i=0} \boldsymbol{x}_i^{\mathrm{T}}(\widehat{\alpha}_{0,\mathrm{t}} - \alpha_{0,\mathrm{t}})\right| \\
&\quad + \left|\frac{1}{n_1}\sum_{z_i=1} \boldsymbol{x}_i^{\mathrm{T}}\alpha_{1,\mathrm{t}} - \frac{1}{n_0}\sum_{z_i=0} \boldsymbol{x}_i^{\mathrm{T}}\alpha_{0,\mathrm{t}} - \tau\right| \\
&\le M_X\left(\|\widehat{\alpha}_{1,\mathrm{t}} - \alpha_{1,\mathrm{t}}\|_1 + \|\widehat{\alpha}_{0,\mathrm{t}} - \alpha_{0,\mathrm{t}}\|_1\right) \\
&\quad + \left|\frac{1}{n_1}\sum_{z_i=1} \boldsymbol{x}_i^{\mathrm{T}}\alpha_{1,\mathrm{t}} - \frac{1}{n_0}\sum_{z_i=0} \boldsymbol{x}_i^{\mathrm{T}}\alpha_{0,\mathrm{t}} - \tau\right|.
\end{aligned}$$

On one hand, by setting the RHS of (33) as $1/(6n)$, we have that, with probability at least $1 - 1/(3n)$, the following holds:

$$\left|\frac{1}{n}\sum_{i=1}^{n} \boldsymbol{x}_i^{\mathrm{T}}\alpha_{1,\mathrm{t}} - \boldsymbol{x}_i^{\mathrm{T}}\alpha_{0,\mathrm{t}} - \tau\right| \le 2\sqrt{\frac{2\sigma_X^2\log(12n)}{n}}.$$

One the other hand, following Lemma 3 and taking λ_{OR} as in (34), we will have that, with probability at least $1 - 2/(3n)$,

$$\|\widehat{\alpha}_{1,\mathrm{t}} - \alpha_{1,\mathrm{t}}\|_1 + \|\widehat{\alpha}_{0,\mathrm{t}} - \alpha_{0,\mathrm{t}}\|_1 \le 5\lambda_{\mathrm{OR}}\left(\frac{1}{2\psi^2} + \frac{2}{\psi} + \frac{s_0}{2\phi_0^2} + \frac{s_1}{2\phi_1^2}\right).$$

Now, combing the above inequalities, we will have that, with probability at least $1 - 1/n$, the following holds:

$$
\begin{aligned}
|\widehat{\tau}_{\mathrm{TLOR}} - \tau| \leq\ & 2\sqrt{\frac{2\sigma_X^2 \log(12n)}{n}} \\
& + 5M_X \left(\frac{1}{m_g} - 1\right) \lambda_{\mathrm{OR}} \left(\frac{1}{2\psi^2} + \frac{2}{\psi} + \frac{s_0}{2\phi_0^2} + \frac{s_1}{2\phi_1^2}\right) \\
& = \mathcal{O}\left((s_0 + s_1)\sqrt{\log d}\left(\frac{1}{\sqrt{rn}} + \frac{d}{\sqrt{rn_{\mathrm{s}}}}\right)\right).
\end{aligned}
$$

To get (35), we only need to notice that, for any constant $\delta > 0$, for large enough n the following holds:

$$
\sqrt{\log(12n)} = \sqrt{\log 12 + \log n} \leq (1 + \delta)\sqrt{\log n}.
$$

We can handle the $\log(12nd)$ term in λ_{OR} (34) in a similar manner and obtain $\sqrt{\log(12nd)} \leq (1 + \delta)\sqrt{\log(nd)}$. Now, we obtain the non-asymptotic result in (35) and complete the proof. □

Non-asymptotic Recovery Guarantee for TLDR

Guarantee for Plug-In TLDR Estimator

We impose another technical assumption as [4] did (see Assumption 1 therein).

Assumption 10 The ground truth target domain OR model parameters are bounded, i.e., for $z \in \{0, 1\}$, there exists $M_\alpha > 0$ such that $\|\alpha_{z,\mathrm{t}}\|_1 < M_\alpha$.

Similarly, due to the doubly robustness of the DR estimator, we have the following non-asymptotic recovery guarantee.

Theorem 3 (Non-asymptotic Recovery Guarantee for $\widehat{\tau}_{\mathrm{TLDR}}$ (14)) *Under Assumptions 1 and 2, as $n, n_{\mathrm{s}} \to \infty$, suppose* (15) *holds. For any constant $\delta > 0$: (I) When the PS model* (4) *is correctly specified and Δ_β* (5) *is s-sparse, if we additionally assume Assumptions 3, 4, 5, 6, 7, and 10 hold, then by taking*

$$
\lambda_{\mathrm{PS}} = \sqrt{\frac{5M_X^2 \log(10nd)}{2n}} \max\left\{25, \frac{nd^2}{n_{\mathrm{s}}}\right\}, \tag{37}
$$

we will have:

$$\mathbb{P}\left(|\widehat{\tau}_{\mathrm{TLDR}}-\tau| \le (1+\delta)\left(C_4 s\sqrt{\frac{\log n+\log d}{n}}\max\left\{1, \frac{25nd^2}{n_{\mathrm{s}}}\right\}\right.\right.$$
$$\left.\left.+C_5\sqrt{\frac{\log n}{n}}\right)\right) \ge 1-\frac{1}{n}. \tag{38}$$

where constants $C_4 = C_4(M_X, M_Y, \psi, \phi; \gamma, m_g, L; M_\alpha)$ *and* $C_5 = C_5(M_X, M_Y; m_g; M_\alpha)$ *are defined as follows:*

$$C_4 = \frac{100\sqrt{5}M_X^2\,(M_X M_\alpha + M_Y/m_g)\,L}{\sqrt{2}m_g\gamma}\left(\frac{1}{8\psi^2}+\frac{1}{\psi}+\frac{1}{\phi^2}\right),$$
$$C_5 = 2\frac{M_Y+\sqrt{10}M_X M_\alpha}{m_g}.$$

(II) When the OR model (10) *is correctly specified and* $\Delta_{z,\alpha}$ (11) *is* s_z*-sparse (for* $z \in \{0, 1\}$*), i.e.,*

$$\|\Delta_{\alpha,0}\|_0 \le s_0, \quad \|\Delta_{\alpha,1}\|_0 \le s_1,$$

under Assumptions 8 and 9, and we further assume the sample balances condition (16) *holds and the covariates in the target domain are sub-Gaussian* (33)*, we strengthen Assumption 6 by assuming the link function* $g(\cdot)$ (4) *takes value on* $[m_g, 1-m_g]$*, then by taking*

$$\lambda_{\mathrm{OR}} = \sqrt{2M_X^2\log(16nd)\max\left\{\frac{100\sigma^2}{rn}, \frac{d^2\sigma_{\mathrm{s}}^2}{rn_{\mathrm{s}}}\right\}}, \tag{39}$$

we will have

$$\mathbb{P}\Bigg(|\widehat{\tau}_{\mathrm{TLDR}}-\tau| \le (1+\delta)\Bigg(C_2\sigma(s_0+s_1)\sqrt{\frac{\log n+\log d}{rn}\max\left\{100, \frac{n\sigma_{\mathrm{s}}^2 d^2}{n_{\mathrm{s}}\sigma^2}\right\}}$$
$$+C_3\sigma\sqrt{\frac{\log n}{n}}+2\sigma_X\sqrt{\frac{2\log n}{rn}}\Bigg)\Bigg) \ge 1-\frac{1}{n}. \tag{40}$$

where constant $C_2 = C_2(M_X, \psi, \phi_0, \phi_1; m_g)$ *is defined in* (36)*, and constant* $C_3 = C_3(m_g) = 2\sqrt{2/m_g}$.

Proof

Proof of Theorem 3 We consider two cases: (i) the PS model is correctly specified and (ii) the OR model is correctly specified.

Case (I): The PS Model Is Correctly Specified This proof closely resembles that of Theorem 1. We only need to show the augmented terms in the DR estimator, i.e.,

$$\frac{1}{n}\sum_{i=1}^{n}\frac{\boldsymbol{x}_i^{\mathrm{T}}\widehat{\alpha}_{1,\mathrm{t}}(z_i-g(\boldsymbol{x}_i^{\mathrm{T}}\widehat{\beta}_{\mathrm{t}}))}{g(\boldsymbol{x}_i^{\mathrm{T}}\widehat{\beta}_{\mathrm{t}})},\quad \frac{1}{n}\sum_{i=1}^{n}\frac{\boldsymbol{x}_i^{\mathrm{T}}\widehat{\alpha}_{0,\mathrm{t}}(z_i-g(\boldsymbol{x}_i^{\mathrm{T}}\widehat{\beta}_{\mathrm{t}}))}{1-g(\boldsymbol{x}_i^{\mathrm{T}}\widehat{\beta}_{\mathrm{t}})},$$

are very close to zero with high probability, which is straightforward since they both have zero means under the correct PS model specification assumption.

To simplify our proof below, we impose Assumption 10, which implies that, when $n, n_{\mathrm{s}} \to \infty$, in regime (15), we will have $\|\widehat{\alpha}_{z,\mathrm{t}}\|_1 \leq M_\alpha$ due to Lemma 3. Similarly, Assumption 6 ensures that $m_g/2 \leq g(\boldsymbol{x}_i^{\mathrm{T}}\widehat{\beta}_{\mathrm{t}}) \leq 1-m_g/2$ for sufficiently large n, n_{s}. Now, we can show that

$$\sum_{i=1}^{n}\frac{\boldsymbol{x}_i^{\mathrm{T}}\widehat{\alpha}_{1,\mathrm{t}}(z_i-g(\boldsymbol{x}_i^{\mathrm{T}}\beta_{\mathrm{t}}))}{g(\boldsymbol{x}_i^{\mathrm{T}}\widehat{\beta}_{\mathrm{t}})}$$

is $(\sqrt{5n}M_X M_\alpha/m_g)$-sub-Gaussian. Notice that Bernoulli r.v. has variance bounded by $1/4$ and

$$\left|\frac{\boldsymbol{x}_i^{\mathrm{T}}\widehat{\alpha}_{1,\mathrm{t}}}{g(\boldsymbol{x}_i^{\mathrm{T}}\widehat{\beta}_{\mathrm{t}})}\right| \leq \frac{2M_X M_\alpha}{m_g}.$$

Thus, we have:

$$\mathbb{P}\left(\left|\frac{1}{n}\sum_{i=1}^{n}\frac{\boldsymbol{x}_i^{\mathrm{T}}\widehat{\alpha}_{1,\mathrm{t}}(z_i-g(\boldsymbol{x}_i^{\mathrm{T}}\beta_{\mathrm{t}}))}{g(\boldsymbol{x}_i^{\mathrm{T}}\widehat{\beta}_{\mathrm{t}})}\right|>t\right)\leq 2\exp\left(-\frac{nm_g^2t^2}{10M_X^2M_\alpha^2}\right). \tag{41}$$

Similarly, we can show that

$$\mathbb{P}\left(\left|\frac{1}{n}\sum_{i=1}^{n}\frac{\boldsymbol{x}_i^{\mathrm{T}}\widehat{\alpha}_{0,\mathrm{t}}(z_i-g(\boldsymbol{x}_i^{\mathrm{T}}\beta_{\mathrm{t}}))}{1-g(\boldsymbol{x}_i^{\mathrm{T}}\widehat{\beta}_{\mathrm{t}})}\right|>t\right)\leq 2\exp\left(-\frac{nm_g^2t^2}{10M_X^2M_\alpha^2}\right). \tag{42}$$

We take RHS of Eqs. 41 and 42 to be $1/(5n)$, and therefore with probability at least $1 - 2/(5n)$, we have:

$$\left| -\frac{1}{n}\sum_{i=1}^{n} \frac{\boldsymbol{x}_i^{\mathrm{T}}\widehat{\alpha}_{1,\mathrm{t}}(z_i - g(\boldsymbol{x}_i^{\mathrm{T}}\widehat{\beta}_{\mathrm{t}}))}{g(\boldsymbol{x}_i^{\mathrm{T}}\widehat{\beta}_{\mathrm{t}})} + \frac{1}{n}\sum_{i=1}^{n} \frac{\boldsymbol{x}_i^{\mathrm{T}}\widehat{\alpha}_{0,\mathrm{t}}(z_i - g(\boldsymbol{x}_i^{\mathrm{T}}\widehat{\beta}_{\mathrm{t}}))}{1 - g(\boldsymbol{x}_i^{\mathrm{T}}\widehat{\beta}_{\mathrm{t}})} \right| \\ \leq \frac{2M_X M_\alpha \sqrt{10\log(10n)}}{m_g\sqrt{n}} + \frac{4LM_X^2 M_\alpha \|\beta_{\mathrm{t}} - \widehat{\beta}_{\mathrm{t}}\|_1}{m_g}. \tag{43}$$

By taking λ_{PS} as in (37) and following the proof of Theorem 1, we have that with probability at least $1 - 1/n$:

$$\begin{aligned}
&|\widehat{\tau}_{\mathrm{TLDR}} - \tau| \\
&\leq \left| \widehat{\tau}_{\mathrm{TLIPW}} - \frac{1}{n}\sum_{i=1}^{n} \frac{z_i y_i}{g(\boldsymbol{x}_i^{\mathrm{T}}\beta_{\mathrm{t}})} - \frac{(1-z_i)y_i}{1 - g(\boldsymbol{x}_i^{\mathrm{T}}\beta_{\mathrm{t}})} \right| \\
&+ \left| \frac{1}{n}\sum_{i=1}^{n} \frac{z_i y_i}{g(\boldsymbol{x}_i^{\mathrm{T}}\beta_{\mathrm{t}})} - \frac{(1-z_i)y_i}{1 - g(\boldsymbol{x}_i^{\mathrm{T}}\beta_{\mathrm{t}})} - \tau \right| \\
&+ \left| -\frac{1}{n}\sum_{i=1}^{n} \frac{\boldsymbol{x}_i^{\mathrm{T}}\widehat{\alpha}_{1,\mathrm{t}}(z_i - g(\boldsymbol{x}_i^{\mathrm{T}}\widehat{\beta}_{\mathrm{t}}))}{g(\boldsymbol{x}_i^{\mathrm{T}}\widehat{\beta}_{\mathrm{t}})} + \frac{1}{n}\sum_{i=1}^{n} \frac{\boldsymbol{x}_i^{\mathrm{T}}\widehat{\alpha}_{0,\mathrm{t}}(z_i - g(\boldsymbol{x}_i^{\mathrm{T}}\widehat{\beta}_{\mathrm{t}}))}{1 - g(\boldsymbol{x}_i^{\mathrm{T}}\widehat{\beta}_{\mathrm{t}})} \right| \\
&\leq \frac{20M_X\left(M_\alpha M_X + \frac{M_Y}{m_g}\right)L\lambda_{\mathrm{PS}}}{m_g\gamma}\left(\frac{1}{8\psi^2} + \frac{1}{\psi} + \frac{s}{\phi^2}\right) \\
&+ \frac{2M_Y\sqrt{\log(20n)} + 2M_X M_\alpha\sqrt{10\log(10n)}}{m_g\sqrt{n}} \\
&= \mathcal{O}\left(s\sqrt{\log d}\left(\frac{1}{\sqrt{n}} + \frac{d}{\sqrt{n_{\mathrm{s}}}}\right)\right).
\end{aligned}$$

To get (38), we only need to notice that, for any constant $\delta > 0$, for large enough n, the following holds:

$$\sqrt{\log(10n)} < \sqrt{\log(20n)} = \sqrt{\log 20 + \log n} \leq (1+\delta)\sqrt{\log n}.$$

We can handle the $\log(10nd)$ term in λ_{PS} (37) in a similar manner and obtain $\sqrt{\log(10nd)} \leq (1+\delta)\sqrt{\log(nd)}$. Now, we obtain the non-asymptotic result in (38) and complete the proof.

Case (II): The OR Model Is Correctly Specified We rewrite our TLDR estimator (14) as follows:

$$\widehat{\tau}_{\mathrm{TLDR}} = \frac{1}{n}\sum_{i=1}^{n} \boldsymbol{x}_i^{\mathrm{T}}\widehat{\alpha}_{1,\mathrm{t}} + \frac{z_i(y_i - \boldsymbol{x}_i^{\mathrm{T}}\widehat{\alpha}_{1,\mathrm{t}})}{g(\boldsymbol{x}_i^{\mathrm{T}}\widehat{\beta}_{\mathrm{t}})} - \boldsymbol{x}_i^{\mathrm{T}}\widehat{\alpha}_{0,\mathrm{t}} - \frac{(1-z_i)(y_i - \boldsymbol{x}_i^{\mathrm{T}}\widehat{\alpha}_{0,\mathrm{t}})}{1 - g(\boldsymbol{x}_i^{\mathrm{T}}\widehat{\beta}_{\mathrm{t}})}.$$

We decompose the estimator error as follows:

$$\begin{aligned}
|\widehat{\tau}_{\mathrm{TLDR}} - \tau| \le & \left|\frac{1}{n}\sum_{i=1}^{n} \boldsymbol{x}_i^{\mathrm{T}}\alpha_{1,\mathrm{t}} - \boldsymbol{x}_i^{\mathrm{T}}\alpha_{0,\mathrm{t}} - \tau\right| \\
& + \left|\frac{1}{n}\sum_{i=1}^{n}\left(1 - \frac{z_i}{g(\boldsymbol{x}_i^{\mathrm{T}}\widehat{\beta}_{\mathrm{t}})}\right)\boldsymbol{x}_i^{\mathrm{T}}(\widehat{\alpha}_{1,\mathrm{t}} - \alpha_{1,\mathrm{t}})\right| \\
& + \left|\frac{1}{n}\sum_{i=1}^{n}\left(1 - \frac{1-z_i}{1-g(\boldsymbol{x}_i^{\mathrm{T}}\widehat{\beta}_{\mathrm{t}})}\right)\boldsymbol{x}_i^{\mathrm{T}}(\widehat{\alpha}_{0,\mathrm{t}} - \alpha_{0,\mathrm{t}})\right| \\
& + \left|\frac{1}{n}\sum_{i=1}^{n}\frac{z_i(y_i - \boldsymbol{x}_i^{\mathrm{T}}\alpha_{1,\mathrm{t}})}{g(\boldsymbol{x}_i^{\mathrm{T}}\widehat{\beta}_{\mathrm{t}})}\right| \\
& + \left|\frac{1}{n}\sum_{i=1}^{n}\frac{(1-z_i)(y_i - \boldsymbol{x}_i^{\mathrm{T}}\alpha_{0,\mathrm{t}})}{1-g(\boldsymbol{x}_i^{\mathrm{T}}\widehat{\beta}_{\mathrm{t}})}\right|.
\end{aligned}$$

Notice that we strengthen the Assumption 6 that link function $g(\cdot)$ only takes value on $[m_g, 1-m_g]$, which gives us

$$\begin{aligned}
\left|\frac{1}{n}\sum_{i=1}^{n}\left(1 - \frac{z_i}{g(\boldsymbol{x}_i^{\mathrm{T}}\widehat{\beta}_{\mathrm{t}})}\right)\boldsymbol{x}_i^{\mathrm{T}}(\widehat{\alpha}_{1,\mathrm{t}} - \alpha_{1,\mathrm{t}})\right| &\le \left(\frac{1}{m_g} - 1\right)\frac{1}{n}\sum_{i=1}^{n}\left|\boldsymbol{x}_i^{\mathrm{T}}(\widehat{\alpha}_{1,\mathrm{t}} - \alpha_{1,\mathrm{t}})\right|, \\
\left|\frac{1}{n}\sum_{i=1}^{n}\left(1 - \frac{1-z_i}{1-g(\boldsymbol{x}_i^{\mathrm{T}}\widehat{\beta}_{\mathrm{t}})}\right)\boldsymbol{x}_i^{\mathrm{T}}(\widehat{\alpha}_{0,\mathrm{t}} - \alpha_{0,\mathrm{t}})\right| &\le \left(\frac{1}{m_g} - 1\right)\frac{1}{n}\sum_{i=1}^{n}\left|\boldsymbol{x}_i^{\mathrm{T}}(\widehat{\alpha}_{0,\mathrm{t}} - \alpha_{0,\mathrm{t}})\right|.
\end{aligned}$$

Combing the above derivations with Assumption 1, we have:

$$\begin{aligned}
|\widehat{\tau}_{\mathrm{TLDR}} - \tau| \le & \left|\frac{1}{n}\sum_{i=1}^{n} \boldsymbol{x}_i^{\mathrm{T}}\alpha_{1,\mathrm{t}} - \boldsymbol{x}_i^{\mathrm{T}}\alpha_{0,\mathrm{t}} - \tau\right| \\
& + M_X\left(\frac{1}{m_g} - 1\right)\left(\|\widehat{\alpha}_{1,\mathrm{t}} - \alpha_{1,\mathrm{t}}\|_1 + \|\widehat{\alpha}_{0,\mathrm{t}} - \alpha_{0,\mathrm{t}}\|_1\right) \\
& + \left|\frac{1}{n}\sum_{i=1}^{n}\frac{z_i(y_i - \boldsymbol{x}_i^{\mathrm{T}}\alpha_{1,\mathrm{t}})}{g(\boldsymbol{x}_i^{\mathrm{T}}\widehat{\beta}_{\mathrm{t}})}\right| + \left|\frac{1}{n}\sum_{i=1}^{n}\frac{(1-z_i)(y_i - \boldsymbol{x}_i^{\mathrm{T}}\alpha_{0,\mathrm{t}})}{1-g(\boldsymbol{x}_i^{\mathrm{T}}\widehat{\beta}_{\mathrm{t}})}\right|.
\end{aligned}$$

(i) Since the OR model is assumed to be correct, we have $\mathbb{E}[Z(Y - X^{\mathrm{T}}\alpha_{Z,\mathrm{t}})] = 0$. Under Assumption 6, we can show:

$$\begin{aligned}
&\mathbb{P}\left(\left|\frac{1}{n}\sum_{i=1}^{n}\frac{z_i(y_i - \boldsymbol{x}_i^{\mathrm{T}}\alpha_{1,\mathrm{t}})}{g(\boldsymbol{x}_i^{\mathrm{T}}\widehat{\beta}_{\mathrm{t}})}\right| > t\right) \\
=&\mathbb{P}\left(\left|\frac{1}{n}\sum_{z_i=1}\frac{y_i - \boldsymbol{x}_i^{\mathrm{T}}\alpha_{1,\mathrm{t}}}{g(\boldsymbol{x}_i^{\mathrm{T}}\widehat{\beta}_{\mathrm{t}})}\right| > t\right) \le 2\exp\left(-\frac{rnm_g^2t^2}{2\sigma^2}\right).
\end{aligned} \tag{44}$$

Similarly, we will get:

$$\begin{aligned}
&\mathbb{P}\left(\left|\frac{1}{n}\sum_{i=1}^{n}\frac{(1-z_i)(y_i - \boldsymbol{x}_i^{\mathrm{T}}\alpha_{0,\mathrm{t}})}{1-g(\boldsymbol{x}_i^{\mathrm{T}}\widehat{\beta}_{\mathrm{t}})}\right| > t\right) \\
=&\mathbb{P}\left(\left|\frac{1}{n}\sum_{z_i=0}\frac{y_i - \boldsymbol{x}_i^{\mathrm{T}}\alpha_{0,\mathrm{t}}}{1-g(\boldsymbol{x}_i^{\mathrm{T}}\widehat{\beta}_{\mathrm{t}})}\right| > t\right) \le 2\exp\left(-\frac{rnm_g^2t^2}{2\sigma^2}\right).
\end{aligned} \tag{45}$$

By setting the RHS of the above two inequalities as $1/(8n)$, we have that, with probability at least $1 - 1/(4n)$, the following holds:

$$\left|\frac{1}{n}\sum_{i=1}^{n}\frac{z_i(y_i - \boldsymbol{x}_i^{\mathrm{T}}\alpha_{1,\mathrm{t}})}{g(\boldsymbol{x}_i^{\mathrm{T}}\widehat{\beta}_{\mathrm{t}})}\right| + \left|\frac{1}{n}\sum_{i=1}^{n}\frac{(1-z_i)(y_i - \boldsymbol{x}_i^{\mathrm{T}}\alpha_{0,\mathrm{t}})}{1-g(\boldsymbol{x}_i^{\mathrm{T}}\widehat{\beta}_{\mathrm{t}})}\right| \le 2\sqrt{\frac{2\sigma^2\log(16n)}{rnm_g^2}}.$$

(ii) Similar to the proof of Theorem 2, by setting the RHS of (33) as $1/(8n)$, we have that, with probability at least $1 - 1/(4n)$, the following holds:

$$\left|\frac{1}{n}\sum_{i=1}^{n}\boldsymbol{x}_i^{\mathrm{T}}\alpha_{1,\mathrm{t}} - \boldsymbol{x}_i^{\mathrm{T}}\alpha_{0,\mathrm{t}} - \tau\right| \le 2\sqrt{\frac{2\sigma_X^2\log(16n)}{n}}.$$

(iii) Finally, by taking λ_{OR} as in (39) as well as following Lemma 3, we will have that, with probability at least $1 - 1/(2n)$:

$$\|\widehat{\alpha}_{1,\mathrm{t}} - \alpha_{1,\mathrm{t}}\|_1 + \|\widehat{\alpha}_{0,\mathrm{t}} - \alpha_{0,\mathrm{t}}\|_1 \le 5\lambda_{\mathrm{OR}}\left(\frac{1}{2\psi^2} + \frac{2}{\psi} + \frac{s_0}{2\phi_0^2} + \frac{s_1}{2\phi_1^2}\right).$$

Now, plugging *(i)*, *(iii)*, *(iii)* back to the decomposition, we will have that, with probability at least $1 - 1/n$, the error $|\widehat{\tau}_{\mathrm{TLDR}} - \tau|$ can be (upper) bounded by

$$2\sqrt{\frac{2\sigma_X^2\log(16n)}{n}} + 5M_X\left(\frac{1}{m_g} - 1\right)\lambda_{\mathrm{OR}}\left(\frac{1}{2\psi^2} + \frac{2}{\psi} + \frac{s_0}{2\phi_0^2} + \frac{s_1}{2\phi_1^2}\right)$$

$$
\begin{aligned}
&+2\sqrt{\frac{2\sigma^2\log(16n)}{rnm_g^2}} \\
&= \mathcal{O}\left((s_0+s_1)\sqrt{\log d}\left(\frac{1}{\sqrt{rn}}+\frac{d}{\sqrt{rn_{\mathrm{s}}}}\right)\right).
\end{aligned}
$$

To get (40), we only need to notice that, for any constant $\delta > 0$, for large enough n, the following holds:

$$\sqrt{\log(16n)} = \sqrt{\log 16 + \log n} \le (1+\delta)\sqrt{\log n}.$$

We can handle the $\log(16nd)$ term in λ_{OR} (39) in a similar manner and obtain $\sqrt{\log(16nd)} \le (1+\delta)\sqrt{\log(nd)}$ when n is large enough. Now, we obtain the non-asymptotic result in (40) and complete the proof. □

Appendix D: Experiments

Additional Details of the GLM-Based Experiments

Here, for the GLM-based parametric approach, we consider the IPW estimator for the demonstration purpose since the focus of our numerical simulation is on NN-based nonparametric approaches (see Sect. 5.2 and Appendix "Additional Details of NN-Based Experiments").

Motivating Toy Example

In the toy example presented in Sect. 2.2, the r.v.s $X_1 \sim N(\mu_1, 1), X_2 \sim N(\mu_2, 1), \epsilon \sim N(0, 1/4)$. We choose $\mu_1 = 0$, $\beta_1 = 0.1$ for both domains; in target domain, we take $\mu_2 = 2$, $\beta_2 = -0.1$ and the causal effects are chosen as $\tau = -2/30 \approx -0.067$ and $\alpha = 0.1$; in source domain, we take $\mu_{2,\mathrm{s}} = 1$, $\beta_{2,\mathrm{s}} = -0.2$.

We randomly generate 2000 samples from the target domain, and the IPW estimate is –0.0531, which is pretty close to the ground truth ATE and validates the effectiveness of the IPW estimator. However, in our TCL setup, we consider limited target domain samples in that we can only observe the first 100 target domain samples, which yields a very biased IPW estimate: $\widehat{\tau}_{\mathrm{TO-CL}} = 0.0002$. Additionally, we observe 1000 randomly generated samples from the source domain, but we "do not know" whether or not the ATEs and the treatment assignment mechanisms are the same across both domains; apparently, in our toy example, treatment assignment mechanisms are different.

In this work, we aim to leverage the abundant source domain data to improve propensity score estimation via TL techniques. Since we do not assume the same ATEs in both domains, we evaluate the IPW estimator only using the target domain data. However, fitting the PS model using the naively merged datasets (i.e., without the TL techniques) would fail since the treatment assignment mechanisms across different domains are different: in our numerical example, this naive approach yields an IPW estimate $\widehat{\tau}_{\texttt{Merge-CL}} = 0.0441$, which is even more biased than only using target domain data. Our proposed ℓ_1-TCL does help yield a more accurate estimated ATE: $\widehat{\tau}_{\text{TLIPW}} = -0.0013$. This toy example tells us that additionally incorporating the source domain data "in a smart way" by using the TL technique does improve the IPW estimator's accuracy—we can now at least infer that there is an inhibiting causal effect from treatment Z to outcome Y.

Synthetic-Data Experiments

Next, we consider experiments with the GLM parametric approach under more settings. The goal is to simply demonstrate the effectiveness of the proposed ℓ_1-TCL framework compared with two baselines: solely using target domain data for causal learning, i.e., TO-CL, and naively merging both domains' datasets for causal learning, i.e., Merge-CL.

Experimental Configurations and Training Details

We generate synthetic data where the treatment assignment follows the GLM-based PS model (4) with randomly generated d-dimensional target domain nuisance parameters as well as s-sparse difference (from Gaussian distribution). The settings we consider include $d \in \{10, 20, 50, 75, 100\}$, $s \in \{1, 3, 5, 7, 10\}$, source domain sample size $n_{\text{S}} \in \{2000, 3000, 5000\}$, and target domain sample size $n \in \{100, 200, 500\}$. For demonstration purposes, the link function is chosen to be a sigmoid function and considered as a prior. This reduces the PS model fitting in the rough estimation step to naive logistic regression; in the ℓ_1 regularized bias correction step, we use gradient descent to optimize the objective function (7) with respect to the (sparse) difference, which has in total 8000 iterations and initial learning rate 0.02 (which decays by half every 2000 iterations). Hyperparameter λ_{PS} is chosen to maximize the treatment prediction area under the ROC curve (AUC) on a validation (target domain) dataset with size 50.

Results

Figure 5 reports the difference between average (over independent 100 trials) ATE estimation errors of our proposed and the baseline frameworks: positive values indicate improved accuracy, whereas negative values are all truncated to zeros for

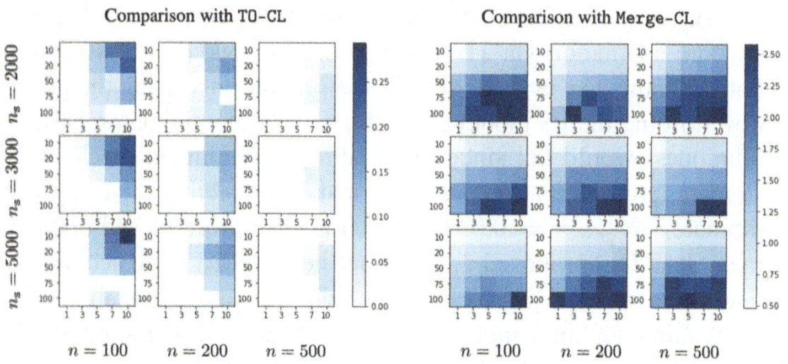

Fig. 5 Comparison between our proposed ℓ_1-TCL with TO-CL (left) and Merge-CL (right) baseline learning frameworks. In each sub-heatmap, the x-axis represents the sparsity s, and the y-axis represents the dimensionality d. We report the difference between the average ATE estimation errors of our proposed and the baseline frameworks: positive values indicate improved accuracy, whereas negative values are all truncated to zeros for better visualization

better visualization From the comparison with TO-CL (left panel), we can observe that ℓ_1-TCL yields more accurate ATEs for most considered experimental settings. Most importantly, we can observe that the benefit from our TL approach is the most significant when we have a limited amount of target domain data, and this benefit gradually disappears when we have an increasing amount of target domain data. From the comparison with Merge-CL (right panel), we can observe improved accuracy for almost all settings, verifying that Merge-CL is inherently flawed due to the different PS models between the target and source domain. In our semisynthetic data (or pseudo-real-data) experiment, we will not consider Merge-CL.

Additional Details of the Real-Data Example

Similar to our synthetic data experiments above, we again consider the GLM-based PS model and use the TLIPW estimator (8) in our ℓ_1-TCL framework; the hyperparameter is selected via a fivefold CV using target domain data based on maximum average treatment classification prediction AUC. As mentioned previously, we use vanilla logistic regression for rough estimation using source domain data, and in the ℓ_1 regularized bias correction step, we use gradient descent to optimize the objective function (7) with respect to the (sparse) difference. In our implementation of the bias correction step, we perform a grid search over `total number of iterations` $\in \{5000, 10000, 20000\}$, `initial learning rate` $\in \{0.05, 0.02, 0.01, 0.005, 0.001\}$, `learning rate decay ratio` $\in \{0.5, 0.8, 0.9, 0.95\}$, and ℓ_1 `regularization strength` $\log_{10} \lambda \in \{-2.5, -2.25, -2, \ldots, 0\}$. The learning rate decays every 1000 iterations.

For the bootstrap uncertainty quantification, we refit the model with a hyper-parameter reselected for each bootstrap sample; then, 90% confidence interval is constructed based on the 5% and 95% quantiles of the 200 bootstrap ATE estimates. Additionally, the mean and median of the bootstrap ATE estimates are reported.

Additional Details of NN-Based Experiments

Description of IHDP Dataset

The IHDP dataset was collected from an observational study in which the goal was to observe the impact of visits from a healthcare provider on children's cognitive development. Patients were placed in the treatment group if they received special care or home visits from a provider. A semisynthetic dataset was created from the original dataset by removing a nonrandom amount of the treatment group in order to induce treatment imbalance. The final cohort consists of 747 subjects, with 139 in the treatment group and 608 in the control group. Each subject contains 25 covariates, 6 of which are continuous, 19 of which are categorical (with 18 being binary and 1 having labels 0, 1, 2). These variables were collected from the child's measurements, the mother's behaviors during pregnancy, and the mother's measurements at the time of birth. The variables are detailed in Table 8. Complete details can be found in the original papers by Brooks-Gunn et al. [7], Hill [18], and the used dataset can be found in the open-source implementation.

Experimental Configurations and Training Details

The source-target domain partition is based on the 4-th categorical covariate, which yields $n_S = 546$ source domain sample (with labels 0) and $n = 201$ target domain samples (with labels 1). The rough estimation step in the nuisance parameter estimation stage is simply done by applying Dragonnet or TARNet fitting on the source domain data; subsequently, in the bias correction step, we randomly select 100 target domain samples as in-sample data, which are (randomly) decomposed into 70 training samples and 30 validation samples, and 101 out-of-sample testing

Table 8 List of covariates in the IHDP dataset

Type	Name
Child's measurements	Birth Weight, Head Circumference, Weeks Born Preterm, Birth Order, First Born, Neonatal Health Index, Sex, Twin Status
Behaviors observed during pregnancy	Smoked Cigarettes, Drank Alcohol, Took Drugs
Mother's measurements at time of birth	Age, Marital Status, Educational Attainment, Worked During Pregnancy, Received Prenatal Care, Resident Site at Start of Intervention

data. Formally, the nuisance parameter estimation stage of, for example, Dragonnet-based ℓ_1-TCL is done by

$$\underline{\text{Rough estimation for Dragonnet}}: \widehat{\theta}_{\text{s}} = \arg\min_{\theta} \mathcal{L}_{\text{Dragon}}(\theta; \mathcal{D}_{\text{s}}),$$

$$\underline{\text{Bias correction for Dragonnet}}: \widehat{\theta}_{\text{t}} = \widehat{\theta}_{\text{s}} + \arg\min_{\Delta} \mathcal{L}_{\text{Dragon}}(\Delta + \widehat{\theta}_{\text{s}}; \mathcal{D}_{\text{t}}) + \lambda \|\Delta\|_1,$$

where the objective function $\mathcal{L}_{\text{Dragon}}$ is defined in (21).

The primary goal is to compare three learning frameworks: `TO-CL`, `WS-TCL`, and our proposed ℓ_1-TCL. Additionally, we use the IPW, OR, and DR estimators for the downstream ATE estimation, which results in a total of nine *estimation procedures*; here, we call a specific learning framework coupled with a specific ATE estimator an estimation procedure (recall that an ATE estimator is defined as a specific nuisance model coupled with a specific plug-in estimator for ATE).

For `WS-TCL` as well as our proposed ℓ_1-TCL frameworks, the rough estimation step uses default NN hyperparameters in the open-source implementation. Notice that those hyperparameters may not be optimal for the rough estimation step using source domain data since the default hyperparameters are optimized using the full data; however, due to limited computational resources, we only consider the following hyperparameter selection based on grid search in the bias correction step: we consider `learning rate` $\in$ {1e-6, 2e-6, 5e-6, 1e-5, 2e-5, 5e-5, 1e-4, 1e-3} and `batch size` $\in$ {1, 3, 6, 16, 32, 64}; in particular, for our proposed ℓ_1-TCL, we also consider `regularization strength` $\lambda \in$ {1e-6, 5e-6, 1e-5, 5e-5, 1e-4, 1e-3, 1e-2, 1e-1, 5e-1, 1e1}. For a fair comparison, we additionally optimize the hyperparameter for the baseline `TO-CL` framework by considering `learning rate` $\in$ {1 e-6, 2e-6, 5e-6, 1e-5, 2e-5, 5e-5, 1e-4, 1e-3} and `batch size` $\in$ {1, 3, 6, 16, 32, 64}. We will show that, even with sub-optimal NN hyperparameters in the rough estimation steps, the TCL frameworks outperform the baseline `TO-CL` framework, verifying the necessity of using source domain data for accurate ATE estimation.

The hyperparameter selection criteria are NN regression loss, NN classification CE loss, and MSE. Again let us take Dragonnet as an example, slightly abuse the notation, and let $(\boldsymbol{x}_i, z_i, y_i)$, $i = 1, \ldots, n$ denote the validation target dataset, then the three aforementioned hyperparameter selection metrics are $\frac{1}{n}\sum_{i=1}^{n}\left(m_{z_i}(\theta; \boldsymbol{x}_i) - y_i\right)^2$, $\frac{1}{n}\sum_{i=1}^{n} \text{CE}\left(e(\theta; \boldsymbol{x}_i), z_i\right)$, and $\frac{1}{n}\sum_{i=1}^{n}\left(e(\theta; \boldsymbol{x}_i) - z_i\right)^2$.

Additional Results

Ablation Study on Hyperparameter Selection Criterion We report additional results using NN classification-based criteria in Table 9, where the column-wise

Table 9 Mean and standard deviation table using other hyperparameter selection criteria (specified on top of each sub-table) with the same source-target domain partition as in Table 6 but with fewer trials (to be precise, 50 trials) due to computing time consideration

Hyperparameter selected based on minimum NN regression loss on validation dataset						
	Dragonnet			3-Headed Variant of TARNet		
In-sample	IPW	OR	DR	IPW	OR	DR
TO-CL	$12.479_{(26.993)}$	$0.868_{(1.47)}$	$0.654_{(0.702)}$	$6.85_{(6.192)}$	$0.567_{(0.446)}$	$0.468_{(0.364)}$
WS-TCL	$6.414_{(9.667)}$	$0.534_{(0.552)}$	$0.572_{(0.636)}$	$3.502_{(4.101)}$	$0.413_{(0.313)}$	$0.359_{(0.22)}$
ℓ_1-TCL	$6.412_{(9.664)}$	$0.543_{(0.557)}$	$0.58_{(0.634)}$	$3.326_{(3.626)}$	$0.36_{(0.312)}$	$\mathbf{0.293}_{(0.222)}$
	Dragonnet			3-Headed Variant of TARNet		
Out-of-sample	IPW	OR	DR	IPW	OR	DR
TO-CL	$35.352_{(75.125)}$	$0.826_{(1.248)}$	$2.009_{(3.397)}$	$5.664_{(6.884)}$	$0.671_{(0.56)}$	$0.367_{(0.318)}$
WS-TCL	$17.684_{(20.993)}$	$0.512_{(0.586)}$	$1.324_{(1.492)}$	$4.204_{(6.092)}$	$0.476_{(0.399)}$	$0.339_{(0.289)}$
ℓ_1-TCL	$17.682_{(20.996)}$	$0.519_{(0.615)}$	$1.337_{(1.494)}$	$4.039_{(4.762)}$	$0.418_{(0.353)}$	$\mathbf{0.308}_{(0.251)}$
Hyperparameter selected based on minimum validation NN classification CE loss						
	Dragonnet			3-Headed Variant of TARNet		
In-sample	IPW	OR	DR	IPW	OR	DR
TO-CL	$11.411_{(30.657)}$	$0.615_{(0.773)}$	$0.675_{(0.649)}$	$3.926_{(4.234)}$	$0.768_{(0.545)}$	$0.464_{(0.365)}$
WS-TCL	$10.455_{(18.907)}$	$0.682_{(0.75)}$	$0.851_{(0.948)}$	$3.418_{(3.428)}$	$0.469_{(0.334)}$	$0.383_{(0.262)}$
ℓ_1-TCL	$11.781_{(27.023)}$	$0.813_{(1.123)}$	$0.907_{(1.135)}$	$4.012_{(6.241)}$	$0.328_{(0.245)}$	$\mathbf{0.326}_{(0.334)}$
	Dragonnet			3-Headed Variant of TARNet		
Out-of-sample	IPW	OR	DR	IPW	OR	DR
TO-CL	$32.228_{(45.735)}$	$0.629_{(0.548)}$	$1.513_{(1.627)}$	$4.144_{(5.009)}$	$0.806_{(0.641)}$	$0.433_{(0.482)}$
WS-TCL	$29.121_{(34.475)}$	$0.629_{(0.816)}$	$2.535_{(4.217)}$	$4.371_{(5.18)}$	$0.529_{(0.484)}$	$\mathbf{0.349}_{(0.339)}$
ℓ_1-TCL	$33.303_{(54.411)}$	$0.746_{(0.951)}$	$2.639_{(3.806)}$	$5.779_{(9.668)}$	$0.426_{(0.33)}$	$0.35_{(0.429)}$
Hyperparameter selected based on minimum validation NN classification MSE						
	Dragonnet			3-Headed Variant of TARNet		
In-sample	IPW	OR	DR	IPW	OR	DR
TO-CL	$10.116_{(24.513)}$	$0.767_{(1.077)}$	$1.033_{(1.075)}$	$4.647_{(5.418)}$	$0.607_{(0.539)}$	$0.474_{(0.322)}$
WS-TCL	$8.342_{(13.545)}$	$0.664_{(0.868)}$	$0.719_{(0.789)}$	$3.77_{(5.429)}$	$0.589_{(0.431)}$	$0.408_{(0.296)}$
ℓ_1-TCL	$8.249_{(13.454)}$	$0.623_{(0.848)}$	$0.704_{(0.759)}$	$4.012_{(6.241)}$	$0.328_{(0.245)}$	$\mathbf{0.326}_{(0.334)}$
	Dragonnet			3-Headed Variant of TARNet		
Out-of-sample	IPW	OR	DR	IPW	OR	DR
TO-CL	$31.608_{(55.768)}$	$0.743_{(0.892)}$	$2.261_{(3.283)}$	$4.764_{(6.154)}$	$0.739_{(0.715)}$	$0.383_{(0.384)}$
WS-TCL	$26.398_{(47.011)}$	$0.663_{(1.014)}$	$1.711_{(2.249)}$	$5.437_{(8.29)}$	$0.73_{(0.698)}$	$0.451_{(0.569)}$
ℓ_1-TCL	$25.786_{(46.738)}$	$0.661_{(0.947)}$	$1.666_{(2.185)}$	$5.779_{(9.668)}$	$0.426_{(0.33)}$	$\mathbf{0.35}_{(0.429)}$

best results are highlighted with a green background color, indicating the best learning framework for the corresponding ATE estimator, and the smallest error is highlighted in bold font, indicating the overall best estimation procedure. Results in Table 9 exhibit similar patterns as shown in Table 9 that TL, especially our proposed ℓ_1-TCL, generally helps improve ATE estimation accuracy, and IPW estimators do not perform well. Furthermore, as we can see from Table 9 in the case where WS-TCL outperforms our proposed ℓ_1-TCL, such as the out-of-sample accuracy for TARNet-DR ATE estimator in the "NN classification CE loss" sub-table, the improvement of WS-TCL is typically marginal; in contrast, when ℓ_1-TCL performs the best, the improvement is significant; see, e.g., the rest TARNet-OR and TARNet-DR ATE estimators in both sub-tables of Tables 9.

Ablation Study on Different Source-Target Domain Partition In addition, we consider another (randomly selected) binary covariate for the source-target domain partition, which is the 8-th categorical covariate and yields $n_s = 642$ source domain sample (with labels 0) and $n = 105$ target domain samples (with labels 1). The (random) train-validation split gives 73 training samples (that is why we choose the largest batch size grid to be 64) and 32 validation samples. We repeat the same experiments and report the results in Table 10.

In Table 10, we can observe similar patterns as mentioned before: the best in-sample performance is 0.352, which is given by TARNet-DR estimator using proposed ℓ_1-TCL, and it is much better than the best WS-TCL in-sample performance, which is 0.375 also given by TARNet-DR estimator. In contrast, even though WS-TCL yields the best out-of-sample performance via TARNet-OR estimator (0.623), there is only a marginal increment compared to that of ℓ_1-TCL (0.627). Additionally, the best out-of-sample performance of ℓ_1-TCL is still given by the NN regression loss selection criterion, which is consistent with previous findings.

Additional Evaluation Metrics Lastly, since both WS-TCL and ℓ_1-TCL are sensitive to the choice of hyperparameters, there will be cases/trials where the optimal empirical option of not covered by the pre-defined grid, leading to unfavorable results. Since our ℓ_1-TCL has one additional hyperparameter, i.e., the regularization strength, such effect will be amplified for ℓ_1-TCL given the limited computation resources when we perform grid search for hyperparameter selections. Therefore, we report the median and interquartile range of the aforementioned experiments using 8-th categorical covariate for source-target domain partition in Table 11, which shows that both the in-sample and out-of-sample best (in terms of median) estimates are given by our ℓ_1-TCL. Overall all results above support the effectiveness of our proposed ℓ_1-TCL framework.

An Alternative Hyperparameter Selection Criterion

Recently, [29] found that proper hyperparameter tuning can sometimes close the performance gap among different ATE estimators. The challenge is that a "golden standard," such as prediction accuracy in classic supervised learning, is largely missing since we cannot evaluate the causal effect estimation accuracy from data due to unobserved counterfactual outcomes. Unfortunately, there is no good solution beyond the recent empirical analysis of some nuisance model prediction

Table 10 Additional absolute error mean and standard deviation table for all aforementioned hyperparameter selection criteria (specified on top of each sub-table) using the different (from that of Table 9) source-target domain partition

Hyperparameter selected based on minimum validation NN regression loss						
	Dragonnet			3-Headed Variant of TARNet		
In-sample	IPW	OR	DR	IPW	OR	DR
TO-CL	5.752 (14.189)	0.572 (0.483)	0.592 (0.775)	5.713 (9.2)	0.466 (0.406)	0.457 (0.434)
WS-TCL	6.448 (10.771)	0.572 (0.463)	0.675 (1.08)	1.703 (2.018)	0.44 (0.362)	**0.375** (0.291)
ℓ_1-TCL	5.376 (9.682)	0.477 (0.526)	0.526 (0.884)	1.697 (2.017)	0.448 (0.362)	0.376 (0.292)
	Dragonnet			3-Headed Variant of TARNet		
Out-of-sample	IPW	OR	DR	IPW	OR	DR
TO-CL	16.704 (24.684)	0.89 (1.05)	1.927 (3.917)	9.916 (12.285)	0.736 (0.811)	0.685 (0.851)
WS-TCL	21.43 (22.895)	0.821 (1.105)	2.252 (2.92)	7.699 (12.458)	**0.623** (0.908)	0.723 (1.089)
ℓ_1-TCL	18.03 (21.948)	0.731 (1.318)	1.661 (2.259)	7.703 (12.46)	0.627 (0.906)	0.724 (1.084)
Hyperparameter selected based on minimum validation NN classification CE loss						
	Dragonnet			3-Headed Variant of TARNet		
In-sample	IPW	OR	DR	IPW	OR	DR
TO-CL	5.752 (14.189)	0.572 (0.483)	0.592 (0.775)	6.302 (12.42)	0.516 (0.47)	0.496 (0.703)
WS-TCL	6.448 (10.771)	0.572 (0.463)	0.675 (1.08)	1.703 (2.018)	0.44 (0.362)	0.375 (0.291)
ℓ_1-TCL	6.442 (10.761)	0.577 (0.466)	0.677 (1.139)	2.056 (2.331)	0.446 (0.449)	**0.352** (0.314)
	Dragonnet			3-Headed Variant of TARNet		
Out-of-sample	IPW	OR	DR	IPW	OR	DR
TO-CL	16.704 (24.684)	0.89 (1.05)	1.927 (3.917)	10.353 (15.414)	0.878 (1.185)	0.782 (1.099)
WS-TCL	21.43 (22.895)	0.821 (1.105)	2.252 (2.92)	7.699 (12.458)	**0.623** (0.908)	0.723 (1.089)
ℓ_1-TCL	21.41 (22.875)	0.822 (1.114)	2.272 (2.948)	8.048 (13.393)	0.632 (0.809)	0.696 (0.917)
Hyperparameter selected based on minimum validation NN classification MSE						
	Dragonnet			3-Headed Variant of TARNet		
In-sample	IPW	OR	DR	IPW	OR	DR
TO-CL	5.752 (14.189)	0.572 (0.483)	0.592 (0.775)	6.302 (12.42)	0.516 (0.47)	0.496 (0.703)
WS-TCL	6.448 (10.771)	0.572 (0.463)	0.675 (1.08)	1.703 (2.018)	0.44 (0.362)	0.375 (0.291)
ℓ_1-TCL	6.441 (10.761)	0.576 (0.465)	0.677 (1.134)	2.056 (2.331)	0.446 (0.449)	**0.352** (0.314)
	Dragonnet			3-Headed Variant of TARNet		
Out-of-sample	IPW	OR	DR	IPW	OR	DR
TO-CL	16.704 (24.684)	0.89 (1.05)	1.927 (3.917)	10.353 (15.414)	0.878 (1.185)	0.782 (1.099)
WS-TCL	21.43 (22.895)	0.821 (1.105)	2.252 (2.92)	7.699 (12.458)	**0.623** (0.908)	0.723 (1.089)
ℓ_1-TCL	21.408 (22.875)	0.822 (1.112)	2.271 (2.946)	8.048 (13.393)	0.632 (0.809)	0.696 (0.917)

performance metrics (which is what we use in the above experiments) as the selection criteria [1, 13, 29].

Here, we "propose" one additional solution by studying the covariate distribution balances via Standard Mean Difference (SMD); indeed, SMD has been used to access the goodness-of-fit of PS models in causal inference in various applications, such as [72]. The SMD is defined using the Cohen's d.

Table 11 Median and interquartile range ([Q1, Q3], where Q1 and Q3 stand for the 25% and 75% quantiles) of absolute errors of estimated causal effects over 50 IHDP datasets for all aforementioned hyperparameter selection criteria (specified on top of each sub-table). The source-target domain partition is the same with that of Table 10

Hyperparameter selected based on minimum validation NN regression loss						
	Dragonnet			3-Headed Variant of TARNet		
In-sample	IPW	OR	DR	IPW	OR	DR
TO-CL	$2.46_{[1.175,5.219]}$	$0.481_{[0.244,0.657]}$	$0.303_{[0.185,0.676]}$	$3.097_{[2.196,5.591]}$	$0.383_{[0.149,0.611]}$	$0.345_{[0.163,0.617]}$
WS-TCL	$3.212_{[1.411,6.828]}$	$0.46_{[0.291,0.717]}$	$0.433_{[0.192,0.731]}$	$1.086_{[0.512,1.851]}$	$0.338_{[0.165,0.662]}$	$0.289_{[0.141,0.547]}$
ℓ_1-TCL	$2.048_{[1.251,5.817]}$	$0.339_{[0.155,0.589]}$	$\mathbf{0.288}_{[0.112,0.593]}$	$1.086_{[0.511,1.784]}$	$0.353_{[0.159,0.659]}$	$0.289_{[0.142,0.542]}$
	Dragonnet			3-Headed Variant of TARNet		
Out-of-sample	IPW	OR	DR	IPW	OR	DR
TO-CL	$9.297_{[3.413,14.861]}$	$0.587_{[0.296,0.979]}$	$0.835_{[0.277,1.876]}$	$5.068_{[2.957,12.122]}$	$0.451_{[0.22,0.87]}$	$0.452_{[0.199,0.825]}$
WS-TCL	$15.119_{[4.856,27.383]}$	$0.513_{[0.286,0.901]}$	$0.979_{[0.547,2.246]}$	$3.636_{[0.973,10.543]}$	$0.425_{[0.121,0.764]}$	$0.399_{[0.157,0.897]}$
ℓ_1-TCL	$12.953_{[5.219,19.517]}$	$\mathbf{0.368}_{[0.183,0.737]}$	$0.862_{[0.457,1.982]}$	$3.636_{[0.97,10.543]}$	$0.426_{[0.127,0.762]}$	$0.395_{[0.163,0.958]}$
Hyperparameter selected based on minimum validation NN classification CE loss						
	Dragonnet			3-Headed Variant of TARNet		
In-sample	IPW	OR	DR	IPW	OR	DR
TO-CL	$2.46_{[1.175,5.219]}$	$0.481_{[0.244,0.657]}$	$0.303_{[0.185,0.676]}$	$2.699_{[2.089,4.958]}$	$0.359_{[0.245,0.586]}$	$0.315_{[0.162,0.58]}$
WS-TCL	$3.212_{[1.411,6.828]}$	$0.46_{[0.291,0.717]}$	$0.433_{[0.192,0.731]}$	$1.086_{[0.512,1.851]}$	$0.338_{[0.165,0.662]}$	$0.289_{[0.141,0.547]}$
ℓ_1-TCL	$3.215_{[1.406,6.861]}$	$0.461_{[0.298,0.719]}$	$0.43_{[0.195,0.702]}$	$1.187_{[0.705,2.253]}$	$0.309_{[0.196,0.55]}$	$\mathbf{0.27}_{[0.096,0.477]}$
	Dragonnet			3-Headed Variant of TARNet		
Out-of-sample	IPW	OR	DR	IPW	OR	DR
TO-CL	$9.297_{[3.413,14.861]}$	$0.587_{[0.296,0.979]}$	$0.835_{[0.277,1.876]}$	$5.103_{[2.116,11.363]}$	$0.541_{[0.362,0.813]}$	$0.51_{[0.258,0.719]}$
WS-TCL	$15.119_{[4.856,27.383]}$	$0.513_{[0.286,0.901]}$	$0.979_{[0.547,2.246]}$	$3.636_{[0.973,10.543]}$	$0.425_{[0.121,0.764]}$	$0.399_{[0.157,0.897]}$
ℓ_1-TCL	$15.117_{[4.856,27.358]}$	$0.514_{[0.266,0.891]}$	$0.976_{[0.593,2.275]}$	$3.781_{[0.832,11.022]}$	$\mathbf{0.361}_{[0.193,0.76]}$	$0.429_{[0.201,0.748]}$

TO-CL	$2.46_{[1.175,5.219]}$	$0.481_{[0.244,0.657]}$	$0.303_{[0.185,0.676]}$	$2.699_{[2.089,4.958]}$	$0.359_{[0.245,0.586]}$	$0.315_{[0.162,0.58]}$
WS-TCL	$3.212_{[1.411,6.828]}$	$0.46_{[0.291,0.717]}$	$0.433_{[0.192,0.731]}$	$1.086_{[0.512,1.851]}$	$0.338_{[0.165,0.662]}$	$0.289_{[0.141,0.547]}$
ℓ_1-TCL	$3.215_{[1.405,6.859]}$	$0.461_{[0.299,0.719]}$	$0.43_{[0.194,0.702]}$	$1.187_{[0.705,2.253]}$	$0.309_{[0.196,0.55]}$	$\mathbf{0.27}_{[0.096,0.477]}$
	Dragonnet			3-Headed Variant of TARNet		
Out-of-sample	IPW	OR	DR	IPW	OR	DR
TO-CL	$9.297_{[3.413,14.861]}$	$0.587_{[0.296,0.979]}$	$0.835_{[0.277,1.876]}$	$5.103_{[2.116,11.363]}$	$0.541_{[0.362,0.813]}$	$0.51_{[0.258,0.719]}$
WS-TCL	$15.119_{[4.856,27.383]}$	$0.513_{[0.286,0.901]}$	$0.979_{[0.547,2.246]}$	$3.636_{[0.973,10.543]}$	$0.425_{[0.121,0.764]}$	$0.399_{[0.157,0.897]}$
ℓ_1-TCL	$15.116_{[4.852,27.351]}$	$0.514_{[0.265,0.892]}$	$0.974_{[0.593,2.275]}$	$3.781_{[0.832,11.022]}$	$\mathbf{0.361}_{[0.193,0.76]}$	$0.429_{[0.201,0.748]}$

Table 12 Absolute error mean and standard deviation for SMD as the hyperparameter selection criterion; the ATE estimator is chosen as the three-headed variant of TARNet coupled with the DR estimator, which has the best performance as shown in Table 6. The above table further establishes the superior performance of our ℓ_1-TCL framework. Moreover, as the above table shows the overall best performance compared with results in Table 6, it also established the potential of SMD as the hyperparameter selection criterion or goodness-of-fit score

	TO-CL	WS-TCL	ℓ_1-TCL
In-sample	$0.415_{(0.385)}$	$0.337_{(0.273)}$	$\mathbf{0.277}_{(0.222)}$
Out-of-sample	$0.421_{(0.467)}$	$0.324_{(0.282)}$	$\mathbf{0.301}_{(0.252)}$

Definition 4 (Cohen's d) Given two sets of samples $\mathcal{A} = \{a_i,\ i = 1, \ldots, m\}$ and $\mathcal{B} = \{b_j,\ j = 1, \ldots, n\}$, the Cohen's d is defined as follows:

$$\mathrm{d}_{\text{Cohen}}(\mathcal{A}, \mathcal{B}) = (\bar{a} - \bar{b}) \Big/ \sqrt{\frac{S_{\mathcal{A}}^2 + S_{\mathcal{B}}^2}{2}},$$

where $\bar{a} = \sum_{i=1}^{m} a_i/m,\ \bar{b} = \sum_{i=1}^{n} b_j/n$, and the pooled sample variance can be calculated as

$$S_{\mathcal{A}} = \frac{1}{m}\sum_{i=1}^{m}(a_i - \bar{a})^2, \quad S_{\mathcal{B}} = \frac{1}{n}\sum_{j=1}^{n}\left(b_j - \bar{b}\right)^2.$$

When the Cohen's d's absolute value is close to zero, the standardized means of two distributions are similar to each other, i.e., the covariates' distributions are balanced. In our multivariate setting, we can simply use the average of the absolute Cohen's d's as the selection criterion. That is, the SMD selection criterion is defined as

$$\mathrm{SMD} = \frac{1}{d}\sum_{j=1}^{d}\left|\mathrm{d}_{\text{Cohen}}\left(\{\boldsymbol{x}(j) : \boldsymbol{x} \in \mathcal{D}_{\boldsymbol{x},\,\text{trt}}\}, \{\boldsymbol{x}(j) : \boldsymbol{x} \in \mathcal{D}_{\boldsymbol{x},\,\text{ctrl}}\}\right)\right|,$$

where $\boldsymbol{x}(j)$ is the j-th element of the vector $\boldsymbol{x} \in \mathbb{R}^d$, and

$$\mathcal{D}_{\boldsymbol{x},\,\text{trt}} = \left\{\frac{\boldsymbol{x}_i}{\widehat{e}(\boldsymbol{x}_i)} : z_i = 1\right\}, \quad \mathcal{D}_{\boldsymbol{x},\,\text{ctrl}} = \left\{\frac{\boldsymbol{x}_i}{1 - \widehat{e}(\boldsymbol{x}_i)} : z_i = 0\right\}.$$

This above metric tells us the average standardized mean difference after propensity score weighting.

Now, we report the results on comparison among different learning frameworks with SMD as the hyperparameter selection metric in Table 12.

Appendix E: Extended Discussion

The successful application of ℓ_1 regularized TL in causal inference suggests its potential in handling real problems with limited data, and our ℓ_1-TCL can benefit from the following improvements:

- As discussed at the end of Sect. 4, developing a principled approach for UQ in the TCL problem can be a future direction. For example, [22] recently introduced a new CI construction approach for GLM using a relatively novel concentration result of vector fields. This may facilitate the construction of CI of the nuisance parameters and, hence, the causal effect through the unbiased plug-in estimators.
- Recently, statistics literature has witnessed a surge of theoretically grounded TL approaches due to their empirical success, and these principled approaches could be readily adapted to the novel TCL problem; for example, TL for nonparametric regression [8, 27] and high-dimensional Gaussian graphical models [25] might be applied to causal effect estimation and causal graph discovery [36, 49], respectively.
- The principled method for multisource TL problem developed by Tian and Feng [54] may help improve our `ParT` approach, as a principled method to verify the transferability of knowledge from the source domains is still missing. This extension is natural when the covariate space is partitioned using a categorical covariate with three or more labels.
- It would be rather interesting to extend the `ParT` framework for CATE estimation (introduced in Sect. 5.1) to "Partition-Transfer-Reconcile": Inspired by the forecasting reconciliation [64], one might be able to develop a reconciliation constraint on the CATEs in the subgroups subject to the ATE of the whole dataset, estimated using some sophisticated models (e.g., NN-based model).
- Lastly, the ℓ_1 regularized TL discussed in this work might be extended to convex causal graph discovery using GLMs [60].

References

1. Athey, S., Imbens, G.: Recursive partitioning for heterogeneous causal effects. Proc. Natl. Acad. Sci. **113**(27), 7353–7360 (2016)
2. Avni, T., Lador, A., Lev, S., Leibovici, L., Paul, M., Grossman, A.: Vasopressors for the treatment of septic shock: systematic review and meta-analysis. PLoS ONE **10**, e0129305 (2015)
3. Bang, H., Robins, J.M.: Doubly robust estimation in missing data and causal inference models. Biometrics **61**(4), 962–973 (2005)
4. Bastani, H.: Predicting with proxies: transfer learning in high dimension. Manage. Sci. **67**(5), 2964–2984 (2021)
5. Bica, I., van der Schaar, M.: Transfer learning on heterogeneous feature spaces for treatment effects estimation. Adv. Neural Inf. Proces. Syst. **35**, 37184–37198 (2022)
6. Bickel, P.J., Ritov, Y., Tsybakov, A.B.: Simultaneous analysis of lasso and dantzig selector. Ann. Stat. **37**, 1705–1732 (2009)

7. Brooks-Gunn, J., Liaw, F.-r., Klebanov, P.K.: Effects of early intervention on cognitive function of low birth weight preterm infants. J. Pediatr. **120**(3), 350–359 (1992)
8. Cai, T.T., Pu, H.: Transfer learning for nonparametric regression: non-asymptotic minimax analysis and adaptive procedure (2022)
9. Candes, E., Tao, T.: The dantzig selector: statistical estimation when p is much larger than n. Ann. Stat. **35**(6), 2313–2351 (2007)
10. Chen, Y., Bühlmann, P.: Domain adaptation under structural causal models. J. Mach. Learn. Res. **22**(1), 11856–11935 (2021)
11. Cole, S.R., Stuart, E.A.: Generalizing evidence from randomized clinical trials to target populations: the actg 320 trial. Am. J. Epidemiol. **172**(1), 107–115 (2010)
12. Curth, A., van der Schaar, M.: Nonparametric estimation of heterogeneous treatment effects: from theory to learning algorithms. In: International Conference on Artificial Intelligence and Statistics, pp. 1810–1818. PMLR (2021)
13. Curth, A., van der Schaar, M.: In search of insights, not magic bullets: towards demystification of the model selection dilemma in heterogeneous treatment effect estimation. In: International Conference on Machine Learning, pp. 6623–6642. PMLR (2023)
14. Daume III, H.: Frustratingly easy domain adaptation. In: Proceedings of the 45th Annual Meeting of the Association of Computational Linguistics, 2007, pp. 256–263 (2007)
15. Evgeniou, T., Pontil, M.: Regularized multi–task learning. In: Proceedings of the Tenth ACM SIGKDD International Conference on Knowledge Discovery and Data Mining, pp. 109–117 (2004)
16. Hartman, E., Grieve, R., Ramsahai, R., Sekhon, J.S.: From sample average treatment effect to population average treatment effect on the treated: combining experimental with observational studies to estimate population treatment effects. J. R. Stat. Soc. Ser. A: Stat. Soc. **178**(3),757–778 (2015)
17. Hatt, T., Berrevoets, J., Curth, A., Feuerriegel, S., van der Schaar, M.: Combining observational and randomized data for estimating heterogeneous treatment effects. Preprint. arXiv:2202.12891 (2022)
18. Hill, J.L.: Bayesian nonparametric modeling for causal inference. J. Comput. Graph. Stat. **20**(1), 217–240 (2011)
19. Horvitz, D.G., Thompson, D.J.: A generalization of sampling without replacement from a finite universe. J. Am. Stat. Assoc. **47**(260), 663–685 (1952)
20. Hosny, K.M., Kassem, M.A., Foaud, M.M.: Skin cancer classification using deep learning and transfer learning. In: 2018 9th Cairo International Biomedical Engineering Conference (CIBEC), pp. 90–93. IEEE, Piscataway (2018)
21. Hu, Y., Li, M., Lu, Q., Weng, H., Wang, J., Zekavat, S.M., Yu, Z., Li, B., Gu, J., Muchnik, S., et al.: A statistical framework for cross-tissue transcriptome-wide association analysis. Nat. Genet. **51**(3), 568–576 (2019)
22. Juditsky, A., Nemirovski, A., Xie, Y., Xu, C.: Generalized generalized linear models: Convex estimation and online bounds. Preprint. arXiv:2304.13793 (2023)
23. Keller, B., Kim, J.-S., Steiner, P.M.: Neural networks for propensity score estimation: simulation results and recommendations. In: Quantitative Psychology Research: The 79th Annual Meeting of the Psychometric Society, Madison, Wisconsin, 2014, pp. 279–291. Springer, Berlin (2015)
24. Künzel, S.R., Stadie, B.C., Vemuri, N., Ramakrishnan, V., Sekhon, J.S., Abbeel, P.: Transfer learning for estimating causal effects using neural networks. Preprint. arXiv:1808.07804 (2018)
25. Li, S., Cai, T.T., Li, H.: Transfer learning for high-dimensional linear regression: prediction, estimation and minimax optimality. J. R. Stat. Soc. Ser. B: Stat. Methodol. **84**(1), 149–173 (2022)
26. Li, S., Zhang, L., Cai, T.T., Li, H.: Estimation and inference for high-dimensional generalized linear models with knowledge transfer. J. Am. Stat. Assoc., pp. 1–12 (2023)
27. Lin, L., Li, W.: Source-function weighted-transfer learning for nonparametric regression with seemingly similar sources. Preprint. arXiv:2302.11222 (2023)

28. Lunceford, J.K., Davidian, M.: Stratification and weighting via the propensity score in estimation of causal treatment effects: a comparative study. Stat. Med. **23**(19), 2937–2960 (2004)
29. Machlanski, D., Samothrakis, S., Clarke, P.: Hyperparameter tuning and model evaluation in causal effect estimation. Preprint. arXiv:2303.01412 (2023)
30. Magliacane, S., Van Ommen, T., Claassen, T., Bongers, S., Versteeg, P., Mooij, J.M.: Domain adaptation by using causal inference to predict invariant conditional distributions. Adv. Neural Inf. Proces. Syst. **31**, 10846–10856 (2018)
31. Mei, S., Fei, W., Zhou, S.: Gene ontology based transfer learning for protein subcellular localization. BMC Bioinf. **12**, 1–12 (2011)
32. Meinshausen, N., Yu, B.: Lasso-type recovery of sparse representations for high-dimensional data. Ann. Stat. **37**(1), 246–270 (2009)
33. Nelder, J.A., Wedderburn, R.W.M.: Generalized linear models. J. R. Stat. Soc.: Ser. A (Gener.) **135**(3), 370–384 (1972)
34. Pan, S.J., Yang, Q.: A survey on transfer learning. IEEE Trans. Knowl. Data Eng. **22**(10), 1345–1359 (2010)
35. Pan, W., Yang, Q.: Transfer learning in heterogeneous collaborative filtering domains. Artif. Intell. **197**, 39–55 (2013)
36. Pearl, J.: Causality. Cambridge University Press, Cambridge (2009)
37. Pirracchio, R., Petersen, M.L., Van Der Laan, M.: Improving propensity score estimators' robustness to model misspecification using super learner. Am. J. Epidemiol. **181**(2), 108–119 (2015)
38. Robins, J.M., Rotnitzky, A., Zhao, L.P.: Estimation of regression coefficients when some regressors are not always observed. J Am. Stat. Assoc. **89**(427), 846–866 (1994)
39. Robins, J.M., Hernan, M.A., Brumback, B.: Marginal structural models and causal inference in epidemiology. Epidemiology **11**, 550–560 (2000)
40. Rojas-Carulla, M., Schölkopf, B., Turner, R., Peters, J.: Invariant models for causal transfer learning. J. Mach. Learn. Res. **19**(1), 1309–1342 (2018)
41. Rosenbaum, P.R., Rubin, D.B.: The central role of the propensity score in observational studies for causal effects. Biometrika **70**(1), 41–55 (1983)
42. Rotnitzky, A., Robins, J.M., Scharfstein, D.O.: Semiparametric regression for repeated outcomes with nonignorable nonresponse. J. Am. Stat. Assoc. **93**(444), 1321–1339 (1998)
43. Rubin, D.B.: Estimating causal effects of treatments in randomized and nonrandomized studies. J. Educ. Psychol. **66**(5), 688 (1974)
44. Scharfstein, D.O., Rotnitzky, A., Robins, J.M.: Adjusting for nonignorable drop-out using semiparametric nonresponse models. J. Am. Stat. Assoc. **94**(448), 1096–1120 (1999)
45. Sevakula, R.K., Singh, V., Verma, N.K., Kumar, C., Cui, Y.: Transfer learning for molecular cancer classification using deep neural networks. IEEE/ACM Trans. Comput. Biol. Bioinf. **16**(6), 2089–2100 (2018)
46. Shalit, U., Johansson, F.D., Sontag, D.: Estimating individual treatment effect: generalization bounds and algorithms. In: International Conference on Machine Learning, pp. 3076–3085. PMLR (2017)
47. Shi, C., Blei, D., Veitch, V.: Adapting neural networks for the estimation of treatment effects. Adv. Neural Inf. Proces. Syst. **32**, 2507–2517 (2019)
48. Shin, H.-C., Roth, H.R., Gao, M., Lu, L., Xu, Z., Nogues, I., Yao, J., Mollura, D., Summers, R.M.: Deep convolutional neural networks for computer-aided detection: CNN architectures, dataset characteristics and transfer learning. IEEE Trans. Med. Imaging **35**(5), 1285–1298 (2016)
49. Spirtes, P., Glymour, C., Scheines, R., Kauffman, S., Aimale, V., Wimberly, F.: Constructing bayesian network models of gene expression networks from microarray data: In Proceedings of the Atlantic Symposium on Computational Biology, Genome Information Systems and Technology, Duke University, Durham, NC, USA (2001)
50. Splawa-Neyman, J., Dabrowska, D.M., Speed, T.P.: On the application of probability theory to agricultural experiments. Essay on principles. Section 9. Stat. Sci. **5**, 465–472 (1990)

51. Sriperumbudur, B.K., Fukumizu, K., Gretton, A., B. Schölkopf, Lanckriet, G.R.G.: On the empirical estimation of integral probability metrics. Electr. J. Stat. **6**, 1550–1599 (2012)
52. Stevenson, E.K., Rubenstein, A.R., Radin, G.T., Wiener, R.S., Walkey, A.J.: Two decades of mortality trends among patients with severe sepsis: a comparative meta-analysis. Crit. Care Med. **42**, 625–631 (2014)
53. Sun, Y.V., Hu, Y.-J.: Integrative analysis of multi-omics data for discovery and functional studies of complex human diseases. Adv. Genet. **93**, 147–190 (2016)
54. Tian, Y., Feng, Y.: Transfer learning under high-dimensional generalized linear models. J. Am. Stat. Assoc. **117**, 1–14 (2022)
55. Torrey, L., Shavlik, J.: Transfer learning. In: Handbook of Research on Machine Learning Applications and Trends: Algorithms, Methods, and Techniques, pp. 242–264. IGI Global, Hershey (2010)
56. Turki, T., Wei, Z., Wang, J.T.L.: Transfer learning approaches to improve drug sensitivity prediction in multiple myeloma patients. IEEE Access **5**, 7381–7393 (2017)
57. Tzeng, E., Hoffman, J., Saenko, K., Darrell, T.: Adversarial discriminative domain adaptation. In: Proceedings of the IEEE Conference on Computer Vision and Pattern Recognition, pp. 7167–7176 (2017)
58. van de Geer, S.A., Bühlmann, P.: On the conditions used to prove oracle results for the Lasso. Electr. J. Stat. **3**, 1360–1392 (2009)
59. Wang, S., Shi, X., Wu, M., Ma, S.: Horizontal and vertical integrative analysis methods for mental disorders omics data. Sci. Rep. **9**(1), 1–12 (2019)
60. Wei, S., Xie, Y., Josef, C.S., Kamaleswaran, R.: Causal graph discovery from self and mutually exciting time series. IEEE J. Select. Areas Inf. Theory **4**, 747–761 (2023). https://doi.org/10.1109/JSAIT.2023.3342569
61. Wei, S., Xie, Y., Josef, C.S., Kamaleswaran, R.: Granger causal chain discovery for sepsis-associated derangements via continuous-time hawkes processes. In: *Proceedings of the 29th ACM SIGKDD Conference on Knowledge Discovery and Data Mining*, pp. 2536–2546 (2023).
62. Weiss, K., Khoshgoftaar, T.M., Wang, D.D.: A survey of transfer learning. J. Big Data **3**(1), 1–40 (2016)
63. Westreich, D., Lessler, J., Funk, M.J.: Propensity score estimation: neural networks, support vector machines, decision trees (cart), and meta-classifiers as alternatives to logistic regression. J. Clin. Epidemiol. **63**(8), 826–833 (2010)
64. Wickramasuriya, S.L., Athanasopoulos, G., Hyndman, R.J.: Optimal forecast reconciliation for hierarchical and grouped time series through trace minimization. J. Am. Stat. Assoc. **114**(526), 804–819 (2019)
65. Wooldridge, J.M.: Inverse probability weighted estimation for general missing data problems. J. Econometr. 141(2), 1281–1301 (2007)
66. Wooldridge, J.M. et al.: Inverse probability weighted m-estimators for sample selection, attrition, and stratification. Portuguese Econ. J. **1**(2), 117–139 (2002)
67. Wu, L., Yang, S.: Transfer learning of individualized treatment rules from experimental to real-world data. J. Comput. Graph. Stat. **31**, 1–10 (2022)
68. Yang, S., Ding, P.: Combining multiple observational data sources to estimate causal effects. J. Am. Stat. Assoc. **115**(531), 1540–1554 (2020)
69. Yang, S., Yu, K., Cao, F., Liu, L., Wang, H., Li, J.: Learning causal representations for robust domain adaptation. IEEE Trans. Knowl. Data Eng. **34**(3), 1430–1442 (2022)
70. Yao, L., Chu, Z., Li, S., Li, Y., Gao, J., Zhang, A.: A survey on causal inference. ACM Trans. Knowl. Discov. Data (TKDD) **15**(5), 1–46 (2021)
71. Zhang, K., Gong, M., Schölkopf, B.: Multi-source domain adaptation: a causal view. In: Proceedings of the AAAI Conference on Artificial Intelligence, vol. 29 (2015)
72. Zhang, Z., Kim, H.J., Lonjon, G., Zhu, Y., et al.: Balance diagnostics after propensity score matching. Ann. Transl. Med. **7**(1), 16:1–6 (2019)
73. Zhuang, F., Qi, Z., Duan, K., Xi, D., Zhu, Y., Zhu, H., Xiong, H., He, Q.: A comprehensive survey on transfer learning. Proc. IEEE **109**(1), 43–76 (2020)

Hybrid Distance for Classification of Complex Biological Data Based on Elastic Shape Analysis of Curves and Topological Data Analysis of Point Clouds

Ye Jin Choi, Karthik Bharath, and Sebastian Kurtek

Abstract Complex data structures are now prevalent in biological applications. Statistical analysis of such data requires sophisticated representations and distances that can be used for their comparison and subsequent modeling. To this end, we propose a hybrid distance for classification of complex biological data objects that is able to capture shape variation of disparate components making up the objects. In particular, the hybrid distance quantifies shape differences in a curve component and topo-geometric differences in a point cloud component composing the complex object under study. For the curve component, we leverage a shape distance originating from the elastic shape analysis framework, which allows for computationally efficient and natural quantification of shape differences. For the point cloud component, we use the bottleneck distance between persistence diagrams, which capture birth and death times of topological features in the point clouds; as such, this distance captures complementary shape features of the data objects under study. To define the hybrid distance, the two individual distances are integrated with an appropriate weight parameter that allows the user to control their contribution in distance-based statistical tasks such as classification or clustering. We demonstrate the utility of the proposed framework for classification using simulations and two real data scenarios: Hawaiian Drosophila fly wings and pyramidal neuron trees.

Keywords Elastic distance · Bottleneck distance · Point clouds · Square-root velocity function · Pyramidal neuron trees

---

Y. J. Choi · S. Kurtek (✉)
Department of Statistics, The Ohio State University, Columbus, OH, USA
e-mail: choi.1577@osu.edu; kurtek.1@stat.osu.edu

K. Bharath
School of Mathematical Sciences, University of Nottingham, Nottingham, UK
e-mail: Karthik.Bharath@nottingham.ac.uk

Y. Zhao, D.-G. Chen (eds.), *Big Data Analytics in Biostatistics and Bioinformatics*, ICSA Book Series in Statistics,
https://doi.org/10.1007/978-3-032-06649-7_13

1 Introduction

Modern technological advancements allow for collection and processing of large amounts of complex data in various applied domains including biology. The geometric and topological complexity of biological data is apparent as objects of interest often contain multiple different types of structures, e.g., curves and point clouds, which must be integrated during analysis. In many cases, researchers are interested in capturing shape or topo-geometric signal in such data for the purposes of classification and statistical modeling. Several examples of complex biological data are displayed in Fig. 1. Panel (a) shows two proteins wherein the three-dimensional backbone can be viewed as a curve component and surrounding atoms form the point cloud component. Both are critical in influencing the stability, structure, dynamics, and function of proteins [1, 28, 36]. In panel (b), we show two sample leafs wherein the shape of the leaf boundary (curve component) as well as the internal vein structure, which can be represented as a point cloud, are informative about the corresponding tree species. Panel (c) displays two examples of Hawaiian Drosophila fly wings; as in the leaf example, both the boundary of the fly wing and the internal vein structure provide information about the corresponding fly species [21, 44]. Finally, panel (d) displays two pyramidal neuron trees with very complex branching structures. Each tree is composed of a main branch (curve component), and apical and basal dendrites, which can be abstracted into a point cloud. The varied shapes of pyramidal neurons correlate with their specific functional roles in the brain [30].

While there are many examples of complex biological data objects associated with many different statistical tasks of interest, our specific focus in this chapter is on distance-based classification of Drosophila fly wings and pyramidal neuron trees. Due to existence of different types of components in such data, i.e., curve and point cloud, sophisticated analytical approaches are necessary to capture their full variation. The complexity of such structures poses challenges for statistical analysis, but also offers an opportunity if one can fully capture both sources of information. In this chapter, we introduce a hybrid distance that integrates information about (i) the shape of a curve component and (ii) topo-geometric properties of a point cloud component in a complex biological object. The proposed distance can then be used for effective classification of such objects as demonstrated later in Sect. 4. In particular, each biological object will be represented as a combination of a curve component and a point cloud component, specifically defined for the object under study, and compared using methods tailored to their specific characteristics. We will use a distance based on the elastic shape analysis framework to capture shape differences between curve components. Similarly, we will use a distance from topological data analysis to capture topo-geometric differences between point clouds. The two sources of variation in biological objects will then be appropriately balanced within the hybrid distance using a weight parameter.

The elastic shape analysis framework [40] for capturing shape differences among curves in d-dimensional Euclidean space is based on an elastic Riemannian metric,

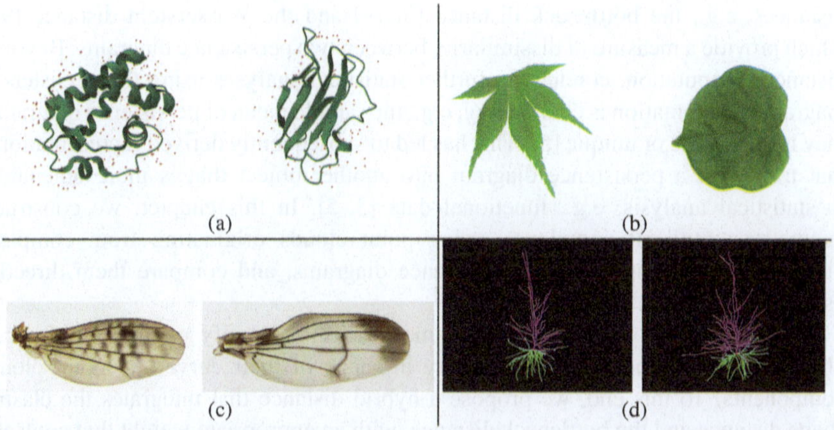

Fig. 1 Examples of complex biological data. (**a**) Two proteins (backbone in green) with ion and water atoms (in red) with PDB IDs 1DLW (left) and 1PLC (right). The data were sourced from the PDB database [25], and images were generated using the Mol* Viewer [39]. (**b**) Images of a Japanese maple leaf (left) and a Chinese redbud leaf (right) [47]. (**c**) Images of fly wings from *Drosophila ornata* (left) and *Drosophila cyrtoloma* (right) [18]. (**d**) Pyramidal neuron trees from the neocortex region, obtained from Neuromorpho.org, of an adult male with epilepsy (left) and an adult male with a tumor (right) [2]

which gives rise to a shape distance that is invariant to all shape-preserving transformations including translation, rotation, reparameterization, and in some cases scale. In this framework, two curves that are within such transformations are deemed equivalent in shape, and the resulting elastic shape distance between them is 0. The term elastic refers to interpretability of the distance as it captures the amount of stretching/compression and bending that is required to deform one shape into another. Furthermore, it allows flexible parameterizations of curves, which yields more natural comparisons across shapes due to a process referred to as registration (see Sect. 2.1 for details). It has been successfully used for capturing shape variation in a number of applications including biology [7, 26, 27, 29] and biometrics [12, 13]. While the form of the elastic Riemannian metric is quite complicated, making the resulting distance difficult to compute in practice directly, there exists an alternative representation, called the square-root velocity function [22, 41], which makes it computable in closed form and allows for its use in large-scale shape analysis of biological data represented as curves.

Topological data analysis [34, 46] is a multipurpose toolbox for discovery, comparison, and statistical analysis of topo-geometric features in point clouds, by summarizing their birth-death times in so-called persistence diagrams [16]. The framework is based on persistence homology [17, 49], which provides a multi-resolution view of the topological and geometric features, e.g., connected components, loops, voids, etc., in data represented as point clouds in $\mathbb{R}^d$. It thus allows one to capture global topo-geometric (shape) differences among point clouds via comparisons of their corresponding persistence diagrams. There exist several distances, e.g., the bottleneck distance [8, 19] and the Wasserstein distance [9], which provide a measure of dissimilarity between two persistence diagrams. Beyond distance computation, conducting further statistical analyses using the persistence diagram representation is challenging, e.g., the sample mean of persistence diagrams may not be stable or unique [5]. This has led to subsequently derived representations that transform a persistence diagram into another object that is more amenable to statistical analysis, e.g., functional data [3, 5]. In this chapter, we construct geometric simplicial complexes, using point clouds originating from complex biological objects, to generate persistence diagrams, and compare them directly using the bottleneck distance.

The main goal of the proposed framework is to classify complex biological objects while accounting for variability in shape of their curve and point cloud components. To this end, we propose a hybrid distance that integrates the elastic shape distance and the bottleneck distance, with an appropriate weight that controls their contributions. The resulting hybrid distance can then be used in conjunction with distance-based classification or clustering methods. We show that the use of diverse shape information derived from complex biological data results in enhanced classification performance.

This chapter is organized as follows. Section 2 introduces concepts from elastic shape analysis (Sect. 2.1) and topological data analysis (Sect. 2.2) that are required to define the proposed hybrid distance for classification of complex biological data (Sect. 2.3). Section 3 presents simulation studies demonstrating the effectiveness of the hybrid distance on binary classification tasks. Finally, Sect. 4 applies the hybrid distance for classification in two real data scenarios: Hawaiian Drosophila fly wings (Sect. 4.1) and pyramidal neuron trees (Sect. 4.2).

2 Methods

The proposed hybrid distance for shape classification of complex biological data objects, composed of a curve component and a point cloud component, relies on mathematical representations based on the elastic shape analysis (ESA) [40] and topological data analysis (TDA) [16] frameworks, which allow for quantification of shape differences between curves and point clouds, respectively. We introduce these two frameworks first. Throughout this chapter, we use $\langle\langle\cdot,\cdot\rangle\rangle$ and $\|\cdot\|$ to denote the $\mathbb{L}^2$ inner product ($\langle\langle f, g\rangle\rangle = \int_0^1 f(t)^\top g(t)dt,$ for $f, g \in \mathbb{L}^2([0,1], \mathbb{R}^d)$) and norm ($\|f\| = \sqrt{\int_0^1 f(t)^\top f(t)dt}$), respectively. On the other hand, $\langle\cdot,\cdot\rangle$ and $|\cdot|$ denote the Euclidean inner product and norm in $\mathbb{R}^d$, respectively. We will use $\langle\langle\langle\cdot,\cdot\rangle\rangle\rangle$ to denote nonstandard inner products. Throughout, we reserve the word "metric" to refer to Riemannian metrics, and not distances, to disambiguate its use.

2.1 Elastic Shape Analysis of Curves

Let $\beta : [0, 1] \to \mathbb{R}^d$ denote an open, absolutely continuous parameterized curve; the representation space of such curves will be denoted by $\mathcal{B}$. Our focus is on $d = 2$ or $d = 3$, which are the typical types of data encountered in biology.

To quantify the shape difference between two curves β_1 and β_2, we require a distance that is invariant to all shape-preserving transformations: scale[1], translation, rotation, and reparameterization. Rotations and reparameterizations are elements of the groups $SO(d) = \{O \in \mathbb{R}^{d\times d} \mid OO^\top = O^\top O = I,\ \det(O) = 1\}$ and $\Gamma = \{\gamma : [0, 1] \to [0, 1] \mid \gamma(0) = 0,\ \gamma(1) = 1,\ 0 < \dot{\gamma} < \infty\}$, respectively. Our focus is on a Riemannian geometric framework, referred to as elastic, which (i) gives rise to a distance that is invariant to all of the aforementioned transformations and (ii) is interpretable by quantifying the amount of bending and stretching/compression needed to deform one shape into another [33].

Any open curve $\beta \in \mathcal{B}$ can be uniquely represented via a pair of functions $(\phi, \theta) \in \Phi \times \Theta$ up to a translation, where $\phi = |\dot{\beta}| : [0, 1] \to \mathbb{R}$ is the speed function and $\theta = \frac{\dot{\beta}}{|\dot{\beta}|} : [0, 1] \to \mathbb{R}^d$ is the angle function. Then, the tangent space $T_{(\phi,\theta)}(\Phi \times \Theta)$ contains all possible perturbations of the speed and angle functions. For two tangent vectors (perturbations) $(\delta\phi_1, \delta\theta_1)$, $(\delta\phi_2, \delta\theta_2) \in T_{(\phi,\theta)}(\Phi \times \Theta)$, the elastic Riemannian metric [33] is then defined as

$$\langle\langle((\delta\phi_1, \delta\theta_1), (\delta\phi_2, \delta\theta_2))\rangle\rangle_{(\phi,\theta)} =$$
$$= w_1 \int_0^1 \delta\phi_1(t)\delta\phi_2(t)\frac{1}{\phi(t)}dt + w_2 \int_0^1 \delta\theta_1(t)^\top \delta\theta_2(t)\phi(t)dt. \quad (1)$$

One can think of the Riemannian metric as an inner product between tangent vectors (functions) in the tangent space at (ϕ, θ). The first term in Eq. (1) measures stretching/compression perturbations via changes in the speed function, whereas the second term measures bending deformations via changes in the angle function (weighted by the speed function). The parameters $w_1,\ w_2 > 0$ are the weights associated with these two terms and allow for control of the amount of elasticity in shape analysis, i.e., the larger the ratio $\frac{w_1}{w_2}$, the more penalization is applied to stretching/compression as compared to bending, and vice versa. An important property of this Riemannian metric is that it is unchanged by simultaneous rotations and reparameterizations of curves, a property that is not satisfied by the simple $\mathbb{L}^2$ metric. However, this metric is difficult to use in practice for shape comparisons. This is due to the fact that the metric changes as one moves from a tangent space to another, and thus, distances cannot be computed in closed form; instead, one must rely on computationally expensive algorithms [33].

The first simplification of the elastic Riemannian metric is due to Younes [48]; however, this simplification is only valid for two-dimensional curves as it is based

[1] In some cases, scale may be a natural property of the objects under study and one is instead interested in size-and-shape analysis. This framework is described in Sect. 2.1.1.

on the complex square-root. Instead, to treat the more general case, we utilize the square-root velocity function (SRVF) transformation introduced in [22, 41]. For a curve $\beta \in \mathscr{B}$, its SRVF $q : [0, 1] \rightarrow \mathbb{R}^d$, is defined via the bijective mapping $Q : \mathscr{B} \rightarrow \mathscr{Q}$ as

$$Q(\beta) = q = \begin{cases} \dot{\beta}/\sqrt{|\dot{\beta}|} & \text{if } |\dot{\beta}| \neq 0, \\ 0 & \text{otherwise,} \end{cases} \tag{2}$$

where $\dot{\beta}$ is the componentwise derivative of β. The space of SRVFs $\mathscr{Q}$ corresponding to absolutely continuous curves is a subset of $\mathbb{L}^2([0, 1], \mathbb{R}^d)$, henceforth simply referred to as $\mathbb{L}^2$. Furthermore, under the SRVF transformation, the complicated elastic Riemannian metric, with $w_1 = 1/4$ and $w_2 = 1$, simplifies to the standard $\mathbb{L}^2$ metric, allowing for efficient computation of distances. Finally, the SRVF is automatically invariant to translations due to the use of a derivative in the representation.

After transforming each curve to its SRVF, we must further account for scale, rotation, and reparameterization variabilities during shape comparisons. Scale variation is removed from the representation space via normalization: all curves are scaled to have unit length resulting in unit $\mathbb{L}^2$ norm SRVFs, i.e., $L(\beta) = \int_0^1 |\dot{\beta}(t)|dt = \int_0^1 |q(t)|^2 dt = \|q\|^2 = 1$. This results in the so-called pre-shape space $\mathscr{C} = \{q : [0, 1] \rightarrow \mathbb{R}^d \mid \|q\| = 1\}$, which is the unit Hilbert sphere. Thus, the $\mathbb{L}^2$ distance between two SRVFs $q_1, q_2 \in \mathscr{C}$ is given by $d_{\mathscr{C}}(q_1, q_2) = \cos^{-1}(\langle\langle q_1, q_2\rangle\rangle) = \cos^{-1}(\int_0^1 q_1^{\top} q_2(t)dt(t))$.

Rotation and parameterization variation is removed from the representation space via the definition of equivalence classes. For a rotated curve $O\beta$, $O \in SO(d)$, the corresponding SRVF is given by Oq. The SRVF of a reparameterized curve $\beta \circ \gamma, \gamma \in \Gamma$, is given by $(q, \gamma) = (q \circ \gamma)\sqrt{\dot{\gamma}}$. Then, the equivalence class $[q] = \{O(q, \gamma) \mid (O, \gamma) \in SO(d) \times \Gamma\}$ represents a shape uniquely, and the task of shape comparison boils down to calculating distances between equivalence classes. The corresponding shape space is the set of all such equivalence classes and is a quotient space: $\mathscr{S} = \mathscr{C}/(SO(d) \times \Gamma) = \{[q] \mid q \in \mathscr{C}\}$. The resulting shape distance between two curves $\beta_1, \beta_2 \in \mathscr{B}$, represented via their SRVFs $q_1, q_2 \in \mathscr{C}$, is defined as

$$\begin{aligned} d_{\mathscr{S}}([q_1], [q_2]) &= \inf_{(O,\gamma)\in SO(d)\times\Gamma} d_{\mathscr{C}}(q_1, O(q_2, \gamma)) = \\ &= \inf_{(O,\gamma)\in SO(d)\times\Gamma} \cos^{-1}(\langle\langle q_1, O(q_2, \gamma)\rangle\rangle). \end{aligned} \tag{3}$$

The optimization problems over $SO(d)$ and Γ in Eq. (3) can be efficiently solved via Procrustes analysis (singular value decomposition) [24] and the dynamic programming algorithm [37], respectively; this process is referred to as the pairwise registration of β_2 to β_1. Registration establishes a nonlinear (optimal) matching of points across curves and results in improved shape comparisons. Figure 2

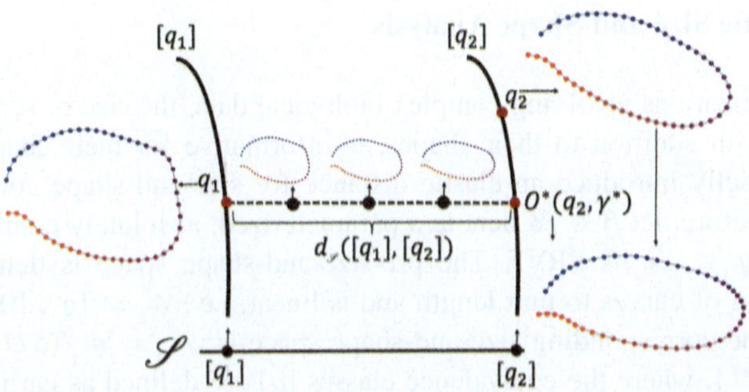

Fig. 2 The distance between two shapes is given by the length of the shortest path between the equivalence classes $[q_1]$ and $[q_2]$. This involves first finding the optimal rotation O^* and reparameterization γ^* through registration of q_2 (β_2) to q_1 (β_1)

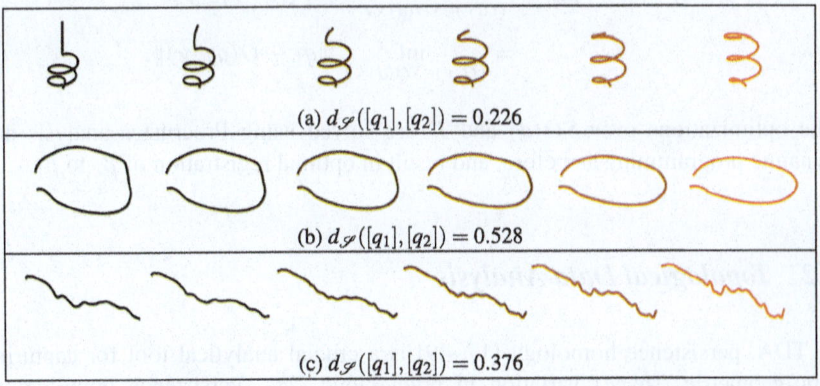

Fig. 3 Shape comparison of curve components: **(a)** simulated 3D spirals, **(b)** outlines of Drosophila fly wings, and **(c)** main branches in neuronal trees. Each panel displays the geodesic (shortest distance) path between two shapes, along with the associated shape distance

visually illustrates the process of registration and computation of the resulting shape distance.

Figure 3 presents three examples of geodesic (shortest distance) paths between shapes, along with the associated shape distances; the shape distances are the lengths of these paths. The first example, shown in panel (a), considers two simulated spiral curves; we use such curves in the simulation study detailed in Sect. 3. The second and third examples, shown in panels (b) and (c), consider 2D outlines of Drosophila fly wings and 3D main branches in pyramidal neuron trees, respectively; these real data examples are considered in Sect. 4. Note that, in all three cases, the geodesic path represents a natural deformation between the two given curves, while the shape distance quantifies differences between them.

2.1.1 Elastic Size-and-Shape Analysis

In some applications involving complex biological data, the size or scale of objects under study, in addition to their shapes, is informative for their characterization. Thus, we briefly introduce an elastic distance for size-and-shape comparisons of curves. As before, let $\beta \in \mathscr{B}$ denote a parameterized, absolutely continuous, open curve, and $q \in \mathscr{Q}$ its SRVF. The pre-size-and-shape space is defined without normalization of curves to unit length and is linear, i.e., $\mathscr{C}' = \{q : [0, 1] \to \mathbb{R}^d \mid q \in \mathbb{L}^2\}$. The corresponding size-and-shape space is $\mathscr{S}' = \mathscr{C}'/(SO(d) \times \Gamma) = \{[q] \mid q \in \mathscr{C}'\}$, where the equivalence classes $[q]$ are defined as earlier. The size-and-shape distance on $\mathscr{S}'$ between two curves $\beta_1, \beta_2 \in \mathscr{B}$, represented via their SRVFs $q_1, q_2 \in \mathscr{C}'$, is thus given by

$$d_{\mathscr{S}'}([q_1], [q_2]) = \inf_{(O,\gamma)\in SO(d)\times\Gamma} d_{\mathscr{C}'}(q_1, O(q_2, \gamma)) = \\ = \inf_{(O,\gamma)\in SO(d)\times\Gamma} \|q_1 - O(q_2, \gamma)\|. \quad (4)$$

The optimizations over $SO(d)$ and Γ are solved using Procrustes analysis and dynamic programming as before, and result in optimal registration of β_2 to β_1.

2.2 *Topological Data Analysis*

In TDA, persistence homology [17, 49] is a crucial analytical tool for capturing topo-geometric (shape) variation in point cloud data. Persistence homology is adept at identifying and tracing, across various levels of resolution, a range of topological features (and their geometric configuration) of a point cloud, e.g., connected components (degree $p = 0$), which represent distinct clusters of points; loops (degree $p = 1$), which are closed paths or cycles; and voids (degree $p = 2$), which refer to hollow spaces enclosed by surfaces [15, 16]. An illustration of these different topological features is presented in Fig. 4.

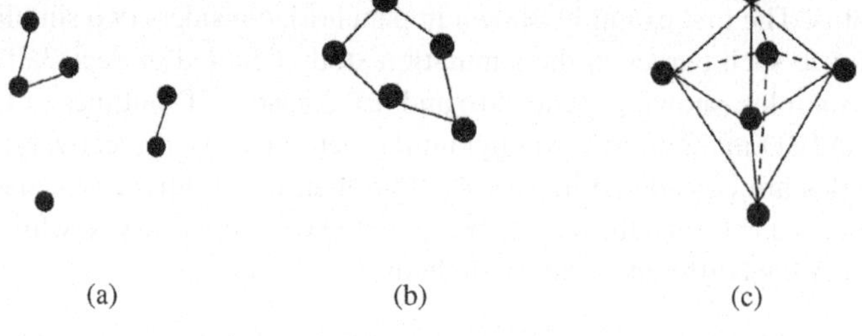

Fig. 4 Illustration of different topological features: (**a**) three connected components, (**b**) one loop, and (**c**) one void

For a set of N points in $\mathbb{R}^d$, $X = \{x_1, \ldots, x_N\}$, the process involves the creation of geometric filtered complexes through the aggregation of balls $\cup_{i=1}^{N} B_{x_i}(t)$ centered around each x_i, all with an identical radius $t > 0$. The two commonly used types of complexes are the Čech complex and the Vietoris-Rips complex, or simply Rips complex [4]. To better understand these complexes, it is essential to grasp the concept of simplices, which are the foundational elements of their structure. A simplex is a generalization of a triangle or tetrahedron to arbitrary dimensions. For instance, a 0-simplex is simply a point, a 1-simplex is a line segment connecting two points, a 2-simplex is a triangle formed by three points, and a 3-simplex is a tetrahedron formed by four points.

The Čech complex, Čech(X, t), consists of k-simplices formed by the intersection of $k + 1$ balls. This approach is computationally intensive due to the requirement to store simplices of various dimensions. In contrast, the Rips complex, a simplification of the Čech complex, is computationally efficient as it forms a simplex whenever all pairs of points in a group of $k+1$ points are within a specified distance of each other. The nature of these complexes ensures invariance to global translation and rotation, but not scaling, of a given point cloud.

In Čech or Rips complexes, as the radius t of the balls increases, several changes occur: new simplices may form and existing ones may disappear, persist further, or grow to include more points. These changes in simplicial structures give rise to topological features, which themselves form, persist, and eventually die as the filtration progresses. This leads to the notion of "birth" and "death" of topological features. Birth and death times of such features, corresponding to specific values of t, are captured in a persistence diagram, where the horizontal axis represents the birth scale, and the vertical axis the death scale. Each topological feature j is mapped to a point (b_j, d_j) corresponding to its birth and death times. The resulting persistence diagram $D^p \in \mathscr{D}$, for a point cloud X and a fixed degree p, thus consists of a multiset of points, $\{s_j = (b_j, d_j) \mid d_j > b_j \geq 0,\ j = 1, \ldots, m\}$, where m is the feature count.

Next, we are faced with defining a distance on the space of persistence diagrams $\mathscr{D}$, which will be used to define the hybrid distance for classification of complex biological data. Given two persistence diagrams $D_1^p,\ D_2^p \in \mathscr{D}$, the bottleneck distance [8, 19] is defined as

$$d_B(D_1^p, D_2^p) = \inf_{\alpha:\ D_1^p \to D_2^p} \ \sup_{s \in D_1^p} |s - \alpha(s)|_\infty, \tag{5}$$

where α is a bijective matching of points in the diagrams D_1^p and D_2^p, including the diagonal $\Delta = \{(y, y) \mid y \in \mathbb{R}\}$, which represents features with zero persistence. The term $|s - \alpha(s)|_\infty$ is the L^∞ norm between a point s in D_1^p and its image $\alpha(s)$ in D_2^p. Consequently, the bottleneck distance is defined as the smallest possible maximum distance required to align each point in one persistence diagram to a counterpart in the other, either through direct pairing or via a connection to the diagonal. The bottleneck distance satisfies all properties of a distance including nonnegativity, symmetry and triangle inequality, as highlighted in [15]. Moreover, it is stable under small perturbations of point clouds [8]. While there are other potential choices of distance on the space of persistence diagrams, e.g., the Wasserstein distance [32], which could be utilized in the definition of the proposed hybrid distance for classification, all results presented in Sects. 3 and 4 were generated using the bottleneck distance to quantify topo-geometric disparities between point cloud components within complex biological objects.

Figure 5 illustrates the construction of persistence diagrams for two simple point clouds in $\mathbb{R}^2$, marked in blue and red, based on the Rips complex. We consider degree $p = 0$ (connected components) first. Figure 5a shows that, at $t = 0.7071$, the original four connected components (born at $t = 0$), corresponding to each of the four points in the blue point cloud, die. This corresponds to four blue filled-in points that overlap perfectly in the persistence diagram in Fig. 5e. Note that at this time, the four connected components also merge to form a new, larger connected component that persists forever and is omitted from the persistence diagram. Similarly, as seen in Fig. 5c, at $t = 1.4142$, the original four connected components (born at $t = 0$), corresponding to each of the four points in the red point cloud, die, which results in four perfectly overlapping red points in the persistence diagram in Fig. 5e; they merge to form a larger connected component that persists forever and is again omitted from the persistence diagram. The resulting bottleneck distance

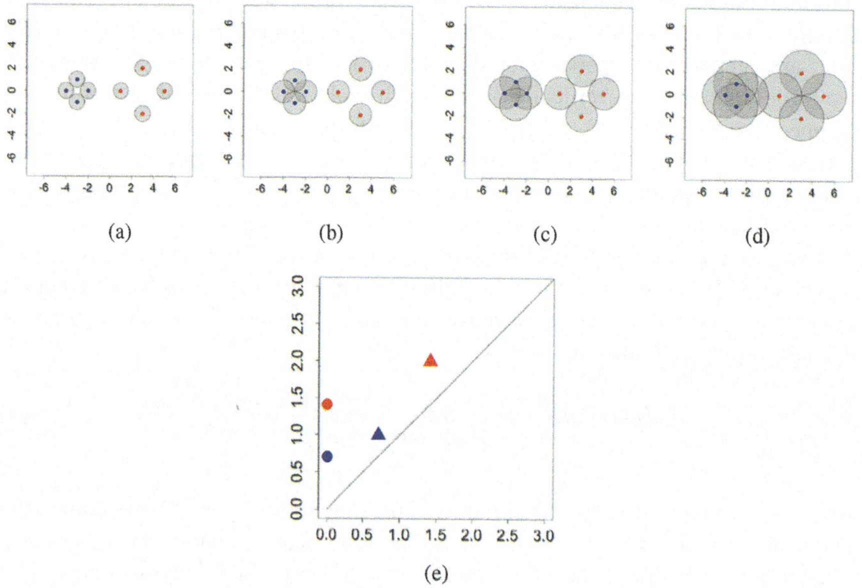

Fig. 5 Construction of Rips filtration for two simulated point clouds, marked in red and blue: (**a**) $t = 0.7071$; (**b**) $t = 1$; (**c**) $t = 1.4142$; (**d**) $t = 2$. (**e**) Degree $p = 0$ (points) and $p = 1$ (triangles) persistence diagrams. For $p = 0$, the bottleneck distance between the red and blue point clouds is 0.7071, and for $p = 1$, it is 0.2929

between these two degree $p = 0$ persistence diagrams (D_1^0, blue, and D_2^0, red) is $d_B(D_1^0, D_2^0) = 0.7071$. Shifting attention to degree $p = 1$ (loops), we see in Fig. 5a and b, that a loop forms in the blue point cloud at $t = 0.7071$, and later dies at $t = 1$, corresponding to the blue filled-in triangle in the persistence diagram in Fig. 5e. In similar fashion, as seen in Fig. 5c and d, a loop forms in the red point cloud at $t = 1.4142$, and dies at $t = 2$, marked by a red triangle in the persistence diagram in Fig. 5e. The resulting bottleneck distance between these two degree $p = 1$ persistence diagrams (D_1^1: blue and D_2^1: red) is $d_B(D_1^1, D_2^1) = 0.2929$.

Figure 6 presents two additional examples of point cloud comparisons, wherein the point clouds correspond to (a) internal vein structures of Drosophila fly wings and (b) apical and basal dendrites in pyramidal neuron trees; these types of data will be used for classification in Sect. 4. In both examples, we report the bottleneck distances based on degree $p = 0$ and $p = 1$ persistence diagrams, which capture and quantify differences between different types of features in the point clouds.

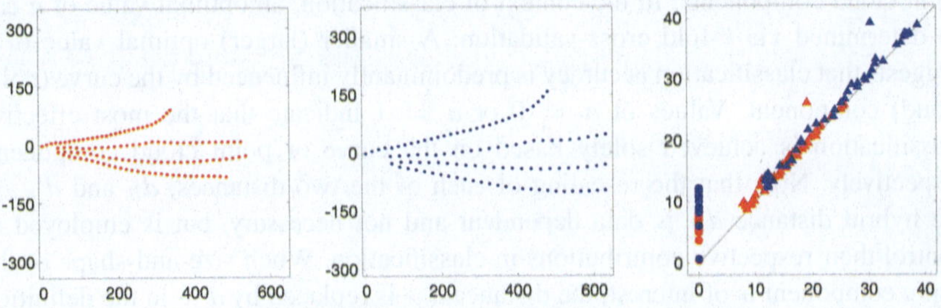

(a) $d_B(D_1^0, D_2^0) = 3.8628, \quad d_B(D_1^1, D_2^1) = 4.4393$

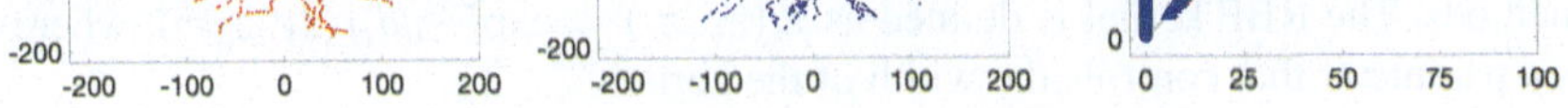

(b) $d_B(D_1^0, D_2^0) = 25.8379, \quad d_B(D_1^1, D_2^1) = 9.0631$

Fig. 6 Comparison of point cloud components: (**a**) internal vein structure in Drosophila fly wings; (**b**) apical and basal dendrites in neuronal trees. Left: Point cloud 1. Middle: Point cloud 2. Right: Degree $p = 0$ (points) and $p = 1$ (triangles) persistence diagrams for the red and blue point clouds

2.3 Hybrid Distance for Classification of Complex Biological Objects

Consider a set of complex biological objects, $\{z_i = (q_i, D_i^p),\ i = 1, \ldots, n\}$ (or equivalently $\{z_i = (\beta_i, D_i^p),\ i = 1, \ldots, n\}$), each of which is represented using the SRVF of its curve component, q_i, and the degree p persistence diagram of its point cloud component, D_i^p. We define a hybrid distance on the product space $\mathscr{S} \times \mathscr{D}$, between two such objects z_1 and z_2, as follows:

$$d_H(z_1, z_2) = \sqrt{a\left(\frac{d_B(D_1^p, D_2^p)}{\max\limits_{i,j} d_B(D_i^p, D_j^p)}\right)^2 + (1-a)\left(\frac{d_{\mathscr{S}}([q_1], [q_2])}{\max\limits_{i,j} d_{\mathscr{S}}([q_i], [q_j])}\right)^2}, \tag{6}$$

where $a \in [0, 1]$ is a constant that controls the contribution of the curve and point cloud components. In the context of classification, an optimal value of a can be determined via k-fold cross-validation. A smaller (larger) optimal value of a suggests that classification accuracy is predominantly influenced by the curve (point cloud) component. Values of $a = 0$ or $a = 1$ indicate that the most effective classification is achieved solely based on the curve or point cloud component, respectively. Note that the rescaling of each of the two distances, d_B and $d_{\mathscr{S}}$, in the hybrid distance d_H is data dependent and not necessary, but is employed to control their respective contributions in classification. When size-and-shape of the curve component is of interest, the distance $d_{\mathscr{S}}$ is replaced by $d_{\mathscr{S}'}$ in the definition of d_H.

Upon constructing the distance matrix D, with entries $D_{i,j} = d_H(z_i, z_j)$, we can apply various distance-based classification or clustering methods. These include k-nearest neighbors, support vector machine (SVM) [10], hierarchical clustering [45], DBSCAN (density-based spatial clustering of applications with noise) [20, 38], and spectral clustering [35, 43], among others. For simulation studies and real data applications in the remainder of this chapter, we will primarily use the nearest neighbor ($k = 1$) and SVM with a Radial Basis Function (RBF) kernel classification methods. The RBF kernel is defined as $K(z_1, z_2) = \exp(-\eta d_H(z_1, z_2)^2)$, where η is a parameter that controls the width of the kernel.

3 Simulation Studies

Before considering real data, we first assess the utility of the proposed hybrid distance for the classification of complex biological objects using simulation studies. In the following sections, we explain the simulation study design, how to generate synthetic datasets used in these simulation studies, and present the simulation results.

3.1 Synthetic Data Generation

Each simulated object is composed of a synthetic 3D spiral curve component and a point cloud component generated from a parametric distribution. The shape variation in the curve components is induced by the number of spirals, controlled by a parameter τ, as well as the width and length of the cycles, which are random. Topo-geometric variation in the point cloud components is induced via changes in parameters in the parametric distribution.

Using previous notation, let z denote the complex geometric data object, composed of (the SRVF of) a curve component and a point cloud component. We use β_τ to denote a spiral curve with τ completed cycles. For each spiral curve with τ completed cycles, the radius of the spiral is sampled uniformly between 0.75 and 2.75, ensuring that the spiral's size varies randomly across observations. Also, X_μ denotes a 3D point cloud generated from a $N([0, 0, \mu]^\top, \sigma^2 I_3)$ distribution, and $Y_\mu = [Y_1, Y_2, Y_{3,\mu}]^\top$ denotes a 3D point cloud with the first two coordinates $(Y_1, Y_2) = (\cos(\theta), \sin(\theta))$, with $\theta \sim Unif(0, 2\pi)$, and the third coordinate $Y_{3,\mu} \sim N(\mu, \sigma^2)$. To illustrate the effect of the weight, a, within the combined distance on classification performance, we designed multiple simulation settings that are presented in Tables 1 and 2. For the settings detailed in Table 1, primary interest is in the use of degree $p = 0$ topological features, i.e., connected components, while for those in Table 2, interest is in degree $p = 1$ features, i.e., loops. Example datasets for a few of the simulation settings are displayed in Fig. 7.

In this study, we only consider binary classification. To distinguish between the shapes of curve components within Class A and Class B, we vary the number of completed cycles, τ, from 2.3 to 2.6 in Class A, and fix $\tau = 2.8$ in Class B. To distinguish between point cloud components within Class A and Class B, components from Class A are generated from one distribution, while those from Class B are generated from two distributions with distinct parameter values μ. This results in a varying number of underlying connected components (Table 1) or loops (Table 2) within each class (with additional Gaussian noise). Consequently, depending on the value of μ, there generally exists one connected component or

Table 1 Simulation settings where degree $p = 0$ topological features (connected components) of point clouds are of interest

Setting	Class A	Class B
1	$z = (\beta_{2.3}, X_0)$	$z = (\beta_{2.8}, X_0, X_{1.5})$
2	$z = (\beta_{2.4}, X_0)$	$z = (\beta_{2.8}, X_0, X_{2.5})$
3	$z = (\beta_{2.5}, X_0)$	$z = (\beta_{2.8}, X_0, X_{3.5})$
4	$z = (\beta_{2.6}, X_0)$	$z = (\beta_{2.8}, X_0, X_{4.5})$

Table 2 Simulation settings where degree $p = 1$ topological features (loops) of point clouds are of interest

Setting	Class A	Class B
1	$z = (\beta_{2.3}, Y_0)$	$z = (\beta_{2.8}, Y_0, Y_1)$
2	$z = (\beta_{2.4}, Y_0)$	$z = (\beta_{2.8}, Y_0, Y_{1.3})$
3	$z = (\beta_{2.5}, Y_0)$	$z = (\beta_{2.8}, Y_0, Y_{1.6})$
4	$z = (\beta_{2.6}, Y_0)$	$z = (\beta_{2.8}, Y_0, Y_{1.9})$

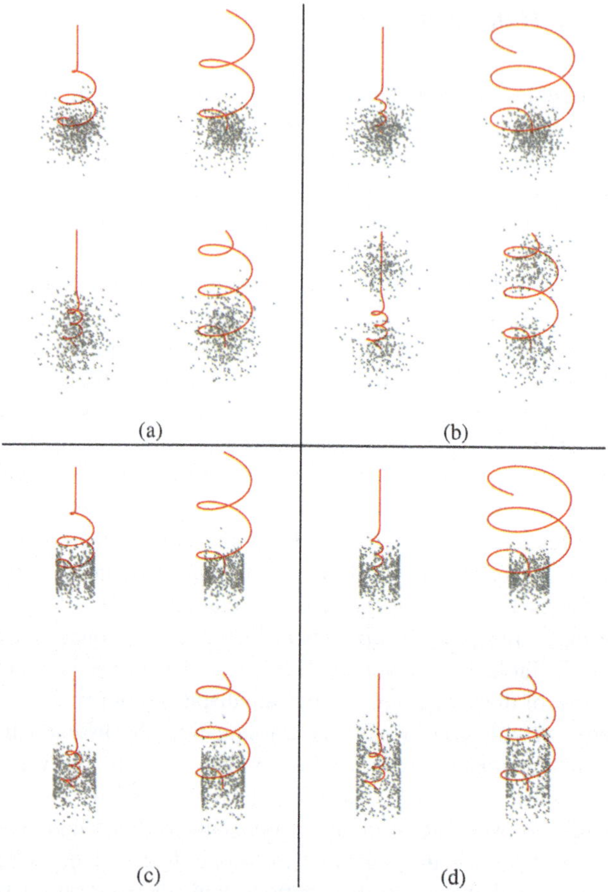

Fig. 7 (**a**) and (**b**) Examples of simulated data for Settings 1 and 4 in Table 1. (**c**) and (**d**) Examples of simulated data for Settings 1 and 4 in Table 2. In each panel, the objects in the top row belong to Class A, and those in the bottom row belong to Class B

loop in Class A and two (or more) in Class B. In both cases, the largest difference in shape between spiral curves and the smallest difference in topology and geometric configuration of point clouds, across Classes A and B, are observed in Setting 1. This pattern gradually reverses as we move from Setting 1 to Setting 4, where point clouds exhibit the largest differences and shapes of spiral curves the smallest differences across Classes A and B.

3.2 Simulation Results

For each class, we generate 50 training observations, split evenly between Classes A and B, with each data object z comprising one spiral curve, β_τ (with SRVF q_τ), and one point cloud, X_μ or Y_μ, with a total of 500 points. In cases where point clouds are generated from 2 distributions, corresponding to Class B, we use equal sample sizes of 250 from each. In this simulation, we use an SVM classifier with an RBF kernel function. During the training stage, for each value of $a \in [0, 1]$ with increments of 0.05, a grid search was conducted over values of the regularization parameter C in SVM and the hyperparameter η in the RBF kernel. For C and η, we consider $\{0.1, 1, 10, 10^2, 10^3, 10^4, 10^5\}$ and $\{10^{-4}, 10^{-3}, 10^{-2}, 10^{-1}, 1, 10\}$, respectively. The optimal combination of C and η for a given value of a was determined via stratified five-fold cross-validation. The SVM, configured with these optimal values, was then used to classify 10 independently generated test sets with 25 objects in each class, for each value of a.

The average accuracy across the ten test sets for each value of a are displayed in Fig. 8a and b, corresponding to the settings detailed in Tables 1 and 2, respectively; the average test accuracy under each setting is marked by a different color: blue for Setting 1, red for Setting 2, orange for Setting 3, and green for Setting 4. When the primary distinction between the two classes originates from the shape of the spiral curve, i.e., Setting 1 in blue, the test accuracy is higher for smaller values of a, with the maximum occurring at or very close to $a = 0$. This indicates that the hybrid distance with most of the emphasis placed on the elastic shape distance yields better classification performance. Conversely, in cases where the primary distinction is in the shape of point clouds, i.e., Setting 4 in green, higher classification accuracy is observed for larger values of a, with the maximum occurring at or close to $a = 1$. For Settings 2 and 3 in red and orange, this pattern is less clear. It appears that the signal in the shape of the curve component is stronger in both settings than the signal in the shape of the point clouds with optimal classification achieved at $a = 0$ and $a = 0.1$ for Settings 2 and 3 in panel (a), respectively, and $a = 0.15$ for

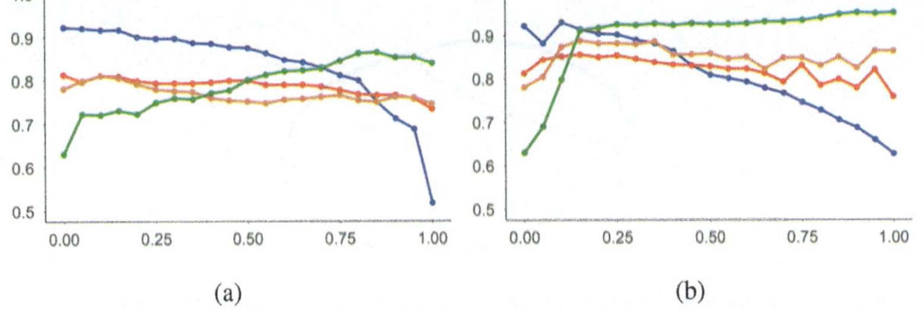

Fig. 8 Average classification accuracy, across ten independent test sets, for different values of a in the hybrid distance d_H. (**a**) Settings corresponding to Table 1. (**b**) Settings corresponding to Table 2. Settings 1–4 are shown in blue, red, orange and green, respectively

Settings 2 and 3 in panel (b). However, in both settings, classification performance is comparable for many values of a. This demonstrates that the hybrid distance provides useful insights when informative signal can be derived from the shape of both the curve component and the point cloud component.

We conducted an additional simulation study using spiral curves generated via principal component analysis, which produced results consistent with those presented here. The details are available in Appendix A.

4 Classification of Real Biological Objects

We apply classification that utilizes the proposed hybrid distance to two different types of complex biological data: Hawaiian Drosophila fly wings and pyramidal neuron trees. In particular, we show that the use of distances based on elastic shape analysis and topological data analysis between appropriately defined curve components and point cloud components, respectively, enhance classification performance in these applications.

4.1 Drosophila Fly Wings

In this application, we consider classification of Hawaiian Drosophila flies into species based on the shape of their wings. The dataset contains 81 observations of fly wings, characterized by their outlines and internal (longitudinal) veins, which are essential for distinguishing between fly species. Figure 9 shows the anatomical structure of a Hawaiian Drosophila fly wing. In particular, we treat the wing outline as an open curve and abstract the vein structure into a point cloud, by sampling each of the 4 veins using 30 equally spaced points. Thus, each fly wing is represented as a complex object z, with a curve component (outline) and a point cloud component (internal veins).

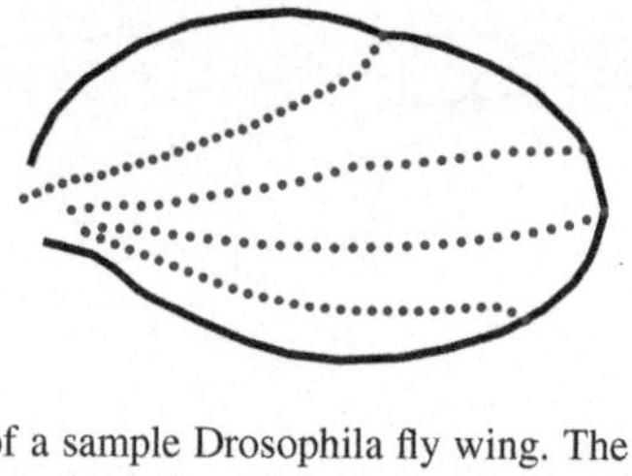

Fig. 9 Anatomical structure of a sample Drosophila fly wing. The boundary of the wing defines the curve component. Each internal vein is sampled using 30 equally spaced points resulting in the point cloud component; there are 4 longitudinal veins, II–V from top to bottom

Table 3 Hierarchical class structure for Drosophila fly species. For each class, we report the corresponding sample size

Subgroup name	Sample size	Primary clusters	Secondary clusters	Tertiary clusters
Adiastola	15	1	1	1
Planitibia	13	1	2	2
Glabriapex	12	1	3	3
Grimshawi	19	1	3	4
Antopocerus	6	2	4	5
Haleakalae	6	3	5	6
Modified Mouthparts	6	3	6	7
Modified Tarsus	4	3	6	8

According to [18], the 81 observations can be classified into 8 subgroups (tertiary class structure), which can be further combined into broader groups in a hierarchical manner, resulting in secondary and primary class structures with 6 and 3 classes, respectively. The subgroups, corresponding sample sizes, and their hierarchical structure are reported in Table 3. Thus, we will consider three classification scenarios based on each of the three different class structures. In this application, we consider the nearest neighbor classifier due to low sample sizes in a few of the classes. To compute the distance matrix for classification, we use the hybrid distance based on the shape distance $d_{\mathscr{S}}$ and bottleneck distance d_B (classification is performed separately using degree $p = 0$ and $p = 1$ persistence diagrams); we consider equally spaced values of the weight $a \in [0, 1]$ with increments of 0.05. Since computation of $d_{\mathscr{S}}$ involves scaling each wing outline to unit length, the point clouds representing internal veins are also scaled by a commensurate amount (recall that the bottleneck distance is not invariant to the scale of the point clouds).

Figure 10 presents the nearest neighbor classification results for different values of the weight a. The results based on degree $p = 0$ topological features (connected components) are shown in panel (a); those based on degree $p = 1$ (loops) are in panel (b). The results based on primary, secondary, and tertiary class structures are

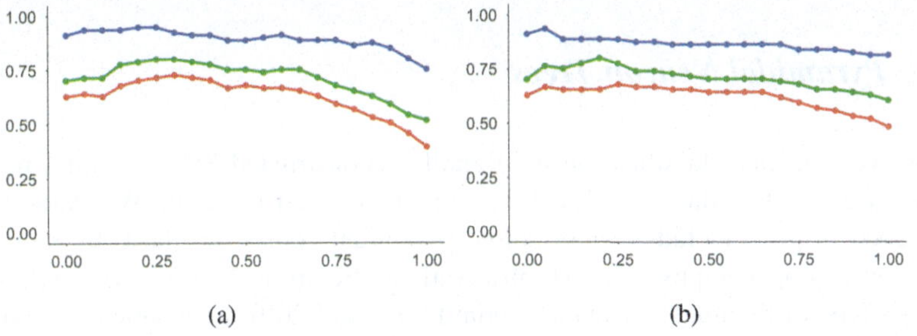

Fig. 10 Nearest neighbor classification accuracy for different values of a. We report separate results based on (**a**) degree $p = 0$ features and (**b**) degree $p = 1$ features. The primary, secondary, and tertiary classification results are shown in blue, green, and red, respectively

Table 4 Classification accuracy under six different scenarios: (i) primary class structure with degree $p = 0$, (ii) primary with $p = 1$, (iii) secondary with $p = 0$, (iv) secondary with $p = 1$, (v) tertiary with $p = 0$, and (vi) tertiary with $p = 1$. Highest classification accuracy for each class structure is italicized and underlined

Class structure	Optimal a	Degree p	Classification accuracy
Primary	0.2	0	<u>*0.951*</u>
	0.05	1	0.938
Secondary	0.25	0	<u>*0.802*</u>
	0.2	1	<u>*0.802*</u>
Tertiary	0.3	0	<u>*0.728*</u>
	0.25	1	0.679

shown in blue, green, and red, respectively. As expected, classification into primary classes resulted in the highest classification accuracy, across all values of a, for both degree $p = 0$ and $p = 1$. This is indeed the simplest scenario with only three classes. As seen in Table 4, the highest classification accuracy of 0.951 is attained at $a = 0.2$ based on degree $p = 0$ in this case; based on degree $p = 1$, the highest accuracy of 0.938 is realized when $a = 0.05$. Next, we shift focus to the more challenging scenarios of secondary and tertiary class structures. The highest secondary classification accuracy of 0.802 is attained at $a = 0.25$ for degree $p = 0$ and $a = 0.2$ for degree $p = 1$. Finally, the highest tertiary classification accuracy of 0.728 is realized for $a = 0.3$ and degree $p = 0$. For degree $p = 1$, the highest accuracy of 0.679 is achieved when $a = 0.25$. Note that in all of the aforementioned results, the optimal value of a is never 0 or 1. Thus, these results demonstrate that integrating information about (i) the shape of the fly wing outline and (ii) topo-geometric characteristics of the internal veins (represented as a point cloud), with a suitable weight a placed on the two distances, enhances classification performance. Overall, in this application, degree $p = 0$ topological features of the veins result in better classification performance as compared to degree $p = 1$ features.

Appendix B presents results for this dataset when the size-and-shape elastic distance is used rather than the shape distance.

4.2 *Pyramidal Neuron Trees*

Next, we consider classification of digitally reconstructed 3D pyramidal neuron trees based on two datasets. The first dataset, referred to as the Wu dataset and described in [42], includes 41 principal pyramidal cells from the CA1 region of the mouse hippocampus. The 41 observations are from 2 groups depending on genetic type of the mice: 21 from standard mice and 20 from genetically modified mice lacking specific protocadherin genes. The second dataset, referred to as the Chen dataset and described in [6], comprises 99 principal pyramidal cells from the hippocampal and layer V of the sensorimotor cortical regions of rat brains. These 99 observations are divided into 3 experimental groups: (i) rats subjected to bile duct ligation (BDL), (ii) rats that underwent BDL and were also fed a diet containing ammonia acetate (BDLHD), and (iii) a control group for baseline comparison. All of the pyramidal neuron trees considered in this section are accessible at NeuroMorpho.org, a publicly available database that gathers neuronal reconstructions and related metadata associated with peer-reviewed research publications.

Figure 11 displays the structure of reconstructed pyramidal neuron trees, including the "main branch" (black), defined as the longest path along the tree starting at the soma (magenta) and ending at the tip of an apical dendrite branch. For each tree, the main branch is identified using Dijkstra's algorithm [11], and serves as the curve component in our analysis. We also display the apical (red) and basal (blue) dendrites, which are sampled to form the point cloud component; the sampling of points on these dendrites is the same as given by the tree reconstruction. As seen in this figure, the pyramidal neuron trees exhibit complex morphologies, making it

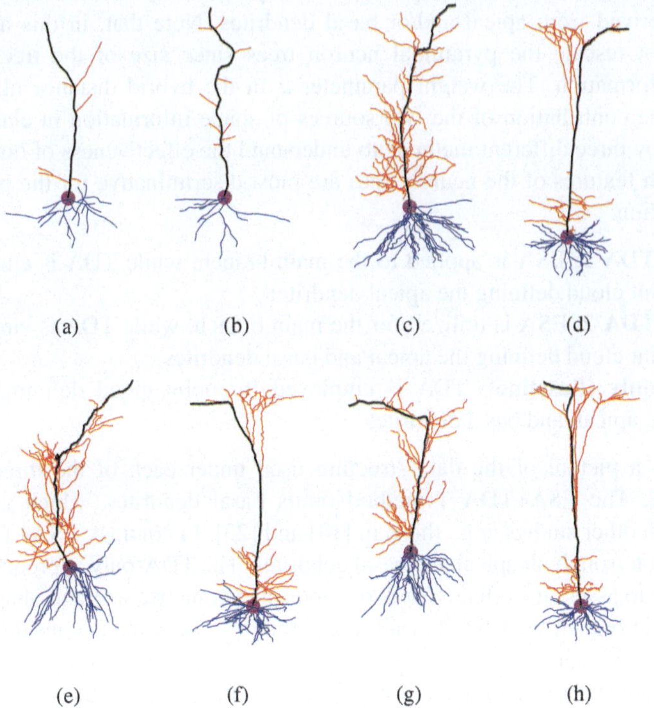

Fig. 11 Pyramidal neuron trees composed of the main branch (black), soma (magenta), and apical (red) and basal (blue) dendrites. Wu dataset: (**a**) and (**b**) show neuron trees from wild-type and knockout mice, respectively. Chen dataset: (**c**) and (**d**) show neuron trees from the control group, (**e**) and (**f**) from the BDL group, and (**g**) and (**h**) from the BDLHD group. Trees in (**c**), (**e**), and (**g**) are samples from the hippocampal region, while those in (**d**), (**f**), and (**h**) are from layer V of the sensorimotor cortical region

very challenging to utilize all available information about the structure (shape) of the trees for classification.

Recently, Duncan et al. [14] introduced a framework for comparison and classification of the shape of (simplified) neuronal trees; their method generalizes the ESA framework allowing for matching of branches across neuronal trees, but first simplifies the tree branching structure through pruning. As a result, this approach leads to significant information loss, especially for trees with many side branches and complex branching structures, e.g., the pyramidal neuron trees shown in Fig. 11. Furthermore, their analysis excludes basal dendrites and only considers primary branches in apical dendrites. On the other hand, Kanari et al. [23] utilized a TDA framework for comparing branching morphologies without pruning. Nevertheless, their method encounters challenges in classifying neuronal trees with subtle topo-geometric differences.

In our analysis, we employ the hybrid distance, which combines elements of ESA and TDA, and is able to capture size-and-shape differences in the main branch, via the distance $d_{\mathscr{S}'}$ defined in Eq. (4), as well as topo-geometric differences in the point clouds derived from apical and/or basal dendrites. Note that, in this application, we do not rescale the pyramidal neuron trees since size of the trees provides useful information. The weight parameter a in the hybrid distance allows us to control the contribution of the two sources of shape information in classification. We employ three different methods to understand the effectiveness of our approach and which features of the neuron trees are most discriminative for the purposes of classification:

- **ESA+TDA 1**: ESA is applied to the main branch, while TDA is employed for the point cloud defining the apical dendrite;
- **ESA+TDA 2**: ESA is utilized for the main branch, while TDA is employed for the point cloud defining the apical and basal dendrites;
- **TDA only (Baseline)**: TDA is employed for point cloud defining the main branch, apical, and basal dendrites.

We show a picture of the data structure used under each of the three methods in Fig. 12. The ESA+TDA 1 method omits basal dendrites, which is common practice in other studies, e.g., those in [14] and [23]. In contrast, ESA+TDA 2 uses information from both apical and basal dendrites. The TDA-only approach serves as a baseline to assess the effectiveness of capturing geometric size-and-shape features of the main branch via ESA. For all three methods, the soma is considered as part of the main branch.

We conduct four classification experiments, one involving the Wu dataset and three involving the Chen dataset. For the Wu dataset, the classes are defined as standard or genetically modified; we do not use the ESA+TDA 1 method in this case due to the sparsity of apical dendrite branches in neuron trees in this dataset, as seen in panels (a) and (b) in Fig. 11. For the Chen dataset, we define classes using the following: (i) the region (two classes), hippocampal or layer V; (ii) the experimental group (three classes), BDL, BDLHD, or control; and (iii) the region and experimental group combination (six classes), hippocampal/BDL,

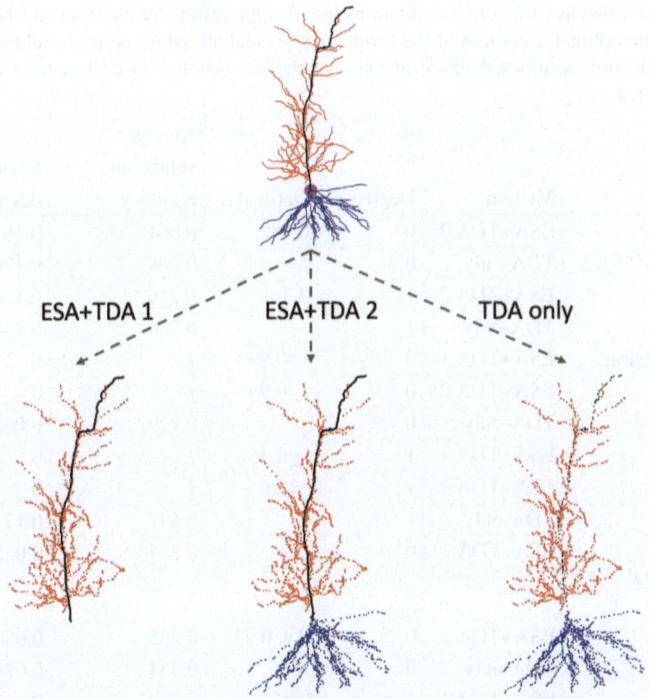

Fig. 12 Data structures used for classification under the ESA+TDA 1, ESA+TDA 2, and TDA-only methods. The presented pyramidal neuron tree is the same as in Fig. 11c. For the first two methods, the curve component (main branch) is shown as a solid black line with red and/or blue point clouds representing the apical and/or basal dendrites, respectively. For the third method, all components of the tree are represented via a point cloud

Table 5 Sample sizes for each subgroup in the Chen dataset [14]

Experimental group	Region Hippocampus CA1	 Neocortex layer V	Total
BDL	15	16	31
BDLHD	15	15	30
Control	18	20	38
Total	48	51	99

hippocampal/BDLHD, hippocampal/control, layer V/BDL, layer V/BDLHD, or layer V/control. The subgroup sample sizes in the Chen dataset are approximately balanced as shown in Table 5.

The classification results for all four experiments are reported in Table 6. We used the hybrid distance in an SVM classifier with an RBF kernel. All parameters were estimated using stratified five-fold cross-validation. The table reports the average and standard deviation of classification rates computed based on the five validation sets. For each case, we also report the estimated optimal weight a in the

Table 6 Stratified five-fold cross-validation classification results for the Wu and Chen datasets. Entries in the optimal a column of the form $\leq x$ represent all values up to x yielding the same average validation accuracy. Highest average validation accuracy for each dataset is italicized and underlined

Dataset	Method	Degree p	Optimal a	Average validation accuracy	Standard deviation
Wu	ESA+TDA 2	0	0.95	0.664	0.161
	TDA-only	0	–	0.606	0.170
	ESA+TDA 2	1	0.3	*0.756*	0.154
	TDA-only	1	–	0.706	0.145
Chen by region	ESA+TDA 1	0	≤0.80	*1*	0
	ESA+TDA 2	0	≤0.95	*1*	0
	TDA-only	0	–	0.929	0.068
	ESA+TDA 1	1	≤0.35	*1*	0
	ESA+TDA 2	1	≤0.6	*1*	0
	TDA-only	1	–	0.697	0.121
Chen by experimental group	ESA+TDA 1	0	≤1	0.384	0.023
	ESA+TDA 2	0	0.9, 0.95	0.585	0.086
	TDA-only	0	–	0.434	0.074
	ESA+TDA 1	1	0.95	0.480	0.167
	ESA+TDA 2	1	1	*0.586*	0.096
	TDA-only	1	–	0.393	0.053
Chen by combination of region and experimental group	ESA+TDA 1	0	0	0.404	0.125
	ESA+TDA 2	0	0.95	*0.656*	0.081
	TDA-only	0	–	0.364	0.099
	ESA+TDA 1	1	0.35	0.426	0.112
	ESA+TDA 2	1	0.35	0.585	0.083
	TDA-only	1	–	0.294	0.074

hybrid distance. For the Wu dataset, we achieve the highest (average) classification accuracy of 0.756 using ESA+TDA 2, with degree $p = 1$ persistence diagrams, and weight $a = 0.3$. In comparison, the TDA-only approach yields the highest average accuracy of 0.706 based on degree $p = 1$. The simplest classification task within the Chen dataset is by region. Both ESA+TDA 1 and ESA+TDA 2 achieve an average classification accuracy of 1, based on both degree $p = 0$ and $p = 1$ persistence diagrams, for multiple values of the weight a. However, the TDA-only approach does not perform nearly as well (0.929 for degree $p = 0$ and 0.697 for degree $p = 1$). Classification by experimental group is much more challenging despite the existence of only three classes. In this case, the highest average classification accuracy is achieved via ESA+TDA 2, with degree $p = 1$ persistence diagrams, and weight $a = 1$. Note that this implies that only point cloud information from the apical and basal dendrites is used for classification (the weight on the elastic size-and-shape distance applied to the main branches is 0). A similar classification accuracy is achieved via ESA+TDA 2, with degree $p = 0$ persistence diagrams, and weights $a = 0.9$ or $a = 0.95$. Finally, the highest average classification accuracy for the Chen dataset, where classes are defined using the combination of region and experimental group, is 0.656; here, degree $p = 0$ persistence diagrams were used with a value of $a = 0.95$. The presented classification results are comparable and, in some cases, better than those reported in [14] on the same data. However, we note that the results are not directly comparable due to different cross-validation settings.

Overall, the highest classification accuracy was consistently achieved using ESA+TDA 2. This implies that

(i) using elastic size-and-shape analysis on the tree main branch combined with topological data analysis applied to the point clouds defining apical and basal dendrites, and integrating the two sources of signal with an appropriate weight offers improved discriminatory power in classification of pyramidal neuron trees;
(ii) the topological structure of basal dendrites plays a significant role in the morphological structure of such trees.

Furthermore, depending on the dataset and classification task, the optimal value of a indicates the strongest source of signal. The lowest classification accuracy is most often obtained using the baseline TDA-only approach, with the only exception being classification of observations in the Chen dataset across experimental groups.

5 Discussion

In this chapter, we introduced a hybrid distance that combines information about the shape of curve components, captured via elastic shape analysis, and topo-geometric variation in point cloud components, captured via topological data analysis. The proposed distance utilizes the elastic shape distance between curves and the bottleneck distance between persistence diagrams, and has the potential to yield detailed insights by fully leveraging the complexities of biological data through its application in various statistical analysis tasks such as classification and clustering. Furthermore, the distance's performance in these tasks is refined by a weight parameter controlling the contribution of each of the two sources of information, whose optimal value can be learned in a data centric manner. Practical applications of our approach, including in classification of Hawaiian Drosophila fly wings and pyramidal neuron trees, highlight the distances's ability to improve classification outcomes. The learned optimal value of the weight parameter in the distance further provides information about the data features that are crucial for effective classification. For example, our analysis revealed that the ESA+TDA 2 method consistently achieved the best average validation accuracy across all datasets. This finding highlights the importance of incorporating basal dendrites into the analysis, as it significantly improves classification rate. Moreover, we observed that in five out of eight cases, the optimal value of the weight parameter a, when using ESA+TDA 2, was greater than or equal to 0.9. This observation further emphasizes that the topo-geometric information from basal dendrites, represented as point clouds, is weighted more heavily and contributes substantially to improving classification accuracy.

We have identified several directions for future work. First, we have chosen to use the bottleneck distance between persistence diagrams to quantify topo-geometric differences in corresponding point clouds. While our results show the effectiveness of this approach in the two real data studies, we will explore the use of other distances derived from topological data analysis for this purpose, e.g., the Wasserstein distance, or a suitable distance between persistence landscapes [31]. Second, in our implementation, persistence diagrams were generated via the Rips filtration. However, in other data scenarios, other types of filtration, e.g., level-set filtrations, may be more appropriate. We will study their performance in classification tasks on different types of data. Finally, we will extend the proposed hybrid distance to incorporate more than two data structures derived from complex biological data.

Acknowledgments This research was partially funded by NIH R37-CA214955 (to SK and KB), NSF DMS-2015374 (to KB), and NSF CCF-1740761, NSF DMS-2015226, NSF CCF-1839252, and NSF DMS-2413747 (to SK). We thank Professor Anuj Srivastava in the Department of Statistics at Florida State University for kindly sharing the pyramidal neuron tree datasets.

Appendix A: Simulation Studies with Different Spiral Curves

We conducted additional simulation studies where the shape components were generated using an alternative method, functional PCA (fPCA), distinct from the approach in Sect. 3. In this approach, we first generated a sample of spiral curves as described in Sect. 3.1. Using these curves, we estimated the shape mean, covariance matrix, and applied singular value decomposition (SVD) to the estimated covariance to extract the first two principal components (PCs). More details on fPCA for shapes can be found in [40]. The variability within each spiral curve belonging to the same class was introduced by generating its two PC coefficients as realizations of i.i.d. random variables distributed as $N(0, 4)$. The generation of 3D point cloud components and the simulation process for training and testing were consistent with the procedures outlined in Sect. 3.1. The results of these simulations are presented in Fig. 13.

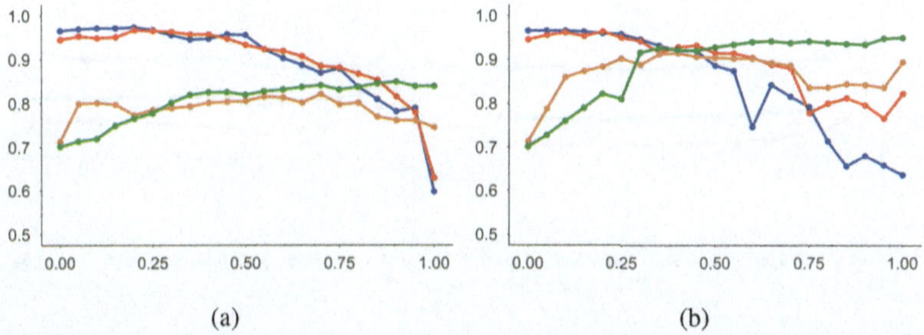

Fig. 13 Average classification accuracy, across ten independent test sets, for different values of a in the hybrid distance d_H. (**a**) Settings corresponding to Table 1, but with the shape component generated as described in Appendix A. (**b**) Settings corresponding to Table 2, but with the shape component generated as described in Appendix A. Settings 1–4 are shown in blue, red, orange, and green, respectively

Let us first consider the case when $p = 0$ (Fig. 13a). Consistent with the findings in Sect. 3.2, the weight $a = 0$ achieves the best performance when the shape signal is the strongest (blue). As the shape signal weakens and the point cloud signal becomes stronger, the optimal weight values shift to $a = 0.2$ (red), $a = 0.4$ (orange) and $a = 1$ (green). For $p = 1$ (Fig. 13b), similar patterns emerge. The optimal weight values of a are 0.2, 0.2, 0.7 and 0.9, corresponding to the blue, red, orange and green curves, respectively.

Appendix B: Analysis of Hawaiian Drosophila Wings with Size-and-shape Elastic Distance

We extended our nearest neighbor classification analysis for the Drosophila wings dataset to include wing size, in addition to the shape-only analysis described in Sect. 4.1. For this analysis, we utilize the size-and-shape elastic distance outlined in Sect. 2.1.1, without rescaling by the length of the wing outline. Figure 14 presents the results for all values of a, while Table 7 reports the best-performing cases. Interestingly, in all cases except the secondary class structure with $p = 1$, the highest classification accuracy is achieved when using curve information only. The inclusion of size information consistently yields lower classification accuracy as compared to the shape-only analysis. This suggests that considering shape without size information allows for improved classification accuracy through optimal integration of topo-geometric information, as modulated by the parameter a.

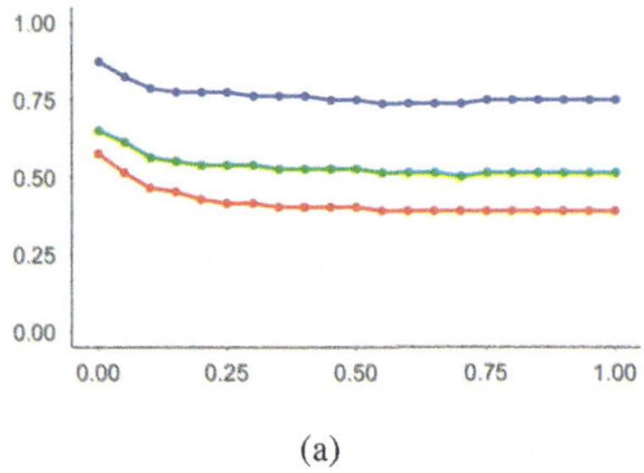

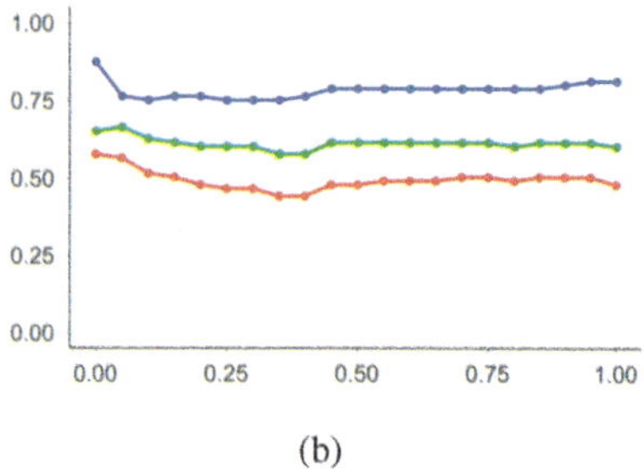

Fig. 14 Nearest neighbor classification accuracy for different values of a, for the Drosophila wings dataset, with size included in the analysis. We report separate results based on (**a**) degree $p = 0$ features, and (**b**) degree $p = 1$ features. The primary, secondary and tertiary classification results are shown in blue, green and red, respectively

Table 7 Classification accuracy under six different scenarios for the Drosophila wings dataset, with size included in the analysis: (i) primary class structure with degree $p = 0$, (ii) primary with $p = 1$, (iii) secondary with $p = 0$, (iv) secondary with $p = 1$, (v) tertiary with $p = 0$, and (vi) tertiary with $p = 1$. Highest classification accuracy for each class structure is italicized and underlined

Class structure	Optimal a	Degree p	Classification accuracy
Primary	0	0	*0.877*
	0	1	*0.877*
Secondary	0	0	0.654
	0.05	1	*0.667*
Tertiary	0	0	*0.580*
	0	1	*0.580*

References

1. Bellissent-Funel, M.-C., Hassanali, A., Havenith, M., Henchman, R., Pohl, P., Sterpone, F., Van Der Spoel, D., Xu, Y., Garcia, A.E.: Water determines the structure and dynamics of proteins. Chem. Rev. **116**(13), 7673–7697 (2016)
2. Berg, J., Sorensen, S., Ting, J., Miller, J., Chartrand, T., Buchin, A., Bakken, T., Budzillo, A., Dee, N., Ding, S.-L., Gouwens, N., Hodge, R., Kalmbach, B., Lee, C., Lee, B., Alfiler, L., Baker, K., Barkan, E., Beller, A., Berry, K., Bertagnolli, D., Bickley, K., Bomben, J., Braun, T., Brouner, K., Casper, T., Chong, P., Crichton, K., Dalley, R., de Frates, R., Desta, T., Dingman Lee, S., D'Orazi, F., Dotson, N., Egdorf, T., Enstrom, R., Farrell, C., Feng, D., Fong, O., Furdan, S., Galakhova, A., Gamlin, C., Gary, A., Glandon, A., Goldy, J., Gorham, M., Goriounova, N., Gratiy, S., Graybuck, L., Gu, H., Hadley, K., Hansen, N., Heistek, T., Henry, A., Heyer, D., Hill, D., Hill, C., Hupp, M., Jarsky, T., Kebede, S., Keene, L., Kim, L., Kim, M.-H., Kroll, M., Latimer, C., Levi, B., Link, K., Mallory, M., Mann, R., Marshall, D., Maxwell, M., McGraw, M., D. McMillen, Melief, E., Mertens, E., Mezei, L., Mihut, N., Mok, S., Molnar, G., Mukora, A., Ng, L., Ngo, K., Nicovich, P., Nyhus, J., Olah, G., Oldre, A., Omstead, V., Ozsvar, A., Park, D., Peng, H., Pham, T., Pom, C., Potekhina, L., Rajanbabu, R., Ransford, S., Reid, D., Rimorin, C., Ruiz, A., Sandman, D., Sulc, J., Sunkin, S., Szafer, A., Szemenyei, V., Thomsen, E., Tieu, M., Torkelson, A., Trinh, J., Tung, H., Wakeman, W., Ward, K., Wilbers, R., Williams, G., Yao, Z., Yoon, J.-G., Anastassiou,

C., Arkhipov, A., Barzo, P., Bernard, A., Cobbs, C., de Witt Hamer, P., Ellenbogen, R., Esposito, L., Ferreira, M., Gwinn, R., Hawrylycz, M., Hof, P., Idema, S., Jones, A., Keene, C., Ko, A., Murphy, G., Ng, L., Ojemann, J., Patel, A., Phillips, J., Silbergeld, D., Smith, K., Tasic, B., Yuste, R., Segev, I., de Kock, C.P., Mansvelder, H., Tamas, G., Zeng, H., Koch, C., Lein, E.; Human cortical expansion involves diversification and specialization of supragranular intratelencephalic-projecting neurons. bioRxiv (2020). https://doi.org/10.1101/2020.03.31.018820
3. Bubenik, P.: Statistical topological data analysis using persistence landscapes. J. Mach. Learn. Res. **16**(1), 77–102 (2015)
4. Carlsson, G.: Topology and data. Bull. Am. Math. Soc. **46**(2), 255–308 (2009)
5. Chazal, F., Fasy, B.T., Lecci, F., Rinaldo, A., Wasserman, L.: Stochastic convergence of persistence landscapes and silhouettes. In: Proceedings of Annual Symposium on Computational Geometry, pp. 474–483 (2014)
6. Chen, J.-R., Wang, B.-N., Tseng, G.-F., Wang, Y.-J., Huang, Y.-S., Wang, T.-J.: Morphological changes of cortical pyramidal neurons in hepatic encephalopathy. BMC Neurosci. **15**(1), 1–12 (2014)
7. Cho, M.H., Asiaee, A., Kurtek, S.: Elastic statistical shape analysis of biological structures with case studies: A tutorial. Bull. Math. Biol. **81**, 2052–2073 (2019)
8. Cohen-Steiner, D., Edelsbrunner, H., Harer, J.: Stability of persistence diagrams. In: Proceedings of Annual Symposium on Computational Geometry, pp. 263–271 (2005)
9. Cohen-Steiner, D., Edelsbrunner, H., Harer, J., Mileyko, Y.: Lipschitz functions have L_p-stable persistence. Found. Comput. Math. **10**(2), 127–139 (2010)
10. Cortes, C., Vapnik, V.: Support-vector networks. Mach. Learn. **20**, 273–297 (1995)
11. Dijkstra, E.W.: A note on two problems in connexion with graphs. Numerische Mathematik **1**, 269–271 (1959)
12. Drira, H., Ben Amor, B., Srivastava, A., Daoudi, M.: A Riemannian analysis of 3D nose shapes for partial human biometrics. In: Proceedings of IEEE International Conference on Computer Vision, pp. 2050–2057 (2009)
13. Drira, H., Ben Amor, B., Daoudi, M., Srivastava, A.: Pose and expression-invariant 3D face recognition using elastic radial curves. In: Proceedings of British Machine Vision Conference, pp. 1–11 (2010)
14. Duncan, A., Klassen, E., Srivastava, A.: Statistical shape analysis of simplified neuronal trees. Ann. Appl. Stat. **12**(3), 1385–1421 (2018)
15. Edelsbrunner, H.: A Short Course in Computational Geometry and Topology. Springer, Berlin (2014)
16. Edelsbrunner, H., Letscher, D., Zomorodian, A.: Topological persistence and simplification. Discrete Comput. Geom. **28**, 511–533 (2002)
17. Edelsbrunner, H., Harer, J., et al.: Persistent homology-a survey. Contemp. Math. **453**(26), 257–282 (2008)
18. Edwards, K.A., Doescher, L.T., Kaneshiro, K.Y., Yamamoto, D.: A database of wing diversity in the Hawaiian Drosophila. PLoS One **2**(5), e487 (2007)
19. Efrat, A., Itai, A., Katz, M.J.: Geometry helps in bottleneck matching and related problems. Algorithmica **31**, 1–28 (2001)
20. Ester, M., Kriegel, H.-P., Sander, J., Xu, X.: A density-based algorithm for discovering clusters in large spatial databases with noise. In: Proceedings of International Conference on Knowledge Discovery and Data Mining, vol. 96, pp. 226–231 (1996)
21. Gilchrist, A., Azevedo, R., Partridge, L., O'Higgins, P.: Adaptation and constraint in the evolution of Drosophila melanogaster wing shape. Evol. Develop. **2**(2), 114–124 (2000)
22. Joshi, S.H., Klassen, E., Srivastava, A., Jermyn, I.H.: A novel representation for Riemannian analysis of elastic curves in $\mathbb{R}^n$. In: Proceedings of IEEE Conference on Computer Vision and Pattern Recognition, pp. 1–7 (2007)

23. Kanari, L., Dłotko, P., Scolamiero, M., Levi, R., Shillcock, J., Hess, K., Markram, H.: A topological representation of branching neuronal morphologies. Neuroinformatics **16**, 3–13 (2018)
24. Kendall, D.G.: Shape manifolds, Procrustean metrics, and complex projective spaces. Bull. London Math. Soc. **16**(2), 81–121 (1984)
25. Kouranov, A., Xie, L., de la Cruz, J., Chen, L., Westbrook, J., Bourne, P.E., Berman, H.M.: The RCSB PDB information portal for structural genomics. Nucleic Acids Res. **34**, D302–D305 (2006)
26. Kurtek, S., Srivastava, A., Klassen, E., Ding, Z.: Statistical modeling of curves using shapes and related features. J. Am. Stat. Assoc. **107**(499), 1152–1165 (2012)
27. Laga, H., Kurtek, S., Srivastava, A., Miklavcic, S.J.: Landmark-free statistical analysis of the shape of plant leaves. J. Theor. Biol. **363**, 41–52 (2014)
28. Levy, Y., Onuchic, J.N.: Water mediation in protein folding and molecular recognition. Ann. Rev. Biophys. Biomol. Struct. **35**, 389–415 (2006)
29. Liu, W., Srivastava, A., Zhang, J.: Protein structure alignment using elastic shape analysis. In: Proceedings of ACM International Conference on Bioinformatics and Computational Biology, pp. 62–70, (2010)
30. Mason, A., Larkman, A.: Correlations between morphology and electrophysiology of pyramidal neurons in slices of rat visual cortex. II. Electrophysiology. J. Neurosci. **10**(5), 1415–1428 (1990)
31. Matuk, J., Kurtek, S., Bharath, K.: Robust persistent homology using elastic functional data analysis. arXiv, 2106.15436v3 (2022)
32. Mileyko, Y., Mukherjee, S., Harer, J.: Probability measures on the space of persistence diagrams. Inverse Probl. **27**(12), 124007 (2011)
33. Mio, W., Srivastava, A., Joshi, S.H.: On shape of plane elastic curves. Int. J. Comput. Vision **73**, 307–324 (2007)
34. Munch, E.: A user's guide to topological data analysis. J. Learn. Analy. **4**(2), 47–61 (2017)
35. Ng, A., Jordan, M., Weiss, Y.: On spectral clustering: Analysis and an algorithm. In: Proceedings of Advances in Neural Information Processing Systems, vol. 14 (2001)
36. Record, M.T., Anderson, C.F., Lohman, T.M.: Thermodynamic analysis of ion effects on the binding and conformational equilibria of proteins and nucleic acids: the roles of ion association or release, screening, and ion effects on water activity. Quart. Rev. Biophys. **11**(2), 103–178 (1978)
37. Robinson, D.T.: Functional Data Analysis and Partial Shape Matching in the Square Root Velocity Framework. The Florida State University, Tallahassee (2012)
38. Schubert, E., Sander, J., Ester, M., Kriegel, H.P., Xu, X.: DBSCAN revisited, revisited: why and how you should (still) use DBSCAN. ACM Trans. Database Syst. **42**(3), 1–21 (2017)
39. Sehnal, D., Bittrich, S., Deshpande, M., Svobodová, R., Berka, K., Bazgier, V., Velankar, S., Burley, S.K., Koča, J., Rose, A.S.: Mol* Viewer: modern web app for 3D visualization and analysis of large biomolecular structures. Nucleic Acids Res. **49**(W1), W431–W437 (2021)
40. Srivastava, A., Klassen, E.P.: Functional and Shape Data Analysis. Springer, Berlin (2016)
41. Srivastava, A., Klassen, E., Joshi, S.H., Jermyn, I.H.: Shape analysis of elastic curves in Euclidean spaces. IEEE Trans. Pattern Analy. Mach. Intell. **33**(7), 1415–1428 (2010)
42. Suo, L., Lu, H., Ying, G., Capecchi, M.R., Wu, Q.: Protocadherin clusters and cell adhesion kinase regulate dendrite complexity through Rho GTPase. J. Mol. Cell Biol. **4**(6), 362–376 (2012)
43. Von Luxburg, U.: A tutorial on spectral clustering. Stat. Comput. **17**, 395–416 (2007)
44. Waddington, C.H.: The genetic control of wing development in Drosophila. J. Genet. **41**, 75–113 (1940)
45. Ward Jr., J.H.: Hierarchical grouping to optimize an objective function. J. Am. Stat. Assoc. **58**, 236–244 (1963)
46. Wasserman, L.: Topological data analysis. Ann. Rev. Stat. Appl. **5**(1), 501–532 (2018)

47. Wu, S.G., Bao, F.S., Xu, E.Y., Wang, Y.-X., Chang, Y.-F., Xiang, Q.-L.: A leaf recognition algorithm for plant classification using probabilistic neural network. In: Proceedings of International Symposium on Signal Processing and Information Technology (2007)
48. Younes, L.: Computable elastic distances between shapes. SIAM J. Appl. Math. **58**(2), 565–586 (1998)
49. Zomorodian, A., Carlsson, G.: Computing persistent homology. In: Proceedings of Annual Symposium on Computational Geometry, pp. 347–356, (2004)

Bifurcation Analysis of an Analog Hopfield Neural Network with Three Time Delays

Vladimir E. Bondarenko

Abstract An analog Hopfield neural network with excitatory and inhibitory connections and three time delays was studied. The neural networks demonstrated synchronous outputs shortly after the initial conditions. The networks with excitatory connections demonstrated either output decay or output growth until saturation at the constant value. The networks with inhibitory connections showed either decaying oscillations or growing oscillations until saturation of their amplitudes. An increase of the time delay in one, two, or three inhibitory subnetworks resulted in various activities, such as the smooth amplitude and period growth, multiresonances of amplitudes, oscillation period jumps, and period-tripling bifurcations. In several cases of subnetwork configurations, oscillation periods demonstrated discrete ranges of changes, similar to the discrete oscillation rhythms in the human and animal electroencephalogram.

Keywords Hopfield neural network · Synchronization · Excitatory and inhibitory neural networks · Bifurcation · Electroencephalogram

1 Introduction

Hopfield neural networks attract attention due to their relative simplicity and capability to store variety of patterns. Two classes of Hopfield neural networks have been studied and continue to study at the present time: discrete Hopfield neural networks [1] and continuous (analog) Hopfield neural networks [2]. Because Hopfield neural networks are used in multiple applications, such as image processing [3–6], speech recognition [7], cryptography [8], and others, it is important to investigate basic

V. E. Bondarenko (✉)
Department of Mathematics and Statistics and Neuroscience Institute, Georgia State University, Atlanta, GA, USA
e-mail: vbondarenko@gsu.edu

Y. Zhao, D.-G. Chen (eds.), *Big Data Analytics in Biostatistics and Bioinformatics*, ICSA Book Series in Statistics,
https://doi.org/10.1007/978-3-032-06649-7_14

properties of Hopfield neural networks, such as stability, different types of outputs (steady-state, periodic, chaotic activities), synchronization, etc. [9–12].

Hopfield neural networks with time delays form a special class of networks that was intensively studied in recent years. As stability properties of the Hopfield neural networks with one time delay established in early studies [9, 13–15], the subsequent investigations were devoted to the neural networks with multiple time delays [12, 16–19]. Conditions for a Hopf bifurcation in Hopfield neural network with two time delays and several examples of the neural network behavior were provided in [16]. In [19], the stability properties of Hopfield neural network with multiple time delays were investigated by the application of geometrical scheme, within which two new angle variables are introduced to develop Hopf bifurcation by varying time delay continuously. Delay-induced synchronization in the coupled memristive Hopfield neural networks was studied in [17]. It was shown that using two time delays had a better effect on the synchronization of the system. Furthermore, synchronization by designing a state feedback controller in the Hopfield network was investigated in Ref. [18]. The proposed method was applied for the image encryption. Synchronization properties, multiresonances, and bifurcations of the Hopfield neural network with two time delays were studied in Ref. [12]. It was shown that such a network demonstrated fast synchronization of all neurons, multiresonances, and period-doubling bifurcation as functions of time delays τ_1 and τ_2.

While significant amount of papers was devoted to the stability analysis and applications of the Hopfield neural network, its behavior in the regions of instability was less studied. Therefore, in this paper, we investigated the behavior of the Hopfield neural network with three time delays and excitatory and inhibitory connections predominantly in the instability regions. In these cases, purely excitatory neural network with all $a_{ij} = +1$ demonstrated synchronous output growth until saturation level, whereas purely inhibitory neural network with $a_{ij} = -1$ showed synchronous oscillation growth until saturation at different levels of amplitudes, depending on the network configuration and stimulation protocols. The stability threshold of purely excitatory neural network did not depend on the time delays and subnetwork configurations. However, if one subnetwork has a much smaller (by an order of magnitude) time delay, the time interval until saturation of the outputs dramatically decreases compared to the neural network composed of the subnetworks with much larger (by an order of magnitude) and identical time delays. Purely inhibitory neural networks with different time delays demonstrated multiresonance activity with period jumps and period-tripling bifurcations that were observed with an increase of time delay in one or two inhibitory subnetworks. They also exhibited transitions between different oscillation shapes as the time delays were varied. In several cases of subnetwork configurations with different time delays, oscillation periods demonstrated discrete ranges of changes, similar to the discrete oscillation rhythms in the human and animal electroencephalogram. This provides potentially an interesting mechanism for the formation of the discrete oscillation spectrum in the neural networks with multiple time delays.

2 Neural Network Model

The neural network model with three time delays studied in this paper (Fig. 1) contains $M = 12$ neurons, which are connected to each other ("all with all" connections). In this network, one-third of the neurons (four neurons) have inputs delayed by time τ_1, one-third of the neurons have inputs delayed by time τ_2, and one-third of the neurons have inputs delayed by time τ_3. Each neuron also has delayed input from itself. The model also considers a leak for each neuron, with identical leak magnitude and without time delay [9].

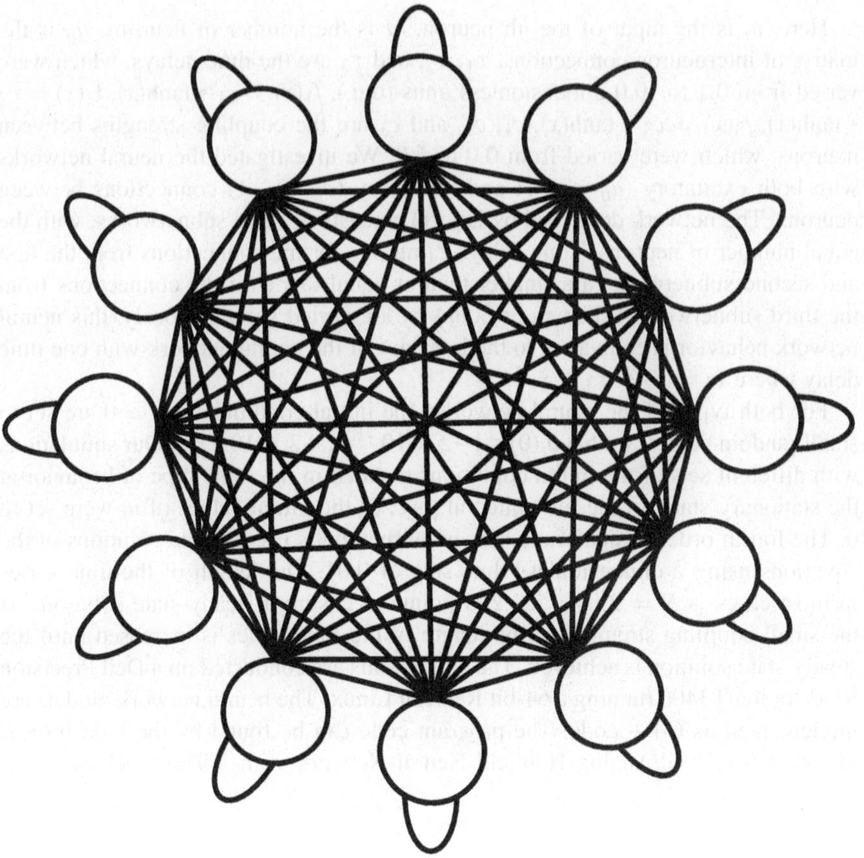

Fig. 1 The Hopfield neural network structure. Twelve neurons are shown by the circles. All neurons in the network are connected to each other with time delay (shown by straight lines). Each neuron has also delayed and non-delayed inputs from itself (curved lines). There are three subnetworks, each of which consists of four neurons

The neural network with three time delays is described by the set of ordinary differential equations:

$$\dot{u}_i(t) = -u_i(t) + \sum_{j=1}^{M/3} a_{ij} f_1\left(u_j\left(t-\tau_1\right)\right) + \sum_{j=M/3+1}^{2M/3} a_{ij} f_2\left(u_j\left(t-\tau_2\right)\right) + \sum_{j=2M/3+1}^{M} a_{ij} f_3\left(u_j\left(t-\tau_3\right)\right), \quad i, j = 1, 2, \ldots, M. \tag{1}$$

Here, u_i is the input of the ith neuron, M is the number of neurons, a_{ij} is the matrix of interneuron connections, τ_1, τ_2, and τ_3 are the time delays, which were varied from 0.1 to 10.0 dimensionless units (d.u.), $f_1(x) = c_1 \bullet \tanh(x)$, $f_2(x) = c_2 \bullet \tanh(x)$, $f_3(x) = c_3 \bullet \tanh(x)$, c_1, c_2, and c_3 are the coupling strengths between neurons, which were varied from 0.0 to 5.0. We investigated the neural networks with both excitatory ($a_{ij} = +1$) and inhibitory ($a_{ij} = -1$) connections between neurons. The network described by Eq. (1) consists of three subnetworks, with the equal number of neurons. Time delays τ_1 and τ_2 for the connections from the first and second subnetworks are smaller than or equal to τ_3 for the connections from the third subnetwork. When τ_1, τ_2, and τ_3 are varied simultaneously, this neural network behavior is equivalent to the behavior of the neural network with one time delay where $\tau_1 = \tau_2 = \tau_3 = \tau$.

For both types of the neural networks, the initial conditions at $t = 0$ are set to small random values, so that $u_i(0) \in [-2 \times 10^{-100}, +2 \times 10^{-100}]$. Our simulations with different sets of the initial conditions resulted in the same type of behavior at the stationary state. In the time interval $[-\tau, 0)$ the initial values of u_i were set to 0. The fourth order Runge-Kutta numerical method is used to find solutions of the equations using a dimensionless time step of 0.01. The length of the time series in most cases is $N = 2^{19} = 524{,}288$ points to ensure a steady-state solution. At the small coupling strengths c, the length of the time series is increased until the steady-state solution is achieved. The simulations are conducted on a Dell Precision Workstation T3400 running a 64-bit Red Hat Linux. The neural network models are implemented as C++ code. The program code can be found by the link: https://github.com/vebond/Analog-Hopfield-Neural-Network-with-3-Time-Delays-

3 Results

3.1 Subthreshold and Suprathreshold Neural Network Outputs

Excitatory neural network displays two types of activities distinguished by a threshold value of c ($c_{\text{th}} \approx 0.08$), which was determined by the method described

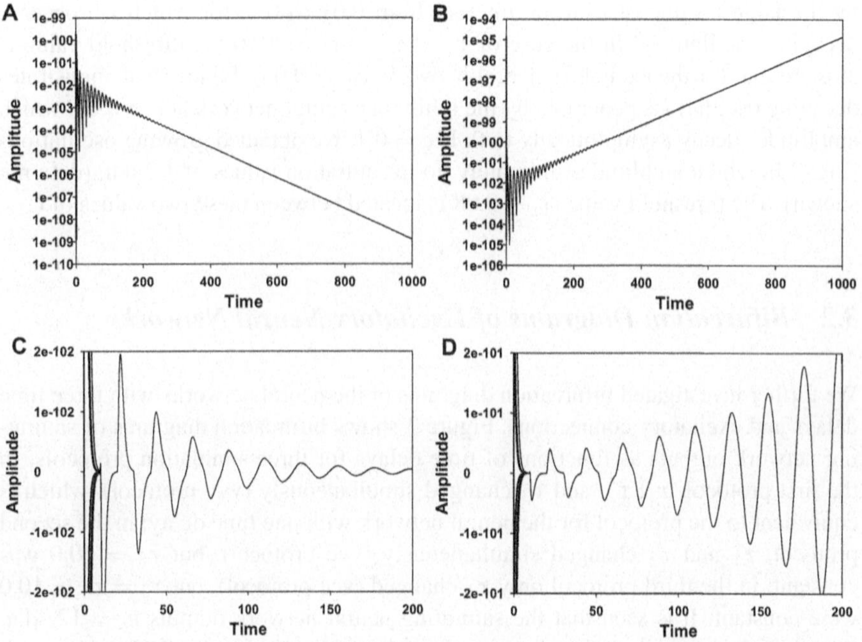

Fig. 2 Activity of the fully connected neural network with excitatory ($a_{ij} = 1$) and inhibitory ($a_{ij} = -1$) connections. (**a**) Excitatory network, subthreshold case ($c = 0.07$). Decaying outputs. (**b**) Excitatory network, suprathreshold case ($c = 0.1$). Growing outputs. (**c**) Inhibitory network, subthreshold case ($c = 0.07$). Decaying oscillations. (**d**) Inhibitory network, suprathreshold case ($c = 0.1$). growing oscillations

in [12]. For this purpose, we simulated the whole network activities from the initial conditions to obtain a time series of $N = 524{,}288$ datapoints as functions of the connection strength c. The parameter c changed from 0.01 to 0.4 with increment 0.01. Figure 2a demonstrates decaying subthreshold neural output oscillations in semilogarithmic plot starting from the initial conditions for all 12 neurons ($c = 0.07$), which become extinct with time. An increase in c to 0.1 results in a growing suprathreshold neural outputs, in which oscillations become extinct in time (Fig. 2b), and the output amplitudes saturate at 1.2 d.u. (data not shown). The threshold value $c_{th} \approx 0.08$ is located between these two values of c and is determined by the largest value of c in the interval from 0.01 to 0.4, for which we observe decaying outputs.

Inhibitory neural network also demonstrates both subthreshold and suprathreshold oscillatory outputs with a threshold value of c. For the inhibitory neural networks, saturation oscillation amplitudes were determined by the calculations of the maxima during the last 65,536 datapoints out of 524,288 datapoints in the time series. The parameter c also changed from 0.01 to 0.4 with increment 0.01, as in case of excitatory neural network. The threshold value c_{th} is determined by the largest value of c in the interval from 0.01 to 0.4, for which we observe decaying oscillations. In the case of $\tau_1 = \tau_2 = \tau_3 = 10.0$ the threshold value is close to that for the excitatory neural network ($c_{th} \approx 0.08$). Figure 2c demonstrates decaying oscillations generated by the inhibitory neural network at $c = 0.07$, which amplitudes decay asymptotically to 0. If $c = 0.1$, we obtained growing oscillations (Fig. 2d), which amplitudes ultimately go to saturation values of 1.2 d.u. (data not shown). The threshold value $c_{th} \approx 0.08$ is located between these two values of c.

3.2 Bifurcation Diagrams of Excitatory Neural Networks

We further investigated bifurcation diagrams of the neural networks with three time delays and excitatory connections. Figure 3 shows bifurcation diagrams of saturating network outputs as functions of time delays for three simulation protocols. In the first protocol, τ_1, τ_2, and τ_3 changed simultaneously (vvv protocol), which is equivalent to the protocol for the neural network with one time delay; in the second protocol, τ_1 and τ_2 changed simultaneously (vvc protocol), but $\tau_3 = 10.0$ was constant; in the third protocol only τ_1 changed (vcc protocol), but $\tau_2 = \tau_3 = 10.0$ were constant. It is seen that the saturating neural network outputs $u_i = 12$ d.u. were identical for all explored protocols and for all 12 neurons. While this result looks trivial, the actual time behavior of the network outputs before saturation was different for different time delay relationships between three subnetworks.

Figure 4 demonstrates the initial parts of the excitatory network activities for different relationships between τ_1, τ_2, and τ_3. All output traces are synchronous after relatively short period of time starting from the initial conditions and represent activities of all 12 neurons. When $\tau_1 = \tau_2 = \tau_3 = 10.0$, the neural outputs of all three subnetworks saturate at time moment ~1055 d.u. (Fig. 4a). Here and further in this paper, the time of the saturation is defined as the time moment when a datapoint differs from the saturating amplitude by less than 0.001 d.u. When the subnetworks have a much smaller time delays ($\tau_1 = \tau_2 = \tau_3 = 1.0$), we observe a dramatical decrease in the growth time to saturation at the amplitude of 12 d.u., which is ~164 d.u. of time (Fig. 4b). In the case, when $\tau_1 = \tau_2 = \tau_3 = 0.1$, our simulations show a further decrease of the time interval until saturation at the amplitude of 12 d.u., which is ~54 d.u. of time (Fig. 4c). The effect of a dramatic decrease in the time interval until saturation was also observed when only time delay in one subnetwork was decreased by 2 orders of magnitude. As an example, we consider the case when $\tau_1 = 0.1$ and $\tau_2 = \tau_3 = 10.0$ (Fig. 4d). In this case, our simulations show a decrease of the time interval until saturation at the amplitude of 12 d.u., which is ~132 d.u. of time. In addition, we also see a saturation sublevel at the amplitude of ~4 d.u. (one-thirds of 12 d.u.), which is ~116 d.u. of time (Fig. 4d), pointing to the more complex excitatory neural output behavior in the networks with inequal time delays.

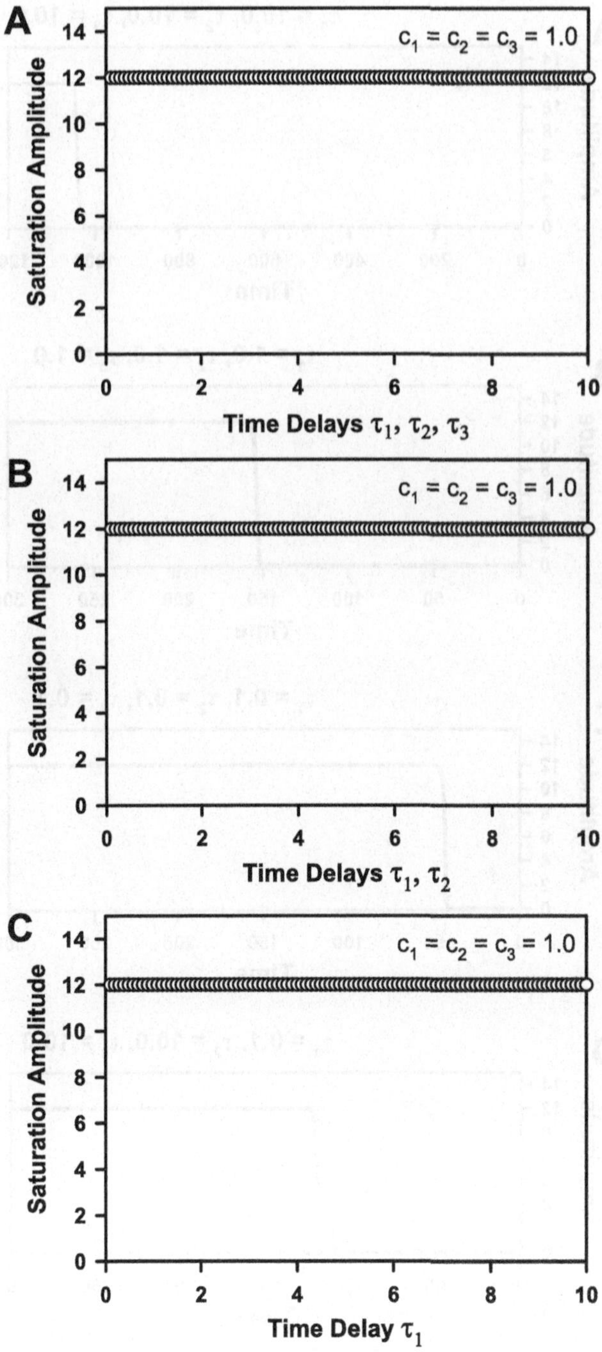

Fig. 3 Saturation amplitudes of the Hopfield neural network with excitatory connections $c_1 = c_2 = c_3 = 1.0$ and three time delays when τ_1, τ_2, and τ_3 (**a**), τ_1 and τ_2 (**b**), or τ_1 (**c**) are varied. In all cases, the outputs saturate at the level of 12 dimensionless units

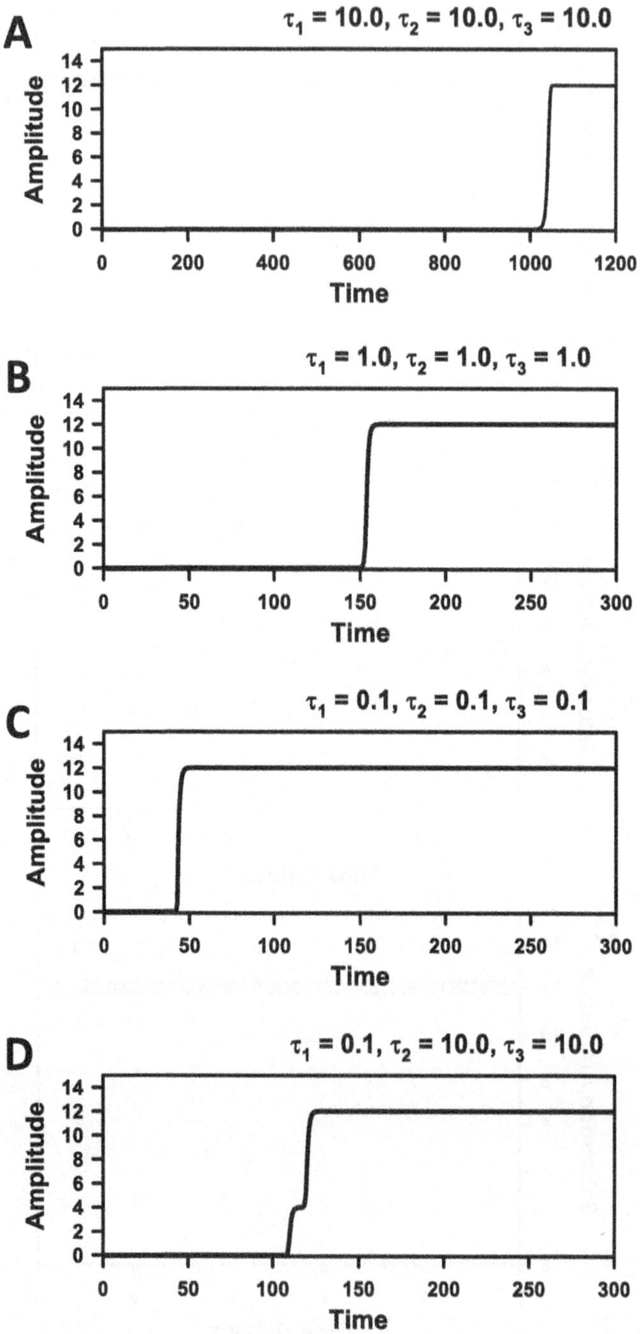

Fig. 4 Excitatory Hopfield neural network output development at different time delays τ_1, τ_2, and τ_3. (**a**) $\tau_1 = 10.0$, $\tau_2 = 10.0$, $\tau_3 = 10.0$; (**b**) $\tau_1 = 1.0$, $\tau_2 = 1.0$, $\tau_3 = 1.0$; (**c**) $\tau_1 = 0.1$, $\tau_2 = 0.1$, $\tau_3 = 0.1$; (**d**) $\tau_1 = 0.1$, $\tau_2 = 10.0$, $\tau_3 = 10.0$. The smaller time delays, the faster output growth to saturation. $c_1 = c_2 = c_3 = 1.0$

3.3 Bifurcation Diagrams of Inhibitory Neural Networks

We also investigated neural networks with three time delays and inhibitory connections. As in the case of excitatory connections, all 12 neural outputs were synchronous after relatively short period of time starting from the initial conditions. Figure 5 shows the bifurcation diagrams of the saturating oscillation amplitudes and oscillation periods as functions of time delays for three simulation protocols (vvv, vvc, and vcc) at the identical connection strengths $c_1 = c_2 = c_3 = 1.0$. In the case, when time delays in all three subnetworks changed simultaneously (vvv protocol, which equivalent to the network with one time delay), the saturation oscillation amplitude grown with time delays until the constant value of 12 d.u. (Fig. 5a). The oscillation periods with the same protocol demonstrated almost linear growth (Fig. 5d).

When the time delays changed only in two subnetworks and the time delay of the third subnetwork was kept constant, $\tau_3 = 10.0$ (vvc protocol), we observed more complex neural network behavior. In this case, we obtained multiple maxima and minima of the saturation oscillation amplitude as a function of time delays τ_1 and τ_2 (Fig. 5b). These changes were accompanied by the relatively small jumps in the corresponding dependence of oscillation period (Fig. 5e), which was close to the linear function. Note that the dependence of the oscillation period of the whole neural network as function of time delays τ_1 and τ_2 (Fig. 5e) closely approximated the dependence of the neural network with one time delay, except for the small-magnitude jumps. Therefore, we can conclude that the third subnetwork with constant time delay $\tau_3 = 10.0$ only slightly affected the oscillation period of the whole network. At the same time, the existence of the third subnetwork with constant time delay clearly indicated by the dramatic change in the behavior of the oscillation amplitude (Fig. 5b).

When we used the third protocol (vcc), where the time delay of one subnetwork τ_1 was changed but the time delays of other two subnetworks were kept constant, $\tau_2 = \tau_3 = 10.0$, we observed different bifurcation diagrams (Fig. 5c, f). At the small time delays τ_1 up to 4.0 d.u., we observed multiple maxima and minima in the saturating oscillation amplitude (Fig. 5c), which were followed by the jumps in the oscillation period (Fig. 5f), from relatively small value of 1.2 d.u. to about 7.5 d.u. When τ_1 changed from 4.0 to 4.6, we observed a period-tripling bifurcation, when the oscillation period changed from ~7.5 d.u. at $\tau_1 = 4.0$ to ~20.6 d.u. at $\tau_1 = 4.6$ (Fig. 5f).

The time series of the oscillations in several characteristic points of bifurcation diagrams of Fig. 5 are shown in Fig. 6. For the vvc protocol, when $\tau_3 = 10.0$, relatively small oscillation amplitudes were obtained at $\tau_1 = \tau_2 = 2.0$ (Fig. 6a), which were increased by almost two-fold at $\tau_1 = \tau_2 = 2.5$ (Fig. 6b). The shape of the oscillations at $\tau_1 = \tau_2 = 2.5$ is of relaxation type, in which first part of the period represented exponential growth and the second part showed exponential decay. Further increase in τ_1 and τ_2 to 4.5 (the last point at the decaying part of the amplitude bifurcation diagram) resulted in a further two-fold amplitude decrease

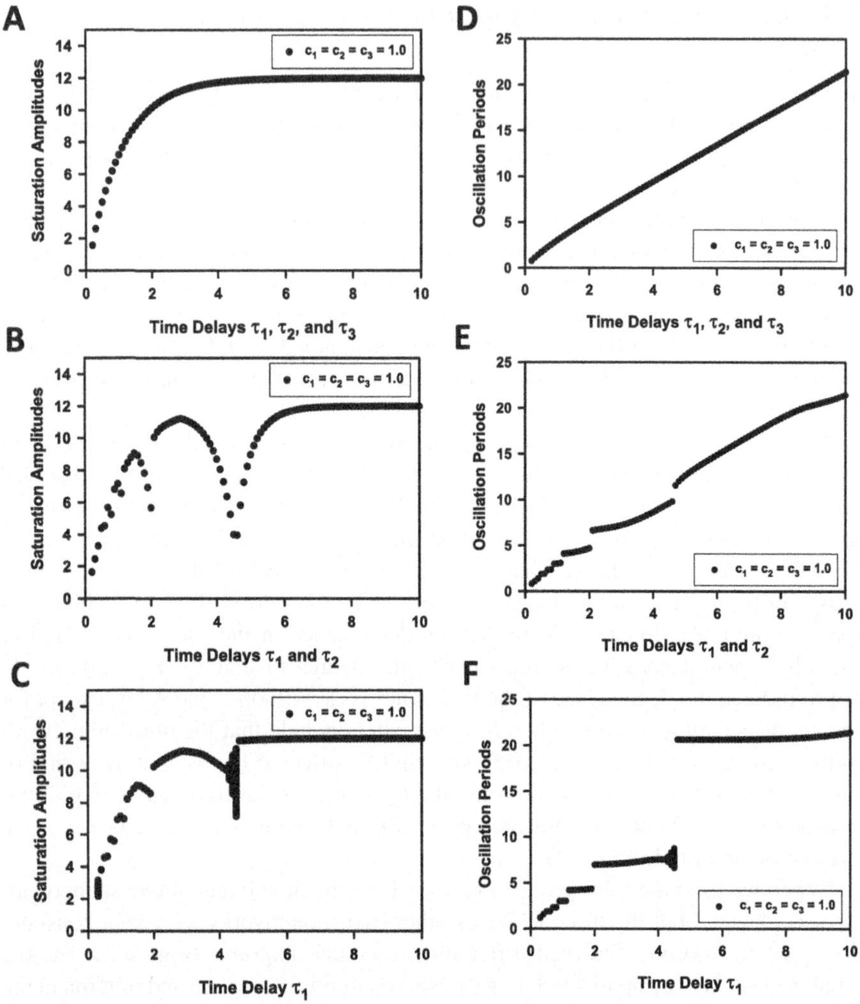

Fig. 5 Bifurcation diagrams of the inhibitory Hopfield neural network when τ_1, τ_2, and τ_3 (**a, d**), τ_1 and τ_2 (**b, e**), or τ_1 (**c, f**) are varied. (**a**) Saturation amplitudes of neural network oscillations as functions of τ_1, τ_2, and τ_3, when they are varied simultaneously. (**b**) Saturation amplitudes of neural network oscillations as functions of τ_1 and τ_2, when they are varied simultaneously. (**c**) Saturation amplitudes of neural network oscillations as functions of τ_1. (**d**) Oscillation period of neural network outputs as functions of τ_1, τ_2, and τ_3, when they are varied simultaneously. (**e**) Oscillation period of neural network outputs as functions of τ_1 and τ_2, when they are varied simultaneously. (**f**) Oscillation period of neural network outputs as functions of τ_1. In all cases, $c_1 = c_2 = c_3 = 1.0$

(Fig. 6c), resulting in trigger-like oscillations (almost instantaneous growth with the following plateau) with the period of 9.6 d.u. Slightly perturbed trigger-like oscillations, similar to those shown in Fig. 6c, but with the period of 9.8 d.u.,

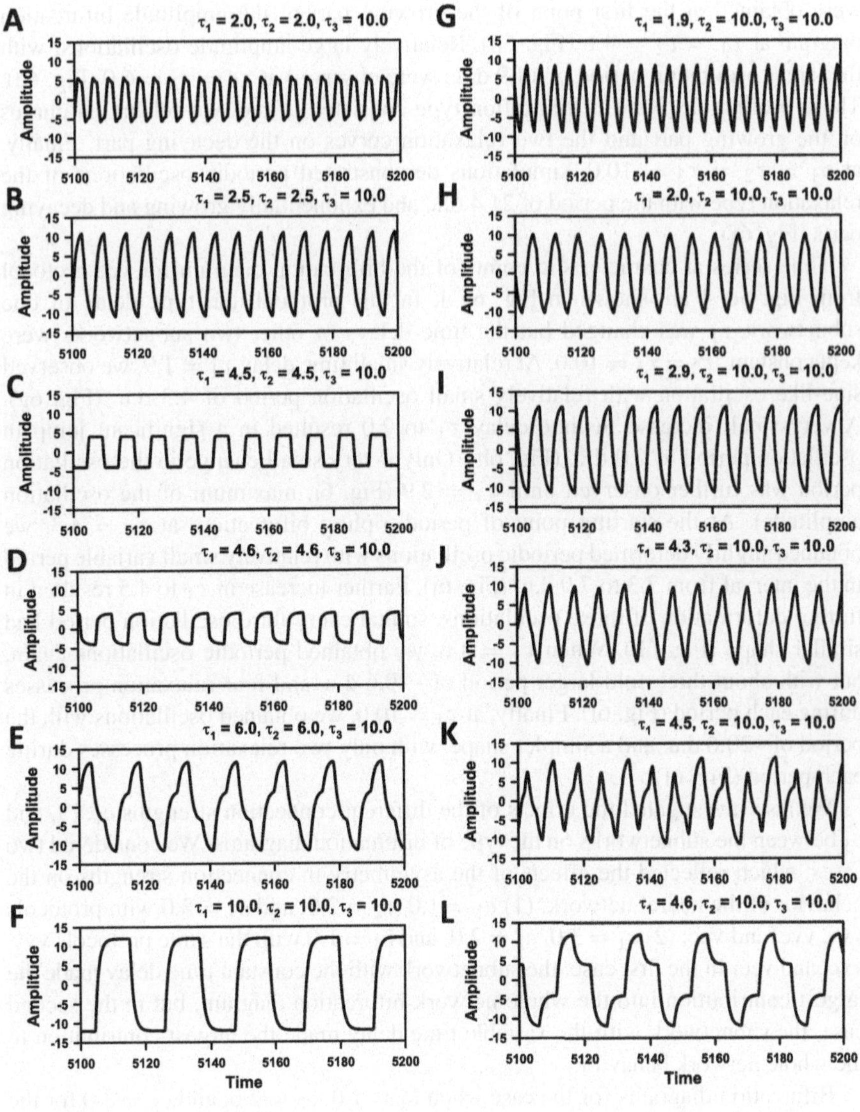

Fig. 6 **(a-f)** Inhibitory Hopfield neural network output time series at characteristics points of bifurcation diagram, when τ_1 and τ_2 are varied simultaneously. **(a)** $\tau_1 = 2.0$, $\tau_2 = 2.0$, $\tau_3 = 10.0$; **(b)** $\tau_1 = 2.5$, $\tau_2 = 2.5$, $\tau_3 = 10.0$; (c) $\tau_1 = 4.5$, $\tau_2 = 4.5$, $\tau_3 = 10.0$; **(d)** $\tau_1 = 4.6$, $\tau_2 = 4.6$, $\tau_3 = 10.0$; **(e)** $\tau_1 = 6.0$, $\tau_2 = 6.0$, $\tau_3 = 10.0$; (f) $\tau_1 = 10.0$, $\tau_2 = 10.0$, $\tau_3 = 10.0$. **(g-l)** Inhibitory Hopfield neural network output time series at characteristic pints of bifurcation diagram during period-tripling bifurcation, when τ_1 is varied. **(g)** $\tau_1 = 1.9$, $\tau_2 = 10.0$, $\tau_3 = 10.0$; **(h)** $\tau_1 = 2.0$, $\tau_2 = 10.0$, $\tau_3 = 10.0$; **(i)** $\tau_1 = 2.9$, $\tau_2 = 10.0$, $\tau_3 = 10.0$; **(j)** $\tau_1 = 4.3$, $\tau_2 = 10.0$, $\tau_3 = 10.0$; **(k)** $\tau_1 = 4.5$, $\tau_2 = 10.0$, $\tau_3 = 10.0$; **(l)** $\tau_1 = 4.6$, $\tau_2 = 10.0$, $\tau_3 = 10.0$. In all cases, $c_1 = c_2 = c_3 = 1.0$

were obtained at the first point of the growing part of the amplitude bifurcation diagram at $\tau_1 = \tau_2 = 4.6$ (Fig. 6d). Relatively large-amplitude oscillations, with the larger oscillation period of 14.9 d.u., were observed at $\tau_1 = \tau_2 = 6.0$ (Fig. 6e). These oscillations were of relaxation type consisted of the two relaxation curves on the growing part and the two relaxation curves on the decaying part. Finally, at $\tau_1 = \tau_2 = \tau_3 = 10.0$, simulations demonstrated periodic oscillations of the relaxation type with the period of 21.4 d.u. and exponentially growing and decaying parts (Fig. 6f).

Time series at characteristic points of the bifurcation diagram for vcc protocol from Fig. 5c, f are shown in Fig. 6g–l. In this protocol, the time delay of one subnetwork τ_1 was changed but the time delays of other two subnetworks were kept constant, $\tau_2 = \tau_3 = 10.0$. At relatively small time delay $\tau_1 = 1.9$, we observed sine-like oscillation with relatively small oscillation period of 4.3 d.u. (Fig. 6g). A very small increase in time delay τ_1 to 2.0 resulted in a significant jump in oscillation period to 7.0 d.u. (Fig. 6h). Only a very small change in the oscillation period was further observed until $\tau_1 = 2.9$ (Fig. 6i, maximum of the oscillation amplitude). At the starting point of period-tripling bifurcation, at $\tau_1 = 4.3$, we obtained slightly deformed periodic oscillations with relatively small variable period in the interval from 7.3 to 7.9 d.u. (Fig. 6j). Further increase in τ_1 to 4.5 resulted in further deformation of those oscillations, so that every third oscillation period had similar shape (Fig. 6k). When $\tau_1 = 4.6$, we obtained periodic oscillations again, but with about three-fold larger period of ~20.6 d.u. and four relaxation processes during each period (Fig. 6l). Finally, at $\tau_1 = 10.0$, we obtained oscillations with the period of ~20.6 d.u. and a simpler shape, with only two relaxation processes during each period (Fig. 6f).

We also investigated the effects of the different connection strengths c_1, c_2, and c_3 between the subnetworks on the type of bifurcation diagrams. We considered two cases, which reflected the effects of the asymmetry in connection strengths on the behavior of the neural network: (1) $c_1 = 1.0$, $c_2 = 2.0$, and $c_3 = 3.0$ with protocols vvv, vvc, and vcc; (2) $c_1 = 3.0$, $c_2 = 2.0$, and $c_3 = 1.0$ with the same protocols vvv, vvc, and vcc. In the first case, the subnetwork with the constant time delay made the largest contribution into the whole network bifurcation diagram, but in the second case, the subnetwork with the variable time delay made the largest contribution to the whole network behavior.

Bifurcation diagrams for the case when $c_1 = 1.0$, $c_2 = 2.0$, and $c_3 = 3.0$ for the three protocols are shown in Fig. 7. When time delays in all three subnetworks changed simultaneously (vvv protocol, equivalent to the network with one time delay), the saturation oscillation amplitude grown with time delays until the saturation value of 24 d.u. (Fig. 7a). The oscillation periods with the same protocol demonstrated almost linear growth (Fig. 7d), and the oscillation periods were similar to those for the network with identical connection strengths $c_1 = 1.0$, $c_2 = 1.0$, and $c_3 = 1.0$ (Fig. 5d).

When we applied the second protocol (vvc), in which the time delays changed only in two subnetworks and the time delay of the third subnetwork was kept constant, $\tau_3 = 10.0$, we observed multiple maxima and minima of the saturation

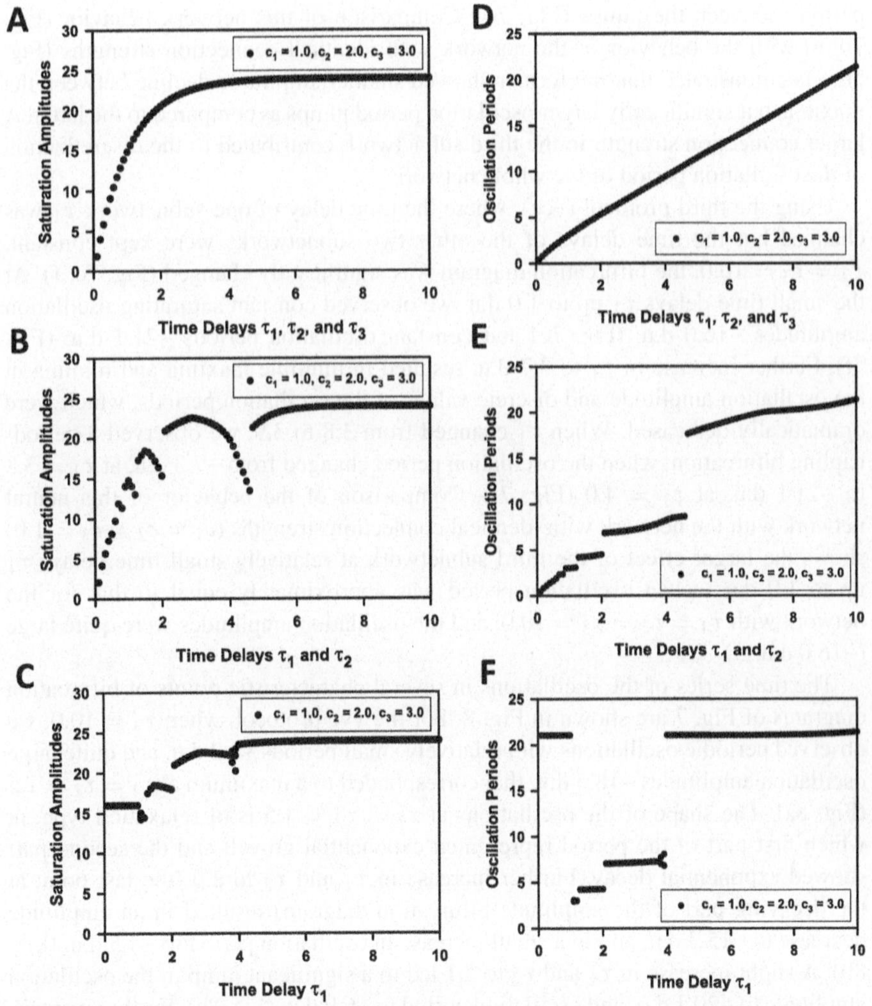

Fig. 7 Bifurcation diagrams of the inhibitory Hopfield neural network when τ_1, τ_2, and τ_3 (**a**, **d**), τ_1 and τ_2 (**b**, **e**), or τ_1 (**c**, **f**) are varied. (**a**) Saturation amplitudes of neural network oscillations as functions of τ_1, τ_2, and τ_3, when they are varied simultaneously. (**b**) Saturation amplitudes of neural network oscillations as functions of τ_1 and τ_2, when they are varied simultaneously. (**c**) Saturation amplitudes of neural network oscillations as functions of τ_1. (**d**) Oscillation period of neural network outputs as functions of τ_1, τ_2, and τ_3, when they are varied simultaneously. (**e**) Oscillation period of neural network outputs as functions of τ_1 and τ_2, when they are varied simultaneously. (**f**) Oscillation period of neural network outputs as functions of τ_1. In all cases, $c_1 = 1.0$, $c_2 = 2.0$, $c_3 = 3.0$

oscillation amplitude as a function of time delays τ_1 and τ_2 (Fig. 7b). The changes in the amplitude were accompanied by quite significant jumps in the corresponding dependence of oscillation period, with relatively weak changes of the oscillation periods between the jumps (Fig. 7e). Comparison of this network behavior (Fig. 7b, e) with the behavior of the network with identical connection strengths (Fig. 5b, e) demonstrated that the former showed smaller amplitude decline between the maxima, but significantly larger oscillation period jumps as compared to the latter. A larger connection strength in the third subnetwork contributed to the discretization of the oscillation period of the whole network.

Using the third protocol (vcc), where the time delay of one subnetwork τ_1 was changed but the time delays of the other two subnetworks were kept constant, $\tau_2 = \tau_3 = 10.0$, the bifurcation diagram was significantly changed (Fig. 7c, f). At the small time delays τ_1 up to 1.0 d.u. we observed constant saturating oscillation amplitudes ~16.0 d.u. (Fig. 7c) and constant oscillation periods ~21.1 d.u. (Fig. 7f). Further increase in τ_1 to 3.7 d.u. resulted in multiple maxima and minima in the oscillation amplitude and discrete values of the oscillation periods, which were dramatically decreased. When τ_1 changed from 3.8 to 3.9, we observed a period-tripling bifurcation, when the oscillation period changed from ~7.3 d.u. at $\tau_1 = 3.8$ to ~21.1 d.u. at $\tau_1 = 4.0$ (Fig. 7f). Comparison of the behavior of this neural network with the network with identical connection strengths ($c_1 = c_2 = c_3 = 1.0$) shows the larger effect of the third subnetwork at relatively small time delays τ_1 up to 1.0 d.u., when oscillation period was approximately equal to that for the network with $\tau_1 = \tau_2 = \tau_3 = 10.0$, and the oscillation amplitudes were quite large (~16.0 d.u.).

The time series of the oscillations in several characteristic points of bifurcation diagrams of Fig. 7 are shown in Fig. 8. For the vvc protocol, when $\tau_3 = 10.0$, we observed periodic oscillations with relatively small periods ~4.2 d.u. and quite large oscillation amplitudes ~18.5 d.u. that corresponded to a maximum at $\tau_1 = \tau_2 = 1.5$ (Fig. 8a). The shape of the oscillations at $\tau_1 = \tau_2 = 1.5$ is of relaxation type, in which first part of the period represented exponential growth and the second part showed exponential decay. Further increase in τ_1 and τ_2 to 2.0 (the last point at the decaying part of the amplitude bifurcation diagram) resulted in an amplitude decrease to ~15.3 d.u. and in a small increase in oscillation period to ~4.5 d.u. (Fig. 8b). A slight increase in τ_1 and τ_2 to 2.1 led to a significant jump in the oscillation amplitude to ~20.1 d.u. and oscillation period to ~6.9 d.u. (Fig. 8c). Further increase in τ_1 and τ_2 to 4.6 (the last point at the decaying part of the amplitude bifurcation diagram) resulted in an amplitude decrease to ~13.5 d.u. and in a moderate increase in oscillation period to ~8.6 d.u. (Fig. 8d). The shape of oscillations demonstrated two exponential increases during the first half of the period and two exponential decreases during the second half of the oscillation period. Yet another slight increase in τ_1 and τ_2 to 4.7 resulted in a significant jump in the oscillation amplitude to ~20.3 d.u. and oscillation period to ~17.6 d.u. (Fig. 8e). The type of the oscillation shape was similar to that in Fig. 8d, but with the larger oscillation period. Finally, at $\tau_1 = \tau_2 = \tau_3 = 10.0$, simulations demonstrated periodic oscillations of relaxation type with the period of 21.4 d.u. and exponentially growing and decaying parts (Fig. 8f).

Time series at characteristic points of the bifurcation diagram for vcc protocol from Fig. 7c, f are shown in Fig. 8g–l. In this protocol, the time delay of one

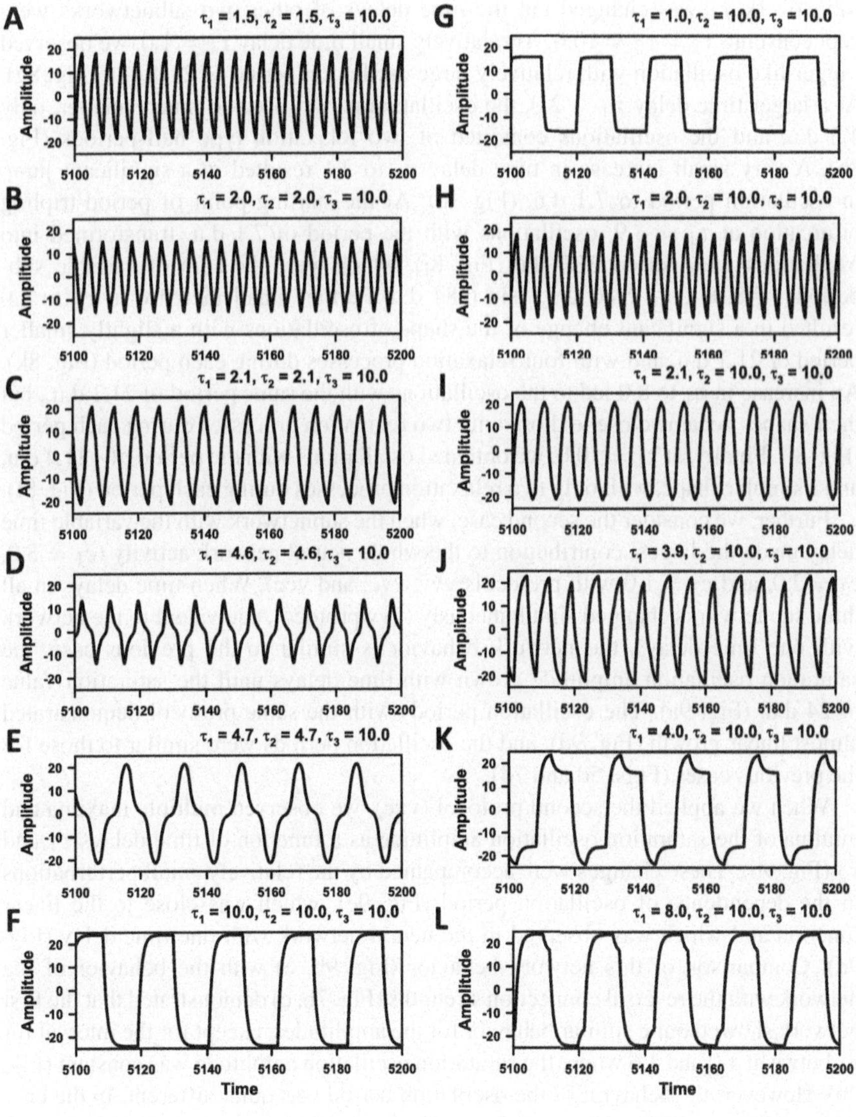

Fig. 8 **(a-f)** Inhibitory Hopfield neural network output time series at characteristics points of bifurcation diagram, when τ_1 and τ_2 are varied simultaneously. **(a)** $\tau_1 = 1.5, \tau_2 = 1.5, \tau_3 = 10.0$; **(b)** $\tau_1 = 2.0, \tau_2 = 2.0, \tau_3 = 10.0$; **(c)** $\tau_1 = 2.1, \tau_2 = 2.1, \tau_3 = 10.0$; **(d)** $\tau_1 = 4.6, \tau_2 = 4.6, \tau_3 = 10.0$; **(e)** $\tau_1 = 4.7, \tau_2 = 4.7, \tau_3 = 10.0$; **(f)** $\tau_1 = 10.0, \tau_2 = 10.0, \tau_3 = 10.0$. **(g-l)** Inhibitory Hopfield neural network output time series at characteristic pints of bifurcation diagram during period-tripling bifurcation, when τ_1 is varied. **(g)** $\tau_1 = 1.0, \tau_2 = 10.0, \tau_3 = 10.0$; **(h)** $\tau_1 = 2.0, \tau_2 = 10.0, \tau_3 = 10.0$; **(i)** $\tau_1 = 2.1, \tau_2 = 10.0, \tau_3 = 10.0$; **(j)** $\tau_1 = 3.9, \tau_2 = 10.0, \tau_3 = 10.0$; **(k)** $\tau_1 = 4.0, \tau_2 = 10.0, \tau_3 = 10.0$; **(l)** $\tau_1 = 8.0, \tau_2 = 10.0, \tau_3 = 10.0$. In all cases, $c_1 = 1.0, c_2 = 2.0, c_3 = 3.0$

subnetwork τ_1 was changed but the time delays of other two subnetworks were kept constant, $\tau_2 = \tau_3 = 10.0$. At relatively small time delay $\tau_1 = 1.0$, we observed trigger-like oscillation with relatively large oscillation period of 21.1 d.u. (Fig. 8g). At a larger time delay $\tau_1 = 2.0$, the oscillation period became much smaller, only 4.3 d.u, and the oscillations consisted of two relaxation type half-periods (Fig. 8h). A very small increase in time delay τ_1 to 2.1 resulted in a significant jump in oscillation period to 7.1 d.u. (Fig. 8i). At the starting point of period-tripling bifurcation at $\tau_1 = 3.9$, oscillations with the period of 7.1 d.u. transformed into oscillations with period 21.7 d.u (Fig. 8j), which were the sum of variable sub-periods of 8.06 d.u., 6.80 d.u., and 6.84 d.u. Further small increase in τ_1 to 4.0 resulted in a significant change of the shape of oscillations with a slightly smaller period of 21.1 d.u. and with four relaxation processes during each period (Fig. 8k). An increase in τ_1 to 8.0 led to the oscillations with the same period of 21.1 d.u., but their shapes became close to those with two relaxation processes during each period (Fig. 8l). Finally, at $\tau_1 = 10.0$, we obtained oscillations with the period of ~21.4 d.u. and a simpler shape, with only two relaxation processes during each period (Fig. 8f).

Further, we consider the second case, when the subnetwork with the variable time delay made the largest contribution to the whole neural network activity ($c_1 = 3.0$, $c_2 = 2.0$, and $c_3 = 1.0$ with protocols vvv, vvc, and vcc). When time delays in all three subnetworks changed simultaneously (vvv protocol, equivalent to the network with one time delay), the network behavior is similar to the previous case, the saturation oscillation amplitude grown with time delays until the saturation value of 24 d.u. (Fig. 9a). The oscillation periods with the same protocol demonstrated almost linear growth (Fig. 9d), and the oscillation periods were similar to those for the previous cases (Figs. 5d and 7d).

When we applied the second protocol (vvc), we observed multiple maxima and minima of the saturation oscillation amplitude as a function of time delays τ_1 and τ_2 (Fig. 9b). These changes were accompanied by the relatively small perturbations in the dependence of oscillation period (Fig. 9e), which was close to the linear function and which was observed in the neural network with one time delay (Fig. 9d). Comparison of this network behavior (Fig. 9b, e) with the behavior of the network with the reversal connection strengths (Fig. 7b, e) demonstrated that the first network showed quite similar behavior for the amplitudes, except for the interval for τ_1 between 4.0 and 4.6 where the saturation oscillation amplitude was constant (Fig. 9b). However, the behavior of the oscillation period was quite different. In the case of $c_1 = 3.0$, $c_2 = 2.0$, and $c_3 = 1.0$, we obtained almost linear growth with τ_1 and τ_2 (Fig. 9e), but in the case of $c_1 = 1.0$, $c_2 = 2.0$, and $c_3 = 3.0$, the oscillation period demonstrated quite significant jumps with the changes in τ_1 and τ_2 (Fig. 7e). Such a behavior of the first network suggests the primary role of the subnetworks with variable time delays, with stronger connection strengths, in the generation of oscillations.

Application of the third protocol (vcc) in the case of $c_1 = 3.0$, $c_2 = 2.0$, and $c_3 = 1.0$ (Fig. 9c, f) resulted in the activity, which was identical to the case of $c_1 = 1.0$, $c_2 = 2.0$, and $c_3 = 3.0$, but with the second protocol (vvc). This identity suggests the equal contributions of the subnetworks with the variable time delays to the network activities due to their equal total connection strengths.

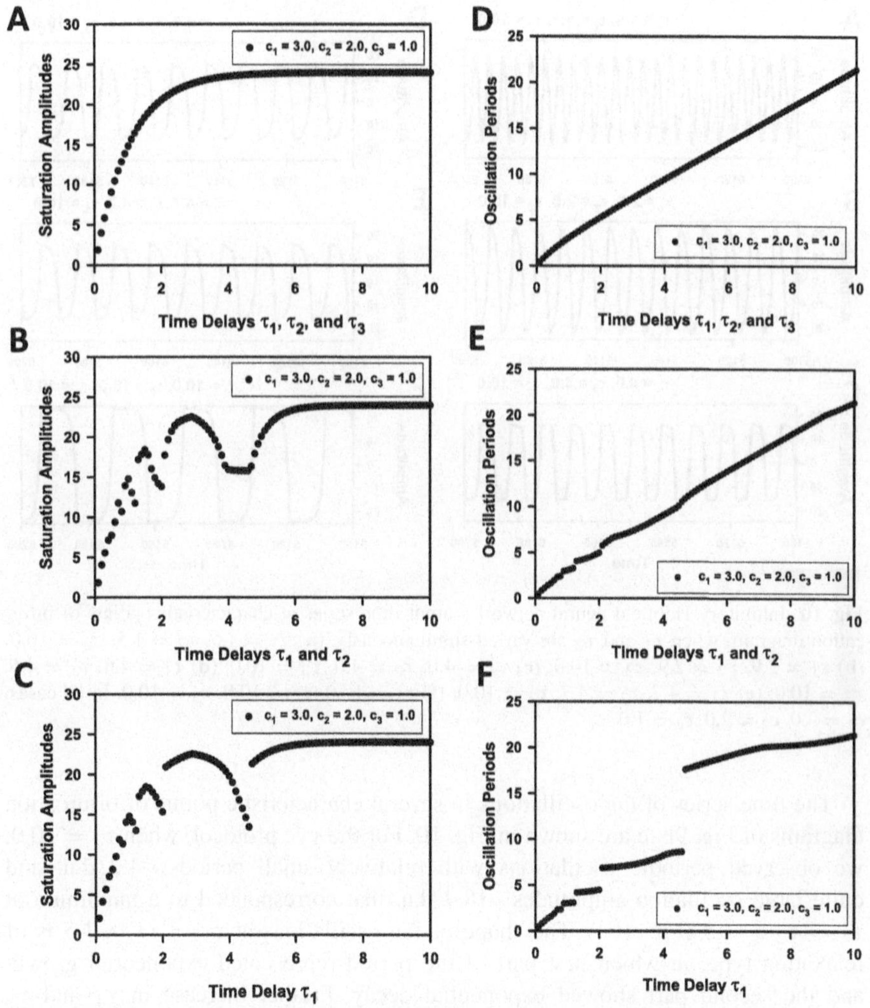

Fig. 9 Bifurcation diagrams of the inhibitory Hopfield neural network when τ_1, τ_2, and τ_3 (**a**, **d**), τ_1 and τ_2 (**b**, **e**), or τ_1 (**c**, **f**) are varied. (**a**) Saturation amplitudes of neural network oscillations as functions of τ_1, τ_2, and τ_3, when they are varied simultaneously. (**b**) Saturation amplitudes of neural network oscillations as functions of τ_1 and τ_2, when they are varied simultaneously. (**c**) Saturation amplitudes of neural network oscillations as functions of τ_1. (**d**) Oscillation period of neural network outputs as functions of τ_1, τ_2, and τ_3, when they are varied simultaneously. (**e**) Oscillation period of neural network outputs as functions of τ_1 and τ_2, when they are varied simultaneously. (**f**) Oscillation period of neural network outputs as functions of τ_1. In all cases, $c_1 = 3.0$, $c_2 = 2.0$, $c_3 = 1.0$

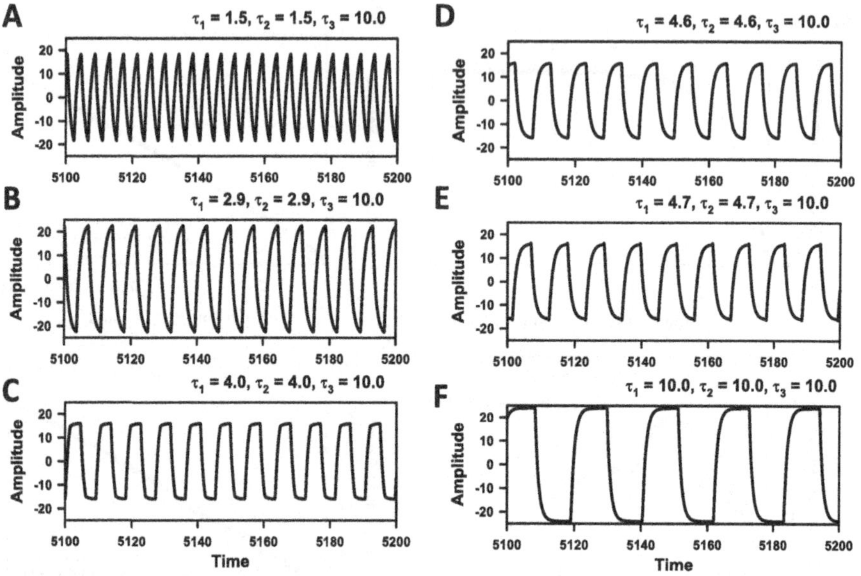

Fig. 10 Inhibitory Hopfield neural network output time series at characteristics points of bifurcation diagram, when τ_1 and τ_2 are varied simultaneously. (**a**) $\tau_1 = 1.5$, $\tau_2 = 1.5$, $\tau_3 = 10.0$; (**b**) $\tau_1 = 2.9$, $\tau_2 = 2.9$, $\tau_3 = 10.0$; (**c**) $\tau_1 = 4.0$, $\tau_2 = 4.0$, $\tau_3 = 10.0$; (**d**) $\tau_1 = 4.6$, $\tau_2 = 4.6$, $\tau_3 = 10.0$; (**e**) $\tau_1 = 4.7$, $\tau_2 = 4.7$, $\tau_3 = 10.0$; (**f**) $\tau_1 = 10.0$, $\tau_2 = 10.0$, $\tau_3 = 10.0$. In all cases, $c_1 = 3.0$, $c_2 = 2.0$, $c_3 = 1.0$

The time series of the oscillations in several characteristic points of bifurcation diagrams of Fig. 9b, e are shown in Fig. 10. For the vvc protocol, when $\tau_3 = 10.0$, we observed periodic oscillations with relatively small periods ~4.2 d.u. and quite large oscillation amplitudes ~18.4 d.u. that corresponded to a maximum at $\tau_1 = \tau_2 = 1.5$ (Fig. 10a). The shape of the oscillations at $\tau_1 = \tau_2 = 1.5$ is of relaxation type, in which first part of the period represented exponential growth and the second part showed exponential decay. Further increase in τ_1 and τ_2 to 2.9 (the next maximum on the amplitude bifurcation diagram) resulted in an amplitude increase to ~22.6 d.u. and in a significant increase in oscillation period to ~7.2 d.u. (Fig. 10b). An increase in τ_1 and τ_2 to 4.0 (the minimum on the amplitude bifurcation diagram) led to a significant decrease in the oscillation amplitude to ~15.9 d.u. and in an increase in oscillation period to ~9.1 d.u. (Fig. 10c). The oscillations become trigger-like oscillations. Further increase in τ_1 and τ_2 to 4.6 (the last point at the plateau part of the amplitude bifurcation diagram) resulted in an approximately the same oscillation amplitude (~15.8 d.u.) and in a moderate increase in oscillation period to ~10.5 d.u. (Fig. 10d). The shape of the oscillations becomes of relaxation type again. A slight increase in τ_1 and τ_2 to 4.7 (the first point on the growing part of the amplitude bifurcation diagram) resulted in a relatively rapid growth in the oscillation amplitude to ~16.3 d.u. and oscillation period to ~10.9 d.u. (Fig. 10e). The type of the oscillation shape was similar to that in Fig. 10d.

Finally, at $\tau_1 = \tau_2 = \tau_3 = 10.0$, simulations demonstrated periodic oscillations of relaxation type with the period of 21.4 d.u. and exponentially growing and decaying parts (Fig. 10f).

4 Conclusions

Our simulation allows for the following conclusions:

1. Excitatory Hopfield neural network with three time delays demonstrated identical saturation outputs regardless of the time delays and their relationships.
2. If one or two subnetworks in the excitatory Hopfield neural network have much smaller delays (one or two orders of magnitude as compared to the larger time delay), the time interval until saturation of the outputs dramatically decreased as compared to the neural network composed of three subnetworks with relatively large and identical time delays.
3. For the inhibitory Hopfield neural network with three time delays, when τ_1, τ_2, and τ_3 changed simultaneously, the networks demonstrated monotonic increase in oscillation amplitude until saturation and almost linear increase in oscillation period with τ_1, τ_2, and τ_3.
4. If we changed time delay τ_1 in only one of three subnetworks of the inhibitory Hopfield neural network, we observed a multiresonance phenomenon, when the amplitude of oscillations demonstrated maxima and minima and the oscillation period changed by jumps with τ_1. We also observed period-tripling bifurcation in this case.
5. If we changed time delays τ_1 and τ_2 in two of three subnetworks of the inhibitory Hopfield neural network, we also observed a multiresonance phenomenon, when the amplitude of oscillations demonstrated maxima and minima and the oscillation period changed by relatively large or small jumps with τ_1 and τ_2. In this case, oscillation periods demonstrated discrete ranges of changes, similar to the discrete oscillation rhythms in the human and animal electroencephalogram.

Thus, the Hopfield neural network with multiple time delays demonstrate rich dynamics that include steady states and oscillations, discrete intervals of oscillation frequency variations, and multiresonances depending on the interneuron connection strengths and relationships between time delays.

We need to note that we have studied only bifurcation diagrams of the Hopfield neural network with three identical subnetworks, with equal and different time delays, purely excitatory and purely inhibitory connections, and with identical and different connection strengths. We also employed only three protocols for the changes of time delay, which have demonstrated quite different types of the neural network behavior. However, such a system can be investigated by the application of virtually infinite number of protocols and mixed connection types, which can potentially show various different bifurcation diagrams as functions of three time delays, τ_1, τ_2, and τ_3.

References

1. Hopfield, J.J.: Neural networks and physical systems with emergent collective computational abilities. Proc. Natl. Acad. Sci. **79**, 2554–2558 (1982)
2. Hopfield, J.J.: Neurons with graded response have collective computational properties like those of two-state neurons. Proc. Natl. Acad. Sci. **81**, 3088–3092 (1984)
3. Egmont-Petersen, M., de Ridder, D., Handels, H.: Image processing with neural networks—a review. Pattern Recogn. **35**, 2279–2301 (2002)
4. Hong, Q., Li, Y., Wang, X.: Memristive continuous Hopfield neural network circuit for image restoration. Neural Comput. & Applic. **32**, 8175–8185 (2020)
5. Isaac, S.D., Njitacke, Z.T., Tsafack, N., Tchapga, C.T., Kengne, J.: Novel compressive sensing image encryption using the dynamics of an adjustable gradient Hopfield neural network. Europ. Phys. J. Special Topics. **231**, 1995–2016 (2022)
6. Pajares, G.: A Hopfield neural network for image change detection. IEEE Trans. Neural Netw. **17**, 1250–1264 (2006)
7. Unnikrishnan, K., Hopfield, J.J., Tank, D.W.: Connected-digit speaker-dependent speech recognition using a neural network. IEEE Trans. Signal Process. **39**, 698 (1991)
8. Bevi, A.R., Monurajan, P., Manjula, J.: Design of Hopfield network for cryptographic application by spintronic memristors. Neural Comput. & Applic. **32**, 9443–9452 (2020)
9. Bélair, J.: Stability in a model of a delayed neural network. J. Dyn. Diff. Equat. **5**, 607–623 (1993)
10. Bondarenko, V.E.: Self-organization processes in chaotic neural networks under external periodic force. Int. J. Bifurcat. Chaos. **7**, 1887–1895 (1997)
11. Bondarenko, V.E.: Control andanticontrol' of chaos in an analog neural network with time delay. Chaos, Solitons Fractals. **13**, 139–154 (2002)
12. Rozier, K., Bondarenko, V.E.: Synchronization, multiresonance phenomena, and discrete oscillation periods in a Hopfield neural network with two time delays. Int. J. Bifurcat. Chaos. **32**, 2250066 (2022)
13. Bélair, J., Campbell, S.A., van den Driessche, P.: Frustration, stability, and delay-induced oscillations in a neural network model. SIAM J. Appl. Math. **56**, 245–255 (1996)
14. Marcus, C., Westervelt, R.: Stability of analog neural networks with delay. Phys. Rev. A. **39**, 347 (1989)
15. Marcus, C., Waugh, F., Westervelt, R.: Nonlinear dynamics and stability of analog neural networks. Physica D: Nonlin. Phenomena. **51**, 234–247 (1991)
16. Cao, J., Xiao, M.: Stability and Hopf bifurcation in a simplified BAM neural network with two time delays. IEEE Trans. Neural Netw. **18**, 416–430 (2007)
17. Wang, Z., Parastesh, F., Rajagopal, K., Hamarash, I.I., Hussain, I.: Delay-induced synchronization in two coupled chaotic memristive Hopfield neural networks. Chaos, Solitons Fractals. **134**, 109702 (2020)
18. Chen, Y., Zhang, X., Xue, Y.: Global exponential synchronization of high-order quaternion Hopfield neural networks with unbounded distributed delays and time-varying discrete delays. Math. Comput. Simul. **193**, 173–189 (2022)
19. Ma, S.: Hopf bifurcation of a type of neuron model with multiple time delays. Int. J. Bifurcat. Chaos. **29**, 1950163 (2019)

Advancing Information Integration Through Empirical Likelihood: Selective Reviews and a New Idea

Chixiang Chen, Jia Liang, Elynn Chen, and Ming Wang

Abstract Information integration plays a pivotal role in biomedical studies by facilitating the combination and analysis of independent datasets from multiple studies, thereby uncovering valuable insights that might otherwise remain obscured due to the limited sample size in individual studies. However, sharing raw data from independent studies presents significant challenges, primarily due to the need to safeguard sensitive participant information and the cumbersome paperwork involved in data sharing. In this article, we first provide a selective review of recent methodological developments in information integration via empirical likelihood, wherein only summary information is required, rather than the raw data. Following this, we introduce a new insight and a potentially promising framework that could broaden the application of information integration across a wider spectrum. Furthermore, this new framework offers computational convenience compared to classic empirical likelihood-based methods. We provide numerical evaluations to assess its performance and discuss various extensions in the end.

Keywords Empirical likelihood · Information integration · Summary data · Weighted estimation

C. Chen (✉)
Division of Biostatistics and Bioinformatics, Department of Epidemiology and Public Health, University of Maryland, School of Medicine, Baltimore, MD, USA
e-mail: chixiang.chen@som.umaryland.edu

J. Liang
Department of Biostatistics, St. Jude Children's Research Hospital, Memphis, TN, USA
e-mail: jia.liang@stjude.org

E. Chen
Department of Technology, Operations, and Statistics, New York University, New York, NY, USA
e-mail: elynn.chen@stern.nyu.edu

M. Wang
Department of Population and Quantitative Health Sciences, School of Medicine, Case Western Reserve University, Cleveland, OH, USA
e-mail: mxw827@case.edu

Y. Zhao, D.-G. Chen (eds.), *Big Data Analytics in Biostatistics and Bioinformatics*, ICSA Book Series in Statistics,
https://doi.org/10.1007/978-3-032-06649-7_15

1 Introduction

Data integration plays a pivotal role in biomedical studies by allowing independent datasets from multiple studies to be combined and analyzed together, thereby unlocking a wealth of insights that would otherwise remain hidden due to the small sample size in an individual study [18, 31]. By synthesizing information, we can improve estimation efficiency, enhance statistical significance, boost prediction accuracy, and detect small signals that may not be apparent when analyzing individual datasets [22, 34]. The improved analysis will inform better decision-making in biomedical studies and promote personalized and precision medicine.

However, sharing raw data from independent studies imposes substantial challenges, primarily due to the need to safeguard sensitive participant information and the cumbersome paperwork involved in data sharing [1, 40]. In biomedical research, raw data frequently encompass detailed medical histories, genetic details, and other personally identifiable information, all subject to rigorous privacy regulations and ethical guidelines. Preserving privacy is fundamental to upholding trust and ethical standards within the research community [28, 37]. Nevertheless, accomplishing this while simultaneously facilitating research utilizing big data across multiple studies poses a complex undertaking.

One of the most popular methods designed to integrate information from different studies without sharing the raw data is meta-analysis [18]. These methods pool the published results of multiple similar scientific studies to produce an enhanced estimate without utilizing the raw individual data from each study [3]. In recent years, many new methods have been developed to integrate summary information under the setting of more complex data structures and modeling strategies: some are based on frequentist inference, such as empirical likelihood-based estimators [4, 7, 9, 17, 20, 30, 35, 39, 43, 44], generalized method of moments [14], generalized-meta estimators [29], communication-efficient distributed estimation [15, 19, 27], and renewal estimation [32, 33], while others are based on Bayesian inference incorporating external information into informative priors [11, 24, 25]. The applications of information integration span over the generalized linear models, survival models, partial linear models, etc., and some methods have been applied to advance medical research, with findings published in esteemed journals, including *Nature Medicine* [26]. Notably, Qin and his colleagues have reviewed some of these works and summarized these into a unified framework of calibration [22, 34].

Given the pivotal role of calibration techniques in unifying numerous existing methods, this article focuses on reviewing empirical likelihood-based methods for information integration. These methods form a crucial foundation for many calibration approaches, and we provide selective reviews highlighting recent updates in this area. Additionally, we introduce a novel insight and a potentially promising framework that could expand the application of information integration across a broader spectrum, such as classic generalized linear model and semi-parametric causal inference. It is noteworthy that this new framework offers computational convenience and stability compared to classic empirical likelihood-based methods.

Furthermore, it holds the potential to flexibly integrate existing techniques, such as density ratio models [12, 23, 39] and penalized regressions [23, 43], and address complex scenarios, such as heterogeneity in covariates/conditional outcome distributions between studies and the incorporation of information from multiple external sources.

The remainder of this article is organized as follows. Section 2 presents selective reviews of information integration methods utilizing empirical likelihood, providing detailed model specifications, algorithms, and recent updates to address data heterogeneity. Section 3 elaborates on the new idea and discusses its advantages in detail. Section 4 offers numerical evidence to illustrate and assess the new concept. Finally, Sect. 5 explores potential extensions and concludes the article. The R codes are available at https://github.com/chencxxy28/reweigtingIB.

2 Information Integration via Empirical Likelihood

2.1 *Basic Setup*

We first introduce the basic setup for the internal and external studies that are widely adopted in the literature. Let n_1 be the number of independent and identically distributed (i.i.d) subjects in the internal study, regarded as our main studied cohort. For each subject i in the internal study, we have individual-level data denoted by $Y_i, \mathbf{X}_i, \mathbf{Z}_i$, where Y_i is the outcome, $\mathbf{X}_i$ is the vector containing well-recognized covariates in the literature, and $\mathbf{Z}_i$ is the vector of extra covariates that are not available in the external study. The conditional density function of the outcome is denoted by $f_1(Y|\mathbf{X}, \mathbf{Z}; \boldsymbol{\beta}_0)$, where $\boldsymbol{\beta}_0$ is the p-dimensional true parameter vector. In literature, one focus of the internal study is to model the conditional mean of the outcome Y_i, i.e., $E_1(Y|\mathbf{X}, \mathbf{Z}; \boldsymbol{\beta}_0)$, with the conditional expectation taken with respect to the internal data.

On the other hand, let n_2 be the number of i.i.d subjects in the external study with the true conditional density function of the outcome denoted by $f_2(Y|\mathbf{X}, \mathbf{Z}; \tilde{\boldsymbol{\beta}}_0)$, which is often assumed to be the same to that from the internal study, i.e., $\tilde{\boldsymbol{\beta}}_0 = \boldsymbol{\beta}_0$. For each subject j from 1 to n_2, only the outcome Y_j and covariates $\mathbf{X}_j$ are assumed to be observed (Fig. 1). This is a reasonable and common setting in research where the external study has a large sample size but does not measure variables in $\mathbf{Z}_j$ from all participants, such as blood biomarkers, metabolic measures, or imaging metrics. These variables are often expensive to measure or are not considered in previous studies, but could be available in the internal study with a smaller sample size [41]. Additionally, suppose the raw data of the external study cannot be easily shared, while the summary information $\hat{\boldsymbol{\theta}}$ could be available, which solves an estimating equation $\sum_{j=1}^{n_2} \boldsymbol{\Psi}(Y_j, \mathbf{X}_j; \boldsymbol{\theta}) = \mathbf{0}$ based on the external data. Here, $\boldsymbol{\Psi}(\cdot)$ can be any regular estimating function, for example, the score function based on a reduced and possibly misspecified model $f_2(Y|\mathbf{X}; \boldsymbol{\theta}_0)$ for the external data, with $\boldsymbol{\theta}_0$ being

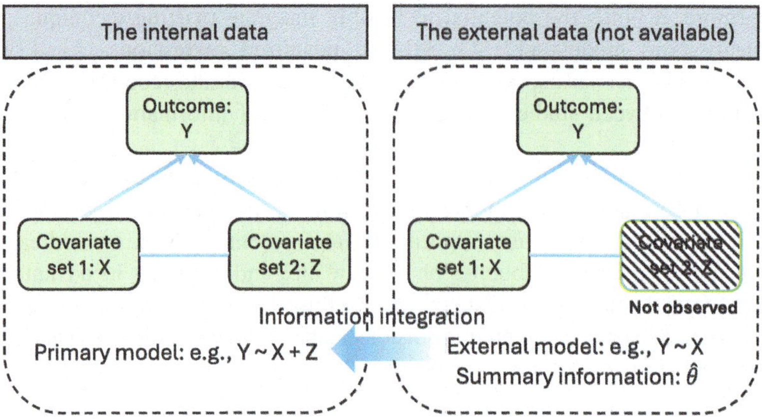

Fig. 1 An illustrative example for data structure and method workflow in existing works

the limiting values of $\hat{\boldsymbol{\theta}}$. The goal of information integration, therefore, is to utilize summary information $\hat{\boldsymbol{\theta}}$ to enhance the precision of estimating $\boldsymbol{\beta}_0$ based on the internally studied data (Fig. 1), when the conditional density $f_1(Y|\mathbf{X}, \mathbf{Z}; \boldsymbol{\beta}_0)$ is of the primary interest. A more general framework will be discussed in Sect. 3.

2.2 Constrained Maximum Likelihood

We start with describing the widely used method, named constrained maximum likelihood (CML) [4]. When the estimation variability of the summary information $\hat{\boldsymbol{\theta}}$ can be ignored, the CML method provides a natural approach to leveraging this summary information to improve the inference of $\boldsymbol{\beta}$ [4, 20]. Specifically, CML is based on a semi-parametric likelihood where the density of the outcome given covariates is modeled by $f_1(Y|\mathbf{X}, \mathbf{Z}; \boldsymbol{\beta})$, whereas the marginal density of covariates $f_1(\mathbf{X}, \mathbf{Z})$ is modeled by a point probability mass $p_i = dF_1(\mathbf{X}, \mathbf{Z})$ defined by the internal data. This probability mass could be $1/n_1$, serving as a nonparametric estimate without incorporating any additional information from the external data. To integrate summary information $\hat{\boldsymbol{\theta}}$ from the external study, the CML estimator $\hat{\beta}_{cml}$ is designed to maximize the following constrained optimization problem:

$$\sum_{i=1}^{n_1} \log f_1(Y_i|\mathbf{X}_i, \mathbf{Z}_i; \boldsymbol{\beta}) + \sum_{i=1}^{n_1} \log p_i, \tag{1}$$

with respect to p_i and is subject to three constraints

$$p_i > 0\,, \forall i, \ \sum_{i=1}^{n_1} p_i = 1, \ \sum_{i=1}^{n_1} p_i \boldsymbol{\Phi}_1(\mathbf{X}_i, \mathbf{Z}_i; \boldsymbol{\beta}, \hat{\boldsymbol{\theta}}) = \mathbf{0}, \tag{2}$$

where $\boldsymbol{\Phi}_1(\mathbf{X}, \mathbf{Z}; \boldsymbol{\beta}, \boldsymbol{\theta}) = E_1\{\boldsymbol{\Psi}(Y, \mathbf{X}; \boldsymbol{\theta})|\mathbf{X}, \mathbf{Z}; \boldsymbol{\beta}\} = \int \boldsymbol{\Psi}(y, \mathbf{X}; \boldsymbol{\theta}) f_1(y|\mathbf{X}, \mathbf{Z}; \boldsymbol{\beta})dy$.

We notice here that the construction of $\boldsymbol{\Phi}_1(\mathbf{X}, \mathbf{Z}; \boldsymbol{\beta}, \boldsymbol{\theta})$ links the internal main model and external reduced model by using the observed likelihood $f_1(Y|\mathbf{X}, \mathbf{Z}; \boldsymbol{\beta})$, which makes the information integration feasible. Moreover, the expression in in (1) involves the logarithm of the joint likelihood of the data $\{Y_i, \mathbf{X}_i, \mathbf{Z}_i\}$, where the marginal marginal density of covariates $\{\mathbf{X}_i, \mathbf{Z}_i\}$ remains unspecified for (2). The following three constraints are then values of p_i's, following the empirical likelihood philosophy [35].

If we exclusively rely on the internal data to estimate $\boldsymbol{\theta}$ and $\boldsymbol{\beta}$, we anticipate little efficiency gains compared to the well-established maximum likelihood (ML) estimator. This is understandable since the ML estimator optimally exploits the internal data, given regularity conditions [13]. However, the CML estimator is shown to be more efficient than the ML estimator by incorporating summary information $\hat{\boldsymbol{\theta}}$ estimated from the external study, without estimating $\boldsymbol{\theta}$ based on the internal data [4]. Intuitively, this additional information capitalizes on the extra degree of freedom from the moment condition $E_1\{\boldsymbol{\Psi}(Y, \mathbf{X}; \boldsymbol{\theta}_0)\} = \mathbf{0}$, leading to a more efficient estimate of $\boldsymbol{\beta}$ compared to the ML estimator.

We also remark here that the CML method considers the setup where the variability of $\hat{\boldsymbol{\theta}}$ can be ignored. This is the case when the sample size n_2 of the external study is much larger than the sample size n_1 of the internal study. However, when n_2 is comparable or even smaller than n_1, the derived variance [4] for the CML estimator will underestimate the true variance [20, 44]. Moreover, the construction of $\boldsymbol{\Phi}_1(\mathbf{X}, \mathbf{Z}; \boldsymbol{\beta}, \boldsymbol{\theta}) = E_1\{\boldsymbol{\Psi}(Y, \mathbf{X}; \boldsymbol{\theta})|\mathbf{X}, \mathbf{Z}; \boldsymbol{\beta}\}$ and the use of covariate probability mass $\hat{p}_i$ imply that the marginal distributions of covariates $\{\mathbf{X}, \mathbf{Z}\}$ between internal and external studies should be the same in general to ensure the consistent estimate of $\boldsymbol{\beta}_0$.

2.3 Generalized Integration Model

When the estimation variability of $\hat{\boldsymbol{\theta}}$ cannot be ignored, a more general and possibly more practical scenario in real applications, the generalized integration model (GIM) should be adopted [44]. Specifically, GIM extended the CML estimation by adding an extra penalty term to the constrained optimization, accounting for the estimation variability of $\hat{\boldsymbol{\theta}}$. This leads to a new constrained optimization problem, which maximizes the following likelihood to obtain the estimator $\hat{\boldsymbol{\beta}}_{gim}$:

$$\sum_{i=1}^{n_1} \log f_1(Y_i|\mathbf{X}_i, \mathbf{Z}_i; \boldsymbol{\beta}) + \sum_{i=1}^{n_1} \log p_i - n_2(\hat{\boldsymbol{\theta}} - \boldsymbol{\theta})^T \hat{\mathbf{V}}^{-1}(\hat{\boldsymbol{\theta}} - \boldsymbol{\theta})/2, \tag{3}$$

with respect to p_i and $\boldsymbol{\theta}$ and is subject to three constraints:

$$p_i > 0, \ \forall i, \ \sum_{i=1}^{n_1} p_i = 1, \ \sum_{i=1}^{n_1} p_i \boldsymbol{\Phi}_1(\mathbf{X}_i, \mathbf{Z}_i; \boldsymbol{\beta}, \boldsymbol{\theta}) = \mathbf{0}, \tag{4}$$

where $\hat{\mathbf{V}}$ is a consistent estimate of the variance-covariance matrix of $n_2^{0.5}(\hat{\boldsymbol{\theta}} - \boldsymbol{\theta}_0)$. Intuitively, the expression in (3) can be regarded as the logarithm of the joint distribution of the data $\{Y_i, \mathbf{X}_i, \mathbf{Z}_i, \hat{\boldsymbol{\theta}}\}$, for $i = 1, \ldots, n_1$. Therefore, the uncertainty of $\hat{\boldsymbol{\theta}}$ is naturally incorporated into the information integration by assuming that $n_2^{0.5}(\hat{\boldsymbol{\theta}} - \boldsymbol{\theta}_0)$ follows a multivariate normal distribution. This estimator is more efficient than both the ML estimator and the CML estimator, and it reaches the semi-parametric efficiency bound [44]. The developed framework also allows the estimation of nuisance parameters, such as the over-dispersion parameter in generalized linear models [44].

Despite advancements, GIM still relies on the assumption that the marginal distributions of covariates are consistent across the two studies.

2.4 The Numerical Procedure

To successfully deliver information, the parameters including p_i, $\boldsymbol{\beta}$, and $\boldsymbol{\theta}$ (only in GIM) should be estimated simultaneously in a constrained optimization procedure. The typical numerical procedure involves the method of Lagrange multipliers to profile out the empirical distribution parameters [4, 35, 44]. Let us take the estimation of GIM for illustration. The Lagrange function will be defined as

$$\begin{aligned} L_{n_1}(p_1, \ldots, p_{n_1}, \boldsymbol{\beta}, \boldsymbol{\theta}, \boldsymbol{\lambda}, t) = & \sum_{i=1}^{n_1} \log p_i + \sum_{i=1}^{n_1} \log f_1(Y_i|\mathbf{X}_i, \mathbf{Z}_i; \boldsymbol{\beta}) \\ & - n_2(\hat{\boldsymbol{\theta}} - \boldsymbol{\theta})^T \hat{\mathbf{V}}^{-1}(\hat{\boldsymbol{\theta}} - \boldsymbol{\theta})/2 - n_1 t\Big(\sum_{i=1}^{n_1} p_i - 1\Big) \\ & - n_1 \sum_{i=1}^{n_1} p_i \boldsymbol{\lambda}^T \boldsymbol{\Phi}_1(\mathbf{X}_i, \mathbf{Z}_i; \boldsymbol{\beta}, \boldsymbol{\theta}), \end{aligned} \tag{5}$$

with $(\boldsymbol{\lambda}^T, t)^T$ being the Lagrange multipliers. Solving the above function using the constraints $\sum_{i=1}^{n_1} p_i = 1$ and $\sum_{i=1}^{n_1} p_i \boldsymbol{\Phi}_1(\mathbf{X}_i, \mathbf{Z}_i; \boldsymbol{\beta}, \boldsymbol{\theta}) = \mathbf{0}$, we have $t = 1$ and $p_i = n_1^{-1}\{1 + \boldsymbol{\lambda}^T \boldsymbol{\Phi}_1(\mathbf{X}_i, \mathbf{Z}_i; \boldsymbol{\beta}, \boldsymbol{\theta})\}^{-1}$. Thus, the function in (5) will be reduced to

$$l_{n_1}(\boldsymbol{\beta}, \boldsymbol{\theta}, \boldsymbol{\lambda}) = -\sum_{i=1}^{n_1} \log\{1 + \boldsymbol{\lambda}^T \boldsymbol{\Phi}_1(\mathbf{X}_i, \mathbf{Z}_i; \boldsymbol{\beta}, \boldsymbol{\theta})\} + \sum_{i=1}^{n_1} \log f_1(Y_i|\mathbf{X}_i, \mathbf{Z}_i; \boldsymbol{\beta}) - n_2(\hat{\boldsymbol{\theta}} - \boldsymbol{\theta})^T \hat{\mathbf{V}}^{-1}(\hat{\boldsymbol{\theta}} - \boldsymbol{\theta})/2. \quad (6)$$

As a result, solving (6) is translated into solving the unconstrained optimization: $\max_{\boldsymbol{\beta}, \boldsymbol{\theta}, \boldsymbol{\lambda}} l_{n_1}(\boldsymbol{\beta}, \boldsymbol{\theta}, \boldsymbol{\lambda})$.

To obtain the estimates of $\boldsymbol{\beta}, \boldsymbol{\theta}, \boldsymbol{\lambda}$, we need to solve the following estimating equations by an iterative manner:

$$\frac{\partial l_{n_1}(\boldsymbol{\mu}, \boldsymbol{\lambda})}{\partial \boldsymbol{\mu}} = \mathbf{0}, \quad \frac{\partial l_{n_1}(\boldsymbol{\mu}, \boldsymbol{\lambda})}{\partial \boldsymbol{\lambda}} = \mathbf{0},$$

with $\boldsymbol{\mu} = (\boldsymbol{\beta}^T, \boldsymbol{\theta}^T)^T$. Note that given the values of $\boldsymbol{\mu}$, the second estimating function is convex, which can be efficiently solved by greedy algorithms [10, 20, 21]. Given the values of $\boldsymbol{\lambda}$, the first equation can be solved by Newton-Raphson method [20, 44].

The variance of the estimator $\hat{\boldsymbol{\beta}}_{gim}$ can be approximated using asymptotic theory [44]. For the detailed variance formula under different scenarios, we refer interested readers to Theorem 1 and Corollary 1 in the original article [44].

2.5 *Various Extensions*

The CML estimator and the GIM estimator establish the theoretical foundation that permits various methodological extensions. We provide a brief overview of several variants designed to tackle the following three challenges: heterogeneous covariate distributions between two studied cohorts, heterogeneous conditional outcome distributions between two studied cohorts, and incorporating summary information from multiple external studies.

Heterogeneous Covariate Distributions The CML and GIM procedures assume homogeneity in the covariate distribution. Given variations in inclusion and exclusion criteria across studies, this assumption may not hold, potentially resulting in biased estimates. To address heterogeneous covariate distributions, one may consider adopting a semi-parametric density ratio model [12, 23, 39], i.e., assume two density functions satisfy the following relationship

$$f_2(\tilde{\mathbf{X}}) = \exp(\alpha_0 + \tilde{\mathbf{X}}^T \boldsymbol{\alpha}) f_1(\tilde{\mathbf{X}}), \quad (7)$$

where $f_1(\tilde{\mathbf{X}})$ and $f_2(\tilde{\mathbf{X}})$ denote the density functions of $\tilde{\mathbf{X}}$ in the internal and external studies, respectively, with $\tilde{\mathbf{X}}$ being a subset vector of $\mathbf{X}$ and unknown parameters in $\boldsymbol{\alpha}$. The scalar α_0 normalizes the function such that $\int f_2(\tilde{\mathbf{x}})d\tilde{\mathbf{x}} = 1$. Based on the above density ratio model, the CML and GIM can be easily modified by adding an additional constraint, i.e., $\sum_{i=1}^{n_2} p_i\{\exp(\tilde{\mathbf{X}}^T\boldsymbol{\alpha}) - 1\} = 0$, into (2) and (4). The rationale of adding this constraint is based upon the fact that $E_1\{\exp(\tilde{\mathbf{X}}^T\boldsymbol{\alpha})\boldsymbol{\Phi}_1(\mathbf{X}_i, \mathbf{Z}_i; \boldsymbol{\beta}, \boldsymbol{\theta})\} = \mathbf{0}$. When $\boldsymbol{\alpha} = \mathbf{0}$, the method will be reduced to CML/GIM estimation. In general case, the parameter vector $\boldsymbol{\alpha}$ is unknown and needs to be estimated. By introducing and jointly estimating extra parameter vector $\boldsymbol{\alpha}$, the estimators derived from the modified constrained optimization is able to calibrate covariate distribution difference and thus unbiased if the density ratio model is correctly specified. This technique has found application in various contexts, including survival data analysis [12] and the setting with label shift/prior probability shift [7]. Two important notes are highlighted: due to the limitedly available external data in summary forms, **(1)** assessing whether the specification of density ratio model in (7) is correct or not is challenging or even impossible; **(2)** Even in the case the density ratio model holds, the identification of the subvector $\tilde{\mathbf{X}}$ is also challenging [23]. In practice, researchers may consider some important covariates, such as race/ethnicity, that are believed to be different between datasets [39].

Heterogeneous Conditional Outcome Distributions In addition to covariate distributions, heterogeneous conditional outcome distributions, $f_1(Y|\mathbf{X}, \mathbf{Z}) \neq f_2(Y|\mathbf{X}, \mathbf{Z})$, will also lead to biased estimators and may impose challenge to calibrate. One promising solution is to introduce a bias term $\mathbf{b}$ into the constraint [23, 43], i.e.,

$$\sum_{i=1}^{n_1} p_i\boldsymbol{\Phi}_1(\mathbf{X}_i, \mathbf{Z}_i; \boldsymbol{\beta}, \boldsymbol{\theta}) - \mathbf{b} = \mathbf{0}. \tag{8}$$

Intuitively, the vector $\mathbf{b}$ models the values of the underlying moment $E_1\{\boldsymbol{\Psi}(Y, \mathbf{X}_i; \boldsymbol{\theta}_0)\}$, where some elements could deviate from zero when conditional outcome distributions are different. We notice here that the values in $\mathbf{b}$ are unknown and need to be estimated using the internal data. Without imposing an extra constraint on estimating the bias term $\mathbf{b}$, there would be no efficiency gain for estimating $\boldsymbol{\beta}_0$. To facilitate information integration, an l_1-based penalty is suggested to be incorporated into the constrained optimization process, effectively estimating $\mathbf{b}$ and shrinking the values in $\hat{\mathbf{b}}$ that are close to zero. The idea using penalty is to shrink the estimated elements of $E_1\{\boldsymbol{\Psi}(Y, \mathbf{X}_i; \boldsymbol{\theta}_0)\}$ that are truly zero and leave the other elements unshrinked. Consequently, the information delivery can be still achievable via the elements $\hat{\mathbf{b}}_* = \mathbf{0}$ with $\hat{\mathbf{b}}_* \subset \hat{\mathbf{b}}$. For a more detailed description of the estimation procedure, we direct readers to the relevant literature [23, 43].

Multiple External Studies Integrating summary information from multiple external studies can be instrumental in further boosting estimation efficiency for $\boldsymbol{\beta}$.

Under the assumption of homogeneous populations, the GIM estimator is able to seamlessly incorporates multiple external estimates $\hat{\boldsymbol{\theta}}_k$ for $k = 2, \ldots, K$ and $K \geq 2$. This modification is achieved by adjusting the last term in the expression in (3) to $\sum_{k=2}^{K} n_k(\hat{\boldsymbol{\theta}}_k - \boldsymbol{\theta})^T \hat{\mathbf{V}}_k^{-1}(\hat{\boldsymbol{\theta}}_k - \boldsymbol{\theta})/2$, where $\hat{\mathbf{V}}_k$ is a consistent estimate of the variance-covariance matrix of $n_k^{0.5}(\hat{\boldsymbol{\theta}}_k - \boldsymbol{\theta}_0)$, with the sample size of n_k in the k-th study.

In addition, in the complex situation where multiple external datasets are believed to exhibit different covariate distributions and conditional outcome distributions, one can adapt techniques from the density ratio model and bias penalty, as described earlier, to facilitate the integration of information from multiple external studies [23].

3 A New Idea

3.1 Method Framework

Despite theoretical advancements, the methods described above involve the conditional distribution $f_1(Y|\mathbf{X}, \mathbf{Z}; \boldsymbol{\beta})$ to link models from internal and external studies, which may not always be applicable to general semi-parametric estimation. Moreover, these methods often necessitate complex computational strategies to jointly estimate all parameters, as described in Sect. 2.4. In this section, we introduce a new perspective and a general framework for information integration that has a significantly lighter computational load and encompasses a possibly broader range of application contexts.

Before describing the proposed method, let us refine the previous notations and consider a broader context. Suppose the quantity of interest $\boldsymbol{\beta}$ can be identified by a generic estimating equation $E_1\{\mathbf{g}(Y, \mathbf{X}, \mathbf{Z}; \boldsymbol{\beta}_0, \boldsymbol{\eta}_0)\} = \mathbf{0}$, with a vector $\boldsymbol{\eta}_0$ consisting of the true values of potential nuisance parameters and an i.i.d estimation function $\mathbf{g}(Y_i, \mathbf{X}_i, \mathbf{Z}_i; \boldsymbol{\beta}_0, \boldsymbol{\eta}_0)$, for $i = 1, \ldots, n_1$. We remark here that the above setting does not require the full specification of the observed likelihood, and the interested parameters in $\boldsymbol{\beta}$ are not limited to the parameters in the conditional outcome distribution. Two examples, but not limited to two, are illustrated below:

Example 1 (Generalized Linear Model (GLM)) In the GLM setting, $\mathbf{g}(Y, \mathbf{X}, \mathbf{Z}; \boldsymbol{\beta}, \boldsymbol{\eta})$ could be the score function with the parameter vector $\boldsymbol{\beta}$ indexed in the conditional mean structure $\mu(\mathbf{X}, \mathbf{Z}; \boldsymbol{\beta})$, i.e., $\mathbf{X}, \mathbf{Z}; \boldsymbol{\beta}, \boldsymbol{\eta}) = (1, \mathbf{X}^T, \mathbf{Z}^T)^T\{Y - \mu(\mathbf{X}, \mathbf{Z}; \boldsymbol{\beta})\}$. Under this GLM framework, CML and GIM estimation procedures are are still applicable to facilitate information integration (Fig. 1).

Example 2 (Causal Inference) Unlike GLM, which allows us directly work on the observed likelihood, causal inference models often rely on the potential outcome framework with calibrated moment conditions [2, 6, 38]. For instance, consider our interest in the marginal and causal odds ratio between two groups (e.g., $A = 0, 1$, a scalar), and let the vector $\mathbf{X}$ defined before contain the the exposure variable A, i.e., $\mathbf{X} = (A, \mathbf{X}_*^T)^T$ with a sub-vector $\mathbf{X}_*$ of $\mathbf{X}$ excluding the variable A. In this context, an unbiased estimator could be identified based on the moment condition $E_1\{\mathbf{g}(Y, \mathbf{X}_*, \mathbf{Z}; \boldsymbol{\beta}_0, \boldsymbol{\eta}_0)\} = \mathbf{0}$ with:

$$\mathbf{g}(Y, \mathbf{X}, \mathbf{Z}; \boldsymbol{\beta}, \boldsymbol{\eta}) = \begin{pmatrix} \frac{1}{\pi(\mathbf{X}_*, \mathbf{Z}; \boldsymbol{\eta})}(1, A)^T\{Y - \mu(\mathbf{A}; \boldsymbol{\beta})\} \\ \mathbf{h}(\mathbf{X}, \mathbf{Z}; \boldsymbol{\eta}) \end{pmatrix}.$$

Here, $\mu(A; \boldsymbol{\beta}) = \{1 + \exp(-\beta_0 - \beta_1 A)\}^{-1}$; the quantity $\pi(\mathbf{X}_*, \mathbf{Z}; \boldsymbol{\eta})$, so-called propensity score (PS), equals the probability of A given the covariates and serves as a calibration weight to balance the confounder distributions between two groups [2, 5, 38]; $\mathbf{h}(\mathbf{X}, \mathbf{Z}; \boldsymbol{\eta})$ is an estimating function solving the parameters in $\boldsymbol{\eta}$, which could be the score function from logistic regression by treating A as the outcome. Stacking two estimating functions together aim to create an i.i.d estimating function $\mathbf{g}(Y, \mathbf{X}, \mathbf{Z}; \boldsymbol{\beta}, \boldsymbol{\eta})$ to ensure efficiency gain in theory theory [30]. Thus, the parameter of interest in this case is the causal odds ratio β_1 based upon the marginal structural model (MSM) under the outcome framework [36]. It is important to note that the CLM and GIM estimators may not be directly applicable in this case for integrating information, as the observed likelihood may no longer represent the distribution of pseudo outcomes in the causal context. Therefore, a new integration method is needed.

To integrate the information from the summary information $\hat{\boldsymbol{\theta}}$ under the above setting, we propose the following weighted estimation procedure: the estimator of $\boldsymbol{\beta}$ and $\boldsymbol{\eta}$ (if exist) could be jointly obtained by solving the weighted estimating equation:

$$\sum_{i=1}^{n_1} \hat{p}_i \mathbf{g}(Y_i, \mathbf{X}_i, \mathbf{Z}_i; \boldsymbol{\beta}, \boldsymbol{\eta}) = \mathbf{0}, \tag{9}$$

where the weight $\hat{p}_i$ is estimated by maximizing the joint log-likelihood l,

$$l = \sum_{i=1}^{n_1} log(p_i) - n_2(\hat{\boldsymbol{\theta}} - \boldsymbol{\theta})^T(\hat{\mathbf{V}})^{-1}(\hat{\boldsymbol{\theta}} - \boldsymbol{\theta})/2, \tag{10}$$

with respect to p_i and $\boldsymbol{\theta}$, and is subject to three constraints:

$$p_i > 0\,, \forall i; \;\; \sum_{i=1}^{n_1} p_i = 1, \;\; \sum_{i=1}^{n_1} p_i \boldsymbol{\Psi}(Y_i, \mathbf{X}_i; \boldsymbol{\theta}) = \mathbf{0}. \tag{11}$$

The new estimator defined by (9)–(11) addresses the general case where the internal model is specified through an estimating function rather than a score function, while the information from the external model is separately transformed into a point probability mass $\hat{p}_i$. Leveraging this probability mass results in greater efficiency compared to not applying such a transformation. Intuitively, the construction of the probability mass $\hat{p}_i$ relies on a semi-parametric joint log-likelihood of the internal data $\{Y, \mathbf{X}\}$ and the summary information $\hat{\boldsymbol{\theta}}$ from the external study, where the external information is delivered through the moment constraint in (11), and the estimation uncertainty is accounted by the quadratic term in (10), analogous to the rationale in the GIM estimator. The external information is expected to be integrated by the constructed semi-parametric joint log-likelihood, where the weight $\hat{p}_i$ is a more efficient estimate of empirical distribution [35]. Thus, the resulting $\hat{p}_i$ serves an informative weight, carrying additional information from the external data and integrating it into the internal estimating equation [8, 9].

Distinct from the GIM procedure, however, the estimation of main parameters in $\boldsymbol{\beta}$ is not involved in the estimation of p_i and $\boldsymbol{\theta}$. This feature decouples the estimation of the main parameter vector $\boldsymbol{\beta}$ and extra parameters p_i and $\boldsymbol{\theta}$ for information integration, which reduces the computational load in comparison with the joint estimation algorithm described in Sect. 2.4. More importantly, the above procedure avoids the specification of observed likelihood to link model systems between two studies, i.e., $\sum_{i=1}^{n_1} \mathbf{g}(Y_i, \mathbf{X}_i, \mathbf{Z}_i; \boldsymbol{\beta}, \boldsymbol{\eta}) = \mathbf{0}$ and $\sum_{i=1}^{n_1} \boldsymbol{\Psi}(Y_i, \mathbf{X}_i; \boldsymbol{\theta}) = \mathbf{0}$. Therefore, the proposed integration framework has larger potential to accommodate broader modeling strategies, particularly in cases where deriving an analytical relationship between internal and external models may prove challenging.

We remark here that the proposed framework has recently been employed to integrate summary information, enhancing estimation efficiency in a partial linear model (PLM) [30]. The theoretical framework has demonstrated that the resulting estimator is more efficient than the typical profile least square estimator [16]. This article extends its application to a more generic setting, including GLM and causal estimation, and we anticipate the same asymptotic properties by following the proof strategy outlined in that literature [30], omitting the detailed proof here. In the subsequent sections of this article, we describe the computational advancements and provide numerical evidence through simulation studies to evaluate the validity of the proposed framework in terms of estimation bias and Monte Carlo standard deviation. Furthermore, we discuss potential extensions of this new framework to handle complex situations as described in Sect. 2.5, such as heterogeneous covariate distributions, heterogeneous conditional outcome distributions, and information integration from multiple external studies.

3.2 *Efficient Computation*

As described from the last section, the proposed estimation requires much less computational load, in comparison with CML- and GIM-based estimators. The decoupled feature leads to more efficient computational strategy to estimate the main parameters in $\boldsymbol{\beta}$ by solving using weighting estimation equation. However, the estimation of weight is still entangled with $\boldsymbol{\theta}$ estimation, which requires iterative updating algorithm from the empirical likelihood framework and could be time-consuming as well. To further release computational load, we advocate the following estimation procedure for estimating $\boldsymbol{\theta}$.

Step 1: Estimate $\boldsymbol{\theta}$ via the meta-analysis, i.e., by minimizing $\sum_{i\in\{0,1\}}(\boldsymbol{\theta} - \hat{\boldsymbol{\theta}}_{(i)})^T\hat{\mathbf{V}}_{(i)}^{-1}(\boldsymbol{\theta} - \hat{\boldsymbol{\theta}}_{(i)})$, where $\hat{\boldsymbol{\theta}}_{(1)} = \hat{\boldsymbol{\theta}}$ and $\hat{\mathbf{V}}_{(1)} = \hat{\mathbf{V}}/n_2$; $\hat{\boldsymbol{\theta}}_{(0)}$ is the estimate solved by the estimating equation $\sum_{i=1}^{n_1}\boldsymbol{\Psi}(Y_i, \mathbf{X}_i; \boldsymbol{\theta}) = \mathbf{0}$ based on the internal data, and $\hat{\mathbf{V}}_{(0)}$ is a consistent estimate of the variance-covariance matrix of $\hat{\boldsymbol{\theta}}_{(0)}$. We denote the resulting estimate as $\hat{\boldsymbol{\theta}}_{meta}$.

Step 2: Using the plug-in estimator from the meta-analysis $\hat{\boldsymbol{\theta}}_{meta}$, the weight $\hat{p}_i = (1/n_1)\{1 + \hat{\boldsymbol{\rho}}^T\boldsymbol{\Psi}(Y_i, \mathbf{X}_i; \hat{\boldsymbol{\theta}}_{meta})\}^{-1}$ is readily calculated, where the estimated Lagrange multiplier $\hat{\boldsymbol{\rho}}$ is obtained by solving $\partial\tilde{l}_{n_1}(\boldsymbol{\rho})/\partial\boldsymbol{\rho} = \mathbf{0}$, with

$$\tilde{l}_{n_1}(\boldsymbol{\rho}) = -\sum_{i=1}^{n_1}\log\{1 + \boldsymbol{\rho}^T\boldsymbol{\Psi}(Y_i, \mathbf{X}_i; \hat{\boldsymbol{\theta}}_{meta})\}. \tag{12}$$

Since $\tilde{l}_{n_1}(\boldsymbol{\rho})$ is a convex function in terms of $\boldsymbol{\rho}$, the estimation of $\boldsymbol{\rho}$ is quick and stable [10, 20, 21]. Two steps above are performed only once, without the need for iterative updating. The above two-step estimation has been demonstrated to be asymptotically equivalent to the empirical likelihood-based estimator by solving the constrained optimization in (10) and (11) under the PLM setting [30]. We expect a similar property in the context discussed in this article.

Finally, using the weights $\hat{p}_i$, the estimator of the parameters $\boldsymbol{\zeta} = (\boldsymbol{\beta}^T, \boldsymbol{\eta}^T)^T$ can be obtained by solving the weighted estimation equations in (9). Moreover, given the homogeneous data assumption between internal and external studies, the asymptotic variance-covariance matrix for the proposed estimator $n_1^{0.5}(\hat{\boldsymbol{\zeta}} - \boldsymbol{\zeta}_0)$ can be calculated by $\hat{\boldsymbol{\Sigma}}^{-1}(\hat{\mathbf{G}} - c\hat{\mathbf{M}}\hat{\boldsymbol{\Omega}}\hat{\mathbf{M}}^T)(\hat{\boldsymbol{\Sigma}}^T)^{-1}$, where $c = \lim_{n_1\to\infty} n_2/(n_1 + n_2)$, assuming to be a constant value between zero and one, and $\hat{\boldsymbol{\Sigma}}$, $\hat{\mathbf{G}}$, $\hat{\mathbf{M}}$, and $\hat{\boldsymbol{\Omega}}$ are sample version estimates for $\boldsymbol{\Sigma}$, $\mathbf{G}$, $\mathbf{M}$, and $\boldsymbol{\Omega}$, respectively, with

$$\begin{aligned}
\boldsymbol{\Sigma} &= E_1\{\partial\mathbf{g}(Y, \mathbf{X}, \mathbf{Z}; \boldsymbol{\zeta}_0)/\partial\boldsymbol{\zeta}^T\}\\
\mathbf{G} &= E_1\{\mathbf{g}(Y, \mathbf{X}, \mathbf{Z}; \boldsymbol{\zeta}_0)\mathbf{g}^T(Y, \mathbf{X}, \mathbf{Z}; \boldsymbol{\zeta}_0)\}\\
\mathbf{M} &= E_1\{\mathbf{g}(Y, \mathbf{X}, \mathbf{X}; \boldsymbol{\theta}_0)\}\\
\boldsymbol{\Omega} &= [E_1\{\boldsymbol{\Psi}(Y, \mathbf{X}; \boldsymbol{\theta}_0)\boldsymbol{\Psi}^T(Y, \mathbf{X}; \boldsymbol{\theta}_0)\}]^{-1}.
\end{aligned}$$

The above formulas can be similarly derived by following the theoretical framework presented in the proof of Theorem 2.2 in Liang et al.'s work [30]. We defer the detailed proof to interested readers.

Besides, it is important to note that the above two-step estimation differs from the existing two-step method [17] in two key aspects. First, the two procedures target different parameters of interest. The existing method [17] obtains an initial estimator in the first step without incorporating auxiliary information and updates the same estimator in the second step by adding extra terms related to auxiliary information.

In contrast, the proposed two-step estimation focuses solely on estimating the parameters in $\boldsymbol{\theta}$, while the primary parameters in $\boldsymbol{\beta}$ are obtained by solving the weighted estimating equations in (9), after estimating $\boldsymbol{\theta}$ and obtaining $\hat{p}_i$. Second, the existing method assumes that the parameters of interest are present in both the estimating equations with and without auxiliary information, while the proposed method does not. In fact, the primary parameters $\boldsymbol{\beta}$ in the internal model could be entirely different from the parameters $\boldsymbol{\theta}$ in the external model, which makes the proposed method more flexible for integrating information from distinct models.

4 Numerical Evidence

4.1 Generalized Linear Model

Data Generation We considered binary outcomes for illustration. Both internal and external data were generated through the model $\xi\{Prob(Y_i = 1|\mathbf{X}_i, Z_i)\} = \beta_0 + \beta_1 X_{1i} + \beta_2 X_{2i} + \beta_3 X_{3i} + \beta_4 Z_i$ with a logit link function $\xi(\cdot)$. To consider potential confounding between covariates, we generated the covariate Z_i following a uniform distribution from 0 to 1, the covariate X_{1i} following a normal distribution with mean equal to Z_i and variance equal to 1, the covariate X_{2i} following a Bernoulli distribution with the probability $exp(Z_i)/\{1+exp(Z_i)\}$, and the covariate X_{3i} following a standard normal distribution. The parameter vector was set to be $\boldsymbol{\beta} = (\beta_0, \beta_1, \beta_2, \beta_3, \beta_4)^T = (1, 1, 1, 1, 1)^T$. We tested two internal sample sizes $n_1 = 200, 600$. The external sample size was set to be proportional to the internal sample size, where $r = n_2/n_1$ equals 0.75, 1.5, and 5.

Following the setting described in Sect. 2.1, we considered the scenario where the variable Z_i was not observed in the external data. Consequently, we assumed that the external study adopted the following model (possibly misspecified): $\xi\{Prob(Y_i = 1|\mathbf{X}_i)\} = \theta_0 + \theta_1 X_{1i} + \theta_2 X_{2i} + \theta_3 X_{3i}$. The estimated vector of parameters $\hat{\boldsymbol{\theta}}$ and its estimated variance-covariance matrix $\hat{\mathbf{V}}$ were assumed to be available, but not the raw external data. We evaluated the performance of the new method, denoted by IB_New, and compared it with GLM and GIM estimators in terms of bias, Monte Carlo standard deviation (MCSD), and relative efficiency (RE), which is the ratio of mean square errors between the GLM estimator and an estimator with data integration (named New_RE for the proposed estimator and GIM_RE for the GIM estimator). All evaluations were conducted in R software under version 4.3.2.

Results The results based on 1000 Monte Carlo runs are summarized in Table 1. Both IB_New and IB_GIM exhibited minimal (even smaller) estimation bias and demonstrated a significant reduction in estimation variability (MCSD) compared to the GLM estimator without information integration across all settings. It is also interesting to note that the IB_New estimator performed very similarly to IB_GIM in terms of RE. These findings suggest that both GIM and the proposed new method effectively integrate information to enhance the analysis of internal studies.

Table 1 Comparison of parameter estimation via the proposed new method, the GIM, and the GLM approach

			0.75			1.5			5		
	Ratio of n_2/n_1		β_1	β_2	β_3	β_1	β_2	β_3	β_1	β_2	β_3
n_1=200	Bias	IB_New	0.013	0.031	0.015	0.017	0.008	0.015	0.018	0.016	0.021
	Bias	GLM	0.078	0.082	0.081	0.056	0.062	0.063	0.067	0.057	0.053
	Bias	IB_GIM	0.024	0.040	0.026	0.023	0.016	0.022	0.016	0.015	0.016
	MCSD	IB_New	0.226	0.399	0.231	0.190	0.338	0.191	0.136	0.226	0.127
	MCSD	GLM	0.316	0.546	0.327	0.306	0.519	0.311	0.315	0.543	0.308
	MCSD	IB_GIM	0.223	0.392	0.228	0.188	0.333	0.190	0.131	0.213	0.122
		New_RE	2.073	1.899	2.125	2.657	2.387	2.739	5.523	5.799	5.900
		GIM_RE	2.115	1.964	2.165	2.717	2.462	2.732	5.996	6.565	6.434
n_1=600	Bias	IB_New	– 0.002	– 0.001	0.002	– 0.000	0.000	0.008	0.005	0.011	0.009
	Bias	GLM	0.020	0.023	0.022	0.015	0.006	0.027	0.027	0.049	0.033
	Bias	IB_GIM	0.001	0.001	0.005	0.003	0.002	0.011	0.006	0.014	0.010
	MCSD	IB_New	0.116	0.213	0.123	0.103	0.188	0.108	0.073	0.130	0.073
	MCSD	GLM	0.158	0.275	0.166	0.162	0.280	0.164	0.161	0.290	0.167
	MCSD	IB_GIM	0.116	0.213	0.121	0.101	0.186	0.106	0.071	0.123	0.070
		New_RE	1.885	1.679	1.836	2.499	2.212	2.365	4.943	5.063	5.394
		GIM_RE	1.905	1.687	1.890	2.574	2.280	2.423	5.321	5.619	5.843

However, the computational difference between GIM and the proposed estimation is significant. The average running time for GIM on one Monte Carlo simulation with an internal sample size of 600 was 27 seconds, while the average time for our new method was only 1.8 seconds, making it 10 times more efficient than the GIM method. Moreover, the GIM method was observed to be more prone to algorithm convergence issues with smaller sample sizes. Therefore, the new method offers a significant computational advantage, which is highly valuable in practice.

4.2 *Causal Inference Model*

Data Generation In this section, we generated the data under the context of causal inference with a binary outcome and a binary exposure. Specifically, for both internal and external data, the exposure was generated based on the Bernoulli distribution, where the probability of success was set to be $\xi\{Prob(A_i = 1|\mathbf{X}_i, Z_i)\} = \gamma_0 + \gamma_1 Z_i + \gamma_2 X_{1i} + \gamma_3 X_{2i} + \gamma_4 X_{3i}$ with a logit link function $\xi(\cdot)$, where all covariates were generated by the same manner described in Sect. 4.1, and $\boldsymbol{\gamma} = (0.5, 0.5, 0.5, 0.5, 0.5)^T$. In the current situation, Z_i was assumed to be observable in both internal and external studies. With the generated exposure, we further generated potential outcomes $(Y_i(A_i))$ from two exposure worlds [36, 38], i.e., $A = 1$ and $A = 0$, based on the outcome conditional mean model, i.e., $\xi\{Prob(Y_i = 1|\mathbf{X}_i, Z_i, A_i = a)\} = \beta_{a0} + \beta_{a1} Z_i + \beta_{a2} X_{1i} + \beta_{a3} X_{2i} + \beta_{a4} X_{3i}$, for $a = 0, 1$, where

$\boldsymbol{\beta}_{a0} = (-0.5, 0.5, -0.5, 0.5, -0.5)^T$, and $\boldsymbol{\beta}_{a1} = (0.5, -0.5, 0.5, -0.5, 0.5)^T$. The observed outcome was then determined by both potential outcomes and the observed exposure label. Moreover, the true causal model of interest was based on pseudo outcomes and MSM: $\xi\{Prob(Y_i(A_i) = 1)\} = \beta_0 + \beta_1 A_i$, where the true parameter value for the logarithm of causal odds ratio β_1 was calculated by computer simulation using generated potential outcomes under 200000 sample size.

On the other hand, we assumed that the external study considered a conventional logistic regression model, i.e., $\xi\{Prob(Y_i = 1|\mathbf{X}_i, A_i)\} = \theta_0 + \theta_1 A_i + \theta_2 Z_i + \theta_3 X_{1i} + \theta_4 X_{2i} + \theta_5 X_{3i}$. The estimated vector of parameter $\hat{\boldsymbol{\theta}}$ and its variance-covariance matrix $\hat{\mathbf{V}}$ were assumed to be available, but not the raw external data. It is worth noting that the external regression model is intrinsically different from the MSM of interest. However, we argue that by integrating information from traditional regression could be still helpful to improve the estimation efficiency in the causal inference model. We evaluated the performance of the new method, denoted by IB_IPTW, and compared it with the classic MSM estimator based on inverse probability treatment weighting (IPTW) [36] using the PS estimated by logistic regression, in terms of bias, MCSD, and RE, which is the ratio of mean square errors between the IPTW estimator and the proposed IB_IPTW estimator with data integration. Note that the GIM-based estimator is not directly applicable in this context.

Results The results based on 1000 Monte Carlo runs are summarized in Table 2, in different settings of internal sample size $n_1 = 200$, 600 and sample size ratio $n_2/n_1 = 0.75$, 1.5, 5. We observed that both IB_IPTW and IPTW estimators had smaller and closer to zero bias as sample size increased. Compared to the IPTW estimator, the IB_IPTW estimator showed smaller MCSD and larger than one RE. These results provide valuable numerical evidence supporting our statement that integrating information from the traditional regression model based on the external data could be still helpful to improve the estimation efficiency in the casual model based on the internal data.

Table 2 Evaluation of the proposed information integration method for estimating the logarithm of causal odds ratio

		$n_1 = 200$			$n_1 = 600$		
Ratio of n_2/n_1		0.75	1.5	5	0.75	1.5	5
Bias	IB_IPTW	– 0.011	0.003	0.003	0.001	0.007	– 0.014
Bias	IPTW	– 0.012	– 0.005	0.003	0.001	– 0.002	0.001
MCSD	IB_IPTW	0.341	0.304	0.271	0.183	0.169	0.143
MCSD	IPTW	0.407	0.405	0.409	0.221	0.215	0.232
RE		1.423	1.774	2.282	1.452	1.602	2.611

5 Discussion

We have provided a selective review of recent and advanced information integration methods via empirical likelihood. Moreover, we provided a new and possibly promising direction to integrate information from a broad context. Compared to existing methods, this new method is computationally more convenient, numerically more stable, and able to integrate summary information from a model that is very different from the main model used for internal analysis. In addition to the simple setting described in Sect. 3.1, the new framework can be extended to handle more complex settings by adapting techniques described in Sect. 2.5: for example, if one has observed the issue of heterogeneous covariate distributions between internal and external data, we may consider adopting the technique of semi-parametric density ratio model [12, 23, 39] described in (7) into the proposed constraint (11); if one has concern about heterogeneous conditional outcome distributions, we may impose a bias term assisted by the technique of penalty, similar to the formula in described in (8), to alleviate potential bias introduced to the internal estimation; when we have summary information from multiple external data, we may change the joint log-likelihood function in (10) to $\sum_{i=1}^{n_1} log(p_i) - \sum_{k=2}^{K} n_k(\hat{\boldsymbol{\theta}}_k - \boldsymbol{\theta})^T(\hat{\mathbf{V}}_k)^{-1}(\hat{\boldsymbol{\theta}}_k - \boldsymbol{\theta})/2$, with $K \geq 2$. Extensive studies are needed to evaluate their validity and utility.

Furthermore, the new framework holds potential for application in various other statistical contexts, including survival analysis, longitudinal data analysis, and analysis of heterogeneous treatment effects, among others, all of which warrant thorough investigation. In terms of applications, the new method has the potential to be applied across diverse disciplines, including the integration of information from multicenter clinical trials, electronic health records from multiple hospitals, and cohort studies from different consortia. In summary, in the era of big data, the authors believe that the framework of information integration and the new idea proposed in this article are poised to play pivotal roles.

Acknowledgments Chen, C's work was supported by National Institutes of Health grants R01 AG089377 and P30 AG028747 and by the Johns Hopkins Institute for Clinical and Translational Research (ICTR) funded under grant 1UM1TR004926 from the National Center for Advancing Translational Sciences (NCATS) a component of the National Institutes of Health (NIH), and NIH Roadmap for Medical Research. The content of this paper is solely the responsibility of the authors and do not necessarily represent the official view of the Johns Hopkins ICTR, NCATS, or NIH.

References

1. Alfonso, F., Adamyan, K., Artigou, J.Y., Aschermann, M., Boehm, M., Buendia, A., ...Lüscher, T.F.: Data sharing: a new editorial initiative of the International Committee of Medical Journal Editors. Implications for the Editors' Network. Archivos de cardiología de México, **87**(2), 101–107 (2017)
2. Austin, P.C., Stuart, E.A.: Moving towards best practice when using inverse probability of treatment weighting (IPTW) using the propensity score to estimate causal treatment effects in observational studies. Stat. Med. **34**(28), 3661–3679 (2015)

3. Borenstein, M., Hedges, L.V., Higgins, J.P., Rothstein, H.R.: Introduction to Meta-Analysis. Wiley, New York (2021)
4. Chatterjee, N., Chen, Y.H., Maas, P., Carroll, R.J.: Constrained maximum likelihood estimation for model calibration using summary-level information from external big data sources. J. Am. Stat. Assoc. **111**(513), 107–117 (2016)
5. Chen, C., Chen, S., Long, Q., Das, S., Wang, M.: Multiple-model-based robust estimation of causal treatment effect on a binary outcome with integrated information from secondary outcomes. In: The American Statistician, pp. 1–11 (2023a)
6. Chen, C., Chen, S., Ye, Z., Shi, X., Ma, T., Shardell, M.: The effect of alcohol intake on brain white matter microstructural integrity: a new causal inference framework for incomplete phenomic data. J. Am. Stat. Assoc. 1–13 (2025)
7. Chen, C., Han, P., Chen, S., Shardell, M., Qin, J.: Integrating external summary information in the presence of prior probability shift: an application to assessing essential hypertension. Biometrics **80**(3), ujae090 (2024)
8. Chen, C., Han, P., He, F.: Improving main analysis by borrowing information from auxiliary data. Stat. Med. **41**(3), 567–579 (2022)
9. Chen, C., Wang, M., Chen, S.: An efficient data integration scheme for synthesizing information from multiple secondary datasets for the parameter inference of the main analysis. Biometrics **79**(4), 2947–2960 (2023c)
10. Chen, J., Variyath, A.M., Abraham, B.: Adjusted empirical likelihood and its properties. J. Comput. Graph. Stat. **17**(2), 426–443 (2008)
11. Cheng, W., Taylor, J.M., Gu, T., Tomlins, S.A., Mukherjee, B.: Informing a risk prediction model for binary outcomes with external coefficient information. J. R. Stat. Soc.: Ser. C: Appl. Stat. **68**(1), 121–139 (2019)
12. Cheng, Y.J., Liu, Y.C., Tsai, C.Y., Huang, C.Y.: Semiparametric estimation of the transformation model by leveraging external aggregate data in the presence of population heterogeneity. Biometrics **79**(3), 1996–2009 (2023d)
13. Daniels, H.E.: The asymptotic efficiency of a maximum likelihood estimator. In: In Fourth Berkeley Symposium on Mathematical Statistics and Probability, vol. 1, pp. 151–163. University of California Press, Berkeley (1961)
14. Lu Deng, S. F., Qin, J., Yu, K.: On combining individual-level data with summary data in statistical inferences. Stat. Sinc. **34**, 1505–1520 (2024)
15. Duan, R., Ning, Y., Chen, Y.: Heterogeneity-aware and communication-efficient distributed statistical inference. Biometrika **109**(1), 67–83 (2022)
16. Fan, J., Li, R.: New estimation and model selection procedures for semiparametric modeling in longitudinal data analysis. J. Am. Stat. Assoc. **99**(467), 710–723 (2004)
17. Gao, F., Chan, K.C.G.: Noniterative adjustment to regression estimators with population-based auxiliary information for semiparametric models. Biometrics **79**(1), 140–150 (2023)
18. Haidich, A.B.: Meta-analysis in medical research. Hippokratia **14**(Suppl 1), 29 (2010)
19. Han, L., Li, Y., Niknam, B.A., Zubizarreta, J.R.: Privacy-Preserving, Communication-Efficient, and Target-Flexible Hospital Quality Measurement. arXiv preprint arXiv:2203.00768 (2022)
20. Han, P., Lawless, J.F.: Empirical likelihood estimation using auxiliary summary information with different covariate distributions. Stat. Sin. **29**(3), 1321–1342 (2019)
21. Han, P.: A further study of the multiply robust estimator in missing data analysis. J. Stat. Plann. Inference **148**, 101–110 (2014)
22. Han, P.: A discussion on "A selective review of statistical methods using calibration information from similar studies" by Qin, Liu and Li. Stat. Theory Relat. Fields **6**(3), 193–195 (2022)
23. Huang, Y., Huang, C.Y., Kim, M.O.: Simultaneous selection and incorporation of consistent external aggregate information. Stat. Med. **42**(30), 5630–5645 (2023)
24. Ibrahim, J.G., Chen, M.H., Gwon, Y., Chen, F.: The power prior: theory and applications. Stat. Med. **34**(28), 3724–3749 (2015)
25. Jiang, L., Nie, L., Yuan, Y.: Elastic priors to dynamically borrow information from historical data in clinical trials. Biometrics **79**(1), 49–60 (2023)

26. Jin, J., Agarwala, N., Kundu, P., Harvey, B., Zhang, Y., Wallace, E., Chatterjee, N.: Individual and community-level risk for COVID-19 mortality in the United States. Nat. Med. **27**(2), 264–269 (2021)
27. Jordan, M.I., Lee, J.D., Yang, Y.: Communication-efficient distributed statistical inference. J. Am. Stat. Assoc. **114**(526), 668–681 (2018)
28. Kisselburgh, L., Beever, J.: The ethics of privacy in research and design: principles, practices, and potential. In: Modern Socio-Technical Perspectives on Privacy, pp. 395–426. Springer International Publishing, Cham
29. Kundu, P., Tang, R., Chatterjee, N.: Generalized meta-analysis for multiple regression models across studies with disparate covariate information. Biometrika **106**(3), 567–585 (2019)
30. Liang, J., Chen, S., Kochunov, P., Hong, L. E., Chen, C.: Integrative data analysis where partial covariates have complex nonlinear effects by using summary information from an external data. Am. Stat. **79**(1), 61–71 (2025)
31. Lapatas, V., Stefanidakis, M., Jimenez, R.C., Via, A., Schneider, M.V.: Data integration in biological research: an overview. J. Biol. Res.-Thessalon. **22**, 1–16 (2015)
32. Luo, L., Song, P.X.K.: Renewable estimation and incremental inference in generalized linear models with streaming data sets. J. R. Stat. Soc. Ser. B Stat Methodol. **82**(1), 69–97 (2020)
33. Luo, L., Wang, J., Hector, E.C.: Statistical inference for streamed longitudinal data. Biometrika **110**(4), 841–858 (2023)
34. Qin, J., Liu, Y., Li, P.: A selective review of statistical methods using calibration information from similar studies. Stat. Theory Relat. Fields **6**(3), 175–190 (2022)
35. Qin, J., Lawless, J.: Empirical likelihood and general estimating equations. Ann. Stat. **22**(1), 300–325 (1994)
36. Robins, J.M., Hernan, M.A., Brumback, B.: Marginal structural models and causal inference in epidemiology. Epidemiology **11**(5), 550–560 (2000)
37. Rothstein, M.A.: Is deidentification sufficient to protect health privacy in research? Am. J. Bioeth. **10**(9), 3–11 (2010)
38. Rosenbaum, P.R., Rubin, D.B.: The central role of the propensity score in observational studies for causal effects. Biometrika **70**(1), 41–55 (1983)
39. Sheng, Y., Sun, Y., Huang, C.Y., Kim, M.O.: Synthesizing external aggregated information in the presence of population heterogeneity: a penalized empirical likelihood approach. Biometrics **78**(2), 679–690 (2022)
40. Vepakomma, P., Gupta, O., Swedish, T., Raskar, R.: Split learning for health: distributed deep learning without sharing raw patient data. arXiv preprint arXiv:1812.00564 (2018)
41. Yang, S., Ding, P.: Combining multiple observational data sources to estimate causal effects. J. Am. Stat. Assoc. **115**(531), 1540–1554 (2019)
42. Zeger, S.L., Liang, K.-Y., Albert, P.S.: Models for longitudinal data: a generalized estimating equation approach. Biometrics **44**(4), 1049–1060 (1988)
43. Zhai, Y., Han, P.: Data integration with oracle use of external information from heterogeneous populations. J. Comput. Graph. Stat. **31**(4), 1001–1012 (2022)
44. Zhang, H., Deng, L., Schiffman, M., Qin, J., Yu, K.: Generalized integration model for improved statistical inference by leveraging external summary data. Biometrika **107**(3), 689–703 (2020)

Part IV
Clinical Trials and Survival Analysis

Hierarchical Semi-parametric Bayesian Modeling in Patient Screening and Enrollment Dynamic Prediction for Multicenter Clinical Trials

Jianmin Chen, Zhaowei Zoe Hua, Qian Meng, Lucie Truffaut-Chalet, Zhaoyang Teng, and Rui Sammi Tang

Abstract Effective recruitment planning is crucial for the success of clinical trials, as inadequate recruitment is a leading cause of trial discontinuation. Such setbacks not only cause delays and incur additional costs but also result in lost market opportunities. In response to this challenge, the development of a predictive tool for recruitment planning has garnered significant interest. Our work focuses on the intricacies of screening and enrollment forecasting for trials involving various disease subtypes or biomarker-defined subgroups within a multi-regional context. We employ a hierarchical semi-parametric Bayesian approach to model recruitment dynamics, which allows for the accommodation of heterogeneity across patient populations attributable to regional or subgroup distinctions. To support ongoing recruitment efforts, we propose a dynamic prediction framework that offers continuous guidance for recruitment planning. This innovative tool, grounded in model-based and data-driven methodologies, demonstrates notable flexibility and precision in projecting enrollment figures. Moreover, it efficiently identifies potential future risks, thereby facilitating informed decision-making in the management of clinical trials.

Keywords Enrollment dynamic prediction · Hierarchical model · Non-parametric Bayesian · Patient screening · Clinical trials

---

J. Chen
University of Pennsylvania, Philadelphia, PA, USA
e-mail: Jianmin.Chen@Pennmedicine.upenn.edu

Z. Z. Hua (✉) · Q. Meng
Servier Bio-Innovation, Boston, MA, USA
e-mail: Zoe.Hua@servier.com

L. Truffaut-Chalet
Institut de Recherche International Servier, Gif-sur-Yvette, France

Z. Teng · R. S. Tang
Astellas Pharma, Cambridge, MA, USA

Y. Zhao, D.-G. Chen (eds.), *Big Data Analytics in Biostatistics and Bioinformatics*, ICSA Book Series in Statistics,
https://doi.org/10.1007/978-3-032-06649-7_16

1 Introduction

Clinical trial is the essential step to investigate the safety and efficacy promise of a new drug following years of costly research and development. Patient recruitment, which is both time-consuming and expensive, is the start of the clinical trial. Optimal recruitment planning plays a vital role in ensuring the success of the trial. As reported in the review paper Fogel [5], poor recruitment is the primary cause for the discontinuation of randomized trials, resulting in numerous negative impacts, including time delay, additional expenses, and missed marketing opportunities. As such, there is a substantial need for a predictive tool to monitor the recruitment process, which supports decision-making and risk management during the drug development process.

Numerous efforts have been made to improve the accuracy in recruitment projection for multicenter clinical trials. One class of methods focuses on estimating the accrual rate at each center and predicting the time required for recruitment completion. The unconditional method is the simplest approach, where the accrual rate at each center is determined based on prior knowledge and assumed to remain constant throughout the entire process [3]. Conversely, the conditional methods are better options to mimic the real recruitment process, as they allow the recruitment rate at each center to vary over time, depending on factors such as the seasonal effects [3]. Another widely discussed class in literature is based on stochastic models, among which the Poisson-Gamma model introduced by Anisimov and Fedorov [1] and its variations are predominately explored [2, 13]. To capture the variations in recruitment among different centers, accrual rates across centers are modeled by a gamma distribution, while the arrival of patients within each center is modeled by a Poisson process. Other methods include the Bayesian approaches proposed in Gajewski et al. [6] and Jiang et al. [10]. Moreover, machine learning methods have been integrated into the prediction task, as proposed in Liu et al. [11]. However, these models often require a relatively larger number of enrolled patients, which can be unrealistic in some trials. For a more thorough review of model-based methods, see Barnard et al. [4] and Gkioni et al. [7].

Nonetheless, recruitment prediction involving multiple groups of patients recruited simultaneously in a clinical trial has not been extensively discussed, with limited literature available. Specifically, we focus on the cases where patients with distinct disease subtypes or biomarker outcomes are recruited in the same trial [9]. Such trials with a heterogenous patient population typically need to recruit patients from a large number of centers to ensure adequate representation of patients across subgroups defined by disease subtype or region, etc. Due to dynamic enrollment process, varying status over time across centers is commonly observed. Heterogeneity across disease subtypes and regions and randomness across centers lead to complexity in modeling recruitment process. To account these factors, we propose a Bayesian model-based approach to capture the uncertainty and simultaneously predict the number of patients screened/enrolled at a future time point, at different center(s), or for different disease subtype(s). The remainder of the paper is organized as follows. Section 2 introduces the model settings and the statistical model employed within the Bayesian hierarchical framework, with detailed explanations. The prediction procedure is discussed in Sect. 3. We conduct simulation studies to explore the performance of the proposed method, and the results are reported in Sect. 4. Further, in Sect. 5, we demonstrate the dynamic prediction strategy within our framework using a synthetic dataset. A summary for the framework is provided in Sect. 6.

2 Multi-stage Modeling

The multicenter trial with centers distributed in several regions is commonly conducted to ensure an adequate number of patients. An example with three centers is shown in Fig. 1, where patients diagnosed with two different disease subtypes are recruited, and the target numbers of patients are set separately for each subtype. As illustrated, centers can have varied times for opening and stopping, and different subtypes may also have specific enrollment completion dates. Moreover, each center can be on different status at the data cutoff point (stopped, opened, opened with no screened patients, or still in planning). In such a scenario, the complexity in modeling patient recruitment increases as the randomness in the process can come from centers, disease subtypes, and patients.

Patient recruitment [12] in most clinical trials can be conceptualized as a four-stage process. Rather than modeling patient arrival with a Poisson process, we focus on the waiting times between two consecutive events, and directly modeling these waiting times using models designed for the time-to-event data, as suggested in Gajewski et al. [6]. Additionally, since there are different disease subtypes involved in the recruitment, we employ joint modeling of screening outcomes and the waiting times in this work. To solve these issues, a multi-stage hierarchical Bayesian modeling approach is adopted. Throughout the paper, we assume that all the patients

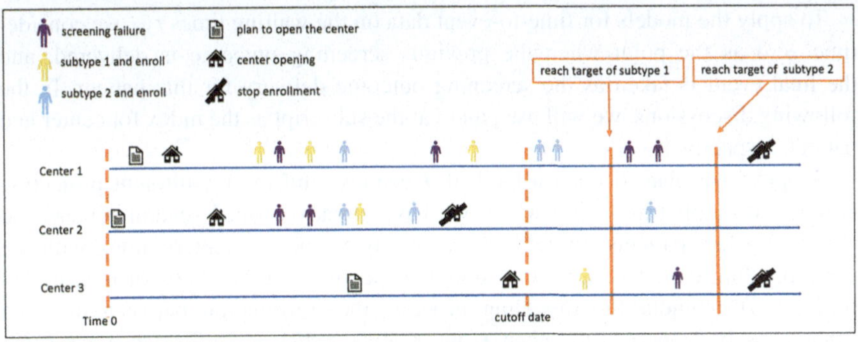

Fig. 1 A multicenter recruitment with two disease subtypes

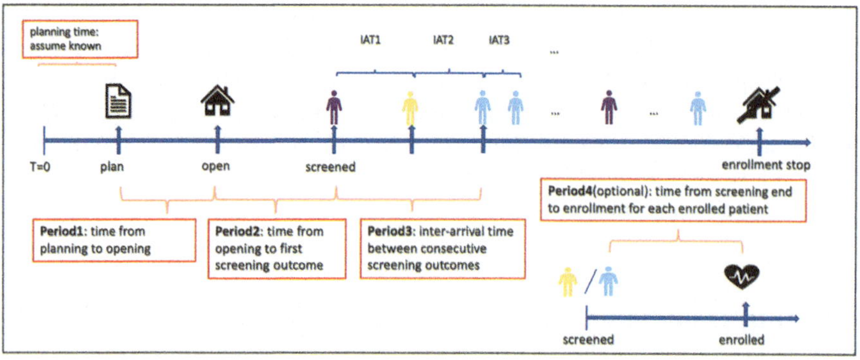

Fig. 2 Four periods in the patient recruitment process. IAT stands for "inter-arrival time"

that pass the screening process will be enrolled, and we do not consider dropout in our settings.

In our study, we assume that the time when a decision is made to open a center or include the center in the recruitment is known. We take this time as the "planning" time for a center and treat the earliest planning time as the start time point of the overall recruitment process. Our target is to predict the final enrollment time of the ith patient at the jth center, t_{ij}. We remark that the patient's index i is defined based on the time of screening outcome delivery. As described in Fig. 2, the process of recruiting a patient into a trial can be divided into four periods: time from planning to center opening (t_{1j}), time from opening to the first screening outcome (t_{2j}), the inter-arrival time (IAT) between consecutive screening outcome deliveries (t_{3ji}), and the time between screening outcome and the final enrollment (t_{4ji}) if the patient passes the screening. We consider four separated models for the four periods and the final predicted enrollment time t_{ij} can be formulated as

$$t_{ij} = t_{1j} + t_{2j} + \sum\nolimits_{k<i} t_{3jk} + t_{4ji}.$$

To apply the models for time-to-event data on the waiting times t_{3ji}, we consider time zero as the point when the previous screening outcome is delivered, and the final event is taken as the screening outcome delivery for this patient. In the following discussions, we will use j and i at the subscript as the index for center and patient, respectively.

Suppose we plan to open a total of J centers, and the recruitment projection is made at cutoff time T, by which we have already opened several centers and recruited a few patients. In Table 1, we list five types of centers along with the corresponding counts observed at time T, depending on the status of recruitment process. Throughout the modeling process, the information between different centers can be leveraged to enhance the overall prediction performance across all the centers.

Table 1 Types of centers at the cutoff date T

Center (index set)	Number of centers
Total centers	J
Not yet opened center (C_1)	J_1
Opened center (C_2)	$J_2 = J - J_1$
Opened center without screened patient (C_3)	J_3
Opened center with screened patient (C_4)	$J_4 = J_2 - J_3$
Enrollment completion center (C_5)	J_5

In the following sub-sections, we introduce the modeling assumption and distribution setup for each stage in the recruitment process.

2.1 t_{1j}: Time from Planning to Opening

As aforementioned, the time for center planning is assumed as a known value. We deploy a uniform distribution to model the waiting times between planning and center opening. The lower limit of the uniform distribution is set as 0, while the upper bound can be estimated based on the data from those already opened centers in C_2.

According to Table 1, at cutoff time T, J_1 centers in C_1 have not yet been opened. We consider

$$t_{1j} \sim U\left(0, T_{1j^*}\right), j \in C_1,$$

where U denotes the uniform distribution, T_{1j^*} is the maximum time gap from planning to opening for centers that have already opened before the cutoff time T in C_2.

2.2 t_{2j}: Time from Opening to the Delivery of the First Screening Outcome

Assume at the cutoff time T, there exist opened centers such that no screening result has been delivered yet, and there are J_3 such centers. Typically, the first inter-arrival time for the screening outcome after center opening is longer than the subsequent waiting times. Consequently, we take the first inter-arrival time as a separate stage in the modeling framework.

Specifically, we assume an exponential distribution with rate parameter $\lambda_1 > 0$ for waiting times t_{2j}, where the likelihood function for the observed data from the opened centers can be formulated as:

$$\prod_j \lambda_1^{\delta_j} e^{-\lambda_1 t_{2j}}, \; j \in C_2,$$

and $\delta_j = 1$ if the jth center has at least one screening outcome and $\delta_j = 0$ otherwise. A Gamma$(1, 1)$ prior is adopted for the rate parameter λ_1. The posterior distribution of λ_1 is given by the Gamma distribution:

$$\text{Gamma}\left(\sum_{j \in C_2} \delta_j + 1, \sum_{j \in C_2, \delta_j = 1} t_{2j} + 1\right).$$

By using the above-mentioned method, the information from those already opened centers with screened patients is borrowed for the predictions in other centers.

2.3 t_{3ji}: *Inter-arrival Time Between Consecutive Screening Outcome Deliveries*

The most important contribution of our work is modeling the screening process, where the screening outcomes can be divided into three subgroups: failure, subtype1, and subtype2. While most of the related discussions in the literature mainly focus on the prediction of the overall enrollment, it is noteworthy that an accurate prediction for the cumulative number of screened patients for each subgroup can be beneficial in budget planning beforehand. In practice, we have observed distinct screening behaviors among centers, mainly from the screening rate and the distribution of the screening outcomes. Some centers may have short inter-arrival times between screening outcome deliveries and a high screening failure rate. In contrast, some centers may be slow in screening but have a higher proportion of patients diagnosed with a specific disease subtype of interest. Building on these findings, joint modeling of screening rate and the outcomes is considered.

We utilize a hierarchical Bayesian modeling framework with four levels, as illustrated in Fig. 3. From top-to-bottom, the structure demonstrates the assumed data generation process, while from bottom-up, it gives the order of parameter estimation/sampling process. We will discuss the four levels in bottom-up order and introduce the corresponding notations in the next sections. We start with Level 3 with the observed data from each center.

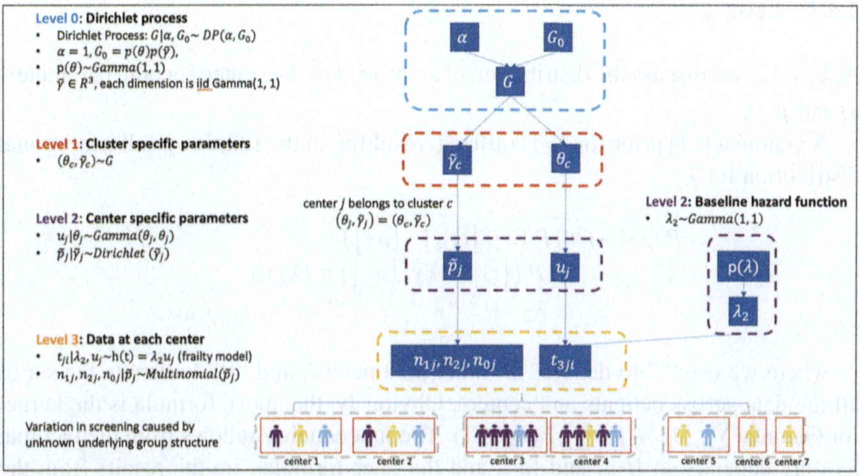

Fig. 3 Hierarchical Bayesian model structure

2.3.1 Level 3

At the bottom level (Level 3), we aggregate the observed inter-arrival times and screening outcomes from each center. We focus on modeling inter-arrival times t_{3ji} and the screening outcome vectors at the jth center, $\tilde{n}_j = (n_{1j}, n_{2j}, n_{0j})$, where n_{1j}, n_{2j}, and n_{0j} are the number of screened patient with disease subtype 1, number of screened patient with disease subtype 2, and the number of screening failure patient.

Here, we include center-specific parameters to account for the heterogeneity. A frailty model is employed for the inter-arrival times t_{3ji}, where we take the hazard function $h(t_{3ji}) = \lambda_2 u_j$ and u_j represents the center-specific random effect. Moreover, for simplicity, we select the exponential baseline hazard function with rate parameter $\lambda_2 > 0$ in our framework. For the screening outcomes $\tilde{n}_j = (n_{1j}, n_{2j}, n_{0j})$, a multinomial distribution with center-specific proportion vector $\tilde{p}_j = (p_{1j}, p_{2j}, p_{0j})$ is considered, where p_{1j}, p_{2j}, and p_{0j} are the event probability for subtype 1, subtype 2, and screening failure with $p_{1j} + p_{2j} + p_{0j} = 1$. Finally, the full observed likelihood of the hierarchical model at the bottom level can be written as

$$L\left(t_{3ji}, \tilde{n_j}\right) \propto \prod_{j \in C_4} \lambda_2^{\sum_i \delta_{ji}} u_j^{\sum_i \delta_{ji}} e^{-\lambda_2 T_{3j} u_j} p_{1j}^{n_{1j}} p_{2j}^{n_{2j}} p_{0j}^{n_{0j}},$$

where $\delta_{ji} = 1$ if the screening outcome of the ith patient has been delivered and 0 otherwise. Also, we use T_{3j} to denote the summation of waiting times at the jth center, i.e., $T_{3j} = \sum_i t_{3ji}$.

2.3.2 Level 2

At Level 2, we discuss the distribution of λ_2 as well as the center-specific parameters u_j and $\tilde{p}_j$.

A Gamma(1, 1) prior for λ_2 is utilized, resulting in the following full conditional distribution for λ_2:

$$\begin{aligned} P(\lambda_2|-) &= P\left(\lambda_2|\left\{t_{3ji}\right\},\left\{u_j\right\}\right) \\ &\propto P\left(\left\{t_{3ji}\right\}|\lambda_2,\left\{u_j\right\}\right)\pi(\lambda_2) \\ &\propto \lambda_2{}^{\sum_{j,i}\delta_{3ji}} e^{-\lambda_2\sum_j T_{3j}u_j} e^{-\lambda_2},\ j \in C_4, \end{aligned}$$

where we use "-" to denote "all other parameters" and "{}" to denote the set of all the data across patients and centers. Obviously, the above formula is the kernel for Gamma($\sum_{j,\,i}\delta_{ji} + 1,\ \ \sum_j T_{3j}u_j + 1$). The first equality follows from the fact that λ_2 only depends on $\{t_{3ji}\}$ and $\{u_j\}$, and the later formulas are the results from the Bayesian rule. The same techniques are used in the derivation of other conditional distributions.

Since the random effect u_j in the frailty model is assumed to be positive, we adopt a Gamma(θ_j, θ_j) distribution for u_j, indexed by the hyper-parameter $\theta_j > 0$. Therefore, the full conditional distribution of u_j given all other parameters can be written as

$$\begin{aligned} P(u_j|-) &= P\left(u_j|\theta_j, \lambda_2, t_{3ji}\right) \propto P\left(t_{3ji}|\lambda_2, u_j\right) P\left(u_j|\theta_j\right) \\ &\propto u_j{}^{\sum_i \delta_{ji}} e^{-\lambda_2 T_{3j}u_j} u_j{}^{\theta_j - 1} e^{-u_j\theta_j},\ j \in C_4. \end{aligned}$$

The posterior distribution of parameter u_j has the kernel of Gamma ($\sum_i \delta_{ji} + \theta_j, \lambda_2 T_{3j} + \theta_j$).

Finally, a Dirichlet-Multinomial model is used to model the screening outcomes, where $\tilde{p}_j \sim$ Dirichlet $\left(\tilde{\gamma}_j\right)$ with $\tilde{\gamma}_j = \left(\gamma_{1j}, \gamma_{2j}, \gamma_{0j}\right)$ being the hyper-parameter of dimension 3. The full conditional distribution of $\tilde{p}_j$ is

$$\begin{aligned} P\left(\tilde{p}_j|-\right) &= P\left(\tilde{p}_j|\tilde{\gamma}_j|n_{1j}|n_{2j}|n_{0j}\right) \\ &\propto P\left(n_{1j}, n_{2j}, n_{0j}, \tilde{p}_j\right) P\left(\tilde{p}_j|\tilde{\gamma}_j\right) \\ &\propto p_{1j}{}^{n_{1j}} p_{2j}{}^{n_{2j}} p_{0j}{}^{n_{0j}} p_{1j}{}^{\gamma_{1j}-1} p_{2j}{}^{\gamma_{2j}-1} p_{0j}{}^{\gamma_{0j}-1}, \end{aligned}$$

which is the kernel for Dirichlet($n_{1j} + \gamma_{1j}, n_{2j} + \gamma_{2j}, n_{0j} + \gamma_{0j}$).

2.3.3 Level 1

We assume that there is an underlying grouping structure among centers. The rationale is that the center variations in screening behavior can result from the intrinsic heterogeneity in the patient population due to region or disease subtype differences. Recall we have the center-specific parameters $\left(u_j, \tilde{p}_j\right)$ relying on the hyper parameters $\left(\theta_j, \tilde{\gamma}_j\right)$. To detect the hidden structure, we assume that $\left(u_j, \tilde{p}_j\right)$ are generated from a mixture distribution where the parameters of the mixture components are linked with the center-specific hyper parameters $\left(\theta_j, \tilde{\gamma}_j\right)$, as shown in Level 1 of Fig. 3. For all centers from the same underlying group c, we have the center-specific hyper parameters equal to the group-specific parameters, that is, $\left(\theta_j, \tilde{\gamma}_j\right) = \left(\theta_c, \tilde{\gamma}_c\right)$, $\forall$ center $j \in$ group c.

2.3.4 Level 0

To enhance flexibility, we treat the number of mixture components as an unknown parameter to be estimated from the data. Under the Bayesian framework, this amounts to first generating the group-specific parameters $\left(\theta_c, \tilde{\gamma}_c\right)$ and group labels from a non-parametric Dirichlet Process denoted as $G \mid \alpha, G_0 \sim DP(\alpha, G_0)$, where we set the concentration parameter $\alpha = 1$ and the baseline joint distribution for $\left(\theta_c, \tilde{\gamma}_c\right)$ as $G_0 = p(\theta)\, p\left(\tilde{\gamma}\right)$. We assume the independence between θ and all three dimensions of $\tilde{\gamma}$, setting their base distributions all to be Gamma(1, 1), that is $p(\theta)\sim$ Gamma(1, 1) and $p\left(\tilde{\gamma}\right) = p(\gamma_1)\ p(\gamma_2)\, p(\gamma_0)$ with $p(\gamma_1) = p(\gamma_2) = p(\gamma_0)\sim$ Gamma(1, 1).

This proposed hierarchical semi-parametric Bayesian model offers high flexibility and is entirely data-driven, as no grouping information is given in advance. We leave the details of the sampling procedure to the Appendix. As we shown in Fig. 3, the Dirichlet process at Level 0 is a non-parametric Bayesian method to model the probability distributions of the latent clusters. On the other hand, parametric Bayesian models are used in Level 2 and Level 3 to model the inter-arrival times and the screening outcomes. Thus, we consider the overall framework to be semi-parametric.

2.4 t_{4ji}: *Time Between Screening Outcome Delivery to Enrollment*

Finally, for the fourth period, our framework allows a time gap between the screening outcome delivery and the final enrollment for patients who pass the screening. The time gap is designed to be sampled from a user-defined uniform distribution according to the trial's specifications. The fourth period is optional. For certain clinical trial, there can be no time gap between screening outcome delivery and the final enrollment. Under such scenario, t_{4ji} is always 0, and the screening projection is equivalent to the enrollment projection.

2.5 *Extension with Piecewise Exponential*

In the frailty model in Level 3, we take the hazard function as $h(t_{3ji}) = \lambda_2 u_j$, in which the exponential model is assumed to have the baseline hazard function as λ_2. There are many other options for the baseline hazard function to enhance flexibility, such as the Weibull and lognormal model. However, by using the baseline function from the exponential model, it is easier to design conjugate prior for the parameters and it benefits the sampling step.

We provide one more option to increase flexibility. The current framework can be easily extended to the piecewise exponential model with slight adjustments in the sampling steps, where we take the baseline hazard function as

$$h_0\left(t_{3ji}\right) = \lambda_s,\ \tau_{s-1} < t_{3ji} < \tau_s,$$

and the $(\tau_1, \tau_2, \ldots)$ are the cutoff points for the piece segments. In real data analysis, the number of segments and the cutoff points can be selected by checking the shape of the Kaplan-Meier curve generated based on the waiting times.

3 Multi-stage Prediction

By working through this four-stage framework, we can predict the screening results and the final screening/enrollment date for each upcoming patient based on the sampled posterior distribution for the parameters. The whole prediction process is conducted multiple times to provide the posterior predictive distribution and give the prediction intervals. In each iteration, a set of parameters is randomly sampled from the MCMC chain, and the prediction is carried out accordingly.

3.1 *Predicting the Center Opening Time*

If the jth center opened before the cutoff date ($j \in C_2$), t_{1j} is known and we use it directly in prediction. If the center is still in planning phase ($j \in C_1$), we randomly draw a value v from $U\left(0, T_{1j^*}\right)$, where T_{1j^*} represents the maximum time gap from the planning date to the opening for centers that have already opened before the cutoff date. Furthermore, we take $t_{1j} = \max(v, w_j)$, where w_j is the waiting time from the planning date to the cutoff time.

3.2 Predicting the Arrival Time and Result of the First Screening Outcome

If the jth center has screened patients before the cutoff date ($j \in C_4$), t_{2j} is known and we can directly use it in prediction. Otherwise, we adopt the following steps for $j \in C_1 \cup C_3$.

- Randomly draw λ_1 from Gamma $\left(\sum_{j \in C_2} \delta_j + 1, \sum_{j \in C_2, \delta_j = 1} t_{2j} + 1\right)$.
- Sample t_{2j}:
  - For $j \in C_1$, sample t_{2j} independently with survival function $S\left(t_{2j}\right) = e^{-\lambda_1 t_{2j}}$.
  - For $j \in C_3$, the waiting time before the first screening outcome delivery is known. The inverse transform sampling method is used with survival function $S\left(t_{2j}\right) = e^{-\lambda_1 t_{2j}}$ conditional on the constraint that the sampled inter-arrival time should be greater than the known waiting time.
- Sample the first screening outcome from {subtype-1, subtype-2, failure}, with probabilities (q_1, q_2, q_0), where q_1, q_2, and q_0 are the proportions of subtype-1, subtype-2, and screening failure patients calculated based on the existing records before the cutoff date.

3.3 Predicting the Consecutive Inter-arrival Times and Outcomes of the Upcoming Patients

For centers that are still operating at the cutoff date ($j \in C_1 \cup C_2 \cup C_3 \cup C_4$), we will sample n_{new} consecutive inter-arrival times and outcomes of the upcoming patients. The following steps are employed based on the posterior distribution of the third stage parameters.

- If the jth center has more than one screened patient before the cutoff date, we use the sampled parameters λ_2, u_j and $\widetilde{p}_j$ to generate n_{new} pairs of t_{3ji} and the screening outcomes.
- If the jth center has fewer than two screened patients, we have no information about the underlying grouping structure of the jth center. Under such scenarios, we take the following steps:
  - Sample the group index c for the jth center, where the selection probability is proportional to the number of existing group members. The hyper-parameter of the center is then set as the hyper-parameter of the corresponding group:

$$\left(\theta_j, \widetilde{\gamma_j}\right) = \left(\theta_c, \widetilde{\gamma_c}\right);$$

- Get the center-specific parameters u_j from Gamma(θ_j, θ_j), and $\widetilde{p}_j$ from Dirichlet $\left(\widetilde{\gamma}_j\right)$.
- Generate n_{new} pairs of t_{3ji} and the screening outcomes.

- Note that, for $j \in C_4$, the waiting time after the last delivered outcome can be collected and the first sampled inter-arrival time needs to be generated from inverse transform sampling with survival function $S\left(t_{3ji}\right) = e^{-\lambda_2 u_j t_{3ji}}$, using the last waiting time as the lower bound constraint. Further details regarding the constrained sampling are left in the Appendix.

3.4 Predicting the Overall Recruitment with Adjustment

If there is a time gap between screening outcome delivery and the final enrollment, the time t_{4ji} can be sampled from a user-defined uniform distribution.

Recall that the final predicted enrollment time of the ith patient at the jth center can be formulated as:

$$t_{ji} = t_{1j} + t_{2j} + \sum\nolimits_{k<i} t_{3jk} + t_{4ji}.$$

By generating predictions for the four stages, we can determine the screening/enrollment time for each upcoming patient. Through aggregating the individual prediction results, we can forecast the number of screened/enrolled patients at a future time point for different centers/subtypes. The probability that the recruitment can be completed on time is obtained based on repeated sampling from the posterior distribution.

Additionally, we implement a rule-based strategy to further enhance the performance of our prediction, which is a novel approach rarely used in the literature. In real patient recruitment for a clinical trial, various types of enrollment caps often exist. For instance, there may be an upper limit for the total number of enrolled patients at a specific center or within a specific region. The final prediction is adjusted to accommodate such prior information, in which we remove any predicted patients after a center reaches its cap during the recruitment process.

4 Simulation Studies

In this section, we conduct a simulation study to illustrate the prediction performance of our method.

4.1 Data Generation

Without the loss of generality, in the simulation study, we assume there is no time gap between screening outcome delivery and the final enrollment. There are two disease subtypes being recruited simultaneously, with enrollment targets of 250 and 270, respectively. We simulate the recruitment data from 50 centers across four regions, with the number of centers in each region being 10, 15, 15, and 10, respectively. Furthermore, we assume that there are three underlying groups among the 50 centers, and the number of centers in each group is 25, 15, and 10, respectively. For the first three regions, we set the enrollment cap for each of the disease subtypes, which are listed in Table 4 of the Appendix. We set the cutoff date as 300/500 days after time 0, and the overall recruitment end date is 1095 days after time 0. The whole process is repeated 100 times. Before the cutoff date, the total number of enrolled patients for subtype-1 and subtype-2 has a mean of 140/215 and 132/223, respectively, over the 100 repetitions. The distribution for the inter-arrival times is shown in Fig. 4, in which the inter-arrival times in period 1 has a larger mean than those of period 2.

To guarantee that we sample enough patients in the prediction process, the number of observations generated at each center is set as 100 × (overall enrollment target − number of enrolled patients until the cutoff date)/number of centers in operation.

4.2 Evaluation Metrics and Results

In our simulation study, we focus on the comparison on the prediction performance between the following models:

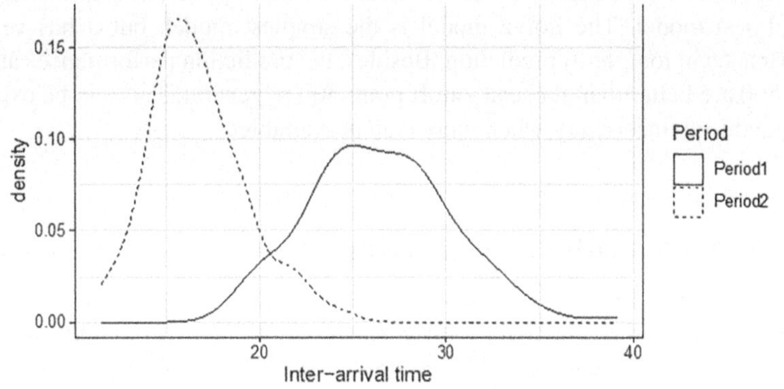

Fig. 4 Distribution of the inter-arrival times before date 300

1. The proposed Bayesian hierarchical model without enrollment cap adjustment (BH).
2. The proposed Bayesian hierarchical model with enrollment cap adjustment (BHA).
3. The Bayesian accrual model introduced in Jiang et al. [10] with a weak informative prior ($P = 0.1$) (Accrual). We used the R package *Accrual* for model fitting.
4. A Bayesian proportional hazard model proposed in [12]. (BMA).
5. Polynomial model with order 2, in which we regressed the cumulative counts of enrolled patients on the date differences with time 0 (Poly 2).

The fourth method BMA uses the same multi-stage modeling as our framework, in which the methods for modeling t_{1j} and t_{2j} are the same, and it sets the fourth period $t_{4ji} = 0$ for all patients. For t_{3ji}, the BMA model does not consider different disease subtypes. A Bayesian proportional hazard model is used to model the inter-arrival times with a shared frailty term to adjust center-to-center variability in the recruitment rate. The baseline hazard function is selected from Weibull, loglogistic, and lognormal model, and the final prediction is provided by a model averaging strategy with equal weights. For the third, fourth, and fifth methods, we fit two separated models for disease subtype-1 and subtype-2, as these models cannot handle the joint modeling of multiple disease subtypes.

The model performance was measured based on the following metrics:

1. AE: absolute difference in days between the true date to complete enrollment and the predicted date to complete enrollment.
2. AE-d: absolute difference between true number of cumulatively enrolled patient and the predicted number of cumulatively enrolled patient at the *d*-day after the cutoff date. Specifically, we focus on $d = 30$, 60, or 90 to compare the short-term prediction performance of the model.

The results are listed in Table 2. We can see that our proposed BHA model has the best performance across all the metrics, followed by the Accrual model as the second-best model. The Poly2 model is the simplest model, but it has very bad performance in long-term prediction. Besides, the prediction performances at cutoff point 500 are better than those at cutoff point 300 in general. This can be explained by the reduced uncertainty when more data is available.

5 Case Study with Synthetic Data

Instead of fitting the model only once at the cutoff date, a dynamic prediction framework is suggested to provide continuous support for recruitment planning. The motivation behind is to keep the predictive model adaptive to the newest recruitment behavior which can be caused by unexpected changes during the long recruiting period. Such changes are commonly seen. For example, the COVID-19 pandemic

Table 2 Prediction performance over 100 repetitions. Reported are the means and standard errors. The best results are marked in bold

Model cutoff = 300	BH	BHA	Accrual	BMA	Poly2
	Subtype-1				
AE (day)	294.44(15.874)	**75.08 (7.663)**	164.37(13.553)	204.96(14.554)	NA*
AE-30 (pts)	11.72(13.395)	**3.27 (0.246)**	11.77(0.729)	4.37(0.360)	17.71 (1.173)
AE-60 (pts)	24.95(0.999)	**4.42 (0.325)**	11.56(0.906)	6.96(0.488)	29.90 (1.815)
AE-90 (pts)	38.52(1.361)	**5.49 (0.438)**	10.56(1.393)	10.09(0.747)	43.54 (2.618)
	Subtype-2				
AE (day)	280.70(14.682)	**96.22 (8.986)**	157.75(12.882)	225.52(14.489)	349.03 (15.359)
AE-30 (pts)	4.84(0.583)	**3.71 (0.253)**	16.02(0.531)	6.42(0.383)	15.62 (0.956)
AE-60 (pts)	10.37(0.921)	**5.20 (0.406)**	20.68(0.893)	9.64(0.685)	29.94 (1.709)
AE (day)	17.31(1.521)	**6.55 (0.480)**	23.93(1.175)	14.29(1.042)	48.43 (2.682)
Cutoff = 500	Subtype-1				
AE (day)	188.26(14.546)	**46.36 (5.174)**	121.66(11.559)	137.37(12.412)	NA*
AE-30 (pts)	12.16(0.453)	**2.106 (0.185)**	16.93(1.614)	3.076(0.242)	10.56 (0.816)
AE-60 (pts)	24.89(0.821)	**2.965 (0.233)**	14.22(1.619)	7.459(0.528)	15.13 (1.193)
AE-90 (pts)	38.17(1.132)	**3.682 (0.290)**	13.66(1.416)	13.212(0.807)	19.69 (1.571)
	Subtype-2				
AE (day)	206.32(13.657)	**53.12 (5.554)**	139.72(11.774)	163.74(12.431)	NA*
AE-30 (pts)	11.02(0.382)	**2.847 (0.227)**	12.15(1.026)	2.747(0.208)	27.27 (1.113)
AE-60 (pts)	23.39(0.623)	**3.676 (0.294)**	8.71(0.797)	8.359(0.496)	38.49 (1.763)
AE-90 (pts)	36.22(0.828)	**4.429 (0.401)**	9.37(0.679)	15.741(0.677)	50.33 (2.413)

1.*: When making prediction from the Poly2 model, the predicted enrollment counts could not reach the targets in some of the repetitions and provided the NA values in Table 2

2. When making predictions with cutoff = 500, the target has been reached in some of the repetitions before the cutoff time. We excluded such repetitions from the model comparison

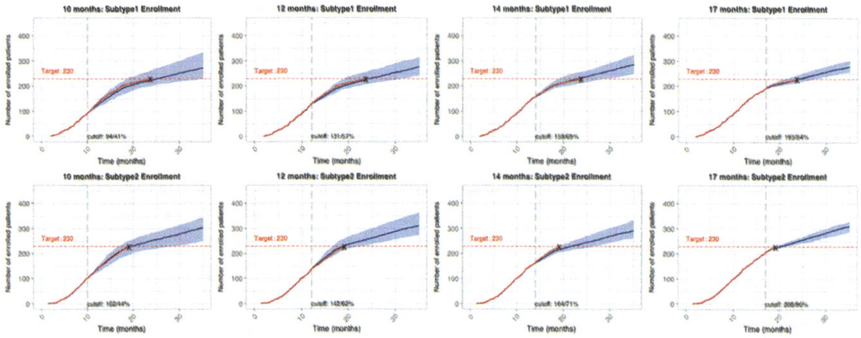

Fig. 5 Dynamic prediction example: The gray dashed line indicates the cutoff date, where the first number is the cumulated patients enrolled for this subtype, and the second number is the percentage of cumulated enrollment count over the enrollment target. The truth is marked with the red solid curve and the prediction is marked with blue curve. The blue region is the 95% prediction interval for prediction based on repeated sampling

has slowed down the recruitment process for many trials. As a result, models built at the early time of recruitment are hopeless to generate accurate predictions. Thus, we suggest updating the model regularly.

We give a prediction example in Fig. 5 with a synthetic dataset, where we fit the model at four cutoff points, 10 months, 12 months, 14 months, and 17 months.

The data was generated with 40 centers, 3 underlying groups and 4 regions. The study has two disease subtypes and each has a target enrollment of 230 patients. The synthetic data generation details are provided in the Appendix. We show the predicted curves for final enrollment in Fig. 5. As suggested by the plots, the blue curves produced by our framework have good capability to predict the nonlinear trend in the true data curves and are adaptive to the change points. Also, as more data is available, the prediction interval gets narrower. Simultaneously, our framework provides region-specific enrollment prediction to facilitate global recruitment management, as demonstrated in Table 3. The completion date is calculated based on pre-specified minimum enrollment requirements for each region. As expected, predictions made at a later stage provide shorter intervals.

6 Discussion

In this work, we propose a novel approach to predict patient enrollment by first dividing the enrollment timeline into four periods and modeling the four periods as waiting times separately. The modeling of periods 1, 2, and 4 are fully parametric, while we consider the method for period 3 to be semi-parametric as the model consists of both non-parametric and parametric components within a Bayesian hierarchical model. This method effectively captures the heterogeneity

Table 3 Dynamic prediction made at consecutive time points. Reported are the medians and the 95% prediction interval of the predicted completion date (in month)

Cutoff	10 month	12 month	14 month	17 month	truth
region1	12.98 (11.59, 15.84)	NA	NA	NA	11.90
region2	17.13 (13.46, 29.60)	17.80 (14.69, 23.48)	15.78 (14.62, 18.18)	NA	14.90
region3	18.42 (15.91, 23.29)	17.76 (16.12, 21.55)	18.04 (16.80, 19.96)	18.04 (17.62, 18.68)	17.87
region4	25.28 (19.91, 35.37)	24.34 (20.10, 31.39)	23.25 (20.32, 28.36)	23.82 (20.82, 27.32)	23.80

NA: True enrollment has been completed before the specific cutoff date

within the patient population and enables simultaneous prediction of multiple recruitment subgroups. Moreover, it offers valuable insights for both the screening and enrollment processes.

The incorporation of prior information in prediction has been shown to largely enhance the prediction accuracy as demonstrated by the simulation studies. Additionally, we suggest a dynamic prediction framework to monitor the recruitment process over time, allowing for timely adjustments.

The proposed method is widely applicable in various real patient recruitment scenarios. Besides the information for the enrollment cap, other extra information such as the new centers' planning times, can also be easily incorporated in the modeling framework.

In summary, this model-based, data-driven, and dynamic prediction tool shows good flexibility and accuracy in patient recruitment projection while highlighting potential risks in the future and supporting decision-making.

Appendix

Inverse Transform Sampling

Here, we describe the sampling steps for t_{2j} as an illustrative example. To get the prediction for t_{2j} when $\delta_j = 0$, we first sample λ_1 from the posterior distribution, then use the inverse transform sampling to get $\hat{t}_{2j}$. The survival function for t_{2j} is $S\left(t_{2j}\right) = e^{-\lambda_1 t_{2j}}$. To guarantee that the predicted time is greater than the observed waiting time (censoring time), we sample $v \sim U(0, c_{2j})$, where c_{2j} is the observed waiting time at the jth center and get $\hat{t}_{2j} = -\log(v)/\lambda_1$. For other predictions that involve the observed waiting time, the same procedure is adopted.

Sampling Strategy for Period 3

In the above hierarchical Bayesian framework, the observed data is (n_{1j}, n_{2j}, n_{0j}) and t_{3ji} at each center. To generate prediction on the future inter-arrival times and the screening outcomes, we try to derive posterior distributions for parameters $G, \theta_j, \tilde{\gamma}_j, u_j, \tilde{p}_j$, and λ_2. We adopt the procedure introduced in Glynn et al. [8].

Based on the above discussion, we consider the following full conditional distribution of the parameters as the following.

$$
\begin{aligned}
&P\left(G, \left\{\theta_j, \tilde{\gamma}_j, u_j, \tilde{p}_j\right\}, \lambda_2 | \left\{t_{3ji}\right\}, \left\{n_{1j}, n_{2j}, n_{0j}\right\}\right) \propto \\
&P\left(G | \left\{\theta_j, \tilde{\gamma}_j, u_j, \tilde{p}_j\right\}, \lambda_2, \left\{t_{3ji}\right\}, \left\{n_{1j}, n_{2j}, n_{0j}\right\}\right) \times \\
&P\left(\left\{\theta_j, \tilde{\gamma}_j, u_j, \tilde{p}_j\right\}, \lambda_2 | \left\{t_{3ji}\right\}, \left\{n_{1j}, n_{2j}, n_{0j}\right\}\right).
\end{aligned}
$$

The sampling process can be decomposed into three steps:

- Step 1: Sample λ_2, u_j and $\tilde{p}_j$.
  Since the closed form of the conditional distribution can be derived, this step can be done by a Gibbs sampler. We have
  - $\lambda_2 \sim \text{Gamma}(\sum_{j,\, i}\delta_{ji} + 1,\ \sum_j T_{3j}u_j + 1)$;
  - $u_j \sim \text{Gamma}(\sum_i \delta_{ji} + \theta_j, \lambda_2 T_{3j} + \theta_j)$;
  - $\tilde{p}_j \sim \text{Dirichlet}\left(n_{1j} + \gamma_{1j}, n_{2j} + \gamma_{2j}, n_{0j} + \gamma_{0j}\right)$.

- Step 2: Update $\left(\theta_j, \widetilde{\gamma}_j\right)$ and the group label for each center.
  - $P\left(\theta_j, \widetilde{\gamma}_j|-\right) = P\left(\theta_j, \widetilde{\gamma}_j|\tilde{p}_j, u_j, \left\{\theta_i, \widetilde{\gamma}_i\right\}_{i\neq j}\right) \propto P\left(u_j|\theta_j\right) P\left(\tilde{p}_j|\widetilde{\gamma}_j\right)$
    $P\left(\theta_j, \widetilde{\gamma}_j|\{\theta_i, \tilde{r}_i\}_{i\neq j}\right)$;
  - $P(u_j|\,\theta_j) \sim \text{Gamma}(\theta_j, \theta_j)$;
  - $P\left(\tilde{p}_j|\widetilde{\gamma}_j\right) \sim \text{Dirichlet}\left(\widetilde{\gamma}_j\right)$;
  - Update by doing
    - Sample r new pairs of $\left(\theta^*_{k^-+h}, \widetilde{\gamma}^*_{k^-+h}\right) \sim G_0, h = 1, \ldots, r$, where $\left(\theta^*_c, \widetilde{\gamma}^*_c\right)$, $\text{c} = 1, \ldots, k^-$ are distinct elements in $\{\theta_i, \tilde{r}_i\}_{i\neq j}$;
    - If $(\theta_j, \widetilde{\gamma}_j) \notin \left\{\left(\theta^*_c, \widetilde{\gamma}^*_c\right) : 1 \le c \le k^-\right\}$, replace the first element of $\left(\theta^*_{k^-+h}, \widetilde{\gamma}^*_{k^-+h}\right)$ with $(\theta_j, \widetilde{\gamma}_j)$;
    - Sample group label c_j from $\{1, \ldots, k^- + r\}$ with probability $p_c \propto s_c$ $P\left(u_j|\theta^*_c\right) P\left(\tilde{p}|\widetilde{\gamma}^*_c\right)$, where $s_c = \begin{cases} n_{-j,c}, \text{c} = 1, \ldots, k^-, \\ \frac{\alpha}{r}, \text{c} = k^- + 1, \ldots, k^- + r. \end{cases}$

- Step 3: Update group-specific parameters $\left(\theta^*_c, \widetilde{\gamma}^*_c\right)$.
  - Denote $S_c = \left\{1 \le j \le J, \left(\theta_j, \widetilde{\gamma}_j\right) = \left(\theta^*_c, \widetilde{\gamma}^*_c\right)\right\}$ as center index set for any group c.
  - Based on S_c, we have

$$P\left(\theta^*_c, \widetilde{\gamma}^*_c|-\right) \propto \prod\nolimits_{j\in S_c} P\left(u_j|\theta^*_c\right)\ P\left(\tilde{p}_j|\widetilde{\gamma}^*_c\right)\pi\left(\theta^*_c\right)\pi\left(\widetilde{\gamma}^*_c\right).$$

  - For θ^*_c, we have

$$P\left(\theta^*_c\,|-\right) \propto \prod\nolimits_{j\in S_c} P\left(u_j|\theta^*_c\right)\ \pi\left(\theta^*_c\right) \propto \prod\nolimits_{j\in S_c} \frac{\theta^{*\theta^*_c}_c}{\Gamma\left(\theta^*_c\right)} u_j^{\theta^*_c - 1} e^{-\theta^*_c u_j} \theta^{*a-1}_c e^{-a\theta^*_c}$$

– Fr $\widetilde{\gamma}_c^*$, we have

$$P\left(\widetilde{\gamma}_c^*|-\right) \propto \prod_{j\in S_c} P\left(\tilde{p}_j|\widetilde{\gamma}_c^*\right)\pi\left(\widetilde{\gamma}_c^*\right)$$

$$\propto \left(\frac{\Gamma\left(\gamma_{1c}^* + \gamma_{2c}^* + \gamma_{0c}^*\right)}{\Gamma\left(\gamma_{1c}^*\right)\Gamma\left(\gamma_{2c}^*\right)\Gamma\left(\gamma_{0c}^*\right)}\right)^{|S_c|} \prod_{j\in S_c} p_{1j}{}^{\gamma_{1c}^*-1} \prod_{j\in S_c} p_{2j}{}^{\gamma_{2c}^*-1}$$
$$\prod_{j\in S_c} p_{0j}{}^{\gamma_{0c}^*-1} e^{-\gamma_{1c}^*} e^{-\gamma_{2c}^*} e^{-\gamma_{0c}^*}$$

Since the closed form distribution in Step 3 is intractable, the adaptive Metropoles sampler is adopted to handle the sampling of $\left(\theta_c^*, \widetilde{\gamma}_c^*\right)$.

Supplement to Simulation Study

Table 4 lists the enrollment cap we used in the simulation study.

The enrollment time (unit: day) and the screening outcomes were generated from the following steps:

(a) Center planning time: The values were sampled from Uniform (0, 180). Additionally, we randomly selected 5 centers and set the planning date as 0.
(b) Center opening time: Time gap from planning to opening was sampled from Uniform (0, 60).
(c) First screening outcome and the delivery time: Time gap from opening to the first screening outcome delivery was sampled from exponential distribution with rate parameter λ_1=0.03, while the screening result was sampled from subtype1, subtype2 and failure with equal probability.
(d) Consecutive screening outcomes and the delivery times:

- Group-specific parameters:

  (i) $\left(\theta_1, \widetilde{\gamma_1}\right) = (0.5, 4, 1, 0.5);$

Table 4 Simulation study: Types of centers at the cutoff date T

Region	Number of centers	Subtype-1 enrollment cap	Subtype-2 enrollment cap
1	10	50	50
2	15	30	30
3	15	80	100
4	10	No cap	No cap

(ii) $\left(\theta_2, \widetilde{\gamma_2}\right) = (5, 3, 5, 1)$;
(iii) $\left(\theta_3, \widetilde{\gamma_3}\right) = (1, 1, 1, 1)$.

- Based on the assumed grouping structure, we sampled the center-specific parameters $u_j \sim Gamma(\theta_c, \theta_c)$ and $\widetilde{p_j} \sim Dirichilet\left(\widetilde{\gamma_c}\right)$ for center j in group c.
- Take $\lambda_2 = 0.04$. For each center, the inter-arrival times were generated from exponential distribution with rate parameter $\lambda_2 u_j$.
- For each center, screening outcome for each patient was generated from multinomial distribution with parameter $\widetilde{p_j}$.

(e) No time gap between screening and enrollment.
(f) Adjust data by region enrollment cap: For each region, the screened patients were sorted by the time of the outcome delivery. We removed extra patients when the region enrollment cap was reached.
(g) Center close time: Close time of a center was considered as the enrollment date of its last patient. If a center had no records after the cutoff date, then the center was considered as a closed center in prediction.

The codes for the proposed method and the code files for data generation are available at the website: https://github.com/jianminc/HSBAM

Supplement to Case Study

In the case study presented in Sect. 5, we adopted the same data generation process as described in Sect. 3 of the Appendix with minor adjustments on the parameters:

(a) Number of centers in each cluster: (15, 15, 10).
(b) The group-specific parameters were set as

(i) $\left(\theta_1, \widetilde{\gamma_1}\right) = (0.5, 2, 1, 0.5)$;
(ii) $\left(\theta_2, \widetilde{\gamma_2}\right) = (1, 2, 4, 1)$;
(iii) $\left(\theta_3, \widetilde{\gamma_3}\right) = (6, 1, 1, 0.5)$.

(c) We took $\lambda_1 = \lambda_2 = 0.03$.

The enrollment target for each subtype is set as 230 each. The number of centers and the enrollment requirements are listed in Table 5.

Table 5 Case study: Types of centers at the cutoff date T

Region	Number of centers	Subtype-1 minimum enrollment requirement/enrollment cap	Subtype-1 minimum enrollment requirement/enrollment cap
1	10	35/50	25/50
2	5	25/30	15/30
3	15	70/100	100/120
4	10	No minimum requirement or cap	No minimum requirement or cap

References

1. Anisimov, V.V., Fedorov, V.V.: Modelling, prediction and adaptive adjustment of recruitment in multicentre trials. Stat. Med. **26**(27), 4958–4975 (2007)
2. Anisimov, V.V.: Using mixed Poisson models in patient recruitment in multicentre clinical trials. Proc World Cong. Eng. **2**, 1046–1049 (2008)
3. Carter, R.E., Sonne, S.C., Brady, K.T.: Practical considerations for estimating clinical trial accrual periods: application to a multi-center effectiveness study. BMC Med. Res. Methodol. **5**, 1–5 (2005)
4. Barnard, K.D., Dent, L., Cook, A.: A systematic review of models to predict recruitment to multicentre clinical trials. BMC Med. Res. Methodol. **10**, 1–8 (2010)
5. Fogel, D.B.: Factors associated with clinical trials that fail and opportunities for improving the likelihood of success: a review. Contemp. Clin. Trials Commun. **11**, 156–164 (2018)
6. Gajewski, B.J., Simon, S.D., Carlson, S.E.: Predicting accrual in clinical trials with Bayesian posterior predictive distributions. Stat. Med. **27**(13), 2328–2340 (2008)
7. Gkioni, E., Rius, R., Dodd, S., Gamble, C.: A systematic review describes models for recruitment prediction at the design stage of a clinical trial. J. Clin. Epidemiol. **115**, 141–149 (2019)
8. Glynn, C., Tokdar, S.T., Zaman, A., Caruso, V.C., Mohl, J.T., Willett, S.M., Groh, J.M.: Analyzing second order stochasticity of neural spiking under stimuli-bundle exposure. Ann. Appl. Stat. **15**(1), 41 (2021)
9. Horwitz, S., O'Connor, O.A., Pro, B., Illidge, T., Fanale, M., Advani, R., Bartlett, N.L., et al.: Brentuximab vedotin with chemotherapy for CD30-positive peripheral T-cell lymphoma (ECHELON-2): a global, double-blind, randomised, phase 3 trial. Lancet. **393**(10168), 229–240 (2019)
10. Jiang, Y., Simon, S., Mayo, M.S., Gajewski, B.J.: Modeling and validating Bayesian accrual models on clinical data and simulations using adaptive priors. Stat. Med. **34**(4), 613–629 (2015)
11. Liu, J., Allen, P.J., Benz, L., Blickstein, D., Okidi, E., Shi, X.: A machine learning approach for recruitment prediction in clinical trial design. arXiv preprint arXiv:2111.07407. (2021)
12. Munda, M., Chen, J., Debard, A., Guilleminot, S., Carlin, B.P., Boulanger, B.: A Bayesian proportional hazards model to predict patient recruitment in multicenter clinical trials. In: Biostatistics in Biopharmaceutical Research and Development: Clinical Trial Analysis, vol. 2, pp. 115–134. Springer, Cham (2024)
13. Mountain, R., Sherlock, C.: Recruitment prediction for multicenter clinical trials based on a hierarchical Poisson–gamma model: asymptotic analysis and improved intervals. Biometrics. **78**(2), 636–648 (2022)

Comparative Effectiveness Analysis of Lobectomy and Limited Resection for Elderly Non-small Cell Lung Cancer Patients via Emulation

Jiping Wang, Rong Wang, and Shuangge Ma

Abstract

Objectives

Lobectomy is a commonly used surgical procedure for early-stage non-small cell lung cancer (NSCLC) patients. Recent studies have suggested that limited resection (segmentectomy or wedge resection) may be a viable alternative for patients as it better preserves lung function. For elderly patients, debates remain on whether limited resection can be used to achieve long-term outcomes that are similar to lobectomy. The goal is to evaluate their relative effectiveness in terms of overall survival.

Methods

An emulation analysis of the Surveillance, Epidemiology, and End Results (SEER)-Medicare data was conducted, in which we constructed an emulated "randomized clinical trial" with rigorously defined inclusion/exclusion criteria, treatment regimens, and analysis procedures.

Results

A total of 13,897 subjects were enrolled, with 10,455 and 3442 in the lobectomy and limited resection arms, respectively. Limited resection was found to be asso-

Supplementary Information The online version contains supplementary material available at https://doi.org/10.1007/978-3-032-06649-7_17.

J. Wang · S. Ma (✉)
Department of Biostatistics, Yale School of Public Health, New Haven, CT, USA
e-mail: Shuangge.ma@yale.edu

R. Wang
Department of Chronic Disease Epidemiology, Yale School of Public Health, New Haven, CT, USA

Yale Cancer Outcomes, Public Policy and Effectiveness Research (COPPER) Center, New Haven, CT, USA

Y. Zhao, D.-G. Chen (eds.), *Big Data Analytics in Biostatistics and Bioinformatics*, ICSA Book Series in Statistics,
https://doi.org/10.1007/978-3-032-06649-7_17

ciated with significantly worse overall survival for the whole cohort (hazard ratio [HR] = 1.26, 95% confidence interval [CI]: 1.19, 1.33), the subgroup without adjuvant chemotherapy (HR = 1.30, 95% CI: 1.22, 1.38), and the subgroup without adjuvant radiotherapy (HR = 1.24, 95% CI: 1.16, 1.32); but not for the subgroup with adjuvant chemotherapy (HR = 1.10, CI: 0.95, 1.27) or with adjuvant radiotherapy (HR = 1.09, 95% CI: 0.92, 1.30).

Conclusions
Compare with limited resection, lobectomy was found to be superior in terms of overall survival for the elderly SEER-Medicare early-stage NSCLC patients. This study can provide new insight into surgical treatment of NSCLC.

Keywords Comparative effectiveness · NSCLC · Lobectomy · Limited resection · Emulation

Abbreviations

NSCLC	Non-Small Cell Lung Cancer
SEER	Surveillance, Epidemiology, and End Results
U.S.	United States
RCT	Randomized Clinical Trial
EMR	Electronic Medical Record
SRP	Surveillance Research Program
DCCPS	Division of Cancer Control and Population Sciences
HMO	Health Maintenance Organization
NY	New York
MA	Massachusetts
ID	Idaho
ICD-9-CM	International Classification of Diseases, Ninth Revision, Clinical Modification
HCPCS	Healthcare Common Procedure Coding System
CPT	Current Procedural Terminology
ITT	Intention-To-Treat
IPT	Inverse Probability Treatment
HR	Hazard Ratio
CI	Confidence Interval
SMD	Standardized Mean Difference
COPPER	Cancer Outcomes, Public Policy and Effectiveness Research
IMS	Information Management Services

Article Summary
Strengths and limitations of this study

- The elderly SEER-Medicare population with early-stage non-small cell lung cancer was of special focus.
- The emulation approach was adopted to explicitly assemble a clinical trial using observational data, and the potential causal conclusion could better inform clinical practice.

– Subgroup analysis for those received or not received adjuvant chemotherapy or radiotherapy were examined, which had been largely neglected in the published comparative effectiveness research studies of non-small cell lung cancer.

1 Introduction

Lung cancer is the leading cause of cancer-related death and makes up about 21% of cancer deaths in the United States (U.S.) [1]. The most common type of lung cancer is non-small cell lung cancer (NSCLC), which accounts for about 82% of all lung cancer diagnoses. With a median age at diagnosis of 70 years, NSCLC poses serious concerns for the elderly [2]. For early-stage NSCLC, surgery is regarded as the curative way [3]. Lobectomy is considered as the standard treatment for the surgical resection of early-stage NSCLC and has a 5-year survival rate of up to 70%. However, it can be associated with considerable morbidity and mortality, particularly among the elderly and patients with multiple comorbidities or poor lung functions. Recent studies have suggested that limited resection (segmentectomy or wedge resection) may be a viable alternative for patients with small-sized tumors as it removes less uninvolved lung tissues and thus may benefit patients by having fewer complications and better postoperative lung functions [4, 5]. However, it requires the division of lung parenchyma across shared lobar vasculature, lymphatics, and bronchi, thus possibly increasing the risk of local recurrence [6].

For small and localized tumors, and elderly patients especially those with chronic conditions, there is controversy as to whether limited resection can be used to achieve long-term outcomes that are similar to lobectomy [7]. One recent study showed that for stage IA patients, histology impacted the association between surgical choice and overall survival. For patients with adenocarcinoma or squamous cell carcinoma, lobectomy was superior to limited resection. However, there was no significant differences for other histology subtypes [8]. For stage I NSCLC patients over 75 years old, Zhang and others (2021) reported the superiority of lobectomy to wedge resection, but not to segmentectomy [5]. A meta-analysis examined only segmentectomy and found that it led to survival comparable to lobectomy for patients with stage I NSCLC [9]. Additionally, for stage I and II NSCLC patients, lobectomy conferred better survival than limited resection after 2 years for young patients, while no difference was found for elderly patients [10].

To objectively quantify the relative effectiveness of lobectomy and limited resection on NSCLC survival, the ideal solution is to conduct a rigorously designed and executed randomized clinical trial (RCT). However, this may not be feasible, as both treatments have been well adopted in clinical practice. For cancer (particularly including lung cancer) and many other diseases, the fast development of electronic medical record (EMR)/insurance claim databases makes it possible to mine a large amount of observational data and effectively and cost-effectively draw conclusions to complement RCTs [11–13]. Among the available observational data analysis techniques that aim to draw RCT-type conclusions, emulation has emerged as an attractive option, given its trial-like architecture, interpretability, and scalability [14–16]. It has been applied to studies of evaluating the effect of initiating fluorouracil on stage II colorectal cancer survival [17], the effect of initiating erlotinib, FOLFIRINOX, or gemcitabine plus nab-paclitaxel on advanced pancreatic cancer survival [17], the effect of screening colonoscopy on colorectal cancer diagnosis [18], and many other clinically highly significant problems [19–24]. However, it is noted that, for our clinical question of interest, there has been a lack of emulation or other causal inference analysis.

In this study, our goal is to address the comparative effectiveness of lobectomy and limited resection in terms of overall survival for elderly early-stage NSCLC patients. It is infeasible to address this using an RCT. Although there are some observational data analyses [5, 8, 25, 26], they focused on different populations and were limited by the lack of generalizability, limited sample sizes, and other factors. This study targets at filling this important knowledge gap by conducting an emulation analysis of the SEER-Medicare data. Additionally, it may also serve as a prototype for studying other lung cancer outcomes/treatments.

2 Methods

2.1 Data and Study Sample

The Surveillance, Epidemiology, and End Results (SEER)-Medicare data provides one of the best resources for studying the US elderly cancer population. SEER is supported by the Surveillance Research Program (SRP) in NCI's Division of Cancer Control and Population Sciences (DCCPS). Data analyzed in this study was obtained through a data use agreement with NCI. The study design has been strongly motivated by relevant RCTs [4, 27, 28] and observational analyses [8, 26, 29], while taking into consideration data availability in SEER-Medicare. The flowchart of emulated trial patient selection is summarized in Fig. 1, and more detailed information is provided in Supplementary Materials. Briefly, the emulated trial enrolled Medicare beneficiaries with first primary NSCLC who were: (1) 66–100 years old at diagnosis, (2) diagnosed between 1/1/07 and 12/31/17, (3) stage I-II, (4) with tumor size $\leq$5 cm, (5) received lobectomy or limited resection within 1 year after diagnosis, and (6) had a continuous enrollment in Medicare Part A and Part B, with no health maintenance organization (HMO) enrollment from 1 year before to 1 year after cancer diagnosis or death, whichever came first. A subject was excluded if he/she (1) was reported from registries in New York (NY), Massachusetts (MA), and Idaho (ID) because of missing cancer-related information, (2) had missing information on month of diagnosis, stage or tumor size, (3) were reported from death certificate or autopsy, and (4) received both lobectomy and limited resection in the same day.

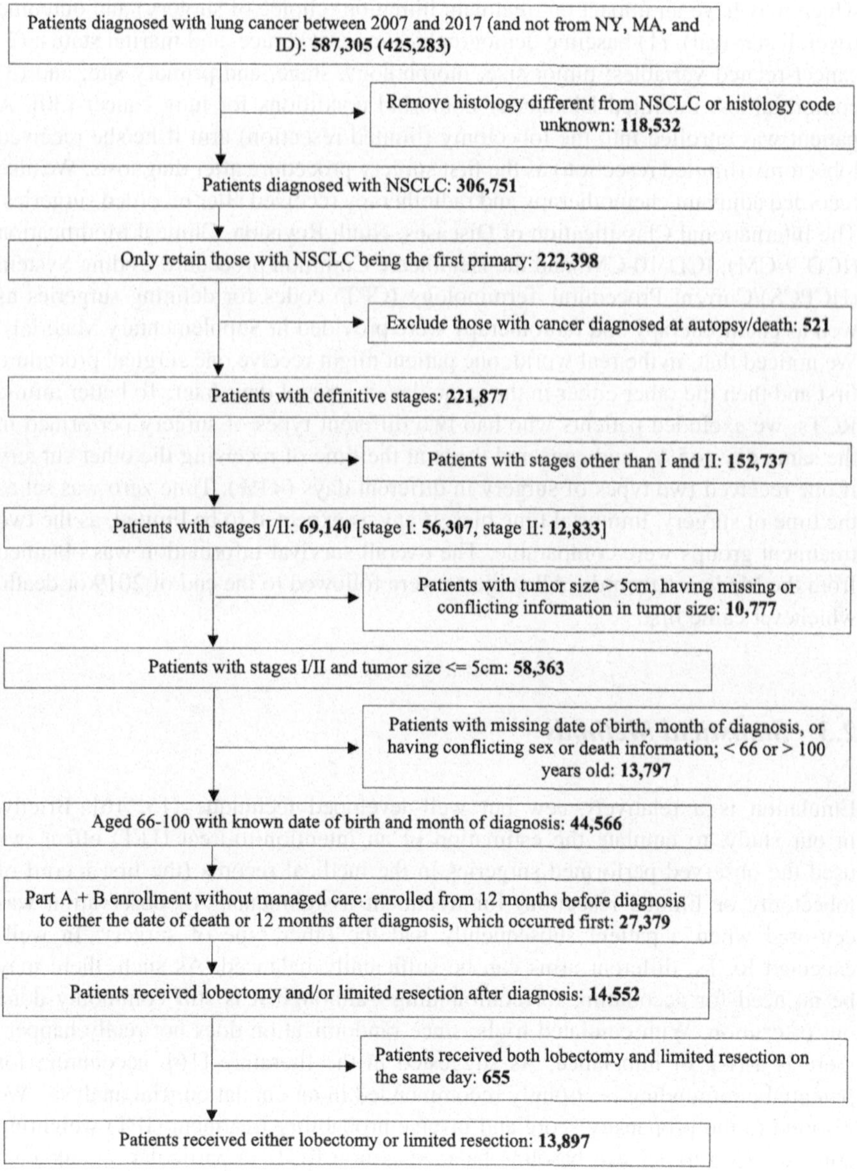

Fig. 1 Flowchart of sample selection

2.2 *Variable Information*

By reviewing the published observational studies, and also taking data availability into consideration, we included the following variables as potential confounders, which may have an impact on treatment initiation (choice of surgery) and outcome (overall survival): (1) baseline demographics: age, sex, race, and marital status; (2) cancer-related variables: tumor size, morphology, stage, and primary site; and (3) comorbidities: modified Elixhauser comorbid conditions for lung cancer [30]. A patient was enrolled into the lobectomy (limited resection) arm if he/she received lobectomy (limited resection) as the first surgery procedure after diagnosis. We also recorded adjuvant chemotherapy and radiotherapy received after recorded surgeries. The International Classification of Diseases, Ninth Revision, Clinical Modification (ICD-9-CM), ICD-10-CM, and the Healthcare Common procedure Coding System (HCPCS)/Current Procedural Terminology (CPT) codes for defining surgeries as well as chemotherapy and radiotherapy were provided in Supplementary Materials. We noticed that, in the real world, one patient might receive one surgical procedure first and then the other either in the same day or several days later. To better mimic RCTs, we excluded patients who had two different types of surgery performed in the same day (<5%), and censored those at the time of receiving the other surgery if one received two types of surgery in different days (<1%). Time zero was set as the time of surgery. Immortal time bias, if any, is expected to be limited, as the two treatment groups were comparable. The overall survival information was obtained from the Medicare records. All subjects were followed to the end of 2019 or death, whichever came first.

2.3 Statistical Methods

Emulation is a relatively new but well-developed technique [15, 16]. Briefly, in our study, to emulate the estimation of an intention-to-treat (ITT) effect, we used the observed performed surgeries in the medical records (the first record of lobectomy or limited resection) for treatment assignments. An observation was censored when a patient subsequently had the other type of surgery. In well-executed RCTs, different arms can be sufficiently balanced. As such, there may be no need for accounting for confounding—although it is still commonly done out of caution. With emulated trials, since randomization does not really happen, there is a risk of imbalance. As suggested in the literature [16], accounting for potential confounding is strongly recommended in an emulation trial analysis. We resorted to the propensity score and inverse probability treatment (IPT) weighting approach [31] to achieve baseline balance as in a RCT. In particular, to calculate the propensity score, we estimated the probability of having a specific treatment using a logistic model and included the baseline confounders described above as covariates. Then the weight was calculated as the inverse of the propensity score for one treatment group and the inverse of one minus the propensity score for the other group. Stabilized weights with a truncation at the upper 99.5th percentile (if a weight was above the 99.5th percentile, it was set as the 99.5th percentile) were adopted for retaining the same group size ratio and avoiding putting extreme weights on a small number of subjects. With such weights, a pseudo-population was created, for which there was no (or very weak) association between the baseline confounders and received treatment. Then the Cox proportional hazards model was fit to derive the desired treatment effect from the weighted pseudo-population. To further adjust for the remaining confounding and improve the precision of estimation, we included all baseline confounders as covariates. Finally, the hazard ratio (HR) and its confidence interval (CI) were obtained to quantify the treatment effect. Analyses were conducted using SAS version 9.4 (SAS Institute Inc., Cary, NC) and R version 4.3. The computer programs for conducting this analysis are available at https://github.com/shuanggema.

Recent studies also suggested that adjuvant chemotherapy and radiotherapy (performed after surgeries) were common for early-stage NSCLC patients [32–34]. To obtain the "net effects" of surgeries, we conducted subgroup analysis of those who received/did not receive either adjuvant chemotherapy or radiotherapy, using the same emulation analysis technique. Details were provided in Supplementary materials.

3 Results

As shown in Fig. 1, a total of 13,897 patients were enrolled in the emulated trial, with 10,455 in the lobectomy arm and 3442 in the limited resection arm. The waiting time from diagnosis to surgery was observed to be short (with a median of 46 days and 90% of surgeries performed within 100 days after diagnosis). The baseline characteristics are summarized in Table 1. It was observed that before IPT weighting, patients treated with limited resection were slightly older and more likely to be stage I and had higher comorbidity scores and smaller tumors.

The unadjusted Kaplan-Meier survival curves by treatment are shown in Fig. 2. For the lobectomy arm, the overall mortality rate and median survival were 50.2% and 7.2 years. For the limited resection arm, they were 55.4% and 5.7 years, respectively. Patients who received lobectomy were observed to have longer overall survival (p-value <0.001 by log-rank test). Figure 3 shows the distributions of the estimated propensity scores and weights. In both arms, the propensity score distributions are centered around 0.25. This is due to the approximate 1–3 sample size ratio between the limited resection arm and the lobectomy arm. The treated arm (the limited resection arm) generally has higher propensity scores, suggesting a higher probability of receiving limited resection. With the imbalance of the two arms, some extreme weights were observed in the limited resection arm. Patients assigned weights above the 99.5th percentile, which indicates a strong inclination toward receiving lobectomy if they actually received limited resection, had several prominent characteristics. They tended to be relatively younger, with an average age of 71.4 (standard deviation: 4.19), and 61.4% of them were male. Notably, 58.6% of them were classified as stage II (compared to 14.0% in the lobectomy arm and 8.9% in the limited resection arm), and their average tumor size was 42.7 mm (this number was 26.0 mm in the lobectomy arm and 22.1 mm in the limited resection

Table 1 Patients' characteristics for the overall cohort and different treatment groups[a]

	Lobectomy ($n = 10{,}455$)	Limited resection ($n = 3442$)	Overall ($n = 13{,}897$)
Demographics			
Age at diagnosis	74.4 (5.45)	75.1 (5.65)	74.6 (5.51)
Sex (female)	5723 (54.7%)	1957 (56.9%)	7680 (55.3%)
Race (non-Hispanic white)	8917 (85.3%)	3027 (87.9%)	11,944 (85.9%)
Marital status (married)	5990 (57.3%)	1857 (54.0%)	7847 (56.5%)
Year of diagnosis			
2007	1060 (10.1%)	467 (13.6%)	1527 (11.0%)
2008	1049 (10.0%)	317 (9.2%)	1366 (9.8%)
2009	1046 (10.0%)	295 (8.6%)	1341 (9.6%)
2010	1002 (9.6%)	280 (8.1%)	1282 (9.2%)
2011	981 (9.4%)	274 (8.0%)	1255 (9.0%)
2012	866 (8.3%)	228 (6.6%)	1094 (7.9%)
2013	956 (9.1%)	269 (7.8%)	1225 (8.8%)
2014	903 (8.6%)	248 (7.2%)	1151 (8.3%)
2015	897 (8.6%)	303 (8.8%)	1200 (8.6%)
2016	831 (7.9%)	375 (10.9%)	1206 (8.7%)
2017	864 (8.3%)	386 (11.2%)	1250 (9.0%)
Tumor characteristics			
Histology			
Adenocarcinoma	6663 (63.7%)	2171 (63.1%)	8834 (63.6%)
Squamous cell carcinoma	3026 (28.9%)	1008 (29.3%)	4034 (29.0%)
Large cell carcinoma	213 (2.0%)	88 (2.6%)	301 (2.2%)
Other carcinoma (other than small cell or neuroendocrine carcinoma)	345 (3.3%)	95 (2.8%)	440 (3.2%)
Unspecified NSCLC	208 (2.0%)	80 (2.3%)	288 (2.1%)
Tumor size (mm)	26.0 (10.7)	22.1 (10.2)	25.0 (10.7)
Stage (II; reference: I)	1462 (14.0%)	305 (8.9%)	1767 (12.7%)
Primary site			
Upper lobe	6231 (59.6%)	2131 (61.9%)	8362 (60.2%)
Middle lobe	615 (5.9%)	119 (3.5%)	734 (5.3%)
Lower lobe	3447 (33.0%)	1135 (33.0%)	4582 (33.0%)
Others (main bronchus, overlapping lesion, NOS)	162 (1.5%)	57 (1.7%)	219 (1.6%)
Elixhauser comorbidities			
Modified comorbidity score	5.33 (3.59)	5.83 (3.58)	5.45 (3.59)

[a] For categorical variables, count (percent); for continuous variables, mean (standard deviation)

arm). These findings align with the observed characteristic difference between the two treatment arms, highlighting that the lobectomy recipients were typically younger and presented with more advanced tumor features. Prior to weighting, some of the absolute standardized mean difference (SMD) values were above the 0.1 threshold. They significantly reduced to be below 0.1 with weighting, with

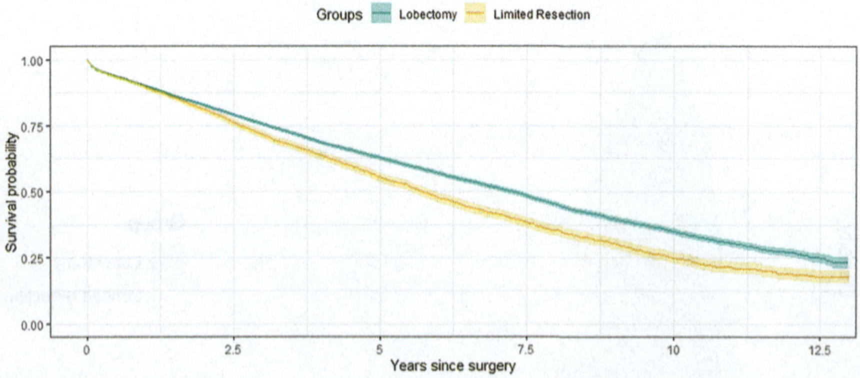

Fig. 2 Kaplan-Meier curves for the unweighted population stratified by treatment

which the two arms could be considered as balanced [35, 36]. Results are visualized in Fig. 4.

As given in Table 2, compared to patients who received lobectomy, those who received limited resection had a significantly higher risk of death. Among the four models, the doubly robust one (with covariates and weights) should serve as the basis for conclusion and decision-making. Under this model, limited resection had an estimated HR = 1.26 with 95% CI: 1.19, 1.33. Additionally, older age, being male, having morphology other than adenocarcinoma, being stage II, a larger tumor size, and having more comorbidities were found as significantly associated with worse survival.

The subgroup analysis results were presented in Supplementary Materials. In the analysis of the subgroup with adjuvant chemotherapy or radiotherapy, no significant difference between lobectomy and limited resection was found (for the subgroup with adjuvant chemotherapy: HR = 1.10, 95% CI: 0.95, 1.27; for the subgroup with adjuvant radiotherapy: HR = 1.09, 95% CI: 0.92, 1.30). In the analysis of the subgroup without adjuvant chemotherapy or radiotherapy, lobectomy was found to be significantly associated with better survival (for the subgroup without adjuvant chemotherapy: HR = 1.30, 95% CI: 1.22, 1.38; for the subgroup without adjuvant radiotherapy: HR = 1.24, 95% CI: 1.16, 1.32). The findings on the confounders were similar to above. Specifically, older age, being male, a larger tumor size, and higher comorbidity score were significantly associated with worse survival, regardless of adjuvant therapy status. Being stage II was significantly associated with worse survival for those without adjuvant chemotherapy or radiotherapy (HR = 1.68, 95% CI: 1.50, 1.89; and 1.47, 95% CI: 1.34, 1.60, respectively). However, it had no significant impact for those who received adjuvant radiotherapy (HR = 0.98, 95% CI: 0.82, 1.18).

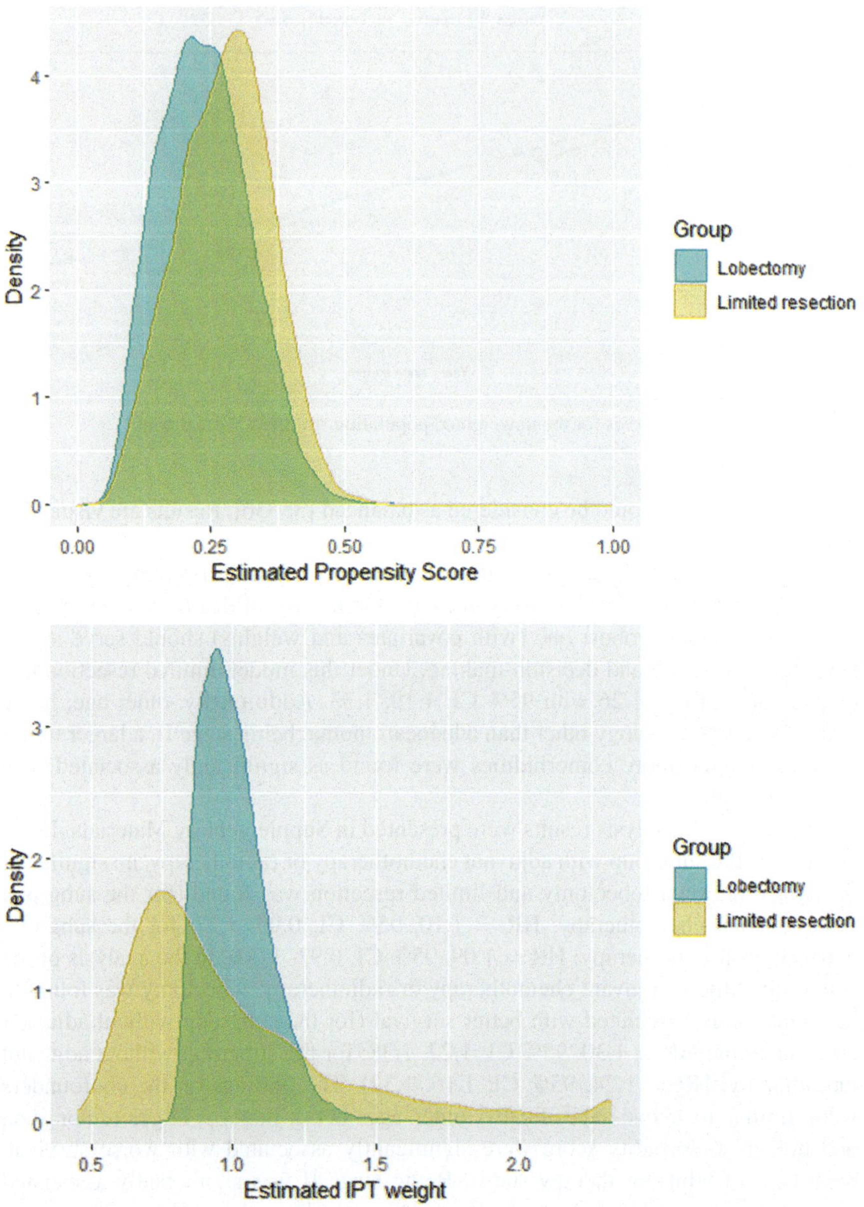

Fig. 3 Distributions of the estimated propensity scores (upper) and IPT weights (bottom)

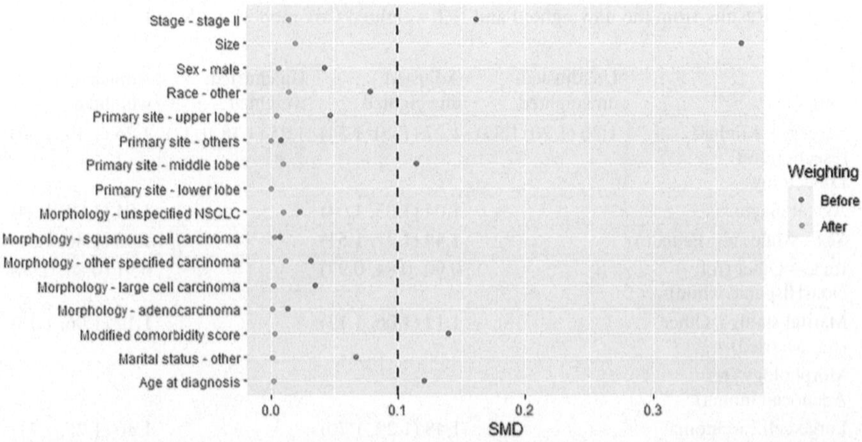

Fig. 4 Absolute standardized mean difference (SMD) for each variable before and after weighting

4 Discussion

It remains a challenging clinical question how to effectively treat early-stage NSCLC. As partly reflected in Sect. 1, there have been extensive debates on the relative effectiveness of different surgical options, and different studies have drawn conflicting conclusions [37]. To further elucidate this question, in this article, we have resorted to real-world evidence contained in SEER-Medicare and evaluated the comparative effectiveness of lobectomy and limited resection (segmentectomy or wedge resection) for stage I-II NSCLC with tumor size ≤5 cm, for elderly patients over 66 years old. To draw findings comparable to RCTs, we have resorted to the emulation technique, whose power has been demonstrated in many recent studies for cancer and other complex diseases. It has been found that lobectomy is significantly superior to limited resection in terms of overall survival. This finding is qualitatively consistent with some published studies [10, 25, 38], but not others [5, 26, 39] which concluded no significant difference. Such discrepancies can be at least partly attributed to differences in target populations (e.g., age, stage, and tumor size), treatment definition (consideration of segmentectomy or wedge resection, or both), and characteristics of cohorts (e.g., histology). Additionally, it is noted that the existing studies have mainly conducted "standard" observational data analysis, and RCT-type analysis has been lacking. Compared to some of the aforementioned and other published studies, the present one may excel with a much larger sample size and hence more power. Another advancement is that we have conducted subgroup analysis, which can better tease out the effects of the two surgical procedures and has been neglected in the literature. The findings specific to the subgroups with/without adjuvant chemotherapy and radiotherapy can provide additional insights into clinical decision-making. Our findings on stage,

Table 2 Results from the unweighted and IPT-weighted Cox models, with and without covariates[a]

Variable	Unadjusted, unweighted	Adjusted, unweighted	Unadjusted, weighted	Adjusted, weighted
Surgery—Limited resection (ref: Lobectomy)	1.26 (1.20, 1.33)	1.27 (1.20, 1.34)	1.25 (1.18, 1.32)	1.26 (1.19, 1.33)
Age at diagnosis		1.04 (1.03, 1.04)		1.04 (1.03, 1.04)
Sex—Male (ref: Female)		1.44 (1.37, 1.51)		1.43 (1.36, 1.51)
Race—Other (ref: Non-Hispanic white)		0.90 (0.84, 0.97)		0.91 (0.84, 0.98)
Marital status—Other (ref: Married)		1.12 (1.06, 1.17)		1.12 (1.06, 1.18)
Morphology (ref: Adenocarcinoma)				
Large cell carcinoma		1.48 (1.29, 1.70)		1.46 (1.25, 1.71)
Squamous cell carcinoma		1.24 (1.18, 1.31)		1.25 (1.18, 1.32)
Other specified carcinoma		1.20 (1.06, 1.36)		1.23 (1.08, 1.41)
Unspecified NSCLC		1.42 (1.24, 1.64)		1.39 (1.19, 1.62)
Primary site (ref: Upper lobe)				
Middle lobe		0.97 (0.88, 1.09)		0.99 (0.88, 1.11)
Lower lobe		1.05 (1.00, 1.10)		1.06 (1.00, 1.11)
Others		1.00 (0.83, 1.19)		1.03 (0.83, 1.28)
Stage—Stage II (ref: Stage I)		1.50 (1.41, 1.61)		1.47 (1.36, 1.59)
Size (in mm)		1.01 (1.01, 1.02)		1.01 (1.01, 1.02)
Modified Elixhauser index		1.13 (1.12, 1.13)		1.13 (1.12, 1.14)

[a]Hazard ratio (95% confidence interval)

comorbidity, age, and other risk factors have been mostly consistently with the published findings [8, 26], providing support to the validity of our analysis.

This study inevitably has limitations in multiple aspects. The SEER-Medicare data has a broad coverage, and our findings can be reasonably extended to the whole U.S. populations with the defined demographic/clinical characteristics. However, their broader generalizability should still be taken with cautions. Emulation is a mature technique and can effectively harvest real-world evidence to complement RCTs—it is noted again that for the clinical question of interest in this study, an RCT is highly unlikely. On the other hand, it has also been well acknowledged that emulation analysis has limitations [14–16, 40], including limited information, possible imbalance in variables not collected, and others. Despite such limitations, similar to many other emulation analyses, our findings are still expected to have high clinical relevance.

Acknowledgments The collection of the California cancer incidence data used in this study was supported by the California Department of Public Health as part of the statewide cancer reporting program mandated by California Health and Safety Code Section 103885; the National Cancer Institute's Surveillance, Epidemiology and End Results Program under contract N01-PC-35136 awarded to the Northern California Cancer Center, contract N01-PC-35139 awarded to the University of Southern California, and contract N02-PC-15105 awarded to the Public Health Institute; and the Centers for Disease Control and Prevention's National Program of Cancer Registries, under agreement #U55/CCR921930-02 awarded to the Public Health Institute. The ideas and opinions expressed herein are those of the author(s) and endorsement by the State of California, Department of Public Health the National Cancer Institute, and the Centers for Disease Control and Prevention or their Contractors and Subcontractors is not intended nor should be inferred. The authors acknowledge the efforts of the Applied Research Program, NCI; the Office of Research, Development and Information, CMS; Information Management Services (IMS), Inc.; and the Surveillance, Epidemiology, and End Results (SEER) Program tumor registries in the creation of the SEER-Medicare database. The interpretation and reporting of the SEER-Medicare data are the sole responsibility of the authors.

Ethics Approval and Consent to Participate Not applicable.

Availability of Data and Materials The SEER-Medicare data produced in this study was obtained through the Yale Cancer Outcomes, Public Policy and Effectiveness Research (COPPER) Center.

Competing Interests The authors declare that they have no competing interests.

Funding This study was supported in part by NIH HL161691 and CA276790.

Author Contributions JW investigated the research question, developed methods, curated, analyzed and interpreted the data, and wrote the original draft. RW facilitated data curation, validated coding, and revised the draft. SM conceptualized and designed the research question and methods, was responsible for supervision, and reviewed and edited the draft. All authors read and approved the final manuscript.

References

1. Siegel, R.L., Miller, K.D., Fuchs, H.E., Jemal, A.: Cancer statistics, 2022. CA Cancer J. Clin. **72**(1), 7–33 (2022)
2. Edwards, B.K., Howe, H.L., Ries, L.A., Thun, M.J., Rosenberg, H.M., Yancik, R., et al.: Annual report to the nation on the status of cancer, 1973–1999, featuring implications of age and aging on US cancer burden. Cancer. **94**(10), 2766–2792 (2002)
3. Howington, J.A., Blum, M.G., Chang, A.C., Balekian, A.A., Murthy, S.C.: Treatment of stage I and II non-small cell lung cancer: diagnosis and management of lung cancer: American College of Chest Physicians evidence-based clinical practice guidelines. Chest. **143**(5), e278S–e313S (2013)
4. Koike, T., Koike, T., Sato, S., Hashimoto, T., Aoki, T., Yoshiya, K., et al.: Lobectomy and limited resection in small-sized peripheral non-small cell lung cancer. J. Thorac. Dis. **8**(11), 3265 (2016)
5. Zhang, X., Lin, G., Li, J.: Comparative effectiveness of lobectomy, Segmentectomy, and wedge resection for pathological stage I non-small cell lung cancer in elderly patients: a population-based study. Front. Surg. **8**, 652770 (2021)
6. Scott, W.J., Howington, J., Feigenberg, S., Movsas, B., Pisters, K.: Treatment of non-small cell lung cancer stage I and stage II: ACCP evidence-based clinical practice guidelines. Chest. **132**(3), 234S–242S (2007)

7. Nakamura, H., Kawasaki, N., Taguchi, M., Kabasawa, K.: Survival following lobectomy vs limited resection for stage I lung cancer: a meta-analysis. Br. J. Cancer. **92**(6), 1033–1037 (2005)
8. Veluswamy, R.R., Ezer, N., Mhango, G., Goodman, E., Bonomi, M., Neugut, A.I., et al.: Limited resection versus lobectomy for older patients with early-stage lung cancer: impact of histology. J. Clin. Oncol. **33**(30), 3447 (2015)
9. Bedetti, B., Bertolaccini, L., Rocco, R., Schmidt, J., Solli, P., Scarci, M.: Segmentectomy versus lobectomy for stage I non-small cell lung cancer: a systematic review and meta-analysis. J. Thorac. Dis. **9**(6), 1615 (2017)
10. Mery, C.M., Pappas, A.N., Bueno, R., Colson, Y.L., Linden, P., Sugarbaker, D.J., et al.: Similar long-term survival of elderly patients with non-small cell lung cancer treated with lobectomy or wedge resection within the surveillance, epidemiology, and end results database. Chest. **128**(1), 237–245 (2005)
11. Takahashi, Y., Nishida, Y., Asai, S.: Utilization of health care databases for pharmacoepidemiology. Eur. J. Clin. Pharmacol. **68**(2), 123–129 (2012)
12. Hu, L., Gu, C., Lopez, M., Ji, J., Wisnivesky, J.: Estimation of causal effects of multiple treatments in observational studies with a binary outcome. Stat. Methods Med. Res. **29**(11), 3218–3234 (2020)
13. Listl, S., Jürges, H., Watt, R.G.: Causal inference from observational data. Community Dent. Oral Epidemiol. **44**(5), 409–415 (2016)
14. Danaei, G., Rodriguez, L.A., Cantero OF, Logan, R., Hernan, M.A.: Observational data for comparative effectiveness research: an emulation of randomised trials of statins and primary prevention of coronary heart disease. Stat. Methods Med. Res. **22**(1), 70–96 (2013)
15. Danaei, G., Garcia Rodriguez, L.A., Cantero OF, Logan, R.W., Hernan, M.A.: Electronic medical records can be used to emulate target trials of sustained treatment strategies. J. Clin. Epidemiol. **96**, 12–22 (2018)
16. Hernan, M.A., Robins, J.M.: Using big data to emulate a target trial when a randomized trial is not available. Am. J. Epidemiol. **183**(8), 758–764 (2016)
17. Petito, L.C., García-Albéniz, X., Logan, R.W., Howlader, N., Mariotto, A.B., Dahabreh, I.J., et al.: Estimates of overall survival in patients with cancer receiving different treatment regimens: emulating hypothetical target trials in the Surveillance, Epidemiology, and End Results (SEER)-Medicare linked database. JAMA Netw. Open. **3**(3), e200452 (2020)
18. García-Albéniz, X., Hsu, J., Hernán, M.A.: The value of explicitly emulating a target trial when using real world evidence: an application to colorectal cancer screening. Eur. J. Epidemiol. **32**(6), 495–500 (2017)
19. Caniglia, E.C., Rojas-Saunero, L.P., Hilal, S., Licher, S., Logan, R., Stricker, B., et al.: Emulating a target trial of statin use and risk of dementia using cohort data. Neurology. **95**, e1322 (2020)
20. Atkinson, A., Zwahlen, M., Barger, D., d'Arminio Monforte, A., De Wit, S., Ghosn, J., et al.: Withholding primary PcP prophylaxis in virologically suppressed HIV patients: an emulation of a pragmatic trial in COHERE. Clin. Infect. Dis. (2020)
21. Mei, H., Xu, Y., Wang, J., Ma, S.: Evaluation of survival outcomes of endovascular versus open aortic repair for abdominal aortic aneurysms with a big data approach. Entropy. **22**(12), 1349 (2020)
22. Admon, A.J., Donnelly, J.P., Casey, J.D., Janz, D.R., Russell, D.W., Joffe, A.M., et al.: Emulating a novel clinical trial using existing observational data. Predicting results of the PreVent study. Ann. Am. Thorac. Soc. **16**(8), 998–1007 (2019)
23. Dickerman, B.A., Garcia-Albeniz, X., Logan, R.W., Denaxas, S., Hernan, M.A.: Avoidable flaws in observational analyses: an application to statins and cancer. Nat. Med. **25**(10), 1601–1606 (2019)
24. Lyu, B., Chan, M.R., Yevzlin, A.S., Gardezi, A., Astor, B.C.: Arteriovenous access type and risk of mortality, hospitalization, and sepsis among elderly hemodialysis patients: a target trial emulation approach. Am. J. Kidney Dis. **79**, 69 (2021)

25. El-Sherif, A., Gooding, W.E., Santos, R., Pettiford, B., Ferson, P.F., Fernando, H.C., et al.: Outcomes of sublobar resection versus lobectomy for stage I non–small cell lung cancer: a 13-year analysis. Ann. Thorac. Surg. **82**(2), 408–416 (2006)
26. Kates, M., Swanson, S., Wisnivesky, J.P.: Survival following lobectomy and limited resection for the treatment of stage I non-small cell lung cancer $\leq$1 cm in size: a review of SEER data. Chest. **139**(3), 491–496 (2011)
27. Nakamura, K., Saji, H., Nakajima, R., Okada, M., Asamura, H., Shibata, T., et al.: A phase III randomized trial of lobectomy versus limited resection for small-sized peripheral non-small cell lung cancer (JCOG0802/WJOG4607L). Jpn. J. Clin. Oncol. **40**(3), 271–274 (2010)
28. Ginsberg, R.J., Rubinstein, L.V., Group LCS: Randomized trial of lobectomy versus limited resection for T1 N0 non-small cell lung cancer. Ann. Thorac. Surg. **60**(3), 615–623 (1995)
29. Wisnivesky, J.P., Henschke, C.I., Swanson, S., Yankelevitz, D.F., Zulueta, J., Marcus, S., et al.: Limited resection for the treatment of patients with stage IA lung cancer. Ann. Surg. **251**(3), 550–554 (2010)
30. Mehta, H.B., Sura, S.D., Adhikari, D., Andersen, C.R., Williams, S.B., Senagore, A.J., et al.: Adapting the Elixhauser comorbidity index for cancer patients. Cancer. **124**(9), 2018–2025 (2018)
31. D'agostino, R.B.: Propensity score methods for bias reduction in the comparison of a treatment to a non-randomized control group. Statist. Med. **17**, 2265–2281 (1998)
32. Veluswamy, R.R., Mhango, G., Bonomi, M., Neugut, A.I., Hershman, D.L., Aldridge, M.D., et al.: Adjuvant treatment for elderly patients with early-stage lung cancer treated with limited resection. Ann. Am. Thorac. Soc. **10**(6), 622–628 (2013)
33. Speicher, P.J., Gu, L., Wang, X., Hartwig, M.G., D'Amico, T.A., Berry, M.F.: Adjuvant Chemotherapy After Lobectomy for T1–2N0 Non–Small Cell Lung Cancer: Are the Guidelines Supported? J. Natl. Compr. Cancer Netw. **13**(6), 755–761 (2015)
34. Alexander, M., Kim, S.Y., Cheng, H.: Update 2020: Management of non-small cell lung cancer. Lung. **198**(6), 897–907 (2020)
35. Zhang, Z., Kim, H.J., Lonjon, G., Zhu, Y.: Balance diagnostics after propensity score matching. Ann. Trans. Med. **7**(1), 16 (2019)
36. Cuijpers, P., Turner, E.H., Koole, S.L., Van Dijke, A., Smit, F.: What is the threshold for a clinically relevant effect? The case of major depressive disorders. Depress. Anxiety. **31**(5), 374–378 (2014)
37. De Zoysa, M.K., Hamed, D., Routledge, T., Scarci, M.: Is limited pulmonary resection equivalent to lobectomy for surgical management of stage I non-small-cell lung cancer? Interact. Cardiovasc. Thorac. Surg. **14**(6), 816–820 (2012)
38. Landreneau, R.J., Sugarbaker, D.J., Mack, M.J., Hazelrigg, S.R., Luketich, J.D., Fetterman, L., et al.: Wedge resection versus lobectomy for stage I (T1 N0 M0) non-small-cell lung cancer. J. Thorac. Cardiovasc. Surg. **113**(4), 691–700 (1997)
39. Okada, M., Koike, T., Higashiyama, M., Yamato, Y., Kodama, K., Tsubota, N.: Radical sublobar resection for small-sized non–small cell lung cancer: a multicenter study. J. Thorac. Cardiovasc. Surg. **132**(4), 769–775 (2006)
40. Hernán, M.A., Sauer, B.C., Hernández-Díaz, S., Platt, R., Shrier, I.: Specifying a target trial prevents immortal time bias and other self-inflicted injuries in observational analyses. J. Clin. Epidemiol. **79**, 70–75 (2016)

Recent Developments in Joint Modeling for Recurrent Gap Times with a Terminal Event

Ming Wang, Yifan Yang, Chixiang Chen, Lijun Zhang, and Menglu Liang

Abstract In clinical and observational studies, recurrent events are frequently encountered, including repeated episodes of hospitalizations, strokes, and others. Throughout the follow-up period, these recurrent events may be censored by a semi-competing risk event (e.g., death), resulting in dependent censoring. While joint modeling of recurrent events with the terminal event has garnered considerable attention, further advancements in analytical methods are necessary to meet real-world application needs. One commonly utilized approach is joint frailty modeling with a shared frailty factor for recurrent and terminal event processes. However, there are limitations, such as the strong assumption of conditional independence, which can be easily violated in practice. Also, handling multiple types of recurrent events, such as repeated occurrences of heart failure, myocardial infarction, stroke, or other cardiovascular diseases, is crucial but has not been thoroughly explored. In this paper, we will provide an overview of existing methods and discuss recently proposed ones to address these gaps, highlighting their advantages and disadvantages. Furthermore, evaluating patient prognosis and dynamically predicting the risk of death are clinically significant, and utilizing developed models considering historical recurrent events is expected to enhance medical decisions and improve healthcare outcomes. Finally, we will discuss current methodological gaps, present an illustrative example using a large-scale dataset and propose directions for future research.

M. Wang (✉) · Y. Yang · L. Zhang
Case Western Reserve University, Cleveland, OH, USA
e-mail: mxw827@case.edu; yxy1423@case.edu; lxz759@case.edu

C. Chen
University of Maryland School of Medicine, Baltimore, MD, USA
e-mail: chixiang.chen@som.umaryland.edu

M. Liang
University of Maryland, College Park, MD, USA
e-mail: mliang23@umd.edu

Y. Zhao, D.-G. Chen (eds.), *Big Data Analytics in Biostatistics and Bioinformatics*, ICSA Book Series in Statistics,
https://doi.org/10.1007/978-3-032-06649-7_18

Keywords Cardiovascular disease · Semi-competing risk · Joint modeling · Recurrent events · Risk prediction

1 Introduction

Recurrent events are commonly encountered in clinical and epidemiological studies, where the subject may experience repeated events over time during follow-up [47, 48, 69]. Examples include successive hospitalized myocardial infarction (MI), acute ischemic strokes, coronary heart disease (CHD), and heart failure, among others [25, 27]. Under such circumstances, events occurring in the same patient should be correlated with each other due to shared patient-level characteristics. However, if correlation within subjects is ignored, the parameter estimates may become biased, and the standard error estimates may be inaccurate, resulting in less reliable interval estimation (compared to the nominal level) and potentially misleading statistical inference and clinic interpretation. For the analysis of recurrent or repeated events, there is tremendous work on ad hoc methods and discussions in the literature [1, 29, 30, 48, 50, 52, 74]. In this paper, we will provide a brief overview of existing approaches in a general context. Additionally, we will discuss several features associated with recurrent events in real-world scenarios, emphasizing the need for more extensive exploration due to limited investigations thus far.

One potential issue is the dependent censoring mechanism, where recurrent events may be censored by a semi-competing risk event (e.g., death) during follow-up [51, 69, 90]. Not only should the correlation between within-subject recurrences be considered but also the correlation between recurrences and terminal events. There are two commonly used models: marginal estimating equation-based modeling [10, 21] and joint frailty modeling [9, 30, 50, 61, 78, 92, 93]. However, these methods may not be appropriate or may still have limitations for particular diseases such as cardiovascular disease, neurological disorders, kidney injuries, etc. Specifically, one strong assumption for joint frailty models is conditional independence, i.e., recurrent events and terminal events (e.g., death) are independent given the observed covariates and the frailty, which could likely be violated in practice due to unobserved (time-varying) covariates. In practice, there are several methods to verify this assumption, including residual diagnostics, goodness-of-fit tests with model comparisons, assessment of frailty variance, and sensitivity analysis. For example, the value of variance estimate for the frailty variable can reflect the association of gap times within subjects [30]. Also, note that previous studies have shown that patients with the first episode of a disease event (e.g., stroke) have a higher risk for subsequent events and death [27, 31]. Thus, the intrinsic correlations might change over time as the subject's health status worsens due to the occurrence of transient ischemic attacks. Consequently, the violation of non-informative censoring as well as the time-varying correlation between the processes of recurrent events and a terminal event could pose challenges for analysis. However, inefficient or improper statistical models are still used to analyze such types of data [9, 14, 29, 88].

The majority of the existing approaches exhibit one or more of the following limitations:

(1) Dependence is naively ignored by treating the terminal event as a censoring event.
(2) The strong conditional independence assumption in regular frailty models, which can be violated in practice.
(3) Vague dependence between processes of recurrent events and a terminal event without estimating their correlation in a straightforward manner or providing a closed-form expression for quantification.
(4) The correlation between processes of the terminal event and recurrent events is assumed to be fixed and constant over time.
(5) While there is considerable research on single-type recurrent events in the presence of a terminal event (e.g., death), multi-type recurrent events may occur in the same individual, and few studies address this context.

Another issue that has garnered more attention is multifaceted effects and symptoms due to the complexity of disease mechanisms (e.g., cancer, Alzheimer's disease) [33, 37]. To quantify the severity of the disease or perform risk prediction, various types of outcomes may be collected over time. Take diabetes mellitus for example; apart from blood glucose levels, diabetes affects various organs and systems in the body, leading to complications such as diabetic retinopathy (affecting vision), diabetic neuropathy (affecting nerves), diabetic nephropathy (affecting kidneys), and cardiovascular diseases. In such contexts, multiple types of recurrent events could be recorded simultaneously, and they are highly likely to be correlated with each other [1, 62, 81]. Evaluating all these outcomes together can provide a holistic picture of the disease's impact and aid in assessing overall disease management and prognosis. However, to date, there has been limited work in the field of multivariate recurrent event analysis, and even less for the scenarios when the terminal event is present.

Besides model fitting, assessing risk prediction is important and clinically impactful. It is without doubt that the history of recurrent disease events embodies substantial information related to patients' health status, which should be invaluable for dynamic risk prediction [13, 20, 40, 62, 91]. Dynamic risk prediction includes classical dynamic prediction, which utilizes recurrent event history (e.g., the number and types of events) as covariates, as well as risk prediction in longitudinal studies through landmarking, which incorporates longitudinal covariates and recurrent event data as predictors. Various metrics of predictive accuracy can be employed to identify the optimal candidate model that incorporates key risk factors and better captures the relationship between recurrent events (whether single-type or multiple-type) and mortality, including their potential evolution over time. This selection process can aid in prognosticating disease progression, devising effective treatment strategies for early detection and intervention, and estimating the medical cost burden for patients. Dynamic prediction based on updated and accumulative recurrent event history is crucial; however, current work remains struggling and limited so far. Several evaluation metrics are employed to assess prediction performance. The Brier score (BS), expressed as the mean squared error between the observed status and its predicted probability, quantifies the accuracy of predictions by evaluating both discrimination and calibration aspects [24]. The receiver operating characteristic (ROC) curve, one of the most frequently used metrics, plots the true positive rate against the false positive rate across different thresholds. It is a rank-order statistic that measures discrimination [28]. The concordance index (C-index) is an extension of the ROC that accounts for censored data, providing a global assessment of discrimination of survival outcomes [26, 71]. In this paper, we emphasize the Brier score for its simplicity and its utility in quantifying the model's ability to predict clinical outcomes.

In this paper, we will provide an overview of existing methods for analyzing recurrent events, both with and without consideration of semi-competing risk events. We will emphasize recently proposed joint hierarchical models for both single-type and multiple-type recurrent events, highlighting their respective advantages and disadvantages. Additionally, we will explore the dynamic prediction of subsequent event occurrence and death using cumulative and historical recurrent event data. Furthermore, we will utilize a large-scale real dataset from the Atherosclerosis Risk in Communities (ARIC) Study to demonstrate their practical application in real-world settings. Specifically, we will summarize these methods and pinpoint current methodological gaps for future research directions.

2 Methods

2.1 Review of the Existing Models for Recurrent Events

In recurrent event analysis, two timescales of interest hold significant value, each with its own merits: (1) time-to-event (calendar time) and (2) time-between-event (gap time). Due to the specific research objectives and the underlying characteristics of the recurrent event data, different approaches and models with their own assumptions and data layouts can be formulated by adopting the basic frameworks of nonhomogeneous Poisson processes (characterized by the occurrence times) or renewal processes (characterized by the distribution of gap times) with extensions for adjusting potential risk factors. For instance, some models assume that future events depend solely on the previous one through a Markov process (e.g., the Prentice, Williams, and Peterson (PWP) model, the multistate model), while others quantify dependency through shared random effects (e.g., frailty models). Specifically, gap times are relevant in applications where understanding the duration between events provides critical insights, such as hospital readmissions, medication refills, and similar scenarios. In our application to cardiovascular disease, the intervals between events have been of clinical interest and widely studied

[56, 60, 86, 89]. Therefore, we focus on modeling recurrent gap times, with the primary goal of understanding the underlying event process, where events occur irregularly over time, and exploring the associated risk predictions. Next, we will provide a brief overview of these commonly used models and describe the most recent developments in model development.

The PWP Models The PWP model is designed for the analysis of recurrent event data, where events are ordered by stratification based on the recurrence index. In this model, all subjects are considered at risk for the first stratum, but only those subjects who have experienced the previous stratum belong to the risk set for the subsequent one. The PWP model incorporates baseline or event-specific covariates in regression as below:

$$h_{ij}(t) = h_{0j}(t - t_{j-1}) \exp\left(\boldsymbol{\beta}_j^\top \boldsymbol{x}_{ij}\right)$$

for the subject i and j-th recurrent event occurred at calendar time t_j, where h_{0j} denotes the baseline hazard function and $\boldsymbol{\beta}_j$ is the regression coefficient corresponding to the covariate $\boldsymbol{x}_{ij}$. It estimates the effects of these covariates on the j-th recurrence since the time from the previous events, which can vary across strata. This model is particularly useful for diseases where the effects of covariates may vary over time or across event recurrences. Of note, the risk sets tend to be smaller for later strata, potentially leading to unreliable estimates and inferences [2].

The Multistate Models The multistate model offers an alternative option to capture the subject transition from one state (recurrence) to another over time, in which the hazard function is given by

$$h^i_{j_1,j_2}(t) = h^0_{j_1,j_2}(t) \exp\left(\boldsymbol{\beta}^\top_{j_1,j_2}(t)\boldsymbol{x}_i(t) + \boldsymbol{\gamma}^\top_{j_1,j_2}\boldsymbol{z}_i(t)\right)$$

for the subject i and j_1- and j_2-th recurrent events, where $h^0_{j_1,j_2}$ denotes the baseline hazard function, $\boldsymbol{\beta}_{j_1,j_2}(t)$ is the time-dependent regression coefficient corresponding to the covariate $\boldsymbol{x}_i(t)$ that change over time, and $\boldsymbol{\gamma}_{j_1,j_2}$ is the time-independent regression coefficient corresponding to the covariate $\boldsymbol{z}_i(t)$ that have constant effects on the event intensities. This model primarily focuses on characterizing the transition probabilities between events. In longitudinal data with recurrences, several key elements need to be modeled and estimated, including transitional probabilities for state movement, hazard rates at which transitions occur from one state to another, and covariate effects on the transition process. Note that transitions are often assumed to be Markovian, and associated probabilities can be obtained using approaches such as maximum likelihood, Bayesian inference, or nonparametric techniques. Hazard rates across recurrences can be analyzed using the PWP model or others. This model enables researchers to investigate the underlying processes driving the occurrence and timing of events over time, as well as associated factors. However, the extension to multi-type recurrent events is still underexplored in the literature [45, 46].

The Frailty Models In addition to the previously mentioned models, the random effects approach via shared frailty models is widely utilized for recurrent event analysis [30, 69, 77]. This model extends traditional survival models to account for the correlation between recurrent events within an individual. Specifically, frailty terms are incorporated into the model to capture unobserved heterogeneity or individual-specific effects that influence both gap times and event occurrence, as shown below:

$$h_0(t|w_i) = h_{00}(t) w_i^{\gamma} \exp\left(\boldsymbol{\beta}_0^\top \boldsymbol{x}_{i0}\right), \quad h_j(t|w_i) = h_{0j}(t) w_i \exp\left(\boldsymbol{\beta}_j^\top \boldsymbol{x}_{ij}\right)$$

for the subject i and j-th recurrent event, where h_{00} and h_{0j} denote the baseline hazard functions of the terminal event and the j-th recurrent event in the gap timescales, respectively, w_i is the frailty term with coefficient γ, and $\boldsymbol{\beta}_0$ and $\boldsymbol{\beta}_j$ are the regression coefficient corresponding to the terminal covariate $\boldsymbol{x}_{i0}$ and the recurrent covariate $\boldsymbol{x}_{ij}$. The frailty is often assumed to follow a prespecified distribution such as (log-) normal or gamma distribution. Given the distribution and the covariates, recurrent events are independent of each other. This model is applied when there is heterogeneous susceptibility to recurrent event risk across subjects. Additionally, shared frailty models demonstrate flexibility and can be expanded to accommodate other data features in the presence of semi-competing risk events and/or multiple-type recurrences, which will be the primary focus of this paper. This enables us to model inter-event times, and various model extensions within this framework can capture the time-dependent nature of recurrent events and the correlation among multiple-type recurrences, thereby improving risk prediction. Next, we will delve into the model development and outline avenues for further refinement.

2.2 Recurrent Events with Semi-Competing Risk

Both marginal and conditional methods have been studied for analyzing recurrent events with dependent censoring [9, 30, 61]. Marginal methods regard the terminating event of death as a censoring event for each recurrent event or estimate the marginal mean of the cumulative number of recurrent events over time. This approach provides inference on the population-level covariate effects without insights into the correlation between two event processes [10, 21, 92, 93]. Conditional methods mainly refer to joint frailty modeling, which utilizes random effects to capture the dependence between event processes [30, 50, 81]. More recent works [4, 69, 90] have extended joint frailty modeling by considering a nonparametric baseline hazard based on a piecewise spline function, incorporating time-dependent coefficients, and/or allowing the hazard functions to be additive. All

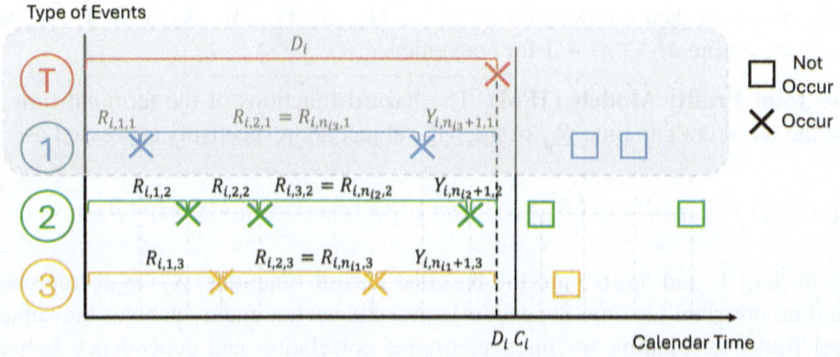

Fig. 1 Example of a schematic plot illustrating recurrent gap times of three-type events and the terminal event for one sample subject, where "T," "1," "2," and "3" represent the terminal event, and the first, second, and third types of recurrent events, respectively. In comparison, the plot in the gray background represents single-type recurrent events and the terminal event

of these approaches are proposed under the conditional independence assumption, that is, the terminal event process and the recurrent event process are conditionally independent of a subject-level frailty term that remains constant over time and the covariates.

Notation For each subject i ($i = 1, 2, \ldots, n$), let D_i denote the time to the terminal event and C_i denote the censoring time. Define $Y_i = \min\{D_i, C_i\}$ as the observed follow-up time and $\Delta_i = I(D_i \le C_i)$ as its indicator for the terminal event. We first focus on a single type of recurrence (i.e., $K = 1$; refer to Fig. 1 for an illustration of a sample subject with single-type recurrent events), and later broaden our analysis to a general framework with $K \ge 1$ types of recurrences in Sect. 2.2.2. We assume a finite but sufficiently large integer J, independent of the data, representing the maximum number of recurrent events of this single type that a subject could experience in the absence of the terminal event.

Suppose subject i experiences a total of n_i recurrences during the follow-up, where $1 \le n_i < J$, $0 < Y_i - T_{i,n_i}$, and $Y_i - T_{i,n_i+1} < 0$, where T_{ij} denotes the calendar time until the j-th recurrence since the origin of follow-up for $j = 0, \ldots, J$ with $T_{i0} = 0$. We define $R_{ij} = T_{ij} - T_{i,j-1}$ as the gap time between the $(j-1)$-th and the j-th recurrences for $j = 1, \ldots, J$. Additionally, let $Y_{ij} = \min\{R_{ij}, C_{ij}\}$ denote the observed gap time with its indicator $\Delta_{ij} = \mathbb{I}\left(R_{ij} \le C_{ij}\right)$, where the censoring time for the j-th gap time is provided by $C_{ij} = \max\{Y_i - T_{i,j-1}, 0\}$ for $j = 1, \ldots, J$. Thus, we note that the first n_i gap times are observed except for the last one, which is censored due to dropout, limited follow-up, or the terminal event, i.e., $Y_{ij} = R_{ij}$ and $\Delta_{ij} = 1$ for $j = 1, \ldots, n_i$; $Y_{ij} = C_{ij} = Y_i - T_{i,j} > 0$ and $\Delta_{ij} = 0$ for $j = n_i + 1$; and $Y_{ij} = C_{ij} = 0$ and $\Delta_{ij} = 0$ for $j = n_i + 1, \ldots, J$. Furthermore, we assume the p-dimensional covariate $\boldsymbol{X}_i = \boldsymbol{X}_{ij}$ (excluding the intercept term 1) remains time-invariant for simplicity; however, this can be generalized to accommodate different sets of covariates if needed. For subject

i, the observed data are denoted as $\mathscr{D}_i = \{Y_i, \Delta_i, Y_{ij}, \Delta_{ij}, \boldsymbol{X}_i, j = 1, \ldots, M_i\}$, where we define $M_i = n_i + 1$ for convenience.

The Joint Frailty Models (JFM) The hazard functions of the terminal time D_i and the recurrent gap time R_{ij} of the i-th subject are respectively expressed as

$$h_D(d|\omega_i) = h_{0D}(d)\exp\left(\boldsymbol{\beta}_D^\top \boldsymbol{x}_i + \psi\omega_i\right), h_R(r|\omega_i) = h_{0R}(r)\exp\left(\boldsymbol{\beta}_R^\top \boldsymbol{x}_i + \omega_i\right), \tag{1}$$

where $h_{0D}(d)$ and $h_{0R}(r)$ are the baseline hazard functions, $\boldsymbol{X}_i = \boldsymbol{x}_i$ represents the time-invariant (or time-dependent) covariate vector, and ω_i denotes the subject-level frailty accounting for inter-recurrence correlation and dependency between recurrent events and the terminal event, quantified by ψ. Given the observed data $\mathscr{D}_i$ for the i-th subject and $\boldsymbol{\omega} = (\omega_1, \ldots, \omega_n)^\top$, the conditional likelihood can be derived for parameter estimation and inference, where the expectation-maximization (EM) algorithm or the Gaussian quadrature method can be used [47, 50, 58, 68]. It's worth noting that the conditional independence assumption is strong and might be violated in practice due to the impossibility of capturing all sufficient recurrence-related covariates over time. In particular, if the models only include baseline factors or consider the same set of covariates for all recurrent gaps, substantial residual dependence may occur, leading to invalid inference if ignored [55, 74, 82]. Additionally, although the dependence between recurrent events and death has been incorporated, it cannot be estimated or interpreted straightforwardly. In clinical practice, it's crucial to report correlations in a direct and quantitative manner, such as Kendall's tau. This enables clinicians and patients to gain a clearer understanding, promoting cost-effective medication and personalized healthcare.

Specifically, various real-data features of epidemiological studies are acknowledged in but not limited to the field of cardiovascular disease:

(1) Long-term follow-up studies where the correlation between these time-to-event processes is likely to be time-varying;
(2) Most recent disease events associated with a higher risk of death compared to the history of previous episodes;
(3) Potential (time-varying) risk factors (i.e., environmental or genetic information) are unknown or unmeasured, leading to invalid inference if completely ignored;
(4) Different types of disease events (i.e., stroke, myocardial infarction, coronary heart disease, peripheral artery disease) could occur concurrently, all contributing to the increase in death risk.

To relax existing model assumptions, address the limitations above, and accommodate clinical needs, several advanced models have been proposed. Next, we will review them with highlights on the most recent ones and discuss various aspects related to their application and potential for further improvement.

2.2.1 Model Advances Within the Joint Frailty Framework

Several extended modeling approaches within the joint frailty framework have been proposed in the literature. For instance, [91] employed dynamic frailty models to incorporate serial dependence in the multivariate recurrent event data, providing additional flexibility compared to the identical models. Pennell and Dunson [62] generalized the shared frailty model, where the frailty is constant over time, to the dynamic frailty model by allowing for multivariate subject-specific time-dependent frailties within a semi-parametric Bayesian framework. Abrams et al. [1] presented an alternative approach to address heterogeneity caused by time-dependent frailties, in which the frailties are assumed to be piecewise or multiplicative on the disjoint subintervals. However, these methods do not yield closed-form solutions for correlation estimates. By extending the local cross-ratio technique, [77] proposed a novel measure for capturing time-dependent correlation in terms of variances of relative frailties, which they applied to copula functions for bivariate event data. Peng and Fine [61] utilized a time-varying parameter in the copula function to model semi-competing events, which can be estimated using both parametric and nonparametric procedures. Although these approaches offer closed-form solutions for correlation estimates, they are restricted to bivariate event data. Most recently, novel joint hierarchical models including joint hierarchical copula modeling (JHCM) and time-varying JHCM (TVJHCM) have been proposed to better capture the time-dependent relationship between recurrent and terminal event processes. These models embed survival copulas into frailty modeling and provide options for assuming constant or recurrence-dependent correlation between the two event processes. Next, we will review TVJHCM including JHCM as a special case to analyze single-type recurrent events with a terminal event.

Time-Varying Joint Hierarchical Copula Modeling (TVJHCM) The joint survival probability of D_i and R_{ij} is

$$\Pr\left(D_i \geq d_i, R_{ij} \geq r_{ij}|\omega_i\right) = C_{\theta_{ij}}\left(S_D\left(d_i|\omega_i\right), S_R\left(r_{ij}|\omega_i\right)\right),$$
$$i = 1, \ldots, n;\ j = 1, \ldots, M_i,$$

where $S_D(\cdot|\omega_i)$ and $S_R(\cdot|\omega_i)$ are the conditional survival functions of D_i and R_{ij} on ω_i, $C_{\theta_{ij}}(\cdot, \cdot)$ is a time-dependent survival copula function with the parameter θ_{ij} quantifying the temporal heterogeneity in the relationship between the terminal event D_i and the j-th recurrent event time R_{ij}, while ω_i provides an overall measure of between-subject heterogeneity induced by time-independent factors. Note that the correlation parameter is modeled at the subject level, indicating that the correlation between the terminal event and the recurrent event could vary across subjects and event recurrences. The conditional survival functions, given the frailty ω_i, can be derived from the hazard functions in (1) ($\psi = 1$ is assumed for simplicity here).

Regarding survival copulas, one important class, called the Archimedean family, is widely used. It includes copulas of the form $C(u, v; \theta) =$

Table 1 $g(\cdot,\cdot)$ function for bivariate copulas

Copula	Correlation	$g(\theta_\mu, \gamma_{ij})$
Clayton	$\theta_{ij} > 0$	$\theta_\mu \exp(\gamma_{ij})$
Frank	$\theta_{ij} \neq 0$	$\theta_\mu \exp(\gamma_{ij})$
Gaussian	$-1 < \theta_{ij} < 1$	$\theta_\mu \left[\exp(2\gamma_{ij}) - 1\right] / \left[\exp(2\gamma_{ij}) + 1\right]$
Gumbel	$\theta_{ij} > 1$	$\theta_\mu [\exp(\gamma_{ij}) + 1]$

$\varphi^{-1}(\varphi(u;\theta) + \varphi(v;\theta))$, where $\varphi(\cdot)$ is a continuous, strictly decreasing convex function, and θ is a parameter that quantifies the association between variables U and V. It's important to note that there are constraints on survival copula coefficients, meaning θ_{ij} may be confined to an interval, which introduces additional challenges for this approach. For example, for the Clayton copula, $\theta_{ij} > 0$, and for the Frank copula, $\theta_{ij} \neq 0$. Initiated by ideas on hierarchical models [17], θ_{ij} can be expressed by an overall correlation between D_i and R_{ij} across recurrence noted as θ_μ and an unrestricted latent effect $\gamma_{ij} \in (-\infty, \infty)$. Thus, $\theta_{ij} = g(\theta_\mu, \gamma_{ij})$, where $g(\cdot,\cdot)$ is a continuous function (see Table 1 for options). The quantity of θ_{ij} and their dependence can be reflected through γ_{ij}. To model γ_{ij}, any correlation structure can be considered. If a Gaussian AR(1) process is used, dependency is more correlated along adjacent times but decreases with increasing distance between time points. Thus, we assume:

$$\gamma_{i1} \sim \mathrm{N}\left(0, \sigma_\epsilon^2 / \left(1 - \rho^2\right)\right), \quad \gamma_{ij} = \rho\gamma_{i,j-1} + \epsilon_{ij}, \quad 2 \leq j \leq M_i,$$

where $0 < |\rho| < 1$ and $\epsilon_{i1}, \ldots, \epsilon_{i,M_i} \overset{\text{i.i.d.}}{\sim} \mathrm{N}\left(0, \sigma_\epsilon^2\right)$. Therefore, $\boldsymbol{\gamma}_i = \left(\gamma_{i1}, \ldots, \gamma_{i,M_i}\right)^\top$ follows a multivariate normal distribution, denoted by $\mathrm{MVN}\left(\mathbf{0}_{M_i\times 1}, \boldsymbol{\Sigma}_i\right)$, with the marginal distribution for $\gamma_{ij} \sim \mathrm{N}\left(0, \sigma_\epsilon^2/\left(1-\rho^2\right)\right)$. Given the parameters for estimation denoted as $\boldsymbol{\Theta} = \left(h_{0D}, h_{0R}, \boldsymbol{\beta}_D, \boldsymbol{\beta}_R, \sigma_\epsilon^2, \sigma_\omega^2, \theta_\mu, \rho\right)$, the conditional likelihood of the observed data $\cup_{i=1}^n \mathcal{D}_i = \{Y_i, Y_{ij}, \Delta_i, \Delta_{ij}, \boldsymbol{X}_j, j = 1, \ldots, M_i; i = 1, \ldots, n\}$ can be derived depending on any prespecified survival copula function. Afterward, a Bayesian augmentation algorithm [75] along with the Metropolis within Gibbs sampling can be invoked for parameter estimation and inference [38, 39].

The Selection of the Copula Various copulas possess different properties [42]. For example, both Clayton and Gumbel copulas can describe asymmetric positive dependence, but the former only exhibits lower-tail dependence, whereas the latter only shows upper-tail dependence. To enhance this model's performance, it is recommended to select an appropriate copula. Several strategies can be considered:

(1) Use an expanded family of copulas and compare and test the results with the assumed one.

(2) Conduct empirical comparisons between the estimated probabilities without considering any covariates and those based on the observed data to learn the sensitivity of the assumed copula.
(3) Consider several information criteria, e.g., the deviance information criteria (DIC) under the Bayesian framework [48, 74].
(4) If no parametric copula demonstrates satisfactory performance, a nonparametric copula is an alternative due to its flexibility [12].

Dependent Coefficient θ_{ij} We can make further generalizations on the model for θ_{ij} by considering potential covariates. In other words, $\theta_{ij} = g\left(\theta_\mu, \gamma_{ij}\right)$, where the overall correlation θ_μ can be represented as $\exp\left(\boldsymbol{Z}^\top \boldsymbol{\theta}\right)$, with $\boldsymbol{Z}$ being potential covariates of clinical interest associated with $\boldsymbol{\theta}$ representing the regression coefficient vector. Thus, the dependency between recurrent events and terminal events can be reported after adjustment for potential covariates of clinical interest such as treatment group, gender, and so on. Additionally, we can extend θ_{ij} by relaxing the index j, which corresponds to event recurrence. In our current model, dependencies are estimated across each event recurrence time point. Therefore, if some subjects only experience a few recurrent events, we have limited information only regarding their time-varying dependency. Based on clinical interest, we can estimate the dependency between two event processes at any particularly pre-identified time point; however, this number can be too high because a larger number of parameters will need to be estimated, which may lead to issues with convergence. For a time-independent case, i.e., the JHCM, the parameter θ_{ij} simplifies to a univariate θ, which quantifies the association between the recurrent event and the terminal event via a specified copula function [34].

2.2.2 Model Extensions to Multiple-Type Recurrent Events

We extend the previous notations for single-type recurrent events to encompass multiple types and introduce some model extensions. The index k is introduced to denote the type of recurrence, with $k = 1, 2, \ldots, K$ and $K \geq 1$ indicating the total number of recurrence types (refer to Fig. 1 for an illustration of a sample subject with multiple-type recurrent events). For simplicity, we designate $k = 0$ to represent the terminal event.

Specifically, for each subject i, D_i, C_i, Y_i, and Δ_i remain the same as stated for the case of $K = 1$. For k-th type of recurrent events, let J_k denote the maximum number of k-th type of recurrent events that a subject could experience in the absence of the terminal event. Let n_{ik} denote the total k-th type of recurrences during the follow-up, satisfying that $1 \leq n_{ik} < J_k$, $0 < Y_i - T_{i,n_{ik},k}$, and $Y_i - T_{i,n_{ik}+1,k} < 0$. Here, T_{ijk} denotes the calendar time until the j-th recurrence since the origin of follow-up for $j = 0, \ldots, J_k$ with $T_{i,0,k} = 0$. Analogously, we define $R_{ijk} = T_{ijk} - T_{i,j-1,k}$ as the gap time between the $(j-1)$-th and the j-th recurrences for $j = 1, \ldots, J_k$. Additionally, let $Y_{ijk} = \min\{R_{ijk}, C_{ijk}\}$

denote the observed gap time with its indicator $\Delta_{ijk} = \mathbb{I}\left(R_{ijk} \le C_{ijk}\right)$, where the censoring time for the j-th gap time is provided by $C_{ijk} = \max\{Y_i - T_{i,j-1,k}, 0\}$ for $j = 1, \ldots, J_k$ and $k = 1, \ldots, K$. We remark that, the first n_{ik} gap times are observed except the last one, i.e., $Y_{ijk} = R_{ijk}$ and $\Delta_{ijk} = 1$ for $j = 1, \ldots, n_{ik}$; $Y_{ijk} = C_{ijk} = Y_i - T_{ijk} > 0$ and $\Delta_{ijk} = 0$ for $j = n_{ik} + 1$; and $Y_{ijk} = C_{ijk} = 0$ and $\Delta_{ijk} = 0$ for $j = n_{ik} + 1, \ldots, J_k$.

We denote $M_i = \max\{n_{i1}, \ldots, n_{iK}\} + 1$ as the maximum observed number of gap times across $K \ge 2$ types of recurrent events. Therefore, the observed data for subject i is $\mathscr{D}_i = \{Y_i, \Delta_i, Y_{ijk}, \Delta_{ijk}, \boldsymbol{X}_i, j = 1, \ldots, M_i, k = 1, \ldots, K\}$. Thus, the hazard functions for the terminal event and K types of recurrences are below:

$$h_0\left(d|\boldsymbol{\omega}_i\right) = h_{00}\left(d\right)\exp\left(\boldsymbol{\beta}_0^\top \boldsymbol{x}_i + \boldsymbol{\phi}^\top \boldsymbol{\omega}_i\right), h_k\left(r|\boldsymbol{\omega}_i\right) = h_{0k}\left(r\right)\exp\left(\boldsymbol{\beta}_k^\top \boldsymbol{x}_i + \omega_{ik}\right) \tag{2}$$

for $k = 1, \ldots, K$, where $h_{00}(d), h_{01}(r), \ldots, h_{0K}(r)$ denote the baseline hazard functions, $\boldsymbol{\beta}_0, \boldsymbol{\beta}_1, \ldots, \boldsymbol{\beta}_K$ denote the regression coefficient vectors for the terminal event and K types of recurrent events, unobserved frailty variables $\boldsymbol{\omega}_i = (\omega_{i1}, \ldots, \omega_{iK})^\top$ follow a multivariate normal distribution $\mathrm{MVN}(\boldsymbol{0}_{K\times 1}, \boldsymbol{\Sigma}_\omega)$, and $\boldsymbol{\phi}$ is a K-dimensional regression coefficient vector for the frailty vector $\boldsymbol{\omega}$. For the cases with $K > 2$, an exchangeable covariance matrix can be considered for parameter dimension reduction. Thus, the joint survival probability of the terminal time D_i and K types of gap times $R_{ij1}, \ldots, R_{ijK}$, conditionally on the frailty vector, are given by

$$\begin{aligned} &\Pr\left(D_i \ge d_i, R_{ij1} \ge r_{ij1}, \cdots, R_{ijK} \ge r_{ijK}|\boldsymbol{\omega}_i\right) \\ &= C_{i,j,\boldsymbol{\theta}_{ij}}\left(S_0\left(d_i|\boldsymbol{\omega}_i\right), S_1\left(r_{ij1}|\boldsymbol{\omega}_i\right), \cdots, S_K\left(r_{ijK}|\boldsymbol{\omega}_i\right)\right), \end{aligned} \tag{3}$$

for $i = 1, \ldots, n$ and $j = 1, \ldots, M_i$, where $S_0(\cdot|\boldsymbol{\omega}_i), \ldots, S_K(\cdot|\boldsymbol{\omega}_i)$ respectively denote the survival functions of the terminal time D_i and K types of gap times R_{ijk} conditional on $\boldsymbol{\omega}_i$, and $C_{i,j,\boldsymbol{\theta}_{ij}}(\cdot, \ldots, \cdot)$ is a $(K+1)$-variate time-dependent survival copula function parameterized by a vector $\boldsymbol{\theta}_{ij} = \boldsymbol{\theta}_{ij}(K+1)$ depending on the terminal event and all K types of recurrent events. Note that the copula function $C_{i,j,\boldsymbol{\theta}_{ij}}(\cdot, \ldots, \cdot)$ could vary across subjects and recurrences, and appropriate copulas can be selected following the above strategies. For example, for a $(K+1)$-variate Clayton copula function

$$C_{i,j,\theta_{ij}}(u, v_1, \ldots, v_K) = \left(u^{-\theta_{ij}} + v_1^{-\theta_{ij}} + \cdots + v_K^{-\theta_{ij}} - K\right)^{-1/\theta_{ij}}, \quad \theta_{ij} > 0,$$

$\boldsymbol{\theta}_{ij}$ reduces to univariate θ_{ij}. Also, we can assume $\boldsymbol{\theta}_{ij} = \left(\theta_{ij0}, \theta_{ij1}, \ldots, \theta_{ijL}\right)^\top$ to be a $(L+1)$-dimensional vector consisting of all unknown parameters in the copula function (e.g., $\theta_{ij0} = \cdots = \theta_{ijL} = \theta_{ij}$ with $L + 1 = 1$ for the above example). We model $\boldsymbol{\theta}_{ij}$ by a function of a $(L+1)$-dimensional vector $\boldsymbol{\theta}_\mu$ and a $(L+1)$-dimensional unrestricted latent vector $\boldsymbol{\gamma}_{ij} = \left(\gamma_{ij0}, \gamma_{ij1}, \ldots, \gamma_{ijL}\right)^\top$. Thus $\boldsymbol{\theta}_{ij} =$

$g(\boldsymbol{\theta}_\mu, \boldsymbol{\gamma}_{ij})$, where $g(\cdot,\cdot)$ is a continuous vector-valued function $\mathbb{R}^{L+1} \times \mathbb{R}^{L+1} \to \mathbb{R}^{L+1}$, depending on the selected copula function.

In this joint modeling, more informative and accurate estimates can be achieved because the information from other types of recurrent events is borrowed via frailty variables and dependent coefficients. With regard to the $((L+1)M_i)$-dimensional latent vector $\boldsymbol{\gamma}_i = \left(\boldsymbol{\gamma}_{i1}^\top, \ldots, \boldsymbol{\gamma}_{i,M_i}^\top\right)^\top$, there are various choices for their joint distribution and the covariance matrix depending on the disease mechanism, clinical experience, or literature. For instance, a multivariate normal distribution with an unknown block-exchangeable structure can be chosen for cardiovascular disease data applications [64, 70]. However, the derivation of the likelihood function depends on the choice of copula function as well as the number of recurrent event types, which can lead to intricate expressions for the likelihood, as well as its gradient and Hessian matrix. In comparison with frequentist approaches for handling unobserved frailties by utilizing the expectation-maximization (EM) method [44] or Gaussian quadrature estimation [43], the Bayesian framework allows for straightforward sampling of frailties, which can be directly incorporated into parameter estimation. Furthermore, estimates under box restrictions are easily obtained with minor algorithmic modifications. Given the complexities of likelihood functions and the challenges in computation, the Bayesian approach is recommended for parameter estimation and inference. For more details on Bayesian approaches in this field, please refer to the review by Sinha et al. [74].

Given parametric (or nonparametric) baseline hazard functions $h_{00}, \ldots, h_{0K}$, a structure of covariance matrix $\boldsymbol{\Sigma}_\omega$, choices of copula function, link function g, distribution and covariance structure for $\boldsymbol{\gamma}_i$, and priors of all unknown qualities, the parameter estimation is straightforward within a full Bayesian framework. First, we impute the unobserved $\boldsymbol{\omega}_i$ and $\boldsymbol{\gamma}_i$ using the random walk Metropolis algorithm, which we denote as the I step. Second, given the imputed $\boldsymbol{\omega}_i$ and $\boldsymbol{\gamma}_i$ along with the priors, we compute the posterior distributions of parameters using the Metropolis-Hastings algorithm, which we denote as the P step. We repeat the I step and P step until convergence is achieved, yielding the Bayesian estimates for all parameters, $\boldsymbol{\omega}_i$, and $\boldsymbol{\gamma}_i$.

2.2.3 Dynamic Risk Prediction

The key feature of the dynamic prediction framework is its ability to dynamically update predictions based on additional information from longitudinal data on recurrences and the longer history of the survival process. However, despite the wealth of patient data available, the majority of prognostic models in the literature provide risk predictions using only a small portion of the recorded information (e.g., considering only the first or last recurrence information [59, 73]), while also ignoring the correlation between recurrent events and terminal events (e.g., assuming conditional independence of recurrent gap times and terminal time [23]). An important limitation is the discarding of valuable information that, if appropriately utilized, could offer better insight into the dynamics of disease progression. In particular, many diseases exhibit an inherent dynamic nature, wherein disease severity and the rate of disease progression dynamically change over time, even within the same patient.

Rizopoulos [66] proposed a Monte Carlo approach to conduct dynamic prediction on time-to-event data, predicting subject-specific survival probabilities using the joint model framework. Other literature on the dynamic prediction problem under the joint model of longitudinal and survival data framework includes works by Blanche [3], Taylor et al. [76]. Regarding the prediction of terminal event risk under the joint modeling framework, [33] extended the usage of joint models of longitudinal data, recurrent events, and a terminal event to the dynamic prediction area. In their paper, they estimated the probability of having a terminal event within a specific time interval, given the previous longitudinal profile and recurrent event history. Papageorgiou et al. [57] proposed a flexible joint model that includes features of the intermediate event as time-varying covariates. Based on these models, they derived dynamic predictions of conditional survival probabilities that are adaptive to different scenarios with respect to the occurrence of the intermediate event. Rizopoulos et al. [67] illustrated a novel approach that weights and combines prediction results based on a class of models simultaneously, employing Bayesian model averaging to utilize various function forms. Li and Luo [37] developed a novel two-stage model that combines multivariate functional principal component analysis with Cox regression to dynamically predict Alzheimer's disease progression using multiple longitudinal markers and time-to-event data.

Specifically in the field of recurrent events prediction, [54] employed the landmark method to handle longitudinal data as a time-fixed covariate at different landmark time points, thereby extending dynamic prediction by landmarking to recurrent event data. Ren et al. [85] developed a dynamic prediction framework for predicting individuals' future outcome trajectories and the risk of the next recurrent event under the Bayesian framework. However, these publications only investigated either the prediction ability of the terminal event or that of a single recurrent event. While it is challenging to specify appropriate parameter distributions when modeling multiple longitudinal trajectories of recurrent events, the major limitation arises in extending the joint modeling approach to incorporate multivariate longitudinal recurrent outcomes while considering the time-varying nature of correlations between recurrent events and the terminal event simultaneously.

Within the joint frailty-copula modeling framework, dynamic prediction of the terminal event (e.g., death) can be performed at a clinically relevant landmark time, alongside the prediction of the next recurrent event if the subject remains alive. Various metrics are available for quantifying predictive accuracy, such as the Brier score [19, 24], the Area Under the Receiver Operating Characteristic curve (AUC-ROC), and others. In this context, we focus on the Brier score for illustration purposes.

Prediction of the Terminal Event Along with similar lines in our recently published paper [38], we can perform subject-level survival prediction for a new subject, indexed as N, by calendar time t' given the cumulative observed recurrent events history data $\mathscr{H}_N(t') = \{Y_N, \Delta_N, Y_{N,j,k}, \Delta_{N,j,k}, \boldsymbol{X}_N, j = 1, 2, \ldots, M_N, k = 1, \ldots, K\}$, where $Y_N = t'$, $\Delta_N = 0$, there exists $n_{N,k}$ satisfying that $\sum_{j=1}^{n_{N,k}} R_{N,j,k} < Y_N$ and $\sum_{j=1}^{n_{N,k}+1} R_{N,j,k} > Y_N$ for all k, and exist $M_N = \max\{n_{N,1}, \ldots, n_{N,K}\} + 1$.

Suppose $\boldsymbol{\Theta}$ consist of all components for estimation in the model (2) with simplifications $C_{i,j,\boldsymbol{\theta}_{ij}} = C_\theta$ and $\boldsymbol{\theta}_{ij} = \theta$ in the joint survival probability (3), i.e., $\boldsymbol{\Theta} = \left(h_{00}, h_{01}, \ldots, h_{0K}, \boldsymbol{\beta}_0^\top, \boldsymbol{\beta}_1^\top, \ldots, \boldsymbol{\beta}_K^\top, \boldsymbol{\phi}^\top, \boldsymbol{\Sigma}_\omega\right)$. Let ω_N denote the frailty for the subject N. For $t > t'$ and data $\cup_{i=1}^n \mathscr{D}_i$, the survival probability for this new subject is $\Pr\left(D_N > t | D_N > t', \mathscr{H}_N(t'), \boldsymbol{\Theta}, \omega_N\right)$, denoted by

$$\pi\left(t|t', \mathscr{H}_N(t'), \boldsymbol{\Theta}, \omega_N\right) = \frac{S_0\left(t|\mathscr{H}_N(t'), \boldsymbol{\Theta}, \omega_N\right)}{S_0\left(t'|\mathscr{H}_N(t'), \boldsymbol{\Theta}, \omega_N\right)},$$

which can be estimated by plugging in the posterior estimates of $\widehat{\boldsymbol{\Theta}}$ and $\widehat{\omega}_N$ based on $\cup_{i=1}^n \mathscr{D}_i$. The predictive accuracy metric of the Bier score is defined as

$$\mathrm{E}\left\{\left[D\left(t|t', \mathscr{H}_N(t'), \widehat{\boldsymbol{\Theta}}\right) - \widehat{\pi}\left(t|t', \mathscr{H}_N(t'), \widehat{\boldsymbol{\Theta}}\right)\right]^2\right\}, \tag{4}$$

where the observed terminal status $D\left(t|t', \mathscr{H}_N(t'), \widehat{\boldsymbol{\Theta}}\right)$ is 1 if the subject has experienced the terminal event in the interval (t', t) and 0 otherwise. The inverse probability of the censored weighted estimate of the Bier score is considered for prediction assessment [19, 24, 38].

Prediction of Next Recurrent Event We can perform subject-level prediction of the next recurrent event for a new subject, conditional on the subject still being alive at calendar time $(t' + r)$, given the cumulative observed recurrent events history data $\mathscr{H}_N(t') = \{Y_N, \Delta_N, Y_{N,j,k}, \Delta_{N,j,k}, \boldsymbol{X}_N, j = 1, 2, \ldots, M_N, k = 1, \ldots, K\}$. The survival probability for the next k-th type of recurrent event for the new subject N can be formulated by $\Pr\left(R_{N,n_{ik}+1,k} > t' + r - \sum_{j=1}^{n_{ik}} R_{N,j,k} | D_N > t' + r, \mathscr{H}_N(t'), \boldsymbol{\Theta}, \omega_N\right)$, denoted by

$$\pi_k\left(r|t', \mathscr{H}_N(t'), \boldsymbol{\Theta}, \omega_N\right) = \frac{S_k\left(r + t' - \sum_{j=1}^{n_{ik}} y_{N,j,k} | \mathscr{H}_N(t'), \boldsymbol{\Theta}, \omega_N\right)}{S_0\left(r + t'|\mathscr{H}_N(t'), \boldsymbol{\Theta}, \omega_N\right)},$$
$$k = 1, \ldots, K,$$

where $y_{N,j,k}$ is the realization of $Y_{N,j,k}$. This can also be estimated by plugging in the posterior estimates of $\widehat{\boldsymbol{\Theta}}$ and $\widehat{\omega}_N$ based on $\cup_{i=1}^n \mathscr{D}_i$. The predictive accuracy metric of the Bier score is defined as

$$\mathrm{E}\left\{\left[R_k\left(r|t', \mathscr{H}_N(t'), \widehat{\boldsymbol{\Theta}}\right) - \widehat{\pi}_k\left(r|t', \mathscr{H}_N(t'), \widehat{\boldsymbol{\Theta}}\right)\right]^2\right\}, \tag{5}$$

where the observed k-th type of recurrence status $R_k\left(r|t', \mathscr{H}_N(t'), \widehat{\Theta}\right)$ is 1 if the subject experiences the next k-th type of recurrent event in the interval $(t', t'+r)$ and 0 otherwise. The estimation of the Brier score is performed along similar lines as above.

3 Real Data Application: The ARIC Study

The ARIC study (1987–2020), a large prospective epidemiological study conducted in four US communities (Forsyth County, North Carolina; Jackson, Mississippi; Minneapolis, Minnesota; and Washington County, Maryland), is being considered for illustration [53]. Originally designed to explore the etiology and natural progression of atherosclerosis, as well as variations in cardiovascular risk factors and diseases, this study recruited $15,792$ adults aged 45–64 years at enrollment. All participants underwent thorough examinations, with particular attention paid to recording the recurrence of cardiovascular events requiring hospitalization during follow-up and monitoring vital status.

Our aim is to conduct recurrent event analysis on the primary event of MI and identify associated risk factors for patients with stage 3–5 chronic kidney disease (the estimated glomerular filtration rate (eGFR) below 60) at baseline. Secondary outcomes such as heart failure (HF) and stroke (SK) are also considered for multiple recurrent event analysis. Throughout the study, all patients have been followed for up to 29 years, with a mortality rate of 48.13% as of 2016. Several baseline risk factors are incorporated into our analysis, including gender (GEN; 1 for male, 0 for female), race (RACE; 1 for white, 0 for non-white), systolic blood pressure (SBP), baseline comorbidity status (COM; indicating presence of MI, heart failure, or stroke at baseline; 1 for yes, 0 for no), baseline diabetes (DIA; 1 for yes, 0 for no), baseline smoking status (SMK; 1 for yes, 0 for no), baseline Body Mass Index (BMI), and baseline age (AGE). For our analysis, participants with missing data in covariates are excluded, resulting in a sample size of 185. Any participants who were still alive at the end of 2016 or were lost to follow-up or refused follow-up during the study period will be considered as censored observations.

In comparison, we fit the PWP model and the JFM to the ARIC data using R packages `survival` and `frailtypack`. We also apply the JHCM to the data. Specifically, they are applied to univariate recurrent event data of MI, HF, and SK, respectively. Then, we apply the multivariate JHCM to the ARIC data using the Metropolis within Gibbs approach. In particular, $K = 3$ in this application, representing the recurrent events of MI, HF, and SK, alongside the terminal event of death. The covariate $\boldsymbol{x}_i$ comprises the above *eight* risk factors: GEN, RACE, SBP, COM, DIA, SMK, BMI, and AGE. Thus, given the observed data $\cup_{i=1}^{n} \mathscr{D}_i$, the hazard functions in the JHCM satisfy the equations in (1) with $\psi = \phi$ for consistent notation, while the multivariate JHCM follows the specifications in (2). For ease of presentation, we consider constant baseline hazard functions h_{00}, h_{01}, h_{02}, and h_{03}.

The copula function for both JHCM and multivariate JHCM is selected as a Clayton copula with time-independent parameter θ. Specifically, for the multivariate JHCM, it is expressed as $C_\theta(u, v_1, v_2, v_3) = \left(u^{-\theta} + v_1^{-\theta} + v_2^{-\theta} + v_3^{-\theta} - 3\right)^{-1/\theta}$ with $\theta > 0$. The covariance matrix $\boldsymbol{\Sigma}_\omega$ for the frailties is designed as below: the diagonal elements are $\sigma_1^2, \ldots, \sigma_K^2$ and the off-diagonal elements are $\rho\sigma_k\sigma_{k'}$ for $k \neq k'$ for $k, k' = 1, \ldots, K$. In practice, the initial values for the JHCM and the multivariate JHCM can either be selected randomly or derived from estimates obtained through other approaches. For instance, in this application, we used the estimates from the JFM as initial values. The findings from fitting both single-type and multiple-type recurrent event models for the ARIC study are presented in Table 2.

The results indicate that, for chronic kidney disease patients, baseline systolic blood pressure, comorbidity status, diabetes status, smoking status, and age exhibit significant associations with the terminal event in both JHCM and multivariate JHCM; baseline gender, systolic blood pressure, comorbidity status, diabetes status, and age exhibit significant associations with the recurrent event of MI in both JHCM and multivariate JHCM. Notably, compared to traditional PWP and JFM models, the JHCM and multivariate JHCM reveal additional disparities, identifying age as a risk factor for MI recurrences. Focused on multivariate JHCM, several risk factors for all-cause mortality are identified. Specifically, male patients have an increased risk for MI (HR = 1.65, 95% CI,1.13, 2.43) and for death (HR = 1.42, 95% CI,1.00, 1.94). Patients with higher SBP also exhibit elevated risks for MI (HR = 1.44, 95% CI:1.18, 1.73) and for death (HR = 1.36, 95% CI,1.15, 1.60). Baseline comorbidity is also significantly associated with MI recurrences (HR = 2.23, 95% CI:1.58, 3.28) and with death (HR = 1.79, 95% CI:1.29, 2.56). Diabetic subjects are more likely to experience MI (HR = 1.50, 95% CI:1.03, 2.29) and death (HR = 1.64, 95% CI:1.17, 2.35). Similarly, the baseline age exhibits increased risk for both MI death (HR = 1.23, 95% CI:1.04, 1.49) and death (HR = 1.54, 95% CI:1.29, 1.82). The estimates of the copula parameter θ are 1.33 for the JHCM and 1.50 for the multivariate JHCM, indicating a relatively moderate to strong positive dependence between the hazards of MI and death in chronic kidney disease patients.

4 Discussion

In this paper, we provide a brief overview of existing models for recurrent gap times and their joint modeling with terminal events, alongside an evaluation of predictive accuracy. Specifically, we emphasize advanced Bayesian joint hierarchical-copula models and their extensions, which incorporate procedures for risk prediction evaluation of subsequent recurrence and death, while addressing subject heterogeneity, covariate effects, time-varying dependence, and multiple types of recurrent events. We illustrate our methodology with a real data example from the ARIC study, demonstrating the superiority of multi-type recurrent modeling in identifying risk

Table 2 Parameter estimates for recurrent MI from various models using the ARIC study, where "PWP" represents the Prentice, Williams, and Peterson model without incorporating the terminal event, "JFM" represents the joint shared frailty model with a normal frailty, "HR," "EST," "LB," and "UB" are hazard ratio, estimate, 95% lower (confidence or Bayesian highest density credible interval) bound for HR or EST, and 95% upper bound for HR or EST, respectively. For the multivariate JHCM, ϕ and σ^2 represent MI's frailty regression coefficient in $\boldsymbol{\phi}$ and variance in $\boldsymbol{\Sigma}_{\omega}$. HRs in bold indicate the statistical significances of the regression coefficients at level of 0.05

		PWP			JFM			JHCM			Multivariate JHCM		
Event	Covariate	HR	LB	UB	HR	LB	UB	HR	LB	UB	HR	LB	UB
Death	GEN				**2.12**	1.29	3.47	**1.45**	1.05	2.00	**1.42**	1.00	1.94
	RACE				**0.54**	0.32	0.90	0.72	0.52	1.04	0.71	0.48	1.01
	SBP				**1.81**	1.38	2.37	**1.37**	1.16	1.61	**1.36**	1.15	1.60
	COM				**3.44**	1.97	6.01	**1.78**	1.27	2.48	**1.79**	1.29	2.56
	DIA				**3.23**	1.84	5.68	**1.67**	1.17	2.39	**1.64**	1.17	2.35
	SMK				**3.20**	1.75	5.85	**1.89**	1.33	2.74	**1.86**	1.30	2.61
	BMI				1.01	0.80	1.30	0.99	0.84	1.15	0.97	0.81	1.14
	AGE				**1.98**	1.49	2.63	**1.54**	1.29	1.82	**1.54**	1.29	1.82
MI	GEN	**1.50**	1.06	2.11	**2.11**	1.27	3.53	**1.68**	1.13	2.50	**1.65**	1.13	2.43
	RACE	0.89	0.61	1.30	0.77	0.44	1.32	0.78	0.54	1.14	0.76	0.53	1.13
	SBP	**1.40**	1.15	1.71	**1.69**	1.28	2.23	**1.47**	1.19	1.77	**1.44**	1.18	1.73
	COM	**1.88**	1.29	2.73	**2.82**	1.63	4.88	**2.21**	1.52	3.37	**2.23**	1.58	3.28
	DIA	**1.63**	1.09	2.46	**1.98**	1.14	3.46	**1.48**	1.00	2.33	**1.50**	1.03	2.29
	SMK	**1.63**	1.08	2.46	1.82	0.98	3.39	1.59	0.98	2.40	1.51	0.96	2.30
	BMI	1.05	0.87	1.27	1.05	0.81	1.35	1.02	0.85	1.22	0.98	0.82	1.18
	AGE	1.16	0.97	1.38	1.25	0.96	1.63	**1.23**	1.02	1.48	**1.23**	1.04	1.49
		EST	LB	UB	EST	LB	UB	EST	LB	UB	EST	LB	UB
	ϕ				0.85	0.40	1.30	− 0.35	− 1.28	0.41	− 0.01	− 1.15	1.50
	σ^2				1.19	0.50	1.88	0.21	0.04	0.51	0.17	0.02	0.39
	θ							1.33	0.70	2.40	1.50	0.94	2.34

factors. It is worth noting that for complex modeling and flexible implementation, Bayesian techniques are utilized. However, the computational burden may be significant due to model complexity and the number of unknown parameters for estimation. Therefore, more efficient algorithms or computing programs (e.g., C/C++, Python) are necessary to overcome these challenges and ensure computational convenience. Moreover, the development of risk prediction tools for both research and clinical practice is essential to identify high-risk patients and deliver more efficient and personalized medication. However, existing literature is limited, often constrained by small sample sizes or statistical limitations resulting from focusing solely on modeling a single event type. While multivariate JHCM holds promise for utilizing multivariate recurrent events in modeling and prediction, addressing the complex dependence structure between multiple-type recurrences and managing intensive computational demands require further efforts and innovation. The R code and additional data analysis will be available at https://github.com/CinemaResearchGroup/ReMRE.

Acknowledgments The authors thank the editors for their invitation to write this review paper. The methods presented in this paper were illustrated using data from the Atherosclerosis Risk in Communities (ARIC) Study, obtained from the National Heart, Lung, and Blood Institute (NHLBI) Biologic Specimen and Data Repository Information Coordinating Center. Wang's work was partially supported by the National Institutes of Health (NIH) grant 1R01HL175410 and by start-up funding from the Department of Population and Quantitative Health Sciences at Case Western Reserve University. Chen's work was partially supported by the NIH grant 1R01AG089377 and by the Johns Hopkins Institute for Clinical and Translational Research, funded under grant 1UM1TR004926. The content is solely the responsibility of the authors and does not necessarily reflect the opinions or views of the National Institutes of Health.

References

1. Abrams, S., Wienke, A., Hens, N.: Modeling time varying heterogeneity in recurrent infection processes: an application to serological data. J. R. Stat. Soc.: Ser. C: Appl. Stat. **67**(3), 687–704 (2018)
2. Amorim, L.D., Cai, J.: Modelling recurrent events: a tutorial for analysis in epidemiology. Int. J. Epidemiol. **44**(1), 324–333 (2014)
3. Blanche, P., Proust-Lima, C., Loubére, L., Berr, C., Dartigues, J.F., JacqminGadda, H.: Quantifying and comparing dynamic predictive accuracy of joint models for longitudinal marker and time-to-event in presence of censoring and competing risks. Biometrics **71**, 102–113 (2015)
4. Che, X., Angus, J.: A new joint model of recurrent event data with the additive hazards model for the terminal event time. Metrika. **79**(7), 763–787 (2016)
5. Chen, C., Shen, B., Liu, A., Wu, R., Wang, M.: A multiple robust propensity score method for longitudinal analysis with intermittent missing data. Biometrics **77**(2), 519–532 (2021)
6. Chen, C., Shen, B., Zhang, L., Xue, Y., Wang, M.: Empirical-likelihood-based criteria for model selection on marginal analysis of longitudinal data with dropout missingness. Biometrics **75**(3), 950–965 (2019)
7. Chen, C., Wang, M., Wu, R., Li, R.: A robust consistent information criterion for model selection based on empirical likelihood. Stat. Sin. **32**(3), 1205–1223 (2022)

8. Chen, Z., Venkat, P., Seyfried, D., Chopp, M., Yan, T., Chen, J.: Brain-heart interaction: cardiac complications after stroke. Circ. Res. **121**(4), 451–468 (2017)
9. Cheng, Y., Fine, J.P.: Cumulative incidence association models for bivariate competing risks data. J. R. Stat. Soc. Ser. B Stat Methodol. **74**(2), 183–202 (2012)
10. Cook, R.J., Lawless, J.F.: Marginal analysis of recurrent events and a terminating event. Stat. Med. **16**(8), 911–924 (1997)
11. Cook, R.J., Lawless, J.F., Lee, K.: A copula-based mixed Poisson model for bivariate recurrent events under event-dependent censoring. Stat. Med. **29**(6), 694–707 (2010)
12. Nelsen, R.B.: An Introduction To Copulas. Springer Science & Business Media, Berlin (2007)
13. Emura, T., Nakatochi, M., Matsui, S., Michimae., H., Rondeau, V.,: Personalized dynamic prediction of death according to tumour progression and high-dimensional genetic factors: meta-analysis with a joint model. Stat. Methods Med. Res. **27**(9), 2842–2858 (2018)
14. Emura, T., Nakatochi, M., Murotani, K., Rondeau, V.: A joint frailty-copula model between tumor progression and death for meta-analysis. Stat. Methods Med. Res. **26**(6), 2649–2666 (2015)
15. Fine, J.P., Jiang, H., Chappell, R.: On semi-competing risks data. Biometrika **88**(4), 907–919 (2001)
16. Fu, H., Wang, Y., Liu, J., Kulkarni, P.M., Melemed, A.S.: Joint modeling of progression free survival and overall survival by a Bayesian normal induced copula estimation model. Stat. Med. **32**(2), 240–254 (2013)
17. Gelman, A., Carlin, J.B., Stern, H.S., Rubin, D.B.: Bayesian data analysis. Chapman and Hall/CRC, New York (1995)
18. Georges, P., Lamy, A.G., Nicolas, E., Quibel, G., Roncalli, T.: Multivariate survival modeling: a unified approach with copulas. Available at SSRN 1032559 (2001)
19. Gerds, T.A., Schumacher, M.: Consistent estimation of the expected Brier score in general survival models with right-censored event times. Biom. J. **48**(6), 1029–1040 (2006)
20. Ghosh, A., Chan, W., Younes, N., Davis, B.R.: A dynamic risk model for multitype recurrent events. Am. J. Epidemiol. **192**(4), 621–631 (2023)
21. Ghosh, D., Lin, D.Y.: Semiparametric analysis of recurrent events data in the presence of dependent censoring. Biometrics **59**(4), 877–885 (2003)
22. Gilks, W.R., Best, N.G., Tan, K.K.C.: Adaptive rejection Metropolis sampling within Gibbs sampling. J. R. Stat. Soc.: Ser. C: Appl. Stat. **44**(4), 455–472 (1995)
23. González, J.R., Fernandez, E., Moreno, V., Ribes, J., Peris, M, Navarro, M, Cambray, M., Borrás, J.M.: Sex differences in hospital readmission among colorectal cancer patients. J. Epidemiol. Community Health **59**(6), 506–511 (2005)
24. Graf, E., Schmoor, C., Sauerbrei, W., Schumacher, M.: Assessment and comparison of prognostic classification schemes for survival data. Stat. Med. **18**(17–18), 2529–2545 (1999)
25. Gunnoo, T., Hasan, N., Khan, M.S., Slark, J., Bentley, P., Sharma, P.: Quantifying the risk of heart disease following acute ischaemic stroke: a meta-analysis of over 50, 000 participants. BMJ Open **6**(1), e009535 (2016)
26. Harrell, F.E., Califf, R.M., Pryor, D.B., Lee, K.L., Rosati, R.A.: Evaluating the yield of medical tests. J. Am. Med. Assoc. **247**(18), 2543–2546 (1982)
27. Hållmarker, U., Åsberg, S., Michaëlsson, K., Ärnlöv, J., Hellberg, D., Lindbäck, J., Wester, P., James, S.: Risk of recurrent stroke and death after first stroke in long-distance ski race participants. J. Am. Heart Assoc. **4**(10), 1–9 (2015)
28. Heagerty, P.J., Zheng, Y.: Survival model predictive accuracy and ROC curves. Biometrics. **61**(1), 92–105 (2005)
29. Huang, C.Y., Wang, M.C.: Joint modeling and estimation for recurrent event processes and failure time data. J. Am. Stat. Assoc. **99**(468), 1153–1165 (2011)
30. Huang, X., Liu, L.: A joint frailty model for survival and gap times between recurrent events. Biometrics **63**(2), 389–397 (2007)

31. Jansen, H., Jänsch, A., Breitling, L.P., Hoppe, L., Dallmeier, D., Schmucker, R., Brenner, H., Koenig, W., Rothenbacher, D.: Hs-cTroponins for the prediction of recurrent cardiovascular events in patients with established CHD–A comparative analysis from the KAROLA study. Int. J. Cardiol. **250**, 247–252 (2018)
32. Jung, T.H., Peduzzi, P., Allore, H., Kyriakides, T.C., Esserman, D.: A joint model for recurrent events and a semi-competing risk in the presence of multi-level clustering. Stat. Methods Med. Res. **28**(10–11), 2897–2911 (2019)
33. Król, A., Ferrer, L., Pignon, J.P., Proust-Lima, C., Ducreux, M., Bouché, O., Michiels, S., Rondeau, V.: Joint model for left-censored longitudinal data, recurrent events and terminal event: predictive abilities of tumor burden for cancer evolution with application to the FFCD 2000–05 trial. Biometrics **72**, 907–916 (2016)
34. Li, Z., Chinchilli, V.M., Wang, M.: A Bayesian joint model of recurrent events and a terminal event. Biom. J. **61**(1), 187–202 (2019)
35. Li, Z., Chinchilli, V.M., Wang, M.: A time-varying bayesian joint hierarchical copula model for analysing recurrent events and a terminal event: an application to the cardiovascular health study. J. R. Stat. Soc. Ser. C. Appl. Stat. **69**(1), 151–166 (2020)
36. Li, D., Hu, X.J., Wang, R.: Evaluating association between two event times with observations subject to informative censoring. J. Am. Stat. Assoc. **118**(542), 1282–1294 (2023)
37. Li, K., Luo, S.: Dynamic prediction of Alzheimer's disease progression using features of multiple longitudinal outcomes and time-to-event data. Stat. Med. **38**(24), 4804–4818 (2019)
38. Li, Z., Chinchilli, M.V., Wang, M.: A Bayesian joint model of recurrent events and a terminal event. Biom. J. **61**(1), 187–202 (2018)
39. Li, Z., Chinchilli, M.V., Wang, M.: A time-varying Bayesian joint hierarchical copula model for analysing recurrent events and a terminal event: an application to the Cardiovascular Health Study. J. R. Stat. Soc.: Ser. C: Appl. Stat. **69**(1), 151–166 (2020)
40. Liang, M., Li, Z., Li, L., Chinchilli, V.M., Zhang, L., Wang, M.: Tackling dynamic prediction of death in patients with recurrent cardiovascular events. Stat. Med. **42**(19), 3487–3507 (2023)
41. Liebscher, E.: Construction of asymmetric multivariate copulas. J. Multivar. Anal. **99**(10), 2234–2250 (2008)
42. Liu, B.Y., Ji, Q., Fan, Y.: A new time-varying optimal copula model identifying the dependence across markets. Quant. Financ. **17**(3), 437–453 (2016)
43. Liu, L., Huang, X.: The use of Gaussian quadrature for estimation in frailty proportional hazards models. Stat. Med. **27**(14), 2665–2683 (2008)
44. Liu, L., Wolfe, R.A., Huang, X.: Shared frailty models for recurrent events and a terminal event. Biometrics. **60**(3), 747–756 (2004)
45. Ma, C., Pan, J.: Multi-state analysis of multi-type recurrent event and failure time data with event feedbacks in biomarkers. Scand. J. Stat. **49**(2), 864–885 (2021)
46. Ma, C., Wang, C., Pan, J.: Multistate modeling and structure selection for multitype recurrent events and terminal event data. Biom. J. **65**(2), e2100334 (2023)
47. Ma, Y.: Analysis of marked recurrent events in the presence of a terminating event. Doctoral Dissertation, The University of Michigan, Michigan (2012)
48. Manda, S.O.M., Meyer, R.: Bayesian inference for recurrent events data using time-dependent frailty. Stat. Med. **24**, 1263–1274 (2005)
49. Mauguen, A., Rachet, B., Mathoulin-Pélissier, S., MacGrogan, G., Laurent, A., Rondeau, V.: Dynamic prediction of risk of death using history of cancer recurrences in joint frailty models. Stat. Med. **32**(30), 5366–5380 (2013)
50. McGilchrist, C.A., Aisbett, C.W.: Regression with frailty in survival analysis. Biometrics **47**(2), 461–466 (1991)
51. McNamara, K., Alzubaidi, H., Jackson, J.K.: Cardiovascular disease as a leading cause of death: how are pharmacists getting involved?. In: Integrated Pharmacy Research and Practice, pp. 1–11 (2019)
52. Meyer, R., Romeo, J.S.: Bayesian semiparametric analysis of recurrent failure time data using copulas. Biom. J. **57**(6), 982–1001 (2015)

53. Johansen, M.C., Wang, W., Zhang, M., Knopman, D.S., Ndumele, C., Mosley, T.H., Selvin, E., Shah, A.M., Solomon, S.D., Gottesman, R.F., Yee Chen, L.Y.: Risk of dementia associated with atrial cardiopathy: the ARIC study. JAHA **11**(16), e025646 (2022)
54. Musoro, J., Struijk, G., Geskus, R., ten Berge, I., Zwinderman, A.: Li, K., Luo, S.: Dynamic prediction of recurrent events data by landmarking with application to a follow-up study of patients after kidney transplant. Stat. Methods Med. Res. **27**(3), 832–845 (2018)
55. Oakes, D.: Bivariate survival models induced by frailties. J. Am. Stat. Assoc. **84**(406), 487–493 (1989)
56. Ozga, A., Kieser, M., Rauch, G.: A systematic comparison of recurrent event models for application to composite endpoints. BMC Med. Res. Methodol. **18**, 1–12 (2018)
57. Papageorgiou, G., Mokhles, M.M., Takkenberg, J.J.M., Rizopoulos, D.: Individualized dynamic prediction of survival with the presence of intermediate events. Stat. Med. **38**, 5623–5640 (2019)
58. Parner, E.: Asymptotic theory for the correlated gamma-frailty model. Ann. Stat. **26**(1), 183–214 (1998)
59. Parast, L., Tian, L., Cai, T.: Landmark estimation of survival and treatment effect in a randomized clinical trial. J. Am. Stat. Assoc. **109**(505), 384–394 (2014)
60. Paulon, G., De Iorio, M., Guglielmi, A., Ieva, F.: Joint modeling of recurrent events and survival: a Bayesian non-parametric approach. Biostatistics **21**(1), 1–14 (2018)
61. Peng, L., Fine, J.P.: Regression modeling of semicompeting risks data. Biometrics. **63**(1), 96–108 (2007)
62. Pennell, M.L., Dunson, D.B.: Bayesian semiparametric dynamic frailty models for multiple event time data. Biometrics **62**(4), 1044–1052 (2006)
63. Peterson, B., Ghahramani, M., Emerich, M., Foy, A.: Frequency of appropriate and low-risk noncardiac preoperative stress testing across medical specialties. Am. J. Cardiol. **122**(5), 744–748 (2018)
64. Quick, H., Waller, L.A., Casper, M.: A multivariate space-time model for analysing county level heart disease death rates by race and sex. J. R. Stat. Soc.: Ser. C: Appl. Stat. **67**(1), 291–304 (2018)
65. Rivest, L.P., Wells, M.T.: A martingale approach to the copula-graphic estimator for the survival function under dependent censoring. J. Multivar. Anal. **79**(1), 138–155 (2001)
66. Rizopoulos, D.: Dynamic predictions and prospective accuracy in joint models for longitudinal and time-to-event data. Biometrics **67**(3), 819–829 (2011)
67. Rizopoulos, D., Hatfield, L.A., Carlin, B.P., Takkenberg, J.J.M.: Combining dynamic predictions from joint models for longitudinal and time-to-event data using Bayesian model averaging. J. Am. Stat. Assoc. **109**(508), 1385–1397 (2014)
68. Rondeau, V., Filleul, L., Joly, P.: Nested frailty models using maximum penalized likelihood estimation. Stat. Med. **25**(23), 4036–4052 (2006)
69. Rondeau, V., Mathoulin-Pelissier, S., Jacqmin-Gadda, H., Brouste, V., Soubeyran, P.: Joint frailty models for recurring events and death using maximum penalized likelihood estimation: application on cancer events. Biostatistics **8**(4), 708–721 (2007)
70. Roy, A., Filipiak, K., Klein, D.: Testing a block exchangeable covariance matrix. Statistics, **52**(2), 393–408 (2018)
71. Schmid, M., Wright, M.N., Ziegler, A.: On the use of Harrell's C for clinical risk prediction via random survival forests. Expert Syst. Appl. **63**, 450–459 (2016)
72. Shih, J.H., Louis, T.A.: Inferences on the association parameter in copula models for bivariate survival data. Biometrics **63**, 1384–1399 (1995)
73. Shi, H., Yin, G.: Landmark cure rate models with time-dependent covariates. Stat. Methods Med. Res. **26**(5), 2042–2054 (2017)
74. Sinha, D., Maiti, T., Ibrahim, J.G., Ouyang, B.: Current methods for recurrent events data with dependent termination: a Bayesian perspective. J. Am. Stat. Assoc. **103**(482), 866–878 (2008)
75. Tanner, M.A., Wong, W.H.: The calculation of posterior distributions by data augmentation. J. Am. Stat. Assoc. **82**(398), 528–540 (1987)

76. Taylor, J.M., Park, Y., Ankerst, D.P., Proust-Lima, C., Williams, S., Kestin, L., Bae, K., Pickles, T., Sandler, H.: Real-time individual predictions of prostate cancer recurrence using joint models. Biometrics **69**, 206–213 (2013)
77. Unkel, S., Farrington, C.P.: A new measure of time-varying association for shared frailty models with bivariate current status data. Biostatistics **13**(4), 665–679 (2012)
78. Unkel, S., Farrington, C.P., Whitaker, H.J., Pebody, R.: Time varying frailty models and the estimation of heterogeneities in transmission of infectious diseases. J. R. Stat. Soc. Ser. C. Appl. Stat. **63**(1), 141–158 (2013)
79. Wang, M., Kong, L., Li, Z., Zhang, L.: Covariance estimators for Generalized Estimating Equations (GEE) in longitudinal analysis with small samples: addressing issues associated with evaluating prediction models for survival endpoints based on the concordance statistic. Stat. Med. **35**(10), 706–721 (2016)
80. Wang, M., Long, Q.: Addressing issues associated with evaluating prediction models for survival endpoints based on the concordance statistic. Biometrics **72**(3), 897–906 (2016)
81. Wang, W., Wells, M.T.: Time varying frailty models and the estimation of heterogeneities in transmission of infectious diseases. J. R. Stat. Soc.: Ser. C: Appl. Stat. **63**(1), 141–158 (1997)
82. Wang, W., Wells, M.T.: Nonparametric estimators of the bivariate survival function under simplified censoring conditions. Biometrika **84**(4), 863–880 (1997)
83. Wilson, P.W.F., D'Agostino S.R., Bhatt, D.L., Eagle, K., Pencina, M.J., Smith, S.C., Alberts, M.J., Dallongeville, J., Goto, S., Hirsch, A.T., others: An international model to predict recurrent cardiovascular disease. Am. J. Med. **125**(7), 695–703 (2012)
84. Xie, C., Huang, X., Li, R., Tsodikov, A., Bhalla, K.: Individual dynamic prediction for cure and survival based on longitudinal biomarkers. Ann. Appl. Stat. **(in press)** (2024)
85. Ren, X., Wang, J., Luo, S.: Dynamic prediction using joint models of longitudinal and recurrent event data: a Bayesian perspective. Biostat. Epidemiol. **5**(2), 250–266 (2021)
86. Rogers, J.K., Yaroshinsky, A., Pocock, S.J., Stokar, D., Pogoda, J.: Analysis of recurrent events with an associated informative dropout time: application of the joint frailty model. Stat. Med. **35**(13), 2195–2205 (2016)
87. Xu, C., Li, Z., Xue, Y., Zhang, L., Wang, M.: An R package for model fitting, model selection and the simulation for longitudinal data with dropout missingness. Commun. Stat. Simul. Comput. **48**(9), 2812–2829 (2019)
88. Yashin, A.I., Vaupel, J.W., Iachine, I.A.: Correlated individual frailty: an advantageous approach to survival analysis of bivariate data. Math. Popul. Stud. **5**(2), 145–159 (1995)
89. Yang, W., Jepson, C., Xie, D., Roy, J.A., Shou, H., Hsu, J.Y., Anderson, A.H., Landis, J.R., He, J., Feldman, H.I.: Statistical methods for recurrent event analysis in cohort studies of CKD. Clin. J. Am. Soc. Nephrol. **12**(12), 2066–2073 (2017)
90. Yu, Z., Liu, L., Bravata, D.M., Williams, L.S.: Joint model of recurrent events and a terminal event with time-varying coefficients. Biom. J. **56**(2), 183–197 (2014)
91. Yue, H., Chan, K.: A dynamic frailty model for multivariate survival data. Biometrics **53**(3), 785–793 (1997)
92. Zeng, D., Chen, Q., Ibrahim, J.G.: Gamma frailty transformation models for multivariate survival times. Biometrika **96**(2), 277–291 (2009)
93. Zheng, M., Klein, J.P.: Estimates of marginal survival for dependent competing risks based on an assumed copula. Biometrika **82**(1), 127–138 (1995)

A Conditional Modeling Approach for Dynamic Risk Prediction of a Survival Outcome Using Longitudinal Biomarkers with an Application to Ovarian Cancer

Yongli Han, Yifan Yang, Zhiwei Zhang, Ming Wang, and Danping Liu

Abstract Longitudinal biomarkers are commonly collected in many observational studies and clinical trials. Dynamic disease risk prediction based on updated longitudinal biomarkers is of increasing interest to both researchers and medical practitioners. In this paper, we propose a novel conditional modeling approach for dynamic risk prediction of a survival outcome using longitudinal biomarkers. The

---

Supplementary Information The online version contains supplementary material available at (https://doi.org/10.1007/978-3-032-06649-7_19).

Y. Han
Biostatistics and Data Management, Daiichi Sankyo, Inc., Basking Ridge, NJ, USA

Biostatistics Branch, Division of Cancer Epidemiology and Genetics, National Cancer Institute, Rockville, MD, USA
e-mail: justin.han@daiichisankyo.com

Y. Yang
Department of Population and Quantitative Health Sciences, School of Medicine, Case Western Reserve University, Cleveland, OH, USA
e-mail: yiorfun@case.edu

Z. Zhang
Biostatistics Branch, Biometric Research Group, Division of Cancer Treatment & Diagnosis, National Cancer Institute, Rockville, MD, USA

Global Biometrics & Data Sciences, Bristol Myers Squib, Lawrenceville, NJ, USA
e-mail: zhiwei.zhang@nih.gov

M. Wang (✉)
Department of Population and Quantitative Health Sciences, School of Medicine, Case Western Reserve University, Cleveland, OH, USA
e-mail: mxw827@case.edu

D. Liu (✉)
Biostatistics Branch, Division of Cancer Epidemiology and Genetics, National Cancer Institute, Rockville, MD, USA
e-mail: danping.liu@nih.gov

Y. Zhao, D.-G. Chen (eds.), *Big Data Analytics in Biostatistics and Bioinformatics*, ICSA Book Series in Statistics,
https://doi.org/10.1007/978-3-032-06649-7_19

idea is to factor the joint density of the biomarkers and the survival time into the product of a conditional density of the biomarkers given the survival time and a marginal density of the survival time, so that the conditional density of the survival time given the biomarkers can be derived. To model the biomarkers conditional on the survival time, we propose a nonlinear mixed model that treats the survival time as an additional covariate via a smooth or a latent changepoint kernel function to account for its effects. The t-year absolute risk prediction and the associated asymptotic variance are derived under two different assumptions for the censoring time. Compared with existing risk prediction methods, such as the joint modeling and the landmark approaches, the proposed conditional modeling approach makes less strict model assumptions, and hence has more robust predictive performance, as demonstrated by the simulation studies. The proposed approach was motivated by and applied to the ovarian cancer risk prediction in the National Cancer Institute Prostate, Lung, Colorectal, and Ovarian (PLCO) Cancer Screening Trial.

Keywords Conditional modeling approach · Longitudinal and survival data analysis · Dynamic risk prediction · Brier score · Time-dependent AUC

1 Introduction

Biomarkers that may be relevant to disease etiology are usually measured repeatedly over time in many cohort studies and clinical trials [15]. Compared to cross-sectional biomarker measurements, longitudinal biomarker trajectories, particularly those with abnormal pattern changes, may contain information that is predictive for disease progression or potential disease onset [29]. Incorporating longitudinal biomarkers into risk prediction of clinical outcomes such as cancer and pregnancy problems is of increasing interest [3, 12, 13, 27]. Dynamic risk prediction of a survival endpoint based on longitudinal biomarkers is helpful for medical practitioners, as it could help to make updated clinical decisions using newly collected biomarker information [34].

An example is the serum marker cancer antigen 125 (CA125), which may be predictive for ovarian cancer detection: in medical practice, CA125 results above 35 U/mL are classified as abnormal or positive, alarming suspicious abnormalities that require additional evaluations by follow-up diagnostic and therapeutic processes [38]. The effects of the CA125 screening test on ovarian cancer mortality have been studied in the ovarian cancer study from the National Cancer Institute Prostate, Lung, Colorectal, and Ovarian (PLCO) Cancer Screening Trial, which is a large randomized controlled trial of 78216 cancer-free women with baseline age between 55 and 74 at 10 screening centers in the USA from 1993 to 2001 [7]. The CA125 screening test was performed on women in the intervention group ($n = 39105$) at baseline visits and then annually for up to 5 years, while usual medical care was given to women in the comparison group ($n = 39111$). After the first 6 years of active screening, women in both groups were followed up without screening tests for additional 7 years [31]. To study the effects of the CA125 screening test, women in the intervention group who developed ovarian cancer are noted as cases and those who did not are controls. In literature, prediction of the ovarian cancer risk based on repeated CA125 measurements is commonly performed using a specifically designed approach, the Risk of Ovarian Cancer Algorithm (ROCA) [37]. However, the ROCA can only predict a binary outcome due to ignoring the survival time [13]. In this paper, we aim to develop a dynamic prediction method for ovarian cancer risk.

Statistical methodologies on dynamic risk prediction have been studied extensively in the statistical literature, and it is widely agreed that a joint distribution is needed to model both the biomarker process and the survival time, e.g., [1, 11, 17, 19, 40]. A popular joint modeling (JM) approach that uses a latent-variable strategy for dynamic risk prediction was developed by Rizopoulos [34]. In specific, a linear mixed-effects model is proposed for the longitudinal biomarkers, while a Cox model is for the survival outcome, and these two models are associated via a shared random effects structure. The risk is then derived from the joint distribution of the longitudinal and the survival data, after integrating out the shared random effects. Effects of the association structure between the longitudinal and the survival processes on risk prediction have been further studied [35]. Other extensions to JM for dynamic risk prediction have been made, for example, subject-level penalized splines [5] and multilevel latent trait model [44] were proposed to flexibly characterize the coevolution of the longitudinal and the survival processes. Desmée [10] developed a nonlinear joint model that uses a Bayesian algorithm to calculate the dynamic risk, while [4] tackled the problem of dynamic risk prediction using joint models for multiple longitudinal biomarkers with competing risk data. While JM appears to be a natural way to describe the joint distribution of the longitudinal and survival data, it has several limitations: (1) it makes a very strong and non-verifiable assumption that the longitudinal and the survival processes are independent conditional on the random effects; (2) it is often difficult to specify a realistic longitudinal model prospectively in time if the biomarker trajectory is not tracking well, for example, with a nonlinear or changepoint structure; and (3) to accommodate the complex longitudinal structure in the joint model, increasing dimension of the random effects needs to be included in the model, resulting in heavy and sometimes prohibitive computational burdens [9].

Another option is the landmark (LM) approach based on the landmark of the survival data [41, 43]. Compared with JM, LM does not assume a structure for the longitudinal biomarkers but estimates an empirical distribution of the residual survival time based on repeatedly cross-sectional biomarker observations at the given landmark time. In specific, LM fits a Cox model to individuals who are event-free at a given landmark time and then calculates the survival probability for a prediction horizon time of interest. More complicated assumptions on the Cox model can be made, for instance, using a polynomial to describe the time-dependent baseline hazard and a parametric model to characterize the time-varying regression parameters [42]. Compared to JM, LM enjoys computational simplicity, particularly when there are multiple biomarkers, time-varying biomarkers, biomarkers with diverse nonlinear longitudinal trajectories, or biomarkers following discrete distributions (e.g., categorical biomarkers) [25, 48]. Though LM often has close performances to JM [39], it does not make full use of the longitudinal information, as the biomarker trajectory is simply left unspecified.

In this paper, we propose a novel conditional modeling (CM) approach for dynamic disease risk prediction. The key idea of the CM approach is to first factor the joint density of the longitudinal biomarkers and the survival time into the product of a conditional density of the biomarkers given the survival time and a marginal density of the survival time. Then, the conditional density of the survival time given the biomarkers is derived to calculate the disease risk. The benefit of the proposed CM approach can be demonstrated using the PLCO ovarian cancer example, where Fig. 1 shows the longitudinal CA125 trajectories. The top row displays the biomarker trajectories in a prospective time axis, with time zero being the study entry, separately for subjects who did and did not develop ovarian cancer during the study window. We can see that a prospective-time longitudinal model, as constructed by the JM approach, is not easy to specify because of the seemingly "random" spikes in the biomarker profiles. As a comparison, the bottom row illustrates the biomarker trajectories in a retrospective-time axis by anchoring every subject's time zero at the time of cancer diagnosis or censoring. In this way, a more apparent biomarker trajectory pattern can be observed: among the subjects who developed ovarian cancer, the spikes in the biomarker profiles often occur at $1 \sim 2$ years before the cancer diagnosis. Therefore, modeling the biomarker process

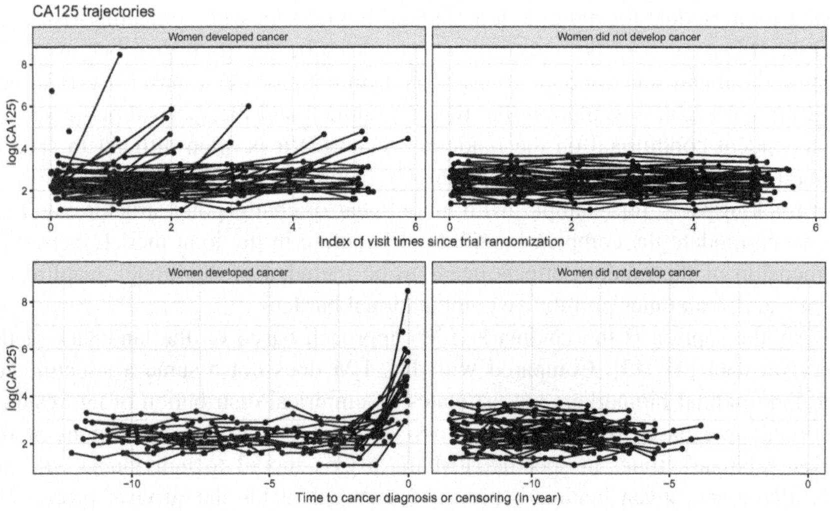

Fig. 1 CA125 trajectories from 50 ovarian cancer women (left) and 50 women who did not develop cancer (right) during the study window. All women were randomly selected from the intervention group of the PLCO Cancer Screening Trial. Top, trajectories in prospective-time axis; bottom, trajectories in retrospective-time axis

conditional on the survival time appears to be a natural and easy way to characterize this feature, as it may be more effective to explore the association between the two processes. Incorporating this important feature into a risk prediction model may help to obtain improved prediction accuracy.

The idea of retrospective-time modeling for longitudinal biomarkers under the CM framework was originally proposed in longitudinal data literature, especially when the longitudinal process is truncated by an informative event such as death. Early works include the terminal-decline model [21] and the reverse-time model [43]. Estimation and application of this type of model have been of growing interest. For example, [8] proposed a nonparametric approach to estimate the medical cost before death of ovarian cancer patients formulated in a backward process; [22] developed a likelihood-based approach for a terminal-decline model on repeated measurements of quality of life in a palliative care study, where a semiparametric approach was further developed [23]. Kong et al. [20] proposed a two-stage semi-parametric likelihood-based approach to estimate the end-of-life cost for patients with end-stage renal disease, while [25] used bivariate penalized splines to estimate the conditional mean medical cost at any month given the terminal event time for stage IV breast cancer patients. Recently, [9] investigated the probabilistic and statistical implications of the time-reversal model in a cirrhosis study. An implicit assumption that [20] and [9] made in their longitudinal models is that subjects with and without the event would essentially have the same longitudinal trajectory when looking retrospectively from the event time. Note that for the subjects without the event, "looking retrospectively" would require a hypothetical follow-up until the event occurs. However, this assumption cannot be verified, since no observed data is available for such follow-ups. Kong et al. [20] further assumed that the longitudinal trajectory a long time before the event is nearly independent of the event. Therefore, their model can only capture the "acute" effects of the longitudinal biomarkers, in the sense that the longitudinal biomarker information useful for predicting the survival event only comes from the measurements close to the event rather than the early-collected ones. Assuming biomarker independence, [36] proposed a joint model to dynamically predict the future risk of an event based on earlier biomarker measurements conditioned on the later event time. We formally define their implicit assumption as the "biomarker independent censoring" assumption and propose a different CM framework when this assumption is violated. In brief, we propose separate longitudinal models for subjects with and without the event and then use these models to derive a dynamic prediction of the event risk. Through separate modeling, our CM framework incorporates both the acute and long-term effects of the longitudinal biomarker trajectory, which will be further elaborated.

The rest of the paper is presented below. Section 2 introduces the proposed CM approach for dynamic risk prediction. Section 3 presents simulation studies with different parameter setups to compare the predictive performances among CM, JM, and LM, while Sect. 4 demonstrates the empirical application of all methods to the PLCO ovarian cancer data. Section 5 ends this paper with a discussion.

2 Methods

Without loss of generality, assume the cohort study of interest has enrolled N participants. Let Y_{ij} denote the jth biomarker measurement of subject i, taken at time t_{ij}, where $i = 1, \ldots, N$, $j = 1, \ldots, n_i$, $0 < t_{i1} < \cdots < t_{in_i} < \infty$, and n_i is the cluster size. When we need to highlight Y_{ij} as a function of the observation time, we also write it as $Y_i(t_{ij})$. Define $\boldsymbol{Y}_i = (Y_{i1}, \ldots, Y_{in_i})^\top$ and $\boldsymbol{W}_i$ as the subject-level baseline covariate vector. In this paper, we only focus on the baseline covariates, but the approach can be generalized to the time-dependent variables as well. Let S_i and C_i be the event time and the censoring time, respectively. Then, the observed survival data for subject i is $(T_i, \Delta_i, \boldsymbol{Y}_i, \boldsymbol{W}_i)$, where $T_i = \min(S_i, C_i)$ is the observed survival time, and the censoring indicator is $\Delta_i = I(S_i \leq C_i)$ with $I(\cdot)$ is the indicator function. We denote the biomarker history data by time s as $\mathscr{Y}_i(s) = \{Y_i(t_{ij}); 0 \leq t_{ij} \leq s\}$. The focus of this paper is to predict the t-year individualized risk of disease beyond a landmark time s, $\Pr(s < S_i \leq s + t | S_i > s, \mathscr{Y}_i(s) = y_i(s), \boldsymbol{W}_i = \boldsymbol{w}_i)$, based on the individual marker measurements available up to the landmark time s, where $y_i(s) = \{y_i(t_{ij}); 0 \leq t_{ij} \leq s\}$, $y_i(t_{ij})$, and $\boldsymbol{w}_i$ are the realizations of $\mathscr{Y}_i(s)$, $Y_i(t_{ij})$, and $\boldsymbol{W}_i$, respectively. Additionally, throughout the paper, we denote $f(\cdot)$, $S(\cdot)$, and $F(\cdot)$ as the density, survival, and cumulative functions, respectively.

2.1 *Conditional Modeling Approach*

We propose a conditional modeling (CM) approach to dynamically calculate the disease risk. The core idea of the CM approach is to factor the joint distribution of $(\mathscr{Y}_i(s), S_i | \boldsymbol{W}_i)$ into the product of the conditional density $f(\mathscr{Y}_i(s) | S_i, \boldsymbol{W}_i)$ and the marginal density $f(S_i | \boldsymbol{W}_i)$. Then, the conditional density $f(S_i | \mathscr{Y}_i(s), \boldsymbol{W}_i)$ is obtained as $f(\mathscr{Y}_i(s) | S_i, \boldsymbol{W}_i) f(S_i | \boldsymbol{W}_i) / f(\mathscr{Y}_i(s) | \boldsymbol{W}_i)$ using Bayes' rule. The risk at a given landmark time s for a prediction horizon time t is

$$
\begin{aligned}
\pi_i(t|s) &\equiv \Pr(s < S_i \leq s + t | S_i > s, \mathscr{Y}_i(s) = y_i(s), \boldsymbol{W}_i = \boldsymbol{w}_i) \\
&= \frac{\Pr(s < S_i \leq s + t | \mathscr{Y}_i(s) = y_i(s), \boldsymbol{W}_i = \boldsymbol{w}_i)}{\Pr(]S_i > s | \mathscr{Y}_i(s) = y_i](s), \boldsymbol{W}_i = \boldsymbol{w}_i)} \\
&= \frac{\int_s^{s+t} f(S_i = u | \mathscr{Y}_i(s), \boldsymbol{W}_i) du}{\int_s^{+\infty} f(S_i = u | \mathscr{Y}_i(s), \boldsymbol{W}_i) du} \\
&= \frac{\int_s^{s+t} f(S_i = u, \mathscr{Y}_i(s) | \boldsymbol{W}_i) du}{\int_s^{+\infty} f(S_i = u, \mathscr{Y}_i(s) | \boldsymbol{W}_i) du} \\
&= \frac{\int_s^{s+t} f(\mathscr{Y}_i(s) | S_i = u, \boldsymbol{W}_i) f(S_i = u | \boldsymbol{W}_i) du}{\int_s^{+\infty} f(\mathscr{Y}_i(s) | S_i = u, \boldsymbol{W}_i) f(S_i = u | \boldsymbol{W}_i) du} \qquad (1)
\end{aligned}
$$

Although the risk calculation depends on the conditional density $f(S_i|\mathscr{Y}_i(s), \boldsymbol{W}_i)$, it actually can be calculated from the joint density $f(S_i, \mathscr{Y}_i(s)|\boldsymbol{W}_i)$, as shown above. The joint density can be factored as a product of the conditional density $f(\mathscr{Y}_i(s)|S_i, \boldsymbol{W}_i)$ and the marginal density $f(S_i|\boldsymbol{W}_i)$. In the following sections, we will discuss the model specifications and the estimation of $f(\mathscr{Y}_i(s)|S_i, \boldsymbol{W}_i)$ under both the biomarker-independent and biomarker-dependent censoring assumptions.

2.1.1 CM with Biomarker-Independent Censoring Assumption

Along with the lines by Kong et al. [20], we include the survival time as a covariate in a nonlinear mixed-effects model for the longitudinal biomarker. $\left(Y_{ij}|S_i, \boldsymbol{W}_i\right)$ is modeled by

$$Y_{ij} = \boldsymbol{X}_i^\top \boldsymbol{\beta} + g(t_{ij} - S_i; \boldsymbol{\eta}_i) + \boldsymbol{Z}_i^\top \boldsymbol{b}_i + \xi_{ij}, \tag{2}$$

where $\boldsymbol{\beta}$ is a vector of fixed effects, $\boldsymbol{b}_i$ is a vector of random effects that follow a multivariate Gaussian distribution with mean $\boldsymbol{0}$ and variance and covariance matrix $\boldsymbol{\Sigma}_b$, random error $\xi_{ij} \sim N\left(0, \sigma_\xi^2\right)$, and $\boldsymbol{X}_i$ and $\boldsymbol{Z}_i$ are design vectors of covariates $\boldsymbol{W}_i$ such as biomarker observation time, baseline age, and other risk factors that may be associated with Y_{ij} and S_i. The kernel function $g(t_{ij} - S_i; \boldsymbol{\eta}_i)$ is parameterized by $\boldsymbol{\eta}_i$ with i indicating the inclusion of both fixed and random effects.

This kernel function characterizes how the survival time S_i would affect the biomarker development: the marker would be barely affected by S_i when measured far away from the occurrence of the event, but it would become increasingly dependent on S_i when measured close to the event. Mathematically, $g(t_{ij} - S_i; \boldsymbol{\eta}_i)$ satisfies below two conditions:

(i) $g(t_{ij} - S_i; \boldsymbol{\eta}_i) \to 0$ (or $= 0$) when $t_{ij} \ll S_i$; and
(ii) $g(t_{ij} - S_i; \boldsymbol{\eta}_i)$ rapidly departs away from 0 as $t_{ij} \to S_i$.

Whether $g(t_{ij} - S_i; \boldsymbol{\eta}_i)$ increases or decreases from 0 as $t_{ij} \to S_i$ depends on the potential etiological relationship between the biomarker and the disease. For example, in the PLCO ovarian cancer study, we require $g(t_{ij} - S_i; \boldsymbol{\eta}_i)$ to increase as time goes on because larger CA125 is often more predictive for the occurrence of ovarian cancer, while in other applications such as the HIV infection, $g(t_{ij} - S_i; \boldsymbol{\eta}_i)$ would be decreasing as $t_{ij} \to S_i$ to characterize the CD4 measurement changes.

We propose the following three forms for $g(t_{ij} - S_i; \boldsymbol{\eta}_i)$, although other forms such as smoothing splines can be utilized:

(a) *Exponential kernel*: $g(t_{ij} - S_i; \boldsymbol{\eta}_i) = \eta_{i1} \exp\{\eta_2(t_{ij} - S_i)\}$, where $\eta_{i1} = \eta_1 + a_i, a_i \sim N(0, \sigma_a^2)$, with both a fixed effect η_1 and a random effect a_i to characterize the slope of the biomarker trajectory. We require $\eta_2 > 0$ for the PLCO ovarian cancer study.
(b) *Gaussian kernel*: $g(t_{ij} - S_i; \boldsymbol{\eta}_i) = \eta_{i1} \exp\left\{-(t_{ij} - S_i + \eta_2)^2/\eta_3\right\}$, where η_3 is positive and $\eta_{i1} = \eta_1 + a_i, a_i \sim N(0, \sigma_a^2)$.

(c) *Latent changepoint kernel*: $g(t_{ij}-S_i;\boldsymbol{\eta}_i)=\eta_{i1}(t_{ij}-S_i+\eta_2)^+$, where $(x)^+=x$ if $x>0$ and 0 otherwise, and $\eta_{i1}=\eta_1+a_i, a_i\sim N(0,\sigma_a^2)$. Unlike the exponential and the Gaussian kernels, this kernel characterizes the relationship between Y_{ij} and S_i in a piecewise linear way via using a changepoint η_2, which indicates the marker trajectory will be elevated η_2 years before the event.

In the above kernel functions, η_2 can be further generalized to be subject-specific by assuming $\eta_{i2}\sim N(\eta_2,\sigma_{\eta_2}^2)$. However, doing so would impose computational complexity on the model estimation of (2). In this paper, we only consider a constant η_2 for the sake of approach demonstration and computational simplicity.

To estimate the parameters in the conditional model (2), [20] made an assumption, indicating that the censoring time C_i and $(\boldsymbol{Y}_i,S_i)$ are conditionally independent given $\boldsymbol{W}_i$, denoted as $C_i \perp\!\!\!\perp (\boldsymbol{Y}_i,S_i)|\boldsymbol{W}_i$. Note that this assumption implies the following assumption, named biomarker-independent censoring assumption (BICA):

$$C_i \perp\!\!\!\perp \boldsymbol{Y}_i|(S_i,\boldsymbol{W}_i) \quad \text{and} \quad C_i \perp\!\!\!\perp S_i|(\boldsymbol{Y}_i,\boldsymbol{W}_i).$$

Since $C_i \perp\!\!\!\perp \boldsymbol{Y}_i|(S_i,\boldsymbol{W}_i)$ in the BICA yields $\Delta_i \perp\!\!\!\perp \boldsymbol{Y}_i|(S_i,\boldsymbol{W}_i)$, we have the following equalities:

$$f(\boldsymbol{Y}_i|S_i,\boldsymbol{W}_i)=f(\boldsymbol{Y}_i|S_i,\Delta_i=1,\boldsymbol{W}_i)=f(\boldsymbol{Y}_i|S_i,\Delta_i=0,\boldsymbol{W}_i) \tag{3}$$

Therefore, the complete case analysis that only uses subjects with the event (i.e., $\Delta_i=1$) would still yield a consistent inference of model (2). If we regard S_i as missing data, this is essentially a missing completely at random assumption. Using model (2) and given the BICA, the likelihood function for the data with the observed event can be given by

$$L(T_i,\Delta_i=1,\boldsymbol{Y}_i,\boldsymbol{W}_i)\propto f(\boldsymbol{Y}_i|S_i=T_i,\boldsymbol{W}_i)f(S_i=T_i|\boldsymbol{W}_i), \tag{4}$$

where the logarithm of the conditional density $f(\boldsymbol{Y}_i|S_i,\boldsymbol{W}_i)$ can be written by

$$\begin{aligned}\log f(\boldsymbol{Y}_i|S_i,\boldsymbol{W}_i) &\propto -\log|\boldsymbol{\Sigma}_i| \\ &-(\boldsymbol{Y}_i-\mathbf{X}_i\boldsymbol{\beta}-\boldsymbol{g}(\boldsymbol{t}_i-S_i\mathbf{1}_{n_i};\boldsymbol{\eta}_i))^\top\boldsymbol{\Sigma}_i^{-1}(\boldsymbol{Y}_i-\mathbf{X}_i\boldsymbol{\beta}-\boldsymbol{g}(\boldsymbol{t}_i-S_i\mathbf{1}_{n_i};\boldsymbol{\eta}_i)),\end{aligned}$$

where $\boldsymbol{g}(\boldsymbol{t}_i-S_i\mathbf{1}_{n_i};\boldsymbol{\eta}_i)=(g(t_{i1}-S_i;\boldsymbol{\eta}_i),\ldots,g(t_{in_i}-S_i;\boldsymbol{\eta}_i))^\top$, $\boldsymbol{\Sigma}_i=\mathbf{R}_i\boldsymbol{\Gamma}_i\mathbf{R}_i^\top+\sigma_\xi^2\mathbf{I}_{n_i}$, $\mathbf{X}_i$ and $\mathbf{Z}_i$ are the design matrices, $\mathbf{R}_i$ is composed of $\mathbf{Z}_i$ and the kernel $\boldsymbol{g}(\boldsymbol{t}_i-S_i\mathbf{1}_{n_i};\boldsymbol{\eta}_i)$, $\boldsymbol{t}_i=(t_{i1},\ldots,t_{in_i})^\top$, $\mathbf{1}_{n_i}$ is the unit vector with the length n_i, and $\mathbf{I}_{n_i}$ is the $n_i\times n_i$ identity matrix. In addition, the conditional density $f(S_i|\boldsymbol{W}_i)$ can be modeled using a Cox proportional hazards model with the hazard function below:

$$h(t|\boldsymbol{W}_i)=h_0(t)\exp\left(\boldsymbol{W}_i^\top\boldsymbol{\alpha}\right), \tag{5}$$

with $h_0(t)$ as a baseline hazard function and $\boldsymbol{\alpha}$ the regression vector.

2.1.2 CM with Biomarker-Dependent Censoring Assumption

While the BICA greatly simplifies the likelihood function (4), several issues are worth noting. First, the assumption in (3) implies the longitudinal marker trajectories of censored subjects are exactly the same as those of event subjects, when looking retrospectively from the event time. Since censored (or control) subjects' biomarkers are often observed a long time before the event, their trajectories would resemble the uncensored (or case) subjects that are measured a long time before the event. Meanwhile, model (2) postulates a flat biomarker trajectory early on and a rapid increase shortly before the event. Therefore, what distinguishes a high-risk from a low-risk subject is whether or not the biomarker trajectory displays an elevated change, which, by the model setup, only occurs shortly before the event. In other words, only the measurements collected close to the event are useful for predicting the event risk, while those collected far away barely contribute any information to the risk prediction. We describe this phenomenon as "acute" effects of the biomarkers described by the prediction model. However, the biomarkers may also have long-term effects on the disease, particularly when the biomarkers are relevant to the disease etiology, e.g., a small elevation of a biomarker at a young age could potentially increase the cancer risk many years later. Second, the estimation of $f(\boldsymbol{Y}_i|S_i, \boldsymbol{W}_i)$ can be based on the event subjects ($\Delta_i = 1$) only [20]. As for the censored subjects ($\Delta_i = 0$), simple extrapolations from the fitted case model could be applied. Nevertheless, validation of such extrapolations is often hard due to the unobserved event times. This assumption may become problematic, especially when the event is a rare disease like ovarian cancer, as there may not be enough case subjects for reliable model estimation and extrapolation. Third, the conditional density of biomarkers given the censoring time and covariates, i.e., $f(\boldsymbol{Y}_i|C_i, \boldsymbol{W}_i)$, is simply left unspecified and not included in the likelihood function, ignoring the potentially useful information from the censored subjects.

To incorporate both the acute and the long-term effects of the biomarkers, as well as to make use of the additional information from the censored subjects, we propose the biomarker-dependent censoring assumption (BDCA), where the conditional independence between C_i and $\boldsymbol{Y}_i$ is violated but the conditional independence between C_i and S_i still holds:

$$C_i \not\perp\!\!\!\perp \boldsymbol{Y}_i|(S_i, \boldsymbol{W}_i) \quad \text{and} \quad C_i \perp\!\!\!\perp S_i|(\boldsymbol{Y}_i, \boldsymbol{W}_i).$$

Because of the above assumptions, we propose to model $(\boldsymbol{Y}_i|C_i, \boldsymbol{W}_i)$ when $\Delta_i = 0$ by

$$Y_{ij} = \boldsymbol{X}_i^\top \boldsymbol{\beta}^{(*)} + g\left(t_{ij} - C_i; \boldsymbol{\eta}_i^{(*)}\right) + \boldsymbol{Z}_i^\top \boldsymbol{b}_i^{(*)} + \xi_{ij}^{(*)}, \tag{6}$$

where the kernel function $g\left(t_{ij} - C_i; \eta_i^{(*)}\right)$ characterizes the potential effects of the censoring time on the biomarker process in a way similar to the case model (2). Other parameter settings are similar by including superscript notations $(*)$. Moreover, modeling the biomarker trajectory for the censored subjects may provide potentially useful information so as to make the risk prediction more efficient. This framework is analogous to the pattern mixture model in the literature [26].

Using models (2) and (6), the likelihood function for the observed data $(T_i, \Delta_i, \boldsymbol{Y}_i, \boldsymbol{W}_i)$ under the BDCA is given by

$$\begin{aligned}
&L(T_i, \Delta_i, \boldsymbol{Y}_i, \boldsymbol{W}_i)\\
&= [f(S_i = T_i|\boldsymbol{Y}_i, \boldsymbol{W}_i)S(C_i = T_i|\boldsymbol{Y}_i, \boldsymbol{W}_i)]^{\Delta_i}\\
&\times [S(S_i = T_i|\boldsymbol{Y}_i, \boldsymbol{W}_i)f(C_i = T_i|\boldsymbol{Y}_i, \boldsymbol{W}_i)]^{1-\Delta_i} f(\boldsymbol{Y}_i|\boldsymbol{W}_i)f(\boldsymbol{W}_i)\\
&\propto \left\{f(S_i = T_i|\boldsymbol{Y}_i, \boldsymbol{W}_i)\left[\int_{T_i}^{\infty} f(\boldsymbol{Y}_i|C_i = u, \boldsymbol{W}_i)\, dF(C_i = u|\boldsymbol{W}_i)\right]\right\}^{\Delta_i} \qquad (7)\\
&\times \left\{\left[\int_{T_i}^{\infty} f(\boldsymbol{Y}_i|S_i = v, \boldsymbol{W}_i)\, dF(S_i = v|\boldsymbol{W}_i)\right] f(C_i = T_i|\boldsymbol{Y}_i, \boldsymbol{W}_i)\right\}^{1-\Delta_i},
\end{aligned}$$

where the first equality holds because of $C_i \perp\!\!\!\perp S_i|(\boldsymbol{Y}_i, \boldsymbol{W}_i)$, the second proportional notation holds by dropping $f(\boldsymbol{W}_i)$ and applying Bayes' rule. Specifically, $f(\boldsymbol{Y}_i|S_i, \boldsymbol{W}_i)$ and $f(\boldsymbol{Y}_i|C_i, \boldsymbol{W}_i)$ are densities provided in (2) and (6), respectively; $F(S_i|\boldsymbol{W}_i)$ is provided in (5), and $F(C_i|\boldsymbol{W}_i)$ can be fitted in a similar manner. Finally, we can calculate $f(S_i|\boldsymbol{Y}_i, \boldsymbol{W}_i) = f(S_i, \boldsymbol{Y}_i|\boldsymbol{W}_i)/f(\boldsymbol{Y}_i|\boldsymbol{W}_i) = f(S_i, \boldsymbol{Y}_i|\boldsymbol{W}_i)/\int_u^{\infty} f(S_i = u, \boldsymbol{Y}_i|\boldsymbol{W}_i)\, du$ and $f(C_i|\boldsymbol{Y}_i, \boldsymbol{W}_i) = f(C_i, \boldsymbol{Y}_i|\boldsymbol{W}_i)/\int_v^{\infty} f(C_i = v, \boldsymbol{Y}_i|\boldsymbol{W}_i)\, dv$ by integrating out S_i and C_i, respectively. Afterward, the parameter estimates can be derived by maximizing the likelihood in (7), and similar strategies in [20] remain applicable.

2.1.3 Risk Calculation and Asymptotic Variance

Calculation of the subject-specific t-year absolute risk in (1) depends on the joint density $f(\boldsymbol{Y}_i, S_i|\boldsymbol{W}_i)$, which can be factored into a product of the density of the biomarker conditional on the survival time $f(\boldsymbol{Y}_i|S_i, \boldsymbol{W}_i)$ and the density of the survival time $f(S_i|\boldsymbol{W}_i)$ using Bayes' rule. Specifically, under the BICA, we can maximize the likelihood function in (4) with specifications (2) and (5), obtaining the estimates of all unknown parameters and estimates $\widehat{f}(\boldsymbol{Y}_i|S_i, \boldsymbol{W}_i)$ and $\widehat{f}(S_i|\boldsymbol{W}_i)$. Under the BDCA, we can maximize the likelihood function in (7) with additional model specifications for censored subjects (6) and censoring times, obtaining the estimates of all unknown parameters, and the estimates $\widehat{f}(\boldsymbol{Y}_i|S_i, \boldsymbol{W}_i)$

and $\widehat{f}(S_i|\boldsymbol{W}_i)$. We evaluate the prediction risk $\pi(t|s)$ in (1) using numerical integral approaches, e.g., the R function `integrate()`.

The variance of the individualized t-year risk $\pi_i(t|s)$ in (1) can be obtained using the Delta method as

$$\sigma^2_{\pi_i(t|s)} = \boldsymbol{q}_i^\top \boldsymbol{\Sigma}_{\boldsymbol{\theta}} \boldsymbol{q}_i. \tag{8}$$

The parameter vector $\boldsymbol{\theta}$ includes all the parameters used in the CM formulation in Sect. 2.1.2, and $\boldsymbol{\Sigma}_{\boldsymbol{\theta}}$ is the associated variance-covariance matrix. The vector $\boldsymbol{q}_i$ is defined as

$$\boldsymbol{q}_i = \{\pi_i^\infty\}^{-2}\{\pi_i^\infty \partial\pi_i^t/\partial\boldsymbol{\theta}^\top - \pi_i^t \partial\pi_i^\infty/\partial\boldsymbol{\theta}^\top\},$$

where $\partial\pi_i^t/\partial\boldsymbol{\theta}^\top = \partial \int_s^{s+t} f(\boldsymbol{Y}_i, S_i = u|\boldsymbol{W}_i)\mathrm{d}u/\partial\boldsymbol{\theta}^\top$ and $\partial\pi_i^\infty/\partial\boldsymbol{\theta}^\top = \partial \int_s^\infty f(\boldsymbol{Y}_i, S_i = u|\boldsymbol{W}_i)\mathrm{d}u/\partial\boldsymbol{\theta}^\top$ are the first-order partial derivatives of the integrals over the joint density $f(\boldsymbol{Y}_i, S_i|\boldsymbol{W}_i)$ in the risk calculation (1) with respect to the parameters involved in each submodel fitting. As the analytical forms of the above derivatives are hard to derive, we calculate these derivatives numerically using the `jacobian` function in the R package `numDeriv`. The estimated standard error is then obtained using plug-in estimates of all model parameters.

2.2 *Joint Modeling and Landmark Approaches*

We compare the proposed CM approach with two commonly used frameworks for dynamic risk prediction: a JM approach that jointly models the longitudinal and the survival data through latent shared random effects [34] and an LM approach based on the landmark or partly conditional model of survival data [41, 43, 47]. The JM approach includes a longitudinal submodel $Y_i(s) = m_i(s) + \xi_i(s) = \boldsymbol{X}_i^\top(s)\boldsymbol{\beta} + \boldsymbol{Z}_i^\top(s)\boldsymbol{b}_i + \xi_i(s)$ and a survival submodel $h_i(s) = h_0(s)\exp\{\boldsymbol{W}_i^\top\boldsymbol{\alpha} + \gamma_1 m_i(s) + \gamma_2 m_i'(s)\}$, where $m_i(s)$ is the true yet unobserved marker value at time s and $m_i'(s)$ is its first derivative. The probability of the survival time falling into $(s, s+t]$ given the observed survival data up to time s can be implemented using the R package `JM` [33].

The LM approach fits a Cox model $h_i(u|s, \boldsymbol{V}(s)) = h_0(u|s)\exp\{\boldsymbol{V}(s)^\top\boldsymbol{\beta}(s)\}$ to each landmark dataset of subjects that are still alive at a landmark time s, where $\boldsymbol{V}(s)$ includes predictive information such as the baseline age and the last marker observation available right before the time s and $\boldsymbol{\beta}(s)$ is a vector of coefficients. Then, the risk of surviving up to a fixed horizon time $s+t$ can be predicted from the Cox model estimated using the R package `survival`.

2.3 Dynamic Prediction Accuracy Evaluation

Comparison of the dynamic prediction accuracy is evaluated using the out-of-sample time-dependent receiving operating characteristic (ROC) curve and the area under the curve (AUC) [16], which will be obtained based on independent testing samples in the simulation study and the ten cross-validation in the empirical data example. The time-dependent ROC curve is constructed using the cumulative sensitivity $\mathrm{Se}^C(c,t) = \Pr(\pi_i > c|s_i \le t)$ and dynamic specificity $\mathrm{Sp}^D(c,t) = \Pr(\pi_i \le c|s_i > t)$, where π_i is the risk calculated from the CM approach in (1), c is an arbitrary threshold for the risks, and t is the specific time of interest. The time-dependent AUC at time t is

$$\begin{aligned}\mathrm{AUC}^{C/D}(t) &= \Pr(\pi_i > \pi_j|s_i \le t, s_j > t)\\ &= \int_{-\infty}^{\infty} \mathrm{Se}^C(c,t)\, d[1 - \mathrm{Sp}^D(c,t)], \quad i \ne j.\end{aligned}$$

The time-dependent AUC at time t is interpreted as the probability that a randomly selected "case," whose cancer onset is before time t, had a larger predicted risk than a randomly selected "control," whose cancer onset is after time t. AUC assesses the discrimination between a case and a control, with a larger AUC value indicating better discrimination ability of a model.

Another metric to compare the dynamic predictive performance is the time-dependent Brier score (BS), which quantifies the difference between the observed data and the predicted risks and is defined as $\mathrm{BS}(t|s) = \mathrm{E}\{(\pi_i(t|s) - d_i(t|s)\}^2$, where $\pi_i(t|s)$ and $d_i(t|s)$ are respectively the predicted risk and the observed disease status of subject i at the given landmark time s and the prediction horizon t [45]. As a prediction error metric, a smaller value of BS implies a better prediction of a model.

3 Simulation Studies

3.1 Simulation One: Compare Overall Dynamic Prediction Accuracy

Three scenarios were performed to compare the overall dynamic prediction accuracy of our proposed CM approach with those of JM and LM in terms of the time-dependent AUC and Brier score. Scenario A simulated data from CM with the BDCA, Scenario B generated data from CM with the BICA, while Scenario C used a JM model to generate data. In Scenario A (or B), we generated data using three different kernel functions, exponential, Gaussian, and latent changepoint kernel, distinguished as A1–A3 (or B1–B3), respectively. Denote the CM with exponential (Exp) kernel, Gaussian (Gau) kernel, and latent changepoint (Lat) kernel under the biomarker-dependent (Dep) and biomarker-independent (Ind) censoring assumptions as CM_Dep_Exp, CM_Dep_Gau, CM_Dep_Lat, CM_Ind_Exp, CM_Ind_Gau, and CM_Ind_Lat, respectively.

In Scenario A, the case model in (2) used the fixed effects of the baseline age Age_i and the screening time t_{ij}, and accounted for both the fixed and the random effects of the kernel function. While the control model in (6) included a fixed effect vector $(1, \text{Age}_i, t_{ij})^\top$ and a random effect vector $(1, t_{ij})^\top$. The survival time had a hazard function $h_i(t) = h_0(t)\exp(\alpha\text{Age}_i)$, where $h_0(t)$ was a piecewise constant baseline hazard, while the censoring time was from an exponential distribution. JM included a longitudinal submodel $Y_{ij} = m_i(t_{ij}) + \xi_{ij} = \beta_0 + \beta_1\text{Age}_i + \beta_2 t_{ij} + b_{i0} + b_{i1}t_{ij} + \xi_{ij}$ and a survival submodel $h_i(t) = h_0(t)\exp(\alpha\text{Age}_i + \gamma_1 m_i(t_{ij}) + \gamma_2 m_i'(t_{ij}))$ with a piecewise constant baseline hazard, while LM was in the form of $h_i(t) = h_0(t)\exp(\alpha\text{Age}_i + \gamma Y_i(t))$ with an unspecified baseline hazard. Scenario B had similar settings as Scenario A except that both case and control subjects were generated from the case model in (2). In Scenario C, the true JM model had a longitudinal submodel $Y_{ij} = m_i(t_{ij}) + \xi_{ij} = \beta_0 + \beta_1\text{Age}_i + \beta_2 t_{ij} + b_{i0} + b_{i1}t_{ij} + \xi_{ij}$ and a survival submodel $h_i(t) = h_0(t)\exp(\alpha\text{Age}_i + \gamma_1 m_i(t_{ij}) + \gamma_2 m_i'(t_{ij}))$ that used a Weibull baseline hazard $h_0(t) = \exp(\lambda_1)\lambda_2 t^{\lambda_2 - 1}$. The LM approach had the same form as the one in Scenarios A and B. As for the CM approach, all settings were kept unchanged except that the case model in (2) only included the fixed effect of the kernel function.

In all scenarios, we mimicked the PLCO ovarian cancer data to establish proper parameter settings. Specifically, in Scenario A, the data was simulated as follows: (i) first generate the baseline age from an empirical distribution fitted from the PLCO data, and then (ii) obtain the survival time S_i under the settings of $h_0(t) = \exp(-5.63)I(t \le 2) + \exp(-5.86)I(t > 2)$ and $\alpha = 0.04$; (iii) generate the censoring time C_i from an exponential distribution with a rate of 0.001 and set an administrative censoring time of 13 to obtain a disease prevalence of 38%; (iv) obtain the observed survival T_i as the minimum between S_i and C_i; (v) set the marker cluster size n_i of the subject i as the minimum value between 6 and the integer part of the observed survival time T_i, and the screening time was hence 0, 1, ..., $n_i - 1$; (vi) finally calculate the marker values using the case model in (2) and the control in (6). The case model in Scenario A1 had fixed coefficients $(\beta_0, \beta_1, \beta_2, \eta_1)^\top = (2.3, 0.0008, 0.007, 2.84)^\top$, $\eta_2 = 1.97$, $\left(\sigma_{b_{i0}}, \sigma_{b_{i1}}, \rho_{b_{i0}b_{i1}}\right)^\top = (0.48, 2.08, -0.28)^\top$ and $\sigma_\xi = 0.24$. While the control model parameters were $\left(\beta_0^{(*)}, \beta_1^{(*)}, \beta_2^{(*)}\right)^\top = (2.03, 0.005, 0.008)^\top$, $\left(\sigma_{b_{i0}}^{(*)}, \sigma_{b_{i1}}^{(*)}, \rho_{b_{i0}b_{i1}}^{(*)}\right)^\top = (0.46, 0.03, -0.14)^\top$, and $\sigma_\xi^{(*)} = 0.2$. In Scenario B, the simulations were implemented in the same steps and used the same parameter settings as Scenario A, except that both case and control markers were generated from the case model in (2) due to the biomarker-independent censoring assumption. As for Scenario C, the parameters of JM were $(\beta_0, \beta_1, \beta_2)^\top = (2.6, 0.2, 0.25)^\top$, $\left(\sigma_{b_{i0}}, \sigma_{b_{i1}}, \rho_{b_{i0}b_{i1}}\right)^\top = (0.4, 0.2, 0.5)^\top, \sigma_\xi = 0.2, \alpha = 1.9, \gamma_1 = 0.2$, and $\gamma_2 = 0.1$.

The Weibull hazard was with $\lambda_1 = -5$ and $\lambda_2 = 2$, such that the disease prevalence is about 45%. Details of parameter settings for all the other scenarios can be found in the Supplementary Material.

In all scenarios, model fittings of all CM and JM models were based on a training dataset of 1000 subjects. As for the LM approach, model fitting was based on a trimmed training dataset, which enforced administrative censoring to the original training samples of 1000 subjects according to the landmark time s and the prediction horizon t. Risk predictions were then obtained by applying the fitted models to a trimmed testing dataset that enforced administrative censoring to an original testing dataset of 1000 subjects. The time-dependent AUC and Brier score for each method were finally calculated based on the predicted risks from two landmark times $s = 2, 5$ and three prediction horizon times $t = 1, 2, 3$, for demonstration purposes. The simulations were repeated 200 times to obtain the averaged time-dependent AUC and Brier scores, as well as their associated standard deviations.

The time-dependent AUC and Brier scores of all methods in Scenario A1, B1, and C are presented in Tables 1 and 2, respectively. The AUC comparison in Table 1 shows that CM significantly outperformed JM and LM when it was the true model. CM could still have close performances to JM even when JM was the true model, regardless of the censoring assumption and the choice of kernel function. The performances of LM were quite similar to JM in all scenarios. As for the effects of the censoring assumption on the performance of CM, we found that when the CM with the BDCA was the true model, a CM with the BICA had deteriorated performance, especially for the circumstances where the landmark time and the prediction horizon are large, e.g., $s = 5$ and $t = 3$. However, a CM with the BDCA could still perform well when the CM with the BICA was true, particularly when the kernels were exponential and Gaussian. As for the choice among the exponential, the Gaussian, and the latent changepoint kernels, it did not affect the predictive accuracy of CM much: all three kernels had similar AUCs in all scenarios. Comparison of Brier scores in Table 2 for all models in these scenarios had similar patterns as the AUC comparison in Table 1. Similar conclusions were obtained for Scenarios A2, A3, B2, and B3 from Tables S5–S8 in the Supplementary Material. We additionally implemented simulations under all scenarios with a smaller disease prevalence (about 6%) and obtained similar comparison results, shown in S9–S13 in the Supplementary Material.

3.2 Simulation Two: Compare Individual Risk Behavior

In this simulation study, we assessed the performances of each approach through the comparison between the estimated risks and the true risks from the aspects of bias and risk pattern. We used the same simulation settings as in Scenarios A, B, and C to generate data and fit all models using 1000 training subjects. As for the testing samples, we employed a fixed set of 100 subjects composed of 50

Table 1 Simulation results for Scenarios A1, B1, C, where CM with the exponential kernel under the BDCA, CM_Dep_Exp, CM with the exponential kernel under the BICA, CM_Ind_Exp, and joint model (JM), are the true models, respectively. The averaged time-dependent AUC and standard deviation (in parentheses) are based on 200 simulated replicates. Two landmark times $s = 2, 5$ and three prediction horizons $t = 1, 2, 3$ are used

		$s = 2$			$s = 5$		
Scenario	Method	$t = 1$	$t = 2$	$t = 3$	$t = 1$	$t = 2$	$t = 3$
A1	CM_Dep_Exp	0.879 (0.041)	0.769 (0.038)	0.704 (0.033)	0.889 (0.041)	0.785 (0.040)	0.725 (0.033)
	CM_Dep_Gau	0.879 (0.041)	0.769 (0.038)	0.703 (0.033)	0.889 (0.041)	0.784 (0.039)	0.724 (0.033)
	CM_Dep_Lat	0.877 (0.041)	0.764 (0.039)	0.701 (0.033)	0.888 (0.041)	0.777 (0.040)	0.721 (0.033)
	CM_Ind_Exp	0.876 (0.043)	0.763 (0.038)	0.694 (0.035)	0.882 (0.042)	0.768 (0.040)	0.696 (0.035)
	CM_Ind_Gau	0.877 (0.043)	0.763 (0.038)	0.694 (0.034)	0.883 (0.042)	0.768 (0.040)	0.697 (0.035)
	CM_Ind_Lat	0.876 (0.043)	0.759 (0.039)	0.690 (0.034)	0.883 (0.042)	0.758 (0.041)	0.687 (0.035)
	JM	0.812 (0.047)	0.710 (0.041)	0.650 (0.036)	0.806 (0.053)	0.698 (0.041)	0.643 (0.031)
	LM	0.818 (0.048)	0.711 (0.039)	0.651 (0.035)	0.817 (0.052)	0.706 (0.040)	0.648 (0.032)
B1	CM_Dep_Exp	0.869 (0.041)	0.756 (0.039)	0.686 (0.034)	0.876 (0.041)	0.762 (0.040)	0.686 (0.034)
	CM_Dep_Gau	0.869 (0.041)	0.756 (0.039)	0.686 (0.034)	0.876 (0.040)	0.762 (0.039)	0.686 (0.033)
	CM_Dep_Lat	0.868 (0.041)	0.751 (0.041)	0.681 (0.035)	0.875 (0.041)	0.753 (0.041)	0.678 (0.034)
	CM_Ind_Exp	0.870 (0.040)	0.758 (0.038)	0.688 (0.032)	0.877 (0.041)	0.765 (0.039)	0.692 (0.034)
	CM_Ind_Gau	0.869 (0.041)	0.757 (0.038)	0.688 (0.033)	0.877 (0.040)	0.764 (0.039)	0.691 (0.035)
	CM_Ind_Lat	0.869 (0.041)	0.750 (0.039)	0.681 (0.034)	0.876 (0.041)	0.753 (0.041)	0.681 (0.034)
	JM	0.798 (0.044)	0.697 (0.036)	0.643 (0.031)	0.798 (0.048)	0.693 (0.040)	0.638 (0.036)
	LM	0.814 (0.044)	0.708 (0.036)	0.651 (0.031)	0.808 (0.047)	0.700 (0.039)	0.643 (0.035)
C	CM_Dep_Exp	0.845 (0.023)	0.857 (0.018)	0.866 (0.017)	0.800 (0.034)	0.811 (0.030)	0.820 (0.028)
	CM_Dep_Gau	0.845 (0.023)	0.857 (0.018)	0.866 (0.017)	0.800 (0.034)	0.811 (0.030)	0.820 (0.028)
	CM_Dep_Lat	0.845 (0.023)	0.857 (0.018)	0.866 (0.017)	0.800 (0.034)	0.812 (0.030)	0.821 (0.028)
	CM_Ind_Exp	0.846 (0.023)	0.858 (0.019)	0.867 (0.018)	0.802 (0.036)	0.814 (0.034)	0.823 (0.033)
	CM_Ind_Gau	0.846 (0.022)	0.859 (0.018)	0.868 (0.017)	0.802 (0.034)	0.817 (0.031)	0.827 (0.029)
	CM_Ind_Lat	0.847 (0.022)	0.859 (0.018)	0.868 (0.016)	0.802 (0.033)	0.818 (0.029)	0.828 (0.028)
	JM	0.849 (0.022)	0.861 (0.018)	0.871 (0.016)	0.811 (0.032)	0.825 (0.028)	0.836 (0.027)
	LM	0.848 (0.023)	0.860 (0.018)	0.871 (0.016)	0.809 (0.033)	0.824 (0.028)	0.835 (0.027)

Table 2 Simulation results for Scenarios A1, B1, C, where CM with the exponential kernel under the BDCA, CM_Dep_Exp, CM with the exponential kernel under the BICA, CM_Ind_Exp, and joint model (JM), are the true models, respectively. The averaged time-dependent Brier score and standard deviation (in parentheses) are based on 200 simulated replicates. Two landmark times $s = 2, 5$ and three prediction horizons $t = 1, 2, 3$ are used

Scenario	Method	$s = 2$			$s = 5$		
		$t = 1$	$t = 2$	$t = 3$	$t = 1$	$t = 2$	$t = 3$
A1	CM_Dep_Exp	0.015 (0.004)	0.043 (0.006)	0.071 (0.007)	0.014 (0.004)	0.042 (0.007)	0.069 (0.007)
	CM_Dep_Gau	0.015 (0.004)	0.043 (0.006)	0.071 (0.007)	0.014 (0.004)	0.042 (0.007)	0.069 (0.007)
	CM_Dep_Lat	0.016 (0.004)	0.044 (0.006)	0.071 (0.007)	0.014 (0.004)	0.042 (0.007)	0.069 (0.007)
	CM_Ind_Exp	0.016 (0.004)	0.044 (0.006)	0.072 (0.007)	0.014 (0.004)	0.043 (0.007)	0.070 (0.008)
	CM_Ind_Gau	0.016 (0.004)	0.044 (0.006)	0.072 (0.007)	0.014 (0.004)	0.043 (0.007)	0.070 (0.008)
	CM_Ind_Lat	0.016 (0.004)	0.045 (0.006)	0.072 (0.007)	0.014 (0.004)	0.044 (0.007)	0.071 (0.008)
	JM	0.029 (0.005)	0.056 (0.007)	0.082 (0.007)	0.027 (0.006)	0.056 (0.007)	0.081 (0.008)
	LM	0.023 (0.005)	0.053 (0.007)	0.081 (0.007)	0.023 (0.005)	0.053 (0.007)	0.080 (0.008)
B1	CM_Dep_Exp	0.017 (0.004)	0.046 (0.006)	0.074 (0.008)	0.015 (0.004)	0.044 (0.007)	0.071 (0.007)
	CM_Dep_Gau	0.017 (0.004)	0.046 (0.006)	0.074 (0.008)	0.015 (0.004)	0.044 (0.007)	0.071 (0.007)
	CM_Dep_Lat	0.017 (0.004)	0.046 (0.007)	0.074 (0.008)	0.015 (0.004)	0.044 (0.007)	0.071 (0.007)
	CM_Ind_Exp	0.017 (0.004)	0.046 (0.006)	0.074 (0.008)	0.015 (0.004)	0.044 (0.007)	0.071 (0.008)
	CM_Ind_Gau	0.017 (0.004)	0.046 (0.006)	0.074 (0.008)	0.015 (0.004)	0.044 (0.007)	0.071 (0.008)
	CM_Ind_Lat	0.017 (0.004)	0.046 (0.007)	0.074 (0.008)	0.015 (0.004)	0.045 (0.007)	0.072 (0.008)
	JM	0.030 (0.005)	0.057 (0.007)	0.084 (0.008)	0.028 (0.006)	0.056 (0.007)	0.082 (0.008)
	LM	0.024 (0.005)	0.054 (0.007)	0.082 (0.008)	0.023 (0.005)	0.054 (0.007)	0.081 (0.008)
C	CM_Dep_Exp	0.076 (0.006)	0.111 (0.007)	0.132 (0.007)	0.082 (0.013)	0.121 (0.012)	0.142 (0.011)
	CM_Dep_Gau	0.076 (0.006)	0.112 (0.007)	0.132 (0.007)	0.082 (0.013)	0.121 (0.012)	0.142 (0.011)
	CM_Dep_Lat	0.076 (0.006)	0.112 (0.007)	0.132 (0.007)	0.082 (0.013)	0.120 (0.012)	0.141 (0.011)
	CM_Ind_Exp	0.076 (0.006)	0.112 (0.007)	0.133 (0.007)	0.082 (0.012)	0.120 (0.012)	0.140 (0.011)
	CM_Ind_Gau	0.076 (0.006)	0.112 (0.007)	0.132 (0.007)	0.082 (0.013)	0.119 (0.012)	0.140 (0.011)
	CM_Ind_Lat	0.076 (0.006)	0.112 (0.007)	0.132 (0.007)	0.082 (0.013)	0.119 (0.012)	0.140 (0.011)
	JM	0.071 (0.006)	0.105 (0.007)	0.126 (0.007)	0.080 (0.011)	0.116 (0.011)	0.140 (0.011)
	LM	0.072 (0.007)	0.105 (0.008)	0.126 (0.007)	0.081 (0.011)	0.118 (0.011)	0.141 (0.011)

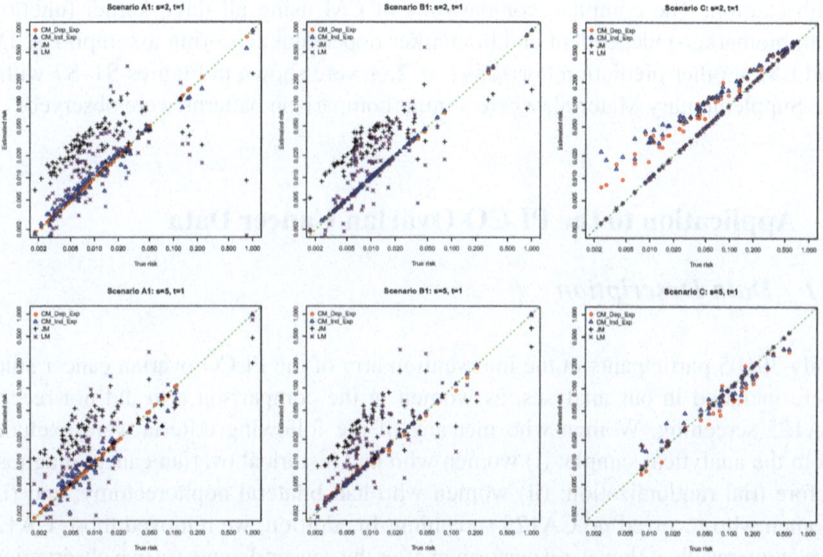

Fig. 2 The averaged predicted risk versus true risks for CM_Dep_Exp, CM_Ind_Exp, JM, and LM in Scenarios A1, B1, and C. The top row displays comparisons at landmark time $s = 2$ and prediction horizon $t = 1$, while the bottom row shows comparisons at $s = 5$ and $t = 1$. Results were based on 200 simulated replicates

cases and 50 controls. In each simulation, we calculated the estimated risks for these testing subjects from each model and the true risks from the true model. We eventually obtained the mean estimated risks of each model based on 200 simulated replicates and plotted them against the true risks. An illustration for CM with an exponential kernel with both biomarker-dependent and biomarker-independent censoring assumptions, JM, and LM in Scenario A1, B1, and C at $s = 2, 5$ and $t = 1$ was demonstrated in Fig. 2. In Scenario A1, CM with dependent censoring had consistent risk estimation; CM with independent censoring generally had a small bias when $s = 2$ and increased bias when $s = 5$. JM and LM both yielded seriously biased risk prediction. Scenario B1, in which CM with independent censoring was the correct model, showed similar patterns as in Scenario A1. The only difference was that CM with independent and dependent censoring both had negligible biases in the risk estimation. In Scenario C where JM was the correct model, JM and LM both estimated the risks consistently. As CM is a misspecified model, it tended to overestimate the risks when $s = 2$, particularly for the low-risk subjects. However, as more biomarker observations became available with $s = 5$, CM resulted in a smaller bias. It is also worth noting that, despite some biases of risk prediction in CM, its AUC was only slightly lower than JM (as in Table 1), suggesting that the estimated risks still maintained the relative ranks of diseased and healthy subjects. Therefore, when CM is severely misspecified, its risk estimation can still be used for developing screening thresholds, although the individual risks should be interpreted with caution. The complete comparisons of CM using all three kernel functions with biomarker-independent and biomarker-dependent censoring assumptions, JM, and LM at other prediction horizons $t = 2, 3$ were shown in Figures S1–S7 within the Supplementary Material, where similar comparison patterns were observed.

4 Application to the PLCO Ovarian Cancer Data

4.1 Data Description

Only 39105 participants in the intervention arm of the PLCO ovarian cancer study were included in our analyses, as women in the comparison arm did not receive CA125 screening. Women who met any of the following criteria were excluded from the analytical sample: (i) women who had historical ovarian cancer diagnosis before trial randomization; (ii) women who had bilateral oophorectomy; and (iii) women who received no CA125 screening. In addition, we removed those CA125 screening results if they were performed after the cancer diagnosis (five observations in total). Our analytic sample eventually includes 30310 women consisting of 208 ovarian cancer cases and 30102 controls. The median numbers of longitudinal CA125 measurements were $four$ for cases and six for controls due to the PLCO trial design. The ovarian cancer cases are older at baseline, have fewer CA125 screenings, and are more likely to have a family history of ovarian or breast cancer [7]. Additional descriptive statistics of the PLCO ovarian cancer data are tabulated in Table S1 in the Supplementary Material.

4.2 Model Specification

From our motivation example of the PLCO ovarian cancer shown in Fig. 1, we can see the longitudinal biomarker trajectories for censored subjects are mainly flat, indicating the trivial effects of the censoring time on the marker profiles. Thus, we additionally propose an approximation of (6) by considering the working model $Y_{ij} = \boldsymbol{X}_i^\top \boldsymbol{\beta}^{(*)} + \boldsymbol{Z}_i^\top \boldsymbol{b}_i^{(*)} + \xi_{ij}^{(*)}$. We expect this model would work well in cases where censoring is mostly administrative, and the biomarkers are not likely to have any increasing patterns near the censoring time. However, if the censoring is due to treatment of conditions such as precancerous lesions, then the biomarker behavior may be more affected, and model (6) could be fitted instead. In our data analysis for the censored subjects, we specifically fit this model with a random intercept and a random slope by considering the baseline age and the screening time as fixed effects and the screening time as a random effect, i.e., $\boldsymbol{X}_i = (1, \text{Age}_i, t_{ij})^\top$ and $\boldsymbol{Z}_i = (1, t_{ij})^\top$.

Further, the case model in (2) for the CM approach used the baseline age and the screening time as fixed effects, and the kernel function had both fixed and random effects. The hazard function for the survival time in (5) used the baseline age as a fixed covariate, while the censoring time distribution was estimated by the Kaplan-Meier estimate. The JM model had a longitudinal submodel that was formulated the same as the above-proposed control model and a survival submodel that used the baseline age, current value, and current slope of the longitudinal submodel as covariates. To better characterize the nonlinear feature in the CA125 profiles, more complicated longitudinal submodels, e.g., using a natural spline basis, have been tried. Unfortunately, the model fitting for the JM approach suffered non-convergence from the R package `JM`. LM was specified as a Cox regression with covariates being the baseline age and the biomarker value right close to the landmark time.

Model fitting and risk calculation were constructed using the tenfold cross-validation technique. Specifically, we randomly separated the ovarian cancer data into ten subsamples, with nine subsamples being used as the training set and the remaining one subsample as the testing set. The cross-validation was repeated ten times so that every subsample would be used once as the testing set. Then, all the predicted risks combined from ten testing sets were used to calculate the time-dependent AUC. At a given landmark time s and a prediction horizon t, the 10-fold cross-validation was repeated 100 times to obtain 100 time-dependent AUC replicates. Finally, the averaged time-dependent AUCs were reported. Other metrics such as the time-dependent Brier score could be obtained in the same fashion.

4.3 Empirical Results

The time-dependent AUCs of all methods at landmark times $s = 2, 5$ years and prediction horizons $t = 1, 2, 3$ years were listed in Table 3. It shows that our proposed CM approach significantly outperformed JM and LM, regardless of the kernel functions and censoring assumptions, indicating the usefulness of the CM approach. As for the comparison of CM with a given kernel function between different censoring assumptions, CM with the BICA outperformed the one with the BDCA at landmark time $s = 2$ years for all $three$ prediction horizons. However, it was outperformed by the latter one at landmark time $s = 5$ years for prediction horizons of 2 and 3 years. This may be due to that the cases at landmark time $s = 2$ provide more information on acute effects, while those at $s = 5$ provide more information on long-term effects. The choice of the kernel function affected the performance of CM, especially the latent changepoint kernel, for risk prediction at $(s = 2, t = 2)$, $(s = 5, t = 1)$, and $(s = 5, t = 2)$, possibly due to the small number of events with complicated biomarker trajectories that may or may not be well characterized by the chosen kernel.

The plots of dynamically predicted risks for two individuals (a case and a control) are shown in Figs. 3 and 4, where risks were made at 1, 2, and 3 years after the last marker observation. When there is no pattern change in the marker trajectory, all

Table 3 Results for the PLCO ovarian cancer data: the averaged time-dependent AUCs are based on 100 replicates calculated using the 10-fold cross-validation technique. Two landmark times $s = 2, 5$ years and three prediction horizons $t = 1, 2, 3$ years are used. The number of events and the number of subjects at risk between s and $s + t$ are also reported

	$s = 2$			$s = 5$		
Method	$t = 1$	$t = 2$	$t = 3$	$t = 1$	$t = 2$	$t = 3$
CM_Dep_Exp	0.794	0.664	0.652	0.793	0.662	0.646
CM_Dep_Gau	0.796	0.661	0.652	0.805	0.668	0.648
CM_Dep_Lat	0.787	0.643	0.645	0.811	0.660	0.639
CM_Ind_Exp	0.815	0.685	0.658	0.791	0.639	0.620
CM_Ind_Gau	0.820	0.682	0.659	0.812	0.655	0.625
CM_Ind_Lat	0.813	0.659	0.653	0.838	0.674	0.622
JM	0.664	0.587	0.563	0.638	0.539	0.553
LM	0.630	0.563	0.571	0.637	0.556	0.532
No. of events	15	36	52	12	24	42
No. of subjects at risk	29326	29305	29289	29208	29196	29178

methods would predict low risks that are very close to zero. However, compared to CM, JM and LM often give slightly higher risks and wider confidence intervals, as shown in Fig. 4. CM with the BICA also has larger estimated risks than the one with the BDCA. When the marker trajectory jumps up, CM would give estimated risks far larger than JM and LM, as shown in Fig. 3, revealing that CM is more sensitive to dramatic marker profile pattern changes.

Though it may be argued that the results of the JM approach may be improved using more complicated model formulations, especially for the longitudinal process, the convergence of model fitting and computational burden in the PLCO example hindered such implementations. We also tried to implement the control model in (6) based on censored subjects, so as to investigate the potential effect of the censoring time on the biomarker trajectories. Unfortunately, model fitting of (6) suffered non-convergence.

5 Discussion

In this paper, we developed a novel CM approach for dynamic risk prediction of ovarian cancer using longitudinal biomarkers and survival information. The idea is to first factor the joint distribution of the longitudinal biomarker and the survival time into the product of the conditional density of the marker given the survival time and the marginal density of the survival time. Then, the conditional density of the survival time given the biomarker is derived using Bayes' rule. Finally, the t-year individual risk given marker measurements up to a landmark time s is calculated. To model the conditional relationship between the marker and the survival time, we used a mixed-effects model that additionally treats the survival time as a covariate

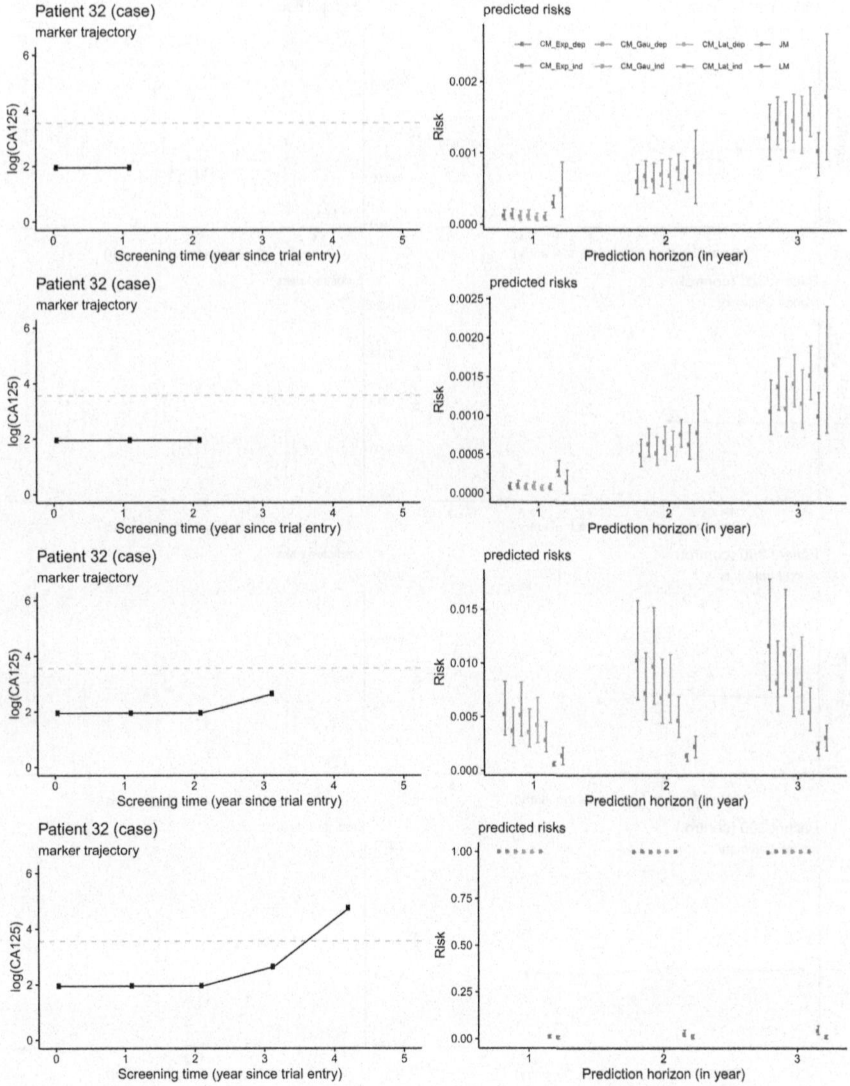

Fig. 3 Biomarker trajectories and predicted risks using 2, 3, 4, and 5 biomarker observations for patient 32, which is a case subject. The dashed line in gray is log(35), below which the marker value is regarded as normal

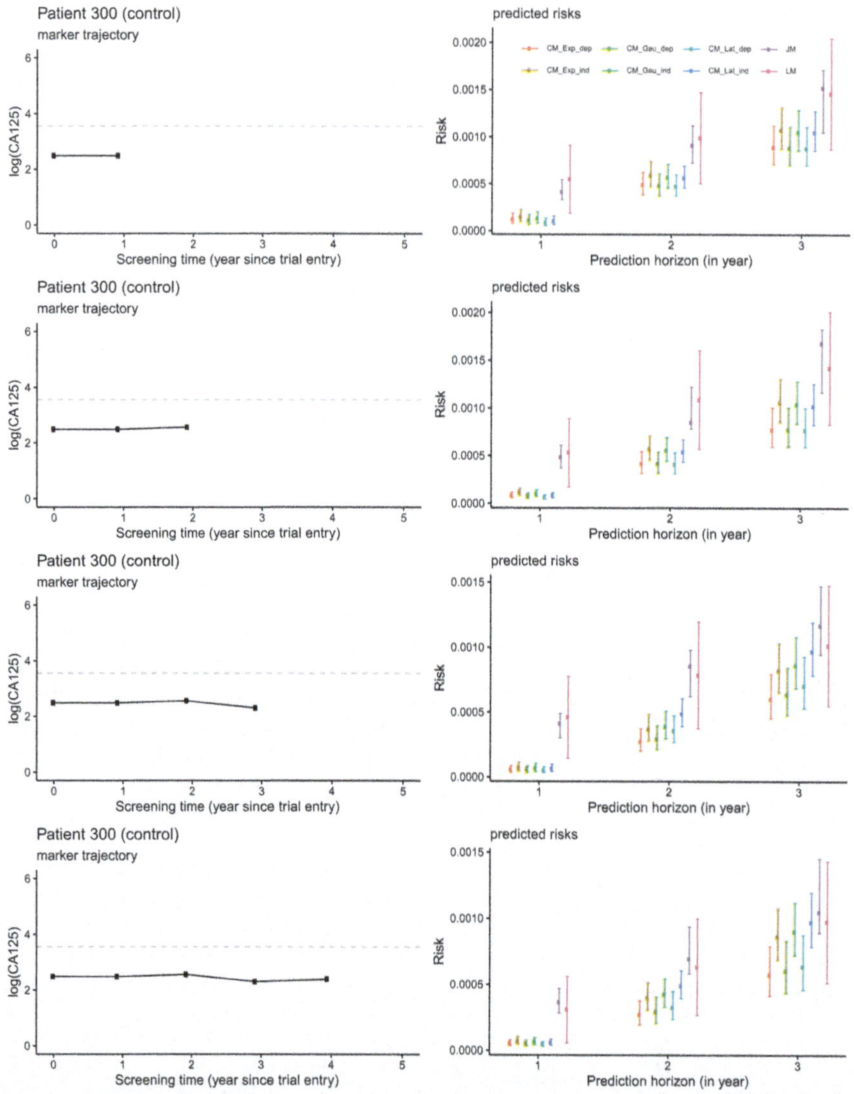

Fig. 4 Biomarker trajectories and predicted risks using 2, 3, 4, and 5 biomarker observations for patient 300, which is a control subject. The dashed line in grey is log(35), below which the marker value is regarded as normal

that has both fixed and random effects. The nonlinear effect of the survival time on the longitudinal marker profile is described using a smooth or piecewise linear kernel function. Risk predictions were performed under two censoring assumptions. Under the BICA where the censoring time is independent of the biomarker and the survival time given observed covariates, the risk calculation only uses a case model that formulates the density of the biomarker conditional on the survival time and a Cox model for the survival time. This assumption only captures the acute effects of the biomarker, i.e., only a rapid increase in the biomarker shortly before the event is indicative of a high disease risk, and suggests that the marker measurements collected far away from the event barely contribute to the risk prediction. As a comparison, the BDCA allows for the incorporation of both the acute and the long-term effects of the biomarker, by separately modeling the subjects with and without the event, and then derives the risk calculation accordingly. The performances of our proposed CM approach were compared with the JM approach and the LM method in extensive simulation studies, where we evaluated the overall performance of the prediction accuracy as well as the behavior of individual risk prediction. Performances of all approaches were further compared in an application to the ovarian cancer data from the PLCO Cancer Screening Trial.

Conceptually, LM, JM, and CM use different model specifications to derive the dynamic risk estimation. LM directly makes an assumption on the conditional distribution of the survival time given the longitudinal data, $f(S|Y)$. Risk estimation using LM is relatively easy to implement and interpret, but it does not make efficient use of the information in the biomarker profiles. As a comparison, JM models the joint distribution $f(S, Y)$ using latent shared random effects b such that $f(S, Y) = \int f(S|b) f(Y|b) f(b)\, db$. This framework is a natural choice for modeling two dependent processes, which describes the dependence structure through shared random effects. However, the model assumption of JM that the two processes become independent given the random effects is quite strong and non-verifiable. In addition, JM poses a heavy computational burden for evaluating the intractable integrals. Although CM also focuses on the joint distribution $f(S, Y)$, it starts from a different factorization: $f(S, Y) = f(Y|S) f(S)$, where the first part $f(Y|S)$ is specified from modeling the cases, and the second part $f(S)$ comes from a Cox regression. The longitudinal model assumption BDCA is based on the observed data and is easy to verify. As we demonstrated in simulation studies, when JM is the true model, CM and JM have similar prediction accuracy; while when CM is the true model, JM has much lower accuracy than CM. These results suggest that CM makes less strict model assumptions and tends to be more robust to misspecified models. We also observed similar robustness for the separate modeling strategy as compared to a joint model in predicting the risk of a binary outcome [27]. What's more, the computational burden is relatively easy for CM. On the other hand, the choices of the kernel function $g(\cdot)$ and the hazard function $h(\cdot)$ will influence the computational burden and the interpretation. With these advantages, we would recommend the use of CM for dynamic risk predictions.

The proposed CM approach may be applied to other applications beyond ovarian cancer risk prediction. Many other diseases also have abnormal marker trajectory changes when the time approaches the terminal event; see, for example, the medical costs in cancer patients incline to increase when patients near death [8, 25] and the menstrual cycles get longer and more changeable when women are closer to menopause [14], though specific model formulations or novel approach development may be needed. We also developed R codes for the convenient implementation of the proposed CM approach for possible clinical applications. Applying the CM approach to dynamic risk prediction using multiple biomarkers would be another possible extension, and we leave it to our future research. The Supplementary Material is available at https://github.com/CinemaResearchGroup/CondModelDRP.

The Data Resource Statement The data generated and/or analyzed for the current study is not publicly available. However, the data can be made available upon reasonable request from the US National Cancer Institute PLCO Cancer Screening Trial Team.

Acknowledgments This work utilized the computational resources of the National Institutes of Health (NIH) HPC Biowulf cluster (http://hpc.nih.gov).

Yongli Han was supported by the NCI Director's Intramural Innovation Award and the NIH Intramural Research Program. Yifan Yang and Ming Wang were supported by the start-up funding from the Department of Population and Quantitative Health Sciences at Case Western Reserve University. Zhiwei Zhang was supported by the NCI Extramural Research Program. Danping Liu was supported by the NIH Intramural Research Program. The content is solely the responsibility of the authors and does not necessarily represent the official views of the NIH.

References

1. Albert, P., Shih, J.: An approach for jointly modeling multivariate longitudinal measurements and discrete time-to-event data. Ann. Appl. Stat. **4**, 1517–1532 (2010)
2. Albert, P., Shih, J.: On estimating the relationship between longitudinal measurements and time-to-event data using a simple two-stage procedure. Biometrics **66**, 983–987 (2010)
3. Albert, P.: A linear mixed model for predicting a binary event from longitudinal data under random effects misspecification. Stat. Med. **31**, 143–154 (2012)
4. Andrinopoulou, E., Rizopoulos, D., Takkenberg, J., Lesaffre, E.: Combined dynamic predictions using joint models of two longitudinal outcomes and competing risk data. Stat. Methods Med. Res. **26**, 1787–1801 (2017)
5. Barrett, J., Su, L.: Dynamic predictions using flexible joint models of longitudinal and time-to-event data. Stat. Med. **36**, 1447–1460 (2017)
6. Barry, M.: Prostate-specific-antigen testing for early diagnosis of prostate cancer. N. Engl. J. Med. **344**, 1373–1377 (2001)
7. Buys, S., Partridge, E., Black, A., Johnson, C., Lamerato, L., Isaacs, C., Reding, D., Greenlee, R., Yokochi, L., Others: Effect of screening on ovarian cancer mortality: the Prostate, Lung, Colorectal and Ovarian (PLCO) cancer screening randomized controlled trial. J. Am. Med. Assoc. **305**, 2295–2303 (2011)
8. Chan, K., Wang, M.: Backward estimation of stochastic processes with failure events as time origins. Ann. Appl. Stat. **4**, 1602–1620 (2010)

9. Dempsey, W., McCullagh, P.: Survival models and health sequences. Lifetime Data Anal. **24**, 550–584 (2018)
10. Desmée, S., Mentré, F., Veyrat-Follet, C., Sé bastien, B., Guedj, J.: Nonlinear joint models for individual dynamic prediction of risk of death using Hamiltonian Monte Carlo: application to metastatic prostate cancer. BMC Med. Res. Methodol. **17**, 1–12 (2017)
11. Ding, J., Wang, J.: Modeling longitudinal data with nonparametric multiplicative random effects jointly with survival data. Biometrics **64**, 546–556 (2008)
12. Han, Y., Liu, D.: Accounting for random observation time in risk prediction with longitudinal markers: an imputation approach. Stat. Methods Med. Res. **29**, 396–412 (2020)
13. Han, Y., Albert, P., Berg, C., Wentzensen, N., Katki, H., Liu, D.: Statistical approaches using longitudinal biomarkers for disease early detection: a comparison of methodologies. Stat. Med. **39**, 4405–4420 (2020)
14. Harlow, S., Mitchell, E., Crawford, S., Nan, B., Little, R., Taffe, J., Collaboration, R., Others: The ReSTAGE Collaboration: defining optimal bleeding criteria for onset of early menopausal transition. Fertil. Steril. **89**, 129–140 (2008)
15. He, B., Luo, S.: Joint modeling of multivariate longitudinal measurements and survival data with applications to Parkinson's disease. Stat. Methods Med. Res. **25**, 1346–1358 (2016)
16. Heagerty, P., Zheng, Y.: Survival model predictive accuracy and ROC curves. Biometrics **61**, 92–105 (2005)
17. Hsieh, F., Tseng, Y., Wang, J.: Joint modeling of survival and longitudinal data: likelihood approach revisited. Biometrics **62**, 1037–1043 (2006)
18. Huang, C., Wang, M.: Joint modeling and estimation for recurrent event processes and failure time data. J. Am. Stat. Assoc. **99**, 1153–1165 (2004)
19. Jewell, N., Nielsen, J.: A framework for consistent prediction rules based on markers. Biometrika **80**, 153–164 (1993)
20. Kong, S., Nan, B., Kalbfleisch, J., Saran, R., Hirth, R.: Conditional modeling of longitudinal data with terminal event. J. Am. Stat. Assoc. **113**, 357–368 (2018)
21. Kurland, B., Johnson, L., Egleston, B., Diehr, P.: Longitudinal data with follow-up truncated by death: match the analysis method to research aims. Stat. Sci. **24**, 211–222 (2009)
22. Li, Z., Tosteson, T., Bakitas, M.: Joint modeling quality of life and survival using a terminal decline model in palliative care studies. Stat. Med. **32**, 1394–1406 (2013)
23. Li, Z., Frost, H., Tosteson, T., Zhao, L., Liu, L., Lyons, K., Chen, H., Cole, B., Currow, D., Bakitas, M.: A semiparametric joint model for terminal trend of quality of life and survival in palliative care research. Stat. Med. **36**, 4692–4704 (2017)
24. Li, L., Luo, S., Hu, B., Greene, T.: Dynamic prediction of renal failure using longitudinal biomarkers in a cohort study of chronic kidney disease. Stat. Biosci. **9**, 357–378 (2017)
25. Li, L., Wu, C., Ning, J., Huang, X., Shih, Y., Shen, Y.: Semiparametric estimation of longitudinal medical cost trajectory. J. Am. Stat. Assoc. **113**, 582–592 (2018)
26. Little, R.: Pattern-mixture models for multivariate incomplete data. J. Am. Stat. Assoc. **88**, 125–134 (1993)
27. Liu, D., Albert, P.: Combination of longitudinal biomarkers in predicting binary events. Biostatistics **15**, 706–718 (2014)
28. Maziarz, M., Heagerty, P., Cai, T., Zheng, Y.: On longitudinal prediction with time-to-event outcome: comparison of modeling options. Biometrics **73**, 83–93 (2017)
29. McIntosh, M., Urban, N.: A parametric empirical Bayes method for cancer screening using longitudinal observations of a biomarker. Biostatistics **4**, 27–40 (2003)
30. Pinsky, P., Zhu, C., Skates, S., Black, A., Partridge, E., Buys, S., Berg, C.: Potential effect of the risk of ovarian cancer algorithm (ROCA) on the mortality outcome of the Prostate, Lung, Colorectal and Ovarian (PLCO) trial. Int. J. Cancer **132**, 2127–2133 (2013)
31. Prorok, P., Andriole, G., Bresalier, R., Buys, S., Chia, D., Crawford, E., Fogel, R., Gelmann, E., Gilbert, F., Others: Design of the prostate, lung, colorectal and ovarian (PLCO) cancer screening trial. Control. Clin. Trials **21**, 273S–309S (2000)

32. Rizopoulos, D., Verbeke, G., Lesaffre, E.: Fully exponential Laplace approximations for the joint modelling of survival and longitudinal data. J. R. Stat. Soc. Ser. B (Stat Methodol.) **71**, 637–654 (2009)
33. Rizopoulos, D.: JM: an R package for the joint modelling of longitudinal and time-to-event data. J. Stat. Softw. **35**, 1–33 (2010)
34. Rizopoulos, D.: Dynamic predictions and prospective accuracy in joint models for longitudinal and time-to-event data. Biometrics **67**, 819–829 (2011)
35. Rizopoulos, D., Hatfield, L., Carlin, B., Takkenberg, J.: Combining dynamic predictions from joint models for longitudinal and time-to-event data using Bayesian model averaging. J. Am. Stat. Assoc. **109**, 1385–1397 (2014)
36. Shen, F., Li, L.: Backward joint model and dynamic prediction of survival with multivariate longitudinal data. Stat. Med. **40**, 4395–4409 (2021)
37. Skates, S., Pauler, D., Jacobs, I.: Screening based on the risk of cancer calculation from Bayesian hierarchical changepoint and mixture models of longitudinal markers. J. Am. Stat. Assoc. **96**, 429–439 (2001)
38. Skates, S., Menon, U., MacDonald, N., Rosenthal, A., Oram, D., Knapp, R., Jacobs, I.: Calculation of the risk of ovarian cancer from serial CA-125 values for preclinical detection in postmenopausal women. J. Clin. Oncol. **21**, 206s–210s (2003)
39. Suresh, K., Taylor, J., Spratt, D., Daignault, S., Tsodikov, A.: Comparison of joint modeling and landmarking for dynamic prediction under an illness-death model. Biom. J. **59**, 1277–1300 (2017)
40. Tsiatis, A., Davidian, M.: Joint modeling of longitudinal and time-to-event data: an overview. Stat. Sin. **14**(3), 809–834 (2004)
41. Van Houwelingen, H.: Dynamic prediction by landmarking in event history analysis. Scand. J. Stat. **34**, 70–85 (2007)
42. Van Houwelingen, H., Putter, H.: Dynamic predicting by landmarking as an alternative for multi-state modeling: an application to acute lymphoid leukemia data. Lifetime Data Anal. **14**, 447–463 (2008)
43. Van Houwelingen, H., Putter, H.: Dynamic Prediction in Clinical Survival Analysis. CRC Press, New York (2011)
44. Wang, J., Luo, S., Li, L.: Dynamic prediction for multiple repeated measures and event time data: an application to Parkinson's disease. Ann. Appl. Stat. **11**, 1787–1809 (2017)
45. Wu, C., Li, L.: Quantifying and estimating the predictive accuracy for censored time-to-event data with competing risks. Stat. Med. **37**, 3106–3124 (2018)
46. Zhang, H., Kelvin, E., Carpio, A., Allen Hauser, W.: A multistate joint model for intervalcensored event-history data subject to within-unit clustering and informative missingness, with application to neurocysticercosis research. Stat. Med. **39**, 3195–3206 (2020)
47. Zheng, Y., Heagerty, P.: Partly conditional survival models for longitudinal data. Biometrics **61**, 379–391 (2005)
48. Zhu, Y., Li, L., Huang, X.: On the landmark survival model for dynamic prediction of event occurrence using longitudinal data. In: New Frontiers of Biostatistics and Bioinformatics, pp. 387–401 (2018)
49. Zhu, Y., Li, L., Huang, X.: Landmark linear transformation model for dynamic prediction with application to a longitudinal cohort study of chronic disease. J. R. Stat. Soc.: Ser. C: Appl. Stat. **68**, 771–791 (2019)
50. Zhu, Y., Huang, X., Li, L.: Dynamic prediction of time to a clinical event with sparse and irregularly measured longitudinal biomarkers. Biom. J. **62**, 1371–1393 (2020)

Index

Y. Zhao, D.-G. Chen (eds.), *Big Data Analytics in Biostatistics and Bioinformatics*, ICSA Book Series in Statistics,
https://doi.org/10.1007/978-3-032-06649-7

The manufacturer's authorised representative in the EU is Springer Nature Customer Service Centre GmbH, Europaplatz 3, 69115 Heidelberg, Germany. If you have any concerns regarding our products, please contact ProductSafety@springernature.com

Printed and bound by CPI Group (UK) Ltd, Croydon, CR0 4YY
05/10/2026
02228016-0015